Diagnosis and Treatment of Hepatocellular Carcinoma

Diagnosis and Treatment of Hepatocellular Carcinoma

Edited by

Tito Livraghi

CHIEF

Department of Radiology,
Ospedale Civile,
Vimercate (Milan), Italy

Masatoshi Makuuchi

CHAIRMAN

Second Department of Surgery,
Faculty of Medicine, University of Tokyo,
Tokyo, Japan

Luigi Buscarini

CHIEF

Department of Gastroenterology
Ospedale Civile,
Piacenza, Italy

GMM

GREENWICH MEDICAL MEDIA
507 The Linen Hall
162-168 Regent Street
London
W1R 5TB

ISBN 1 900151 308

First Published 1997

British Library Cataloguing in Publication Data
A catalogue record for this book is available from the British Library

Distributed worldwide by
Oxford University Press

Designed and Produced by
Derek Virtue, DataNet

Printed in Hong Kong by
Dah Hua

Contents

Part IV

Contributors

E Angeli, MD
STAFF RADIOLOGIST
Department of Radiology,
Scientific Institute, San Raffaele
University Hospital,
Milan, Italy.

A D'Antoni, MD
REGISTRAR IN GASTROENTEROLOGY
Division of Medicine
Hospital V. Cervello,
Palermo, Italy.

C Balsano, MD
ASSOCIATE PROFESSOR OF INTERNAL MEDICINE
Department of Internal Medicine,
University of L'Aquila,
L'Aquila, Italy.

C Bartolozzi, MD
PROFESSOR AND CHAIRMAN
Department of Radiology,
University of Pisa,
Pisa, Italy.

KP Batts, MD
Department of Diagnostic Radiology,
Mayo Clinic, Rochester,
Minnesota, USA

L Bolondi, MD
ASSOCIATE PROFESSOR
Department of Internal Medicine and
Gastroenterology
S. Orsola University Hospital,
Bologna, Italy.

C Bru, MD
Department of Radiology,
University Hospital,
Barcelona, Spain

E Buscarini, MD
ASSISTANT
Department of Gastroenterology,
General Hospital,
Piacenza, Italy.

L Buscarini, MD
PROFESSOR AND CHIEF
Department of Gastroenterology,
General Hospital,
Piacenza, Italy.

D Caramella, MD
STAFF RADIOLOGIST
Department of Radiology,
University of Pisa,
Pisa, Italy.

BI Carr, MD, PhD, FRCP
PROFESSOR
Hepatobiliary Tumor Service,
Thomas E Starzl Transplantation
Institute,
University of Pittsburgh,
Pittsburgh, Pennsylvania, USA

JW Charboneau, MD
PROFESSOR OF RADIOLOGY
Department of Diagnostic Radiology.
Mayo Medical School,
Mayo Clinic, Rochester,
Minnesota, USA

P Chirillo, MD
Department of Pharmacology,
University of California School
of Medicine,
San Diego, California, USA.

BI Choi, MD
PROFESSOR
Department of Radiology,
Seoul National University Hospital,
Seoul, Korea.

F De Cobelli, MD
STAFF RADIOLOGIST
Department of Radiology,
Scientific Institute San Raffaele
University Hospital,
Milan, Italy.

M Colombo, MD
PROFESSOR OF MEDICINE
Institute of Internal Medicine,
University of Milan,
Liver Cancer Unit,
Milan, Italy.

M Cottone, MD
RESEARCH FELLOW IN INTERNAL MEDICINE
Division of Internal Medicine,
Hospital V. Cervello,
Palermo, Italy.

LF Frigerio
STAFF RADIOLOGIST
National Institute for the Study and
Treatment of Tumors,
Milan, Italy

T Gabata, MD
LECTURER
Department of Radiology
Kanazawa University Hospital
Kanazawa, Japan.

F Garbagnati, MD
STAFF RADIOLOGIST
National Institute for the Study and
Treatment of Tumors,
Milan, Italy.

H Higashihara, MD
ASSISTANT PROFESSOR
Department of Radiology,
Fukuoka University,
Fukuoka, Japan.

K Isono, MD
Second Department of Surgery,
Chiba University School of Medicine,
Chiba, Japan.

M Kadoya, MD
LECTURER
Department of Radiology,
Kanazawa University Hospital,
Kanazawa, Japan.

M Kojiro, MD, PhD
PROFESSOR AND CHAIRMAN
First Department of Pathology,
Kurume University School of Medicine,
Kurume, Japan.

K Kubota, MD, PhD
ASSISTANT PROFESSOR
Second Department of Surgery
Faculty of Medicine University of Tokyo,
Tokyo, Japan.

M Kudo, MD, PhD
CHIEF
Division of Hepatology,
Department of Internal Medicine,
Kobe City General Hospital,
Kobe, Japan.

S Lazzaroni, MD
Department of Internal Medicine,
Hospital San Biagio,
Clusone (Bergamo), Italy.

R Lencioni, MD
STAFF RADIOLOGIST
Department of Radiology,
University of Pisa,
Pisa, Italy.

M Levrero, MD
ASSOCIATE PROFESSOR OF INTERNAL MEDICINE
Department of Internal Medicine,
University of Cagliari,
Cagliari, Italy.

Tito Livraghi, MD
CHIEF
Department of Radiology,
General Hospital,
Vimercate (Milan), Italy.

JM Llovett, MD
Liver Unit,
University Hospital,
Barcelona, Spain.

M Makuuchi, MD, PhD
CHAIRMAN AND PROFESSOR
Second Department of Surgery,
Faculty of Medicine University of Tokyo,
Tokyo, Japan.

A Del Maschio, MD
CHIEF
Department of Radiology,
Scientific Institute San Raffaele
University Hospital,
Milan, Italy.

O Matsui, MD
ASSOCIATE PROFESSOR
Department of Radiology,
Kanazawa University Hospital,
Kanazawa, Japan.

F Meloni, MD
STAFF RADIOLOGIST
Department of Radiology,
General Hospital,
Vimercate (Milan), Italy.

T Nagashima, MD
Second Department of Surgery,
Chiba University School of Medicine,
Chiba, Japan.

DM Nagorney, MD
PROFESSOR OF SURGERY
Department of Geneal Surgery
Mayo Clinic, Rochester,
Minnesota, USA

G Natoli, MD
Genetic Expression Laboratory,
A. Cesalpino Foundation,
Hospital Umberto I,
Rome, Italy.

T Ogino, MD
Department of Radiotherapy
National Cancer Center Hospital East,
Chiba, Japan.

M Okazaki, MD, PhD
PROFESSOR
Department of Radiology,
Fukuoka University,
Fukuoka, Japan.

K Okuda, MD, PhD
EMERITUS PROFESSOR OF MEDICINE
Department of Medicine,
Chiba University Hospital,
Chiba, Japan.

AJ Roche, MD
CHIEF
Section of Interventional Radiology,
Department of Medical Imaging
Institute Gustave-Roussy,
Villejuif (Paris), France.

J Rodés, MD
PROFESSOR OF MEDICINE
Liver Unit,
University Hospital,
Barcelona, Spain.

S Rossi, MD
ASSISTANT
Department of Gastroenterology,
General Hospital,
Piacenza, Italy.

M Ryu, MD
CHIEF
Department of Surgery,
National Cancer Center
Hospital East,
Chiba, Japan.

G Sangalli, MD
ASSOCIATE PATHOLOGIST
Department of Anatomical Pathology,
General Hospital,
Busto Arsizio(Varese), Italy

A Sangiovanni, MD
ASSISTANT PROFESSOR OF MEDICINE
Institute of Internal Medicine,
Valduce Hospital,
Como, Italy.

Hiroshi Shijo, MD
ASSISTANT PROFESSOR
First Department of Internal Medicine
Fukuoka University,
Fukuoka, Japan.

MD Simms, MD, FRCP(C)
Department of Diagnostic Radiology,
Erlang Medical Center, Chattanooga,
Tennessee, USA

S Sironi, MD
STAFF RADIOLOGIST
Department of Radiology,
Scientific Institute San Raffaele
University Hospital,
Milan, Italy.

C Spreafico, MD
STAFF RADIOLOGIST
National Institute for the Study and Treatment of Tumors, Milan, Italy.

M Di Stasi, MD
Department of Gastroenterology, General Hospital, Piacenza, Italy.

DH Stephens, MD
PROFESSOR OF RADIOLAGY
Department of Diagnostic Radiology, Mayo Clinic, Rochester, Minnesota, USA

T Takayama, MD PhD
ASSISTANT PROFESSOR
Second Department of Surgery, Faculty of Medicine University of Tokyo, Tokyo, Japan.

S Tanaka, MD PhD
Liver Cancer Mass Survey, Center for Adult Diseases, Osaka, Japan.

Z-Y Tang, MD
PROFESSOR OF SURGERY AND CHAIRMAN
Institute of Liver Cancer, Zhong Shan Hospital, University of Shanghai, Shanghai, China.

G Torzilli, MD
ASSISTANT
Department of Surgery, General Hospital, Lodi, Italy

A Vanzulli, MD
STAFF RADIOLOGIST
Department of Radiology, Scientific Institute San Raffaele University Hospital, Milan, Italy.

C Vettori, MD
STAFF RADIOLOGIST
Department of Radiology, General Hospital, Vimercate (Milan), Italy.

A Yasuhisa, MD
Second Department of Surgery, Chiba University School of Medicine, Chiba, Japan.

J Yoshikawa, MD
LECTURER
Department of Radiology, Kanazawa University Hospital, Kanazawa, Japan.

X-D Zhou, MD
PROFESSOR OF SURGERY AND VICE CHAIRMAN
Institute of Liver Cancer, Zhong Shan Hospital, University of Shanghai,

Introduction

Hepatocellular carcinoma (HCC) is one of the most frequently occurring human cancers. It has long been recognised as having an extremely high incidence in certain regions (eg parts of the African sub-continent), but it is also common in countries where HBV and HCV are prevalent. For example, approximately 20,000 people in Japan and 12,000 in Italy develop the tumor each year.

Before the introduction of ultrasound, and especially before its application in the screening of high risk populations, early diagnosis of HCC was impossible. Now, however, small and treatable lesions are routinely detected, and their precise staging can be ascertained using a wide range of advanced imaging techniques, including enhanced color flow Doppler, spiral CT, contrast MRI, digital angiography and intraoperative ultrasound. Because of the high risk and contraindications of surgical resection to many patients, a variety of alternatives treatments such as chemoembolisation, ethanol injection and other ablation procedures, have also been developed, whilst, in carefully selected patients, liver transplantation remains an effective alternative.

Given the wide range of diagnostic and therapeutic options, and the number of variables involved, the choice of the optimum strategy is not always straightforward. Prognostic factors related to the cancer, such as grading, type, size, number, location, invasiveness and level of serological markers, interact with those relating to hepatic disease, for example, Child's classification and viral activity. When considering the best approach, economic resources and the expertise within individual centers may also often exert a considerable influence on the choice of treatment. Therefore, the diagnosis and treatment of HCC is sufficiently complex to justify a multidisciplinary team approach, a factor reflected in the wide range of specialties represented by the editors and contributors to this book: surgery, radiology, hepatology, pathology, oncology and basic sciences.

The book itself is divided into five parts. Part I deals with epidemiology, etiology and pathology, placing particular emphasis on multistep histologic changes, from cirrhotic nodule to overt cancer. Part II describes the clinical aspects of hepatocellular carcinoma and stresses the paramount importance of screening. In Part III diagnostic imaging, including discussion of all relevant modalities, both established and innovative, are exhaustively described, compared and evaluated. Part IV discusses therapies, including, surgical resection, liver transplantation, chemoembolization, percutaneous ablation procedures and radiation. In both Part III and IV, guidelines for diagnosis and treatment are given. The final part covers the fibrolamellar variant, from both a diagnostic and therapeutic standpoint.

T Livraghi,
Vimercate (Milan), Italy

M Makuuchi,
Tokyo, Japan

L Buscarini,
Piacenza, Italy

Abbreviations

AAH = Atypical adenomatous hyperplasia
AFP = Serum alpha-feto-protein
AH = Adenomatous hyperplasia
AHN = Adenomatous hyperplastic nodule
AI = Acceleration index
ALT = Serum alanine transaminase
ALP = Alkaline phosphatase
AST = Serum aspartate transaminase
CC = Cholangiocarcinoma
CEA = Carcino embryonic antigen
CNR = Contrast-to-noise ratio
CT = Computed tomography
CTA = CT arteriography
CTAP = CT arterial portography
DCP = Des-γ-carboxy prothrombin
DSA = Digital subtraction angiography
EGF = Epidermal growth factor
FNB = Fine needle biopsy
FNH = Focal nodular hyperplasia
GCT = Gamma glutamyl transpeptipase
GRE = Gradient echo
HA = Hepatocellular adenoma
HBsAg = Hepatitis B surface antigen
HBV = Hepatitis B virus
HCC = Hepatocellular carcinoma
HCV = Hepatitis C virus
HGF = Hepatocyte growth factor
ICG = Indcyanine green retention rate
IOUS = Intraoperative ultrasound
IVC = Inferior vena cava
MH = Microhistology
MR/MRI = Magnetic resonance imaging
OLT = Orthotopic liver transplantation
PAS = Periodic acid-schiff stain
PEI = Percutaneous ethanol injection
PFOB = Perfluorooctylbromide
PMCT = Percutaneous microwave coagulation therapy
PH = Partial hepatectomy
PT = Prothrombin time
PTT = Partial thromboplastin time
PVTT = Portal vein tumor thrombus
RI = Resistance index
RITA = Percutaneous radiofrequency interstitial thermal ablation
SC = Smear cytology
SNR = Signal-to-noise ratio
TACE = Transarterial chemoembolization
TAE = Transarterial embolization
TGF = Transforming growth factor
TNF = Tumor necrosis factor
US = Ultrasonography /ultrasound
VIP = Vasoactive intestinal peptide
WHV = Woodchuck hepatitis virus

PART I
BASIC ASPECTS

1

Epidemiology

K Okuda

Hepatocellular carcinoma (HCC) is one of the commonest malignancies throughout the world, but its weight among all cancers varies greatly with the country. In males, primary liver cancer ranks first among all malignancies in Mozambique and some African countries where the age-standardized cancer ratio is greater than 20%, and third in Japan and China.

The relative significance of primary liver cancer among all malignancies may be appreciated from the age-adjusted cancer rates shown in Tables 1.1 and 1.2, the former taken from the paper by Munoz and Bosch,[1] and the latter from the statistics compiled by the Ministry of Health and Welfare of Japan.[2]

Table 1.1 – Age-standardized cancer ratios for primary liver cancer in developing countries

Country (Registry)	Males (%)	Females (%)
Uganda, West Nile	21.0	9.2
Zambia, Kuska	15.9	17.0
Kenya, National Registry	8.8	4.7
Sudan	6.4	2.6
Tunisia	0.6	0.2
Malaysia, Kuala Lumpur		
Malaysians	13.8	0.4
Chinese	12.9	3.6
Indian	6.0	0
Iraq, Baghdad	2.1	1.1
Bangladesh	1.3	1.3
Sri Lanka, Colombo	0.8	0.5
Argentina, Santa Fe	1.3	1.3
Uruguay, Montevideo	0.2	0.2

Types of registry are not the same.
(From Munoz and Bosch[1] with permission)

In 1980, liver cancer represented 4% of the total number of malignancy cases worldwide. It was the 7th most common cancer in males and the 8th when both sexes were combined. In 1980, the absolute number of new cases per year was about 251,000, of which 192,000 occurred in developing countries and about 60,000 in developed countries.[3] In China alone, 100,000 people die from liver cancer, mostly HCC, every year.[4]

GEOGRAPHIC PREVALENCE

The incidence of HCC varies considerably with the geographic region perhaps due to differences in the major etiologic factors. Whereas the incidence of HCC is low among caucasians in north Europe, the United States, and Australia, it is much higher among the black populations in Mozambique and sub-Saharan Africa, and Asians in the Far East.[1,3,5,6]

It is difficult to grasp the exact incidence rate of HCC because the vital statistics are based on diagnoses made by physicians which mostly lack histologic confirmation, and which list HCC and cholangiocarcinoma (CC) together as 'primary liver cancer'. However, liver tumors associated with cirrhosis are almost invariably HCC in areas where the incidence rate is high. In our case control study in Japan based on autopsy, 369 of 391 liver cancers associated with cirrhosis were found to be primary as contrasted by 88 out of 226 cirrhosis-associated liver cancers being primary in Trieste, Italy.[7] CC is far less common compared with HCC, and the error caused by CC is not large. As far as histologic diagnosis is concerned,

Table 1.2 – Frequency (%) of primary liver cancer among all malignancies and relative to other major cancers in developed countries

Organ	Males			Females		
	Japan	USA	England-Wales	Japan	USA	England-Wales
Stomach	21.1	3.3	7.8	18.3	2.5	5.6
Lung	21.5	34.3	33.8	11.5	19.5	15.3
Liver	13.7 (3rd)	1.7	0.9	8.0 (4th)	1.3	0.8
Pancreas	5.7	4.5	4.1	6.6	5.5	4.6

These figures were quoted from reference (2).
Japan: Vital statistics, 1993, Japan
USA: Vital statistics of the United States, Vol II, Part A, 1987
England-Wales: Mortality statistics Cause, 1987

Table 1.3 – Age-adjusted incidence rates of liver cancer in various countries, cities, and ethnic groups

Country	Incidence rate (per 100,000/yr)	
	Males	**Females**
Mozambique, Lourenco Marques	112.9	30.8
Zimbabwe, Bulawayo	64.6	25.4
Gambia	33.1	12.6
Senegal	25.6	9.0
Cape		
Bantu	26.3	8.4
Colored	1.5	0.7
White	1.2	0.6
Algeria	1.6	1.4
Nigeria, Ibadan	15.4	3.2
Argentina,Tandil	9.9	5.8
Brazil, Fortaleza	3.5	3.7
Peru, Lima	4.0	2.9
Jamaica	6.1	2.1
United States, San Francisco		
Chinese	19.1	3.6
Black	3.9	1.8
Japanese	3.0	0.4
White	2.9	1.1
Canada		
Eskimos	6.9	3.7
Alberta	1.3	0.5
Switzerland, Geneva	10.2	1.5
Italy, Parma	8.6	3.3
Spain, Zaragoza	7.2	5.5
France, Doubs	3.7	1.0
Germany, Hamburg	4.5	1.7
Denmark	3.6	2.3
Yugoslavia, Slovenia	2.0	1.2
Czechoslovakia, Slovakia	5.1	2.8
United Kingdom, England and Wales	1.6	0.8
Ireland	0.1	0.3
China, Shanghai	34.4	11.6
Singapore		
Chinese	31.6	7.2
Malay	15.6	5.3
Indian	14.1	2.8
Korea	13.8	3.2
Japan		
Miyagi	11.2	4.0
Nagasaki	25.8	7.9
India, Bombay	4.9	2.5
Philippines, Manila	19.9	6.2
Hong Kong	32.3	7.4
Pakistan	0.7	0.8
New Zealand		
Maori	11.2	4.2
Non-Maori	2.4	1.1
Pacific Polynesian Islands	26.6	2.3
Australia, South	2.0	0.7
Hawaii, Chinese	7.8	2.4

(From Munoz and Bosch[1] and Bosch and Munoz [3] with permission)

autopsy studies are reliable, but only a relative frequency of HCC among all autopsies or malignancies may be calculated; there is a considerable bias at the time of hospital admission and autopsy, due to the socioeconomic state of the society and patients, and changing interest on the part of physicians. A well-established cancer registry with frequent histologic diagnosis is more reliable, yet the statistics based on a cancer registry are often different from vital statistics which depend on death certificates.[8]

The highest incidence rate of HCC is known in Mozambique because so many young Mozambican workers come down with HCC while working in gold mines around Johannesburg through the agreement between the South African Republic and Mozambique. These young patients are mostly noncirrhotic. It was Berman[9] and later Higginson[10] who called world attention to the extremely high incidence among the male blacks (Shangaan tribe) from Mozambique. Table 1.3 gives the age-adjusted incidence rates of primary liver cancer per 100,000/year in various countries, areas and ethnic groups. They may be roughly divided into the high incidence areas/peoples (>20/100,000/yr) which include Mozambique, Zimbabwe, Senegal, Gambia, Nigeria, Singapore Chinese, South African blacks, Hong Kong, China, Taiwan, Polynesian islands, and Japan (after 1976); intermediate incidence areas/peoples (5-20/100,000/yr) including Switzerland, Italy, Spain, Argentina, Jamaica, Canadian Eskimos, New Zealand Maori, Singapore Malay, Singapore Indian, Korea, Hawaii Chinese, etc; and low incidence areas/peoples (<5/100,000/yr) such as Sweden, United Kingdom, Ireland, Norway, Germany, Denmark, France, Yugoslavia, Algeria, Brazil, Peru, US blacks and whites, Pakistan, Australia, Canadian whites, Israel, India (Bombay), etc.[1,3-5] In Table 1.3, different ethnic groups are compared within the same country or area, and considerable differences are apparent. Although African blacks have high incidence rates, the incidence is much lower among the blacks in the United States who originally came from Africa. A similar difference exists between the Chinese in Hawaii and those in the Far East. The Chinese in the San Francisco Bay area who still have a relatively high incidence may not have lived in the United States long enough for the incidence rate to be reduced as much as in the black population in the

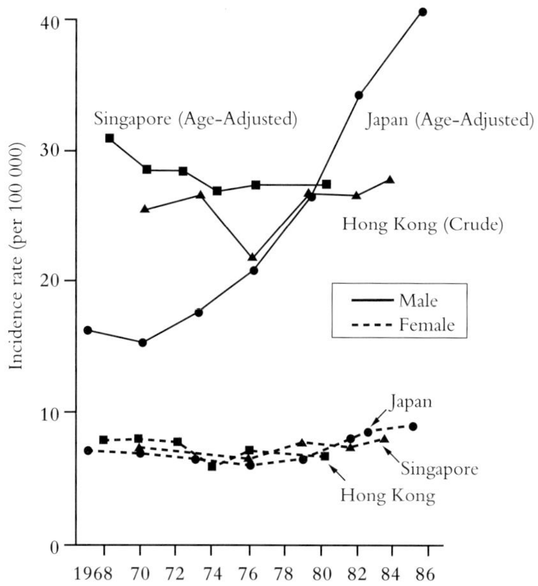

Figure 1.1 – Time trends in the incidence rate of primary liver cancer in Japan, Singapore, and Hong Kong. The incidence rate has been rising at a remarkable pace among men in Japan, and no parallel has been observed elsewhere (quoted from reference (15) with permission).

States. Chinese in San Francisco are known to have a high carrier rate for the hepatitis B surface antigen (HBsAg) which may be an important etiologic factor among them. Even within the same ethnic group, the incidence differs because of the difference in eating habit and living conditions. In Mozambique, for instance, the coast region has a nine-fold greater incidence compared with that in the inland region.[11]

China has a unique history of cancer epidemiology study. After the founding of the People's Republic of China, the central government set out to determine the regional incidences of various cancers. From 1972 to 1977, 250,000 physicians and more than 600,000 assistants (bare-foot doctors) were mobilized in a mass survey on cancer incidence in 2,392 counties where 840 million people were chosen as the study population. With a special census, the causes of 18 million deaths were studied retrospectively from the medical records and by interview of the relatives. Prospectively, 71% of the cancers were diagnosed either by histology, exploratory surgery, or laboratory assay.[12] For liver cancer, the alpha-fetoprotein (AFP) tests were used.[13] Based on this survey, it became clear that the main endemic areas for liver cancer in this country are along the southeast seacoast, and particularly deltas, valleys, and islands. The hyperendemic areas such as Fusui and Qidong counties have standardized mortality of more than 60/100,000/yr whereas low incidence areas have mortalities of about 6/100,000/yr.[14] A mortality of 60/100,000/yr for both sexes combined may be nearly as high as that in Mozambique, considering an M:F ratio of 2-3:1 in China.

SEX AND AGE

HCC is more common in males than in females regardless of geography, but the male:female (M:F) ratio differs with the country, as well as with the year of survey beause of changing time trends. It appears that the M:F ratio of incidence is greater in the high prevalence regions such as Africa, China, Hong Kong, Singapore and Japan, and lower in the low-incidence regions such as Latin America and Europe. This ratio rises as the incidence rate increases, as is the case in Japan, because the increase occurs mainly in males (Fig. 1.1).[15] The greater susceptibility of males may be hormonal or genetic, or due to a greater exposure to environmental carcinogens. The age-specific incidence rate of cancer generally increases in proportion to age with a tendency to level off in the very advanced years. In most countries, the peak age of HCC cases is in the 60's, but in Japan it is in the

Table 1.4 – Age distribution in histologically-proven patients in Japan (1978-1987)*

Age (years)	HCC	CCC
1-9	27	1
10-19	43	0
20-29	91	12
30-39	420	37
40-49	1,365	104
50-59	4,183	191
60-69	3,628	276
70-79	1,423	163
80-	125	18
Total	11,305	802

* Liver Cancer Study Group of Japan

50's (Table 1.4). In the high-incidence areas such as Mozambique and Zimbabwe, the age curve shifts toward the younger age groups. The crude incidence among Mozambican males aged 25 to 34 years is more than 500 times that of the equivalent white population in the United Kingdom or the USA. because HCC under age 40 years is very rare in these countries. The difference becomes smaller (15 times) in the aged populations above 65 years.[1,5] HCC can occur in childhood and adolescence, but primary liver cancer in the young is often fibrolamellar carcinoma[16] among caucasians, a variant of HCC which is extremely rare in the Far East, and under age 5 years it is mostly hepatoblastoma.[17] The M:F ratio tends to decrease with younger ages,[18,19] and frequency of underlying cirrhosis is also low.[20-22] Our study[23] based on autopsies comparing Chiba and Trieste, Italy, demonstrated a significant difference in the age of patients. The average age of patients at death was nearly 20 years older in Trieste. This age difference is presumably due to different underlying cirrhosis, posthepatitic vs alcoholic.

Table 1.5 – Relative frequencies of primary liver cancer in autopsy series

Country	Period	No. of autopsies	No. of primary liver cancers	%
Europe				
Denmark[24]	1938-59	14,881	50	0.34
Finland[25]	1952-62	15,545	93	0.60
Sweden[18]	1957-64	8,837	121	1.47
France[19]	1959-66	2,540	42	1.65
Federal Republic of Germany[26]	1961-70	4,411	47	1.06
Scotland[27]	1949-58	26,158	96	0.38
	1959-65	29,160	178	0.61
Switzerland[28]	1901-66	86,549	300a	0.35
Bulgaria[29]	1901-67	50,361	306	0.60
Italy-Trieste[23]	1980-84	12,340	205a	1.66
Italy-Florence[30]	1958-62			0.30
		8,514	113	
	1978-82			2.56
Africa				
Lagos[31]	1957	2,000	26	1.30
Uganda[32]	?	5,728	108	1.90
Asia				
Japan (Autopsy Registry of Jpn)	1958-59	19,356	369	1.92
	1968-69	49,128	1,278a	2.60
	1978-79-	62,565	3,113a	4.98
	1986-87	79,420	6,081a	7.66
Thailand[33]	1954-66	1,480	100	6.76
Pakistan[34]	1960-65	5,450	11	0.20
India-Bombay[35]	1947-68	12,616	45	0.36
China[36]	?	3,498	107	3.06
North America				
Boston[37]	1917-68	14,000	84a	0.60
Los Angeles[38]	1918-53	49,915	75a	0.15
	1954-63	23,476	79a	0.34
	1964-83	6,427	95a	1.48
Latin America				
Mexico[39]	1935-66	6,558	37	0.56
Costa Rica[40]	?	3,000	25	0.83
Chile[41]	1960-70	4,140	25	0.60
Argentina[42]	1905-67	22,170	64	0.28

a= HCC only, not including CCC.

Table 1.6 – Relative frequency of hepatocellular carcinoma among all autopsies and all autopsied malignancies in Japan (National Autopsy Registry)

Year	All autopsies	All malignancies	HCC	Percent	
				All autopsies	Malignancies
1961,62	26,445	9,821	443	1.68	4.51
1963,64	30,479	12,359	610	2.00	4.94
1965,66	35,342	17,695	779	2.20	4.40
1967,69	44,806	24,203	1,115	2.49	4.61
1970,71	43,728	22,250	1,376	3.15	6.18
1972,73	46,201	24,748	1,516	3.28	6.13
1974,75	45,744	23,960	1,758	3.84	7.34
1976,77	49,965	27,389	2,270	4.54	8.29
1978,79	62,565	32,720	3,113	4.98	9.51
1980,81	64,821	42,045	4,131	6.37	9.83
1982,83	78,341	45,052	4,921	6.28	10.92
1984,85	80,072	48,514	5,584	6.97	11.51
1986,87	79,420	46,765	6,082	7.66	13.01
1988,89	77,946	46,235	6,147	7.88	13.28
1990,91	75,020	43,938	6,238	8.32	14.20
1992,93	77,946	46,185	6,147	7.89	13.31

TIME TRENDS

Studies on time trends are subject to error due to changing diagnostic capability, and classification as exemplified by the repeated revisions in the International Classification of Diseases (ICD), and because of registration artifacts. Statistics based on autopsy[18,19,23-42] give relative frequency of histologically proven HCC among all autopsies, and a comparison of various countries is given in Table 1.5. From this table, time trends are apparent in the areas where old and new data are available. In the National Autopsy Registry published annually by the Japan Pathological Society, which records nearly 90% of all individual autopsy cases compiled by major hospitals throughout the country, HCC constituted 1.68% among 26,445 necropsies in 1961-62, and this rate steadily increased in the ensuing 30 years to the current (1992-93) 7.89%, demonstrating an indisputable 5-fold increase as shown in Table 1.6. In this study, the incidence rate was found to have risen from 16.3/100,000/yr in 1966-68 to 40.9/100,000/yr in 1984-86 among males, but peculiarly the increase among females was almost unrecognizable. This increase is now attributed to the increase in hepatitis-C associated HCC as discussed below. Thus, there is a distinct sex difference not only in the incidence rate but also in the time trends. In Los Angeles, the rate of HCC among all autopsies was 0.15% in 1918-53, and it rose to 1.48% in 1964-83,[37] again the increase being remarkable. In the Florence area of Italy, an 8-fold increase has been reported.[29] A less dramatic but significant increase was also noted in west Scotland.[27] According to the study of Saracci and Repetto[43] in 1980 based on cancer registries, there was an increase in incidence rate among males in 24 out of 37 countries. Analysis of more recent data is needed. Liver cancer mortality increased about 2-fold from 1959 to 1976 in Shanghai, China.[14]

ETIOLOGIC FACTORS

Cirrhosis

The vast majority of patients with HCC have chronic liver diseases, notably cirrhosis.[44] It is the underlying disease in more than 80% of HCC patients in most countries, and nonalcoholic posthepatitic cirrhosis is more frequently associated with HCC than is alcoholic micronodular cirrhosis. It is known, as already discussed, that among African blacks who have a high incidence of HCC, the association of cirrhosis with HCC is weaker and cirrhosis is mild, if present, whereas in low-incidence areas cirrhosis is more frequently associated with HCC.[31,45-48] However, if one compares young and old patients with HCC, cirrhosis is less common and HBsAg much more frequently positive in younger patients.[49] Studies of Miyaji[50] and Shikata[51] in Japan clearly showed that cirrhotic livers with large nodules and thin stromas are more commonly associated with HCC than livers with small nodules and thick stromas. The former type is assumed to have greater regenerative activities of hepatocytes with increased DNA synthesis, hence more frequent rearrangements of DNA sequences in the chromosomes. In a study in London, there was a higher incidence of HCC among patients with alcoholic cirrhosis who had abstained and whose micronodular cirrhosis had turned macronodular.[52] With abstinence, there is a surge of regenerative activity, transforming small nodules to larger ones. Clinically, patients with alcoholic cirrhosis seldom develop HCC while they are imbibing. While alcoholic cirrhosis is the predominant type in the western countries, posthepatitic cirrhosis is much more common in the Far East, and there is a considerable difference in the frequency of HCC and age of onset for patients who develop HCC.[23]

The death rate is higher for cirrhosis than for HCC in areas where HCC is uncommon, such as Chile, Mexico, Portugal, France, Puerto Rico, Ireland and Austria, as contrasted by reported lower death rates for cirrhosis in Thailand, Hong Kong, Greece and Switzerland which have relatively high rates for HCC.[53] It is generally thought that macronodular cirrhosis is more commonly associated with hepatitis B virus (HBV) infection and is more prone to hepatocarcinogenesis.[50] However, association of HBV and HCC is even stronger among young HCC patients without cirrhosis in Japan.[49] In Senegal, it was estimated that in 62% of HCC cases positive for HBsAg cancer arose in noncirrhotic livers and that the degree of association with HBV was similar for HCC with cirrhosis and HCC without.[54] In certain countries like Japan, the role of HBV infection is becoming less important due to the recent surge of hepatitis C virus (HCV) infection and HCV-associated cirrhosis.[55] HCV-associated cirrhosis is distinctly different from HBV-associated macronodular thin stromal cirrhosis; it is mixed micro- and mesonodular cirrhosis with wide stromas with active inflammation.[56] Under experimental conditions in animals, high doses of hepatocarcinogens induce cirrhosis and HCC,[57] but in humans there is no evidence that aflatoxins or other hepatocarcinogens are responsible for the development of cirrhosis that underlies HCC.

HEPATITIS VIRUS INFECTIONS

Hepatitis B

Numerous epidemiologic and biologic studies have suggested an important role of HBV infection in hepatocarcinogenesis. When the close relationship between HBV infection and HCC incidence was discovered, it was thought that the age-old enigma of close association of HCC with cirrhosis was resolved, namely, both cirrhosis and HCC were caused by HBV infection. However, HBV is not an oncovirus, having no oncogene in its genome, and the exact mechanism whereby HCC is induced by this virus has yet to be elucidated. Nevertheless, evidence is strong that chronic HBV infection or HBsAg carriage is intimately associated with HCC. Worldwide, there is a considerable parallel between HBsAg carrier rate and HCC incidence rate among various populations or ethnic groups.[58] There are areas where such parallel is not found, however. The estimated risk of HBsAg carriers for developing HCC is 100-fold that of non-carriers according to the study made in Taiwan,[59] where 90% of HCC cases are positive for HBsAg.[60] Our study in Tokyo showed a relative risk of about 30 among adult carriers.[61] As a result of improved living conditions and vaccination, the prevalence of HBV infection is sharply declining in Japan and elsewhere. HBV associated HCC is set to decrease.

Hepatitis C

Around 1975, the relative proportion of HBsAg positive cases among all HCCs began declining, slowly but noticeably, in Japan with increasing HBV unassociated cases (Fig. 1.2). The decline was steady, and the HBsAg positivity of more than 40% in HCC cases before 1978 in the national study[62] was reduced to 17.8 % in the 1990, 91 survey.[63] We in 1982 predicted that non-A, non-B hepatitis virus could account for this trend.[64] As already discussed and shown in Fig. 1.1, this particular time trend was due to increasing HCV-associated HCC. When HCV was identified in 1989, and an antibody test system was developed,[65] many countries almost simultaneously found out that positivity for anti-HCV is significantly high in HCC cases. In Italy, Spain and Japan among others, around 70% of HCC cases are associated with HCV infection as shown in Table 1.7[66-88]; this rate is lower in areas where HBV infection is

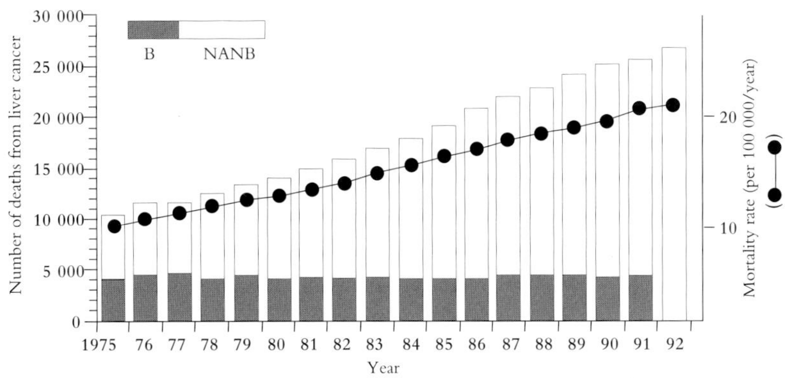

Figure 1.2 – Time trends in liver cancer mortality in Japan. Relation between HBsAg-positive and -negative (non-A, non-B) patients based on vital statistics for Japan 1992 (Statistics & Information Department 1993). The number of deaths of HBsAg-positive patients (shaded) was calculated from HBsAg positivity rates among HCC patients published by the Liver Cancer Study Group of Japan. Note that the number of deaths related to HBV is unchanged in the past 18 years,while deaths of patients with non-A, non-B hepatitis have more than tripled.

endemic and a large proportion of HCC cases are HBsAg carriers.[55] Yet, among HBsAg negative cases, HCV infection is just as frequent as in Italy, Spain and Japan.[79]

Clearly, HCV infection is etiologically involved in HCC in a manner yet to be elucidated. HCV virus is an RNA virus, not reverse transcribed and is not integrated into hepatocyte DNA. It is transmitted mainly through skin wounds. It is assumed that the prevalence of this virus has undergone remarkable temporal changes, due in part to the new medical practice evolved in the past century or so, including surgical operation using blood, injection, vaccination, blood transfusion, use of plasma and its products, etc. There was a time after the end of World War II when more than 60% of patients developed posttransfusion hepatitis after major surgery requiring blood transfusion in Japan. In fact, in several areas in China, anti-HCV positivities among professional blood

Table 1.7. – Prevalence of anti-HCV among patients with HCC in selected countries

Country/Area	Year	Anti-HCV positivity percent (no./total)	Control value	Reference
Italy	1989		0.87	66
Padua	1989	76 (152/200)		67
France	1989		0.68	68
Paris	1991	58 (32/55)		69
Spain/Barcelona	1989	75 (72/96)	7.3	70
UK	1990	11 (1/9)	0.18	71
Greece/Athens	1991	39 (72/185)		72
USA	1995		1.4	73
Miami	1990	53 (31/59)		74
S.Africa/Johannesburg	1990	29 (110/380)	0.7	75
Mozambique	1990	46 (69/150)		76
Japan	1991		1.15	77
Matsumoto	1991	68 (74/109)		78
Taiwan/Taipei	1990	33 (22/66)	0.95	79
Hong Kong	1992	7 (31/414)	0.64	80
China/South	1993	25 (64/261)		81
Korea/Seoul	1993	28 (28/100)	1.3	82
Thailand	1990	6 (3/47)	2.6	83
Singapore	1991	15 (7/47)	0	84
India/New Delhi	1992	15 (8/53)		85
Indonesia/Jakarta	1991	34 (24/70)		86
Nepal/Kathmandu	1994	10 (6/62)	3.5	87
Saudi Arabia/Riyadh	1992	26 (11/42)	1.5	88

Most studies used C100-3 test, and these figures would have been greater if the 2nd generation test were used.

donors is more than 60%, and on Fiji island where blood transfusion is rarely carried out, none of 2,000 people tested positive (Yoshihara N, personal communication). It is now apparent that patients who received blood bought from professional donors and had posttransfusion hepatitis in the 1950s and 1960s are coming down with HCC in Japan. Similar situations are expected to exist in other countries where medicine progressed in a similar manner and disposable needles were introduced only after 1970. It is also established that it takes an average of 30 years from acute HCV infection through chronic hepatitis and cirrhosis to the development of HCC.[89] A time trend is expected along with the reduction of incidence of transfusion-associated hepatitis in recent years, with the number of HCC cases declining after a lapse of 30 years or so. It is not predictable at the moment whether after reduction of HCV-associated HCC, hepatitis G or GB virus[90,91] associated HCC will increase in relative proportion.

Budd-Chiari syndrome

It was Nakamura *et al*,[92] Japan, who first documented frequent HCC among patients who had an occlusion of the hepatic portion of the inferior vena cava (idiopathic type of Budd-Chiari syndrome). This disorder is commonly referred to as membranous obstruction of the inferior vena cava. The etiology is unknown.[93] It is endemic among southern African blacks,[94,95] in Nepal[96] and India.[97] More than 47% of such African blacks develop HCC.[94] In Japan, the incidence of HCC among such patients was 10 out of 156 patients (6.4%).[98] HCC is a common complication of Budd-Chiari syndrome in Nepal,[96] yet it is not a major complication in India, the neighboring country. In the USA, Rector *et al*[99] described 2 cases of HCC among 8 patients with membranous obstruction of the inferior vena cava. Such geographic differences in the frequency of HCC as a complication of Budd-Chiari syndrome may reflect differing hepatocarcinogenic factors or the degree of exposure to them.

Chemical carcinogens

Many organic chemical compounds are known to produce HCC in rodents under experimental conditions. Of all these substances, aflatoxin B1 is the best documented and perhaps the most hepatocarcinogenic. Aflatoxins have been found to be a food contaminant in many sub-Saharan areas of Africa, notably Mozambique, and South East Asian countries, such as Indonesia, and there is a crude parallel between the degree of aflatoxin contamination and HCC incidence.[100] The molecular events that ensue exposure to aflatoxin may not be the same as those in which viral infection but not aflatoxin is involved.[101] Perhaps aflatoxin and hepatitis virus infection are the two most important carcinogenic factors that may determine the frequency of HCC in specified areas of the world.

REFERENCES

1. Munoz N, Bosch X. Epidemiology of hepatocellular carcinoma. In: Okuda K, Ishak KG, eds. *Neoplasms of the liver.* Tokyo: Springer, 1987: 3-19
2. Ministry of Health and Welfare of Japan, Health and Welfare Statistics Association. *Trends in the health of nation* (in Japanese). *Kosei no Shihyo* 1995;**42**:50-55
3. Bosch X, Munoz N. Hepatocellular carcinoma in the world: epidemiologic questions. In: Tabor E, Di Bisceglie AM, Purcell RH, eds. *Etiology, pathology, and treatment of hepatocellular carcinoma in North America.* Woodlands, TX: Portofolio Publ. Co, 1991: 35-54
4. Yu SZ. Epidemiology of primary liver cancer. In: Tang ZY ed. *Subclinical hepatocellular carcinoma.* Beijin: China Academic Publishers, 1985:189-211
5. Munoz N, Linsell A. Epidemiology of primary liver cancer. In: Correa P, Haenszel W, eds. *Epidemiology of cancer of the digestive tract.* Jague: Martinus Nijhoff, 1982:161-195
6. Waterhouse JAH, Nuir CS, Correa P, Powell J. *Cancer incidence in five continents, Vol III.* Lyon: International Agency for Research on Cancer, 1976
7. Melato M, Laurino L, Mucli E, *et al.* Relationship between cirrhosis, liver cancer, and hepatic metastases. An autopsy study. *Cancer* 1989; **64**:455-459
8. Okuda K, Beasley RP. Epidemiology. In: Okuda K, Mackay I, eds. *Hepatocellular carcinoma.* Geneva:UICC, 1982:9-30
9. Berman C. *Primary carcinoma of the liver.* London: Lewis, 1951:5-14
10. Higginson J. The geographic pathology of primary liver cancer. *Cancer Res* 1963; **23**:1624-1633
11. Harrinton JS, McGlashan ND, Bradshaw E, *et al.* A spatial and temporal analysis of four cancers in African gold miners from southern Africa. *Br J Cancer* 1975; **31**:665-678
12. Li EP, Shiang EL. Cancer mortality in China. *J Natl Cancer Inst* 1980; **65**:217-221
13. Tang ZY. Subclinical hepatocellular carcinoma - historical aspects and general considerations. In: Tang ZY, ed. *Subclinical hepatocellular carcinoma.* Beijing: China Acad Publ, 1985: 1-11
14. Yu SZ. Epidemiology of primary liver cancer. In: Tang ZY, ed. *Subclinical hepatocellular carcinoma.* Beijing: China Acad Publ, 189-211
15. Okuda K, Fujimoto I, Hanai A, Urano Y. Changing incidence of hepatocellular carcinoma in Japan. *Cancer Res* 1987; **47**:4967-4972

16. Craig JR, Peters RL, Edmondson HA, Omata M. Fibrolamellar carcinoma of the liver: a tumor of adolescents and young adults with distinctive clinicopathologic features. *Cancer* 1980; **46**:372-379

17. The Liver Cancer Study Group of Japan. Primary liver cancer in Japan. Sixth report. *Cancer* 1987; **60**:1400-1411

18. Ohlsson EGH, Noden JG. Primary carcinoma of the liver. A study of 121 cases. *Acta Pathol Microbiol Immunol Scand* 1965; **64**:430-440

19. Pequignot H, Ethiene JP, Delavierre P, Petite JP. Cancers primitifs du foie sur cirrhose. Augmentation de frequence et observation chez des cirrhotiques connus et suivis. *Presse Med* 1967; **75**:2595-2600

20. Lack EE, Neave C, Vawters GF. Hepatocellular carcinoma. Review of 32 cases in childhood and adolescence. *Cancer* 1983; **52**:1510-1515

21. Farhi DC, Shikes RH, Maurari PJ, Silverberg SG. Hepatocellular carcinoma in young people. *Cancer* 1983; **52**:1516-1545

22. Okuda K, Nakashima T, Sakamoto K, *et al.* Hepatocellular carcinoma arising in noncirrhotic and highly cirrhotic livers: a comparative study of histopathology and frequency of hepatitis markers. *Cancer* 1982; **49**:450-455

23. Tiribelli C, Melato M, Croce LS, Giarelli L, Okuda K, Ohnishi K. Prevalence of hepatocellular carcinoma and relation to cirrhosis: comparison of two different cities of the world - Trieste, Italy, and Chiba, Japan. *Hepatology* 1989; **10**:998-1002

24. Glennert J. Primary carcinoma of the liver. A post-mortem study of 104 cases. *Acta Pathol Microbiol Immunol Scand* 1969; **53**:50-60

25. Evrasti J. Primary carcinoma of the liver. A pathologic and clinical study of 100 cases. *Acta Chir Scand, Suppl* 1964; **334**:1-65

26. Sievers BU. Leberzirrhose und Leberkarzinom in 10 Yahren einer Prosektur. *Acta Hepatogastroenterol* 1969; **20**:483-490

27. Manderson WG, Patrick RS, Peters EE. Incidence of primary carcinoma of the liver in the west of Scotland between 1949 and 1965. *Gut* 1968; **9**:480-484

28. Fierz L. Das Hepatom in Sektionsgut des Zuricher Pathologischen Instituts der Jahre 1901-1966 (86,549 Autopsien). *Acta Hepatol-Splenol* 1969; **16**:383-389

29. Brailski C. Primary liver carcinoma in Bulgaria. In: Remmer H, Bolt HM, Bannasch P, Popper H, eds. *Primary liver tumors*. Lancaster: NTP Press, 1978:137-139

30. Bartoloni ST, Omer F, Giannini A, Napoli P. Hepatocellular carcinoma and cirrhosis: a review of their relative incidence in a 25-year period in the Florence area. *Hepato-Gastroenterol* 1984; **31**:215-217

31. Steiner PE. Cancer of the liver and cirrhosis in trans-Saharan Africa and the United States of America. *Cancer* 1960; **13**:1085-1145

32. Davies JN. Primary liver carcinoma in Uganda. *Acta Un Int Cancer* 1961; **17**:787-792

33. Stitnimankarn T. Primary hepatic carcinoma in Thailand. In: Hirayama T, ed. *Cancer in Asia*. Tokyo: Univ Park Press, 1976:123-127

34. Islam AKN. Primary carcinoma of the liver. *E Pak Med J* 1969; **13**:92-96

35. Patwardhan JR, Kshirsagar VH, Gadgil PK. Primary carcinoma of the liver in Bombay. *Indian J Cancer* 1970; **7**:113-118

36. Ying UY, Ma CC, Hsu UT, Lei HH, Liang SF, Liu CH, Ku CY. Primary carcinoma of the liver. *Chin Med J* 1963; **82**:279-294

37. Purtilo DT, Gottlieb LS. Cirrhosis and hepatoma occurring at Boston City Hospital (1917-1968). *Cancer* 1973; **32**:458-462

38. Craig JR, Peters RL, Edmondson HA. *Tumors of the liver and intrahepatic bile ducts*. Washington DC: AFIP, 1989:6-7

39. Lopez-Corella E, Ridaura-Sanz C, Abares-Savedra J. Primary carcinoma of the liver in Mexican adults. *Cancer* 1968; **22**:678-685

40. Mena Solera H. Freceuencia cancer en Costa Rica. *Acta Med Cost* 1964; **7**:26-33

41. Ugarte G, Donos S. Primary hepatic tumors in Chile. In: Remmer H, Bolt HM, Bannach P, Popper H, eds. *Primary liver tumors*. Lancaster: MTP, 1978:165-169

42. Elsner B, Jauregui EM. Autopsy study of primary liver carcinoma in Buenos Aires, Argentina. *Acta Hepato Gastroenterol* 1974; **21**:26-34

43. Sarraci R, Repetto F. Time trends of primary liver cancer: indication of increased incidence in selected cancer registry populations. *J Natl Cancer Inst* 1980; **65**:241-247

44. Okuda K, Nakashima T, Kojiro M, Kondo Y, Wada K. Hepatocellular carcinoma without cirrhosis in Japanese patients. *Gastroenterology* 1989; **97**:40-46

45. Kew MC. Clinical pathologic, and etiologic heterogeneity in hepatocellular carcinoma: evidence from southern Africa. *Hepatology* 1981; **1**:366-369

46. Kew MC, Geddes EW. Hepatocellular carcinoma in rural southern African blacks. *Medicine* 1982; **61**:98-108

47. Okuda K, Peters RL, Simson IW. Gross anatomical features of hepatocellular carcinoma from three disparate geographic areas. Proposal of new classification. *Cancer* 1984; **54**:2165-2173

48. Kashala LO, Conne B, Kalengayi MMR, Kapanchi Y, Frei PC, Lambert PH. Histopathologic features of hepatocellular carcinoma in Zaire. *Cancer* 1990; **65**:130-134

49. Furuta T, Kanematsu T, Matumata T, Shirabe K, Yamagata M, Utsunomiya T, Sugimachi K. Clinicopathologic features of hepatocellular carcinoma in young patients. *Cancer* 1990; **66**:2395–2398

50. Miyaji T. Association of hepatocellular carcinoma with cirrhosis among autopsy cases in Japan during 14 years from 1958 to 1971. *Gann Monogr* 1976; **18**:129–149

51. Shikata T. Primary liver carcinoma and liver cirrhosis. In: Okuda K, Peters RL, eds. *Hepatocellular carcinoma*. New York: Wiley, 1976:53-95

52. Lee FK. Cirrhosis and hepatoma in alcoholics. *Gut* 1966; **7**:77-95

53. World Health Organization. World health statistics annual, 1978-1982. Vital statistics and causes of death. Geneva: WHO, 1982

54. Prince AM, Szmuness W, Michon J, Demaille J, Dieblt G, Linhard J, Quenum C, Sankale M. A case-control study of the association betwen primary liver cancer and hepatitis B infection in Senegal. *Int J Cancer* 1975; **16**:376-383

55. Okuda K. Hepatitis C virus and hepatocellular carcinoma. In: Tabor E, DiBiscegli A, eds. *Etiology, pathology and treatment of hepatocellular carcinoma in North America*. Woodlands: Portfolio Publ Co, 1991:119-126

56. Shimamatsu K, Kage M, Nakashima O, Kojiro M. Pathomorphological study of HCV antibody-positive liver cirrhosis. *J Gastroenterol Hepatol* 1994; **9**:624-630

57. Wogan GN. Aflatoxins and their relationship to hepatocellular carcinoma. In: Okuda K, Peters RL, eds. *Hepatocellular carcinoma*. New York: Wiley, 1976:25-42

58. Szmuness W. Hepatocellular carcinoma and the hepatitis B virus: evidence for a causal association. *Prog Med Virol* 1978; **24**:40-69

59. Beasley RP. Hepatitis B virus. The major etiology of hepatocellular carcinoma. *Cancer* 1988; **61**:1942-1956

60. Sung JL. Hepatitis B virus infection and its sequelae in Taiwan *Proc Natl Sci Counc Republ China* 1981; **5**:385-399

61. Sakuma K, Saitoh N, Kasai M, *et al.* Relative risks of death due to liver disease among Japanese male adults having various statuses for hepatitis B s and e antigen/antibody in serum: a prospective study. *Hepatology* 1988; **8**:1642-1646

62. Okuda K, Liver Cancer Study Group of Japan. Primary liver cancers in Japan. *Cancer* 1980; **45**:2663-2669

63. Liver Cancer Study Group of Japan. Follow-up primary liver cancer patients. Report 11 (1990-1991). *Acta Hepatol Jpn* 1995; **36**:208-217

64. Iwama S, Ohnishi K, Nakajima Y, *et al.* A clinical study of hepatocellular carcinoma (HCC) in relation to hepatitis B seromarkers: implication of non-A, non-B hepatitis (NANB). *Hepatology* 1982; **2**:117 (Abstract)

65. Kuo G, Choo QL, Alter HJ, *et al.* An assay for circulating antibodies to a major etiologic virus of human non-A non-B hepatitis. *Science* 1989; **244**:362-364

66. Sirchia G, Bellobuono A, Giovanetti A, Marconi M. Antibodies to hepatitis C virus in Italian blood donors. *Lancet* 1989;**ii**:797

67. Simonetti R, Cottone M, Craxi A, *et al.* Prevalence of antibodies to hepatitis C virus in hepatocellular carcinoma. *Lancet* 1989;**ii**:1338

68. Janot C, Courouce AM, Maneiz M. Antibodies to hepatitis C virus in French blood donors. *Lancet* 1989;**ii**:796-797

69. Nalpas B, Driss F, Pol S, *et al.* Association between HCV and HBV infection in hepatocellular carcinoma and alcoholic liver disease. *J Hepatol* 1991; **12**:70-74

70. Bruix J, Barrera JM, Calver X, *et al.* Prevalence of antibodies of hepatitis C virus in Spanish patients with hepatocellular carcinoma and hepatic cirrhosis. *Lancet* 1989;**ii**:1004-1006

71. Brind AM, Codd AA, Cohen DG, *et al.* Low prevalence of antibody to hepatitis C virus in north east England. *J Med Virol* 1990; **32**:242-248

72. Kaklamani E, Trichopoulos D, Tzonou A, *et al.* Hepatitis B and C viruses and their interaction in the origin of hepatocellular carcinoma. *JAMA* 1991; **265**:1974-1976

73. Alter MJ, Epidemiology of hepatitis C in the west. *Semin Liver Dis* 1995; **15**:15-32

74. Hasan F, Feffers LJ, Madina M, et al. Hepatitis C-associated hepatocellular carcinoma. *Hepatology* 1990; **12**:589-591

75. Kew MC, Houghton M, Choo QL, Kuo G. Hepatitis C virus antibodies in southern African blacks with hepatocellular carcinoma. *Lancet* 1990;**i**:873-874

76. Dazza M-C, Meneses L-V, Girard P-M, *et al.* Hepatitis C virus antibody and hepatocellular carcinoma. *Lancet* 1990;**335**:1216

77. Nishioka K. Hepatitis C virus infection in Japan. *Gastroenterol Jpn* 1991; **26**:Suppl. 3, 152-155.

78. Kiyosawa K, Furuta S. Review of hepatitis C in Japan. *J Gastroenterol Hepatol* 1991; **6**:383-391

79. Chen DS, Kuo GC, Sung L, *et al.* Hepatitis C virus infection in an area hyperendemic for hepatitis B and chronic liver disease: the Taiwan experience. *J Infect Dis* 1990; **162**:817-822

80. Leung NWY, Tam JS, Lai JY, *et al.* Does hepatitis C virus infection contribute to hepatocellular carcinoma in Hong Kong? *Cancer* 1992; **70**:4044

81. Ito S, Yao DF, Nii C, *et al.* Epidemiological characteristics of the incidence of hepatitis C virus (C100-3) antibodies in patients with liver diseases in the Inshore area of the Yangtze river. *J Gastroenterol Hepatol* 1993; **8**:232-237

82. Kim BS, park YM. Prevalence of hepatitis C virus related to liver diseases in Korea. *Gastroenterol Jpn* 1993; **28**:Suppl. 17-22

83. Boonmar S, Pojanagaroon B, Watanabe Y, *et al.* Prevalence of hepatitis C virus antibody among healthy blood donors and non-A, non-B hepatitis patients in Thailand. *Jpn J Med Sci Biol* 1990; **43**:29-36

84. Oon CJ, Chia SC, Fock KM. Prevalence of hepatitis C in liver diseases and in a random population in Singapore. *Proc. 3rd International Symp on Viral Hepatitis and Hepatocellular Carcinoma, Taipei*. Gastroenterological Society of the Republic of China, Taipei, 1991:p.141

85. Ramesh R, Muhshi A, Panda SK. Prevalence of hepatitis C virus antibodies in chronic liver disease and hepatocellular carcinoma patients in India. *J Gastroenterol Hepatol* 1991; **7**:393-395

86. Sulaiman HA, Noer S, Endardjo S, Hoyaranda E. The prevalence of antibody to hepatitis C virus (anti-HCV) in patients with acute and chronic liver disease in Jakarta, Indonesia. *Gastroenterol J* 1991; **26**:Supp. 3, 179-183

87. Shrestha SM, Tsuda F, Okamoto H, et al. Hepatitis B virus subtypes and hepatitis C virus genotypes in patients with chronic liver disease in Nepal. *Hepatology* 1994;**19**:805-809

88. Al Karawi MAA, Shariq S, El Shiekh Mohamed AR, *et al.* Hepatitis C virus infection in chronic liver disease and hepatocellular carcinoma in Saudi Arabia. *J Gastroenterol Hepatol* 1992; **7**:237-239

89. Kiyosawa K, Sodeyama T, Tanaka E, *et al.* Interrelationship of blood transfusion, non-A, non-B hepatitis and hepatocellular carcinoma: analysis by detection of antibody to hepatitis C virus. *Hepatology* 1990; **12**:671-675

90. Anonymous. New hepatitis viruses in the blood supply. *Blood Bank Week* 1995; **12**:1-2

91. Simons JN, Pilot-Matias TM, Leary TP, *et al.* Identification of two flavivirus-like genomes in the GB hepatitis agent. *Proc Natl Acad Sci USA* 1995; **92**:3401-3405

92. Nakamura T, Nakamura S, Aikawa T, *et al.* Obstruction of the inferior vena cava in the hepatic portion and the hepatic veins. Report of 18 cases and review of the Japanese literature. *Angiography* 1968; **19**:479-498

93. Okuda K. Membranous obstruction of the inferior vena cava: etiology and relation to hepatocellular carcinoma. *Gastroenterology* 1982; **82**:376-379

94. Simson IW. Membranous obstruction of the inferior vena cava and hepatocellular carcinoma in South Africa. *Gastroenterology*1982; **68**:171-178

95. Kew MC, McKnight A, Hodkinson J, Bukofzer S, Esser JD. The role of membranous obstruction of the inferior vena cava in the etiology of hepatocellular carcinoma in Southern African blacks. *Hepatology* 1989; **9**:121-125

96. Shrestha SM, Okuda K, Uchida T, *et al.* Endemicity and clinical picture of liver disease due to obstruction of the hepatic portion of the inferior vena cava. *J Gastroenterol Hepatol* 1996; **11**:170-179

97. Datta DV, Saha S, Singh SA, Gupta BB, Aikat BK, Chhutani PN. Clinical spectrum of Budd-Chiari syndrome in Chandigarh with particular reference to obstruction of intra-hepatic portion of inferior vena cava. *Ind J Med Res* 1972; **60**:385-402

98. Okuda H, Yamagata H, Obata H, *et al.* Epidemiological and clinical features of Budd-Chiari syndrome in Japan. *J Hepatol* 1995; **22**:1-9

99. Rector WG Jr, Xu Y, Goldstein L, Peters RL, Reynolds TB. Membranous obstruction of the inferior vena cava in the United States. *Medicine* 1985; **64**:134-143

100. Van Rensburg SJ, Cook-Mozaffari P, Van Schalkwy DJ, *et al.* Hepatocellular carcinoma and dietary aflatoxin in Mozambique and Transkai. *Br J Cancer* 1985; **51**:713-726

101. Okuda K. Hepatocellular carcinoma: recent progress. *Hepatology* 1992; **15**:948-963

2

Etiology

M Colombo and A Sangiovanni

The identification of risk factors for hepatocellular carcinoma (HCC) has provided insight into the etiology of this tumor, and has made prevention and screening campaigns aimed at early detection of the tumor possible.[1,2]

HCC is a multistage disease whose occurrence is linked to environmental, dietary and life-style factors. The great variations in levels of carcinogenic factors account for the different incidences of the tumor.[3] Recent advances in molecular biology and genetics have initiated a whole new field, the molecular epidemiology of HCC.

Risk factors for HCC have been grouped into two clusters, physiologic and pathologic factors (Table 2.1). Much evidence indicates that these risk factors may interact with each other either as a group or as single factors to modulate development of liver cancer.

PHYSIOLOGIC FACTORS

In all populations, regardless of the risk, HCC rates increase progressively with age, and men have been more prone to develop liver cancer than women. In high incidence areas, there is a shift toward younger age groups which could be due to the many cases of HCC developing in patients with perinatally acquired hepatitis B infection. In these areas, the male to female risk ratio is between 4 to 1 and 8 to 1, whereas the male predominance is less marked in the low-risk populations of North America and Europe. It is unclear whether male preponderance of HCC reflects increased susceptibility of men to the tumor or their greater exposure to the environmental risk factors for HCC. Race has no direct pathogenetic role in HCC. Studies of immigrants clearly indicate that the risk of HCC for an ethnic group largely depends on that population's exposure to environmental factors, in particular to hepatitis viruses.[1,2] The rates of HCC are lower for Oriental people born in the USA than for those who emigrated to the USA. The latter have lower incidence than those living in their countries of origin. These findings could be accounted for by better standards of hygiene in the USA than in Asian countries, resulting in reduced exposure to alimentary carcinogens, and diminished intrafamilial spread of HBV.

Table 2.1 – Major risk factors associated with HCC

Physiologic:	
	Age
	Sex
	Race
Pathologic:	
	Hepatitis B
	Hepatitis C
	Alcohol
	Dietary Aflatoxin
	Rare Metabolc Disorders
	Sex Hormones
	Chemical
	Cirrhosis
Interaction	

VIRAL FACTORS

Hepatitis B virus

Epidemiological, clinical and experimental studies link HCC to HBV. The prevalence of HBV was found to be high in the areas of the world in which there is also a high incidence of HCC (Africa, South Pacific, Asia) and the risk for HCC for HBV carriers is substantially greater than the risk for non-carriers.[4]

In Taiwan, the risk of 3,454 HBsAg carriers developing HCC was 102 times greater than that of 19,253 non-carriers (Table 2.2). The carriers at especially high risk of developing HCC were those with actively replicating infection (HBeAg/HBV-DNA+) and those with cirrhosis.[4] The strict association between HBV and HCC was confirmed in a study of 824 native Alaskan male carriers, in whom the annual incidence rate of HCC was 387/100,000 men.[5] In the pre-screening era, this tumor was the most common sequela of cirrhosis in the Alaskan native

Table 2.2 – Prospective study of HCC in 22,707 Chinese male government employees

Study duration 1978-89

	HBsAg(+)	**HBsAg(-)**
No of Patients	3,454	19,253
No of HCC	184	10
No of Cases/10^5/yr	473.5	4.6

Relative Risk = 102

Table 2.3 – Anti-HCV as a risk factor for HCC

Location		Case/Control (No)	Relative Risk	Author
USA				
	Miami	87/200	134.0	Hasan[15]
	Los Angeles	51/128	10.5	Yu[16]
Africa				
	South Africa	380/152	61.5	Kew[17]
	Senegal	80/136	19.8	Coursaget[18]
Europe				
	Italy	212/212	68.1	Simonetti[19]
	Greece	185/467	6.3	Kaklamani[20]
Asia				
	Japan	91/410	52.3	Tanaka[21]
	Taiwan	128/384	6.9	Chuang[22]

HBV carriers, accounting for 57% of fatal cancers, as compared to the non-carrier Alaskan native population, in which HCC accounted for approximately 2% of cancer-related deaths. In a prospective cohort study of 1,069 chronic carriers of HBsAg in Toronto, 11 cases of HCC were identified in a 26 month period, giving an annual HCC incidence of 470/100,000. [6]

In all studies the incidence of HCC was greater in men than in women and in patients with chronic hepatitis or cirrhosis than in carriers with persistently normal transaminases.[4-6] Thus, the differences in the HCC risk among HBsAg carriers that have been reported in different studies, i.e., from 155 to 3,000/100,000/year[7,8] probably reflect differences in the patients' demography. In a prospective study of 349 European patients with HBV-related cirrhosis, the probability of developing HCC was 6% in 5 years, with preference for aged patients and those with more advanced liver disease.[9] The higher incidence of HCC in Asian carriers in these studies could be due to the fact that most Asians have acquired HBV in childhood and may therefore have more advanced liver disease than Caucasian patients, who often acquired HBV later. In fact, the time in life when infection occurs seems to be important for subsequent development of the tumor. Infection early in life or during pregnancy often becomes persistent and frequently results in HCC. This was clearly shown with the woodchuck model, in which animals that were either naturally or experimentally infected at birth with woodchuck hepatitis virus developed HCC after 17-36 months of persistent infection.[10] In the clinical setting, neonates to HBV-infected mothers have progressed to chronic infection and HCC, while infection of adults with HBV carries a far lower risk of carrier state and subsequent HCC development.[11] Thus, HBV is an important carcinogen in most Asian and African countries, in which high endemicity is maintained by infection occurring early in life, but not in the Western World, in which other environmental factors are major risk factors for HCC. One main point in HBV-associated liver carcinogenesis that has emerged from both animal and human studies is the coexistence of persistent viremia and significant liver disease. However, carriers with persistently normal liver enzyme are also at risk for HCC, but the level of risk is yet undefined. The risk of HCC was low in 92 such Italian carriers, who were followed prospectively for more than 10 years.[11] However, HBV carriers are a heterogeneous group of patients that also includes cases with an indolent progression to cirrhosis. This is the situation for many carriers of pre-core HBV mutants (anti-HBe+/HBV-DNA+), who are common in southern Europe. Liver disease in pre-core mutant carriers causes a fluctuating pattern of serum transaminases. During the pauses between biochemical flare-ups, these patients are indistinguishable from "healthy" carriers of HBsAg.[12]

Hepatitis C virus

The sequential development of cirrhosis and HCC in patients with post-transfusion hepatitis was a clue leading to the identification of HCV as a risk factor for HCC.[13] The average time-lag between transfusion-associated infection and cancer development was 30 years, but with a 15 to 45 yr range. HCC patients chronically infected with HCV prevailed in Japan, Italy and Spain, but not in other high-risk areas for HCC.[14] There are important variations in the HCC risk for anti-HCV patients even in the same geographical area[15-22] (Table 2.3). Interestingly, almost all patients with HCC had cirrhosis and up to 30% of them had coexisting serological evidence of HBV or alcohol abuse, further supporting the idea that both HCC and cirrhosis might result from the interplay of several risk factors. Anedoctal observation, however, indicates that patients with chronic HCV infection and normal livers have also developed HCC.[23] Using the polymerase chain reaction technique, HCV-RNA has been almost invariably detected in serum and tumor tissue of anti-HCV patients with HCC. In many patients, HCV-RNA was found to belong to the more pathogenic type 1b,[21] suggesting that this virus strain could be more pathogenic than others. However, data showing similar prevalences of genotypes in patients with HCC militate against the pathogenetic importance of HCV1b.[24,25]

The association between HCV1b and HCC could be a cohort effect due to the recruitment in referral centers of patients with long-standing infections, who are at higher risk for HCV1b and advanced liver disease than patients with more recent infections.[26]

It is unlikely that HCV plays a direct role in liver tumorigenesis, since no reverse transcriptase activity has been found in infected livers. One current opinion is that HCV may promote cancer through cirrhosis, which is "per se" an important risk factor for this tumor. However, development of HCC in HCV carriers without chronic hepatitis or cirrhosis has been reported. It is possible that truncated fragments of core region (p22) migrate into liver cell nuclei, as has been shown experimentally to occur, and act as cancer promoters through interaction with cell regulatory genes.

LIVER DISEASES

Cirrhosis

Approximately 20% of all patients who died of cirrhosis had associated HCC, and HCC was found to be associated with cirrhosis in more than 90% of all reported cases.[2] The association between these two conditions was confirmed by close follow-up studies of cirrhotic patients. The yearly conversion rates from cirrhosis to HCC were approximately 3% in both Western and Japanese patients[27-29] (Table 2.4). Liver cell regeneration in cirrhotic livers could be the crucial oncogenic event, in that it promotes selection and clonal expansion of committed liver cells after damage by genotoxic agents. Whatever the biological meaning of the association between cirrhosis and HCC, this association provides a formidable tool for screening for patients who are at risk for liver cancer. Certain histologic features and metabolic alterations of liver cells that are connected with hepatic carcinogenesis could help to identify patients who have excess risk of HCC. HCC would appear within adenomatous hyperplastic nodules in post-hepatitis cirrhotic livers.[2]

Extremely well differentiated tumors (grade 1 of the Edmondson-Steiner classification) are also often seen in benign macroregenerative nodules, with cells arranged in layers of nearly normal cell thickness, showing occasional microacinar formation, nuclear crowding, increased cytoplasmic basophilia and increased nucleus/cytoplasm ratio (small cell dysplasia). Adenomatous hyperplastic nodules containing small cell dysplasia are defined as atypical nodules and

Table 2.4 – Detection of HCC according to different screening intervals in prospectively studied cohorts of patients with cirrhosis

Author	Year	Screening Intervals (months)	No.	Hepatocellular carcinoma			
				Annual Rate(%)	Single Node(%)	<3cm (%)	AFP(-) (%)
Sato *et al*[30]	1993[28]	3	33	3.0	88	64	41
Cottone *et al*[31]	1994[29]	6	30	4.4	87	53	60
Colombo *et al* unpublished	1994	12	65	3.2	55	29	32

are considered precursors of HCC.[2] In a cohort study of 307 consecutive Italian patients with viral cirrhosis who were followed for an average of 46 months, HCC was demonstrated in 45 (15%). Multivariate analysis showed that liver small cell dysplasia was the most important risk factor correlated with tumor development.[30]

Serum AFP is another marker which might potentially help identify patients with cirrhosis who are at increased risk for HCC. Elevated serum levels of AFP are, indeed, a predictor of the development of HCC and rapidly growing tumors. In a prospective study of 447 Italian cirrhotics, the cumulative hazard of the development of HCC during follow up was higher among those with consistently elevated serum levels of AFP than among those with fluctuating levels or those with consistently normal levels.[27]

Patients with chronic hepatitis and persistently elevated levels of AFP are another group of patients at "special" risk for HCC, for whom aggressive screening programs are justified. [31]

Another approach to identifying patients who are at particularly high risk for cancer is to measure the microheterogeneity of the sugar component of AFP. Using lectin-affinity electrophoresis, a high percentage of atypical AFP was detected in patients with HCC or in those who developed HCC within 12-18 months.[28] Thus, patients with altered profiles of serum AFP might be another "high" risk group of patients for whom more aggressive screening is justified. The US pattern of hepatic parenchyma could be another predictor of HCC development. In 38 anti-HCV positive patients with Child's A cirrhosis, 9 of 10 with a coarse-nodular pattern developed HCC, compared to only 1 of 20 patients with a fine pattern and 3 of 7 with a coarse pattern.[31] In this study, the risk of development of HCC was somehow associated with greater hepatocyte proliferation, measured by the bromodeoxyuridine labeling assay.

Rare diseases

HCC has developed in patients with rare metabolic conditions. Patients with porphyria cutanea tarda, genetic hemochromatosis, tyrosinemia, hypercitrullinemia and alpha_1 antitrypsin deficiency are at high risk.[2] Patients with glycogenosis types I and III, Wilson's disease and hereditary fructose intolerance may also develop HCC, but are at substantially lower risk. HCC was also reported in 1983 among patients with primary biliary cirrhosis, and this could reflect treatment-related improvements in patient survival. During a 15-year period, HCC occurred in 64% of 160 Japanese patients with Budd-Chiari syndrome, the majority of whom had idiopathic obstructing lesions in the inferior vena cava.[2] The incidence of Budd-Chiari syndrome among all cases of HCC was less than 1% in the survey made by the Liver Cancer Study Group in Japan. In a study in South Africa, 48 of 101 patients with Budd-Chiari syndrome attributed to congenital malformation developed HCC. However, in that study the cooperation with so far unidentified cocarcinogens could not be properly excluded.[32]

DIETARY FACTORS

Aflatoxin

Aflatoxin B_1, the most toxic member of a family of difurano-coumarins produced as secondary metabolites by strains of Aspergillus flavus and related fungi, has been associated with liver cancer. Humans can be exposed to aflatoxin by ingestion of contaminated foodstuffs or by products of animals fed aflatoxin-contaminated cereals. There is strong evidence of carcinogenic effects of aflatoxin in many animal species. Rats treated with aflatoxin B_1 have developed HCC in a dose-dependent fashion; treatment with aflatoxin B_1 of transgenic mice carrying integrated HBV-DNA greatly enhanced the development of HCC over that of mice not treated with aflatoxin.[33]

The evidence for an association between aflatoxin and HCC in humans is less conclusive. This evidence is based primarily on many population correlation surveys, case-control studies and molecular epidemiology surveys. Aflatoxin B_1 is a frequent contaminant of grains and legumes, particularly in Asia and sub-Saharan Africa, where climate and food storage techniques allow for higher quantities of aflatoxins in the food supply. The world-wide incidences of HCC parallel the prevalence of aflatoxin-contaminated food products, supporting a strong epidemiological link between aflatoxin ingestion and liver cancer. However, such an association between HCC and aflatoxin was not consistently detected in studies in which biological markers of exposure to aflatoxin were used[1,2]. Discrepancies are probably due not only to the lack of appropriate methods for assessing the past exposure of individuals, but also to confusion about the interplay of such environmental factors as alcohol and hepatitis viruses which are not distributed homogeneously in the various geographical areas.

Recently, a specific mutation at codon 249 of the tumor-suppressor gene p53 in HCC tissue from patients at risk of aflatoxin ingestion, has been reported.[34] Mutations were found only in patients (12/72) from Africa and South East China, but not in any of the 95 specimens of HCC collected from the USA, Europe and Japan. Interestingly, all the patients with HCC and p53 mutations at codon 249 had also been infected with HBV, suggesting that this virus or other hepatotoxic agents could be necessary prerequisites for aflatoxin-mediated HCC. The prevalence of p53 mutations in Mozambique was found to be higher than that in the neighboring Transkei. Both countries have similar rates of HCC and infection with HBV, but the estimated aflatoxin intake in Mozambique is four times greater than in Transkei. Thus, HCC might result from the interplay between aflatoxin, HBV and individual susceptibility to these procarcinogens.

Alcohol

Ethanol has no mutagenic properties. However, chronic alcohol consumption is associated with an increased risk for cancer in several organs, including the oral cavity, pharynx, larynx and esophagus. The association between ethanol and liver cancer has been investigated in thousands of patients. The effect of alcohol was dose-dependent and cirrhosis could be the basis for ethanol-associated HCC cases. In areas such as the USA in which the prevalence of HBV carriers is low, risk for HCC was increased up to 40% by heavy alcohol consumption. In California, a survey in alcoholics showed that moderate alcohol intake was not associated with an increased risk of HCC, whereas a daily intake of 80 g or more was, by a four-fold factor.[35] In Italy, a multicenter study of cirrhotics revealed that the risk of HCC was 13 times greater in drinkers than in abstainers.[36] In a retrospective study the 10-yr cumulative occurrence of HCC in Japanese patients with alcoholic cirrhosis was calculated to be 18.5%.[37] In that study and others in Europe, alcohol was found to promote liver cancer when the patient was positive for anti-HCV.[2,38] HBV seems to be another agent which promotes liver cancer in alcoholics, even when serum markers of infection are not detectable. In Japan, alcohol abusers with HBsAg-related cirrhosis were 10 years younger than patients with HBsAg cirrhosis who did not drink alcohol (38.8 *vs* 49.3).[39] In one study[40], integrated HBV-DNA was detected in the hepatocytes of HBsAg seronegative alcoholics with HCC, and thought to be a sign of occult infection promoting liver carcinogenesis.

OTHER FACTORS

The potential carcinogenic role of dietary vegetables is debated. Vegetables that have been shown to cause HCC in animals include alkaloids of Senecio and Felce,[41] to which humans are also exposed. In a prospective cohort study of 8,436 men in Taiwan, a lower vegetable intake measured by personal interviews and assays for serum retinol, was associated with an increased risk of HCC.[42] In Northern Italy, the risk of HCC was found to be lower in individuals with large intakes of milk, eggs, vegetables and fruits.[43] Thus, overall composition of the diet and the overall alimentary standards may influence the risk of developing HCC.

HORMONES AND CHEMICALS

Exposure to exogenous steroidal sex hormones may enhance the risk for liver adenomas and HCC.[44] Several case-control studies which have been conducted in areas not endemic for HBV and HCC revealed a positive correlation between use of oral contraceptives and HCC, with a relative risk of 3.8-13.5 and an association with long-term use. Two studies that were limited to short-term users living in endemic HBV areas gave negative results. The fact that the increase in HCC risk attributable to contraceptives was detectable only in areas non endemic for HCC and the rare occurrence of this tumor in young women worldwide, suggests that sex hormones most likely enhance the tumor risk by only a small absolute number. There are also reports of HCC developing in patients who have been treated with androgenic or anabolic steroids.[45]

The association between tobacco smoking and human HCC is also biologically plausible, since the liver is a natural target of the many potential carcinogens in tobacco and data exist for experimental liver carcinogenesis.[39] However, there is no epidemiological evidence for a pathogenic role of tobacco smoking in human HCC. In fact, existence of this association, especially in HBsAg-negative patients with HCC who had been long-term and heavy smokers, has been proven in only three of 20 studies performed (see ref 1). The available data do not support interaction of tobacco with alcohol consumption. However, important methodological problems in the designs of these studies might explain some of the discrepancies. Several dietary constituents may be genotoxic after metabolic activation by the liver and, theoretically, promote HCC.[47] Small amounts of these substances might cause enough initiation of tumors as long as there is a concomitant condition to cause persistent liver cell proliferation.

Thorotrast, a colloidal solution of thorium dioxide with the isotope radiothorium, which was formerly used as contrast medium in radiology, has been associated with development of HCC.[48] Due to the long half-life of the isotope, hepatic tumors have developed after a latent period of about 20 years after intravascular administration of Thorotrast. Although many cases of HCC associated with Thorotrast administration have been associated with cirrhosis, tumors have also been found in non-cirrhotic livers. Characteristically, refractile granules of Thorotrast are trapped in the phagocytes in the portal tracts.

Exposure at work, e.g., employment in the rubber or PVC industry, and contact with oil products and hydrocarbons is another potential risk factor for HCC.[49] In Hanoi, a case control study of 152 men with HCC disclosed an association between risk of tumor and exposure to organophosphorous pesticides, in addition to such well known risk factors as alcohol and HBV.[50] The slight increase in mortality from HCC observed among young adults in the USA could reflect increased exposure to chemical carcinogens.

CONCLUSIONS

There is convincing evidence for a causal association between HCC and hepatitis viruses, alcohol and aflatoxin. Thus, primary prevention of HCC is possible: eradication of the HBV carrier state is now possible with programs of universal vaccination of newborns; spread of HCV has been consistently reduced with programs of donor screening and use of disposable syringes; educational programs and new regulations could help to decrease alcoholism; and food contamination with aflatoxin could be reduced by improved agricultural and storage methods. Secondary prevention through screening campaigns is also possible, but it is a matter of controversy whether such a strategy is cost-effective. For other factors, such as hormones, tobacco and chemicals, it has not been established whether or not they play a role in human hepatocarcinogenesis.

REFERENCES

1. Colombo M. Hepatocellular Carcinoma *J Hepatol* 1992; **15**: 225-36
2. Okuda K. Hepatocellular Carcinoma. Recent Progress. *Hepatology* 1992; **15**:948-55
3. Parkin DM, Stjernward J, Muir CS. Estimates of the worldwide frequency of twelve major cancers. *BuletinWHO* 1984; **62**:163-82
4. Beasley RP. Hepatitis B virus. The major etiology of hepatocellular carcinoma. *Cancer* 1987; **61**: 184-56
5. McMahon BJ, Alberts SR, Wainwright RB, Bulkow L, Lanier AP. Hepatitis-B sequelae: Prospective study in 1400 hepatitis-B surface antigen-positive Alaska native carriers. *Arch Intern Med* 1990;**150**: 1051-1054
6. Sherman M, Peltekian KM, Lee C. Screening for hepatocellular carcinoma in chronic carriers of hepatitis B virus: Incidence and prevalence of hepatocellular carcinoma in North American urban population. *Hepatology* 1995;**22**: 432-438
7. London WT, Atleson J, Eto M, Hwang C. Early detection of hepatocellular carcinoma among Asians living in the United States. In: Tabor E, Di Bisceglie AM, Purcell RH, eds. *Etiology, pathology, and treatment of hepatocellular carcinoma in North America*. Houston: Gulf Publishing, 1991: p243-253
8. Tony MJ, Schwindt RR, Lo GH, Co RL. Chronic hepatitis and hepatocellular carcinoma in Asian Americans In: Tabor E, Di Bisceglie AM, Purcell RH, eds. *Etiology, pathology, and treatment of hepatocellular carcinoma in North America*. Houston: Gulf Publishing, 1991: p15-24
9. Fattovich G, Giustina G, Schalm SW *et al.* Occurrence of hepatocellular carcinoma and decompensation in Western European patients with cirrhosis type B. *Hepatology* 1995, **21**: 77-82
10. Rogler CE. Recent advances in hepatitis B viruses and hepatocellular carcinoma. *Cancer Cell-Mon Rev* 1990; **2**: 366-70.
11. de Franchis R, Meucci G, Vecchi M *et al.* The natural history of asymptomatic hepatitis B surface antigen carriers. *Ann Intern Med* 1993, **118**: 191-194
12. Bonino F, Brunetto MR. Hepatitis B virus heterogeneity, one of the many factors influencing the severity of hepatitis B. *Hepatology* 1991; **18**: 5-8
13. Tabor E. Hepatocellular Carcinoma: possible etiologies in patients without serologic evidence of hepatitis B virus infection. *J Med Virol* 1989; **27**: 1-6

14. Colombo M, Kuo G, Choo QL *et al.* Prevalence of antibodies to hepatitis C virus in Italian patients with hepatocellular carcinoma. *Lancet* 1989; **2**: 1006-9

15. Hasan F, Jeffers LJ, De Modina M *et al.* Hepatitis C-associated hepatocellular carcinoma. *Hepatology* 1990; **12**: 589-591

16. Yu MC, Tong MJ, Corsaget P, *et al.* Prevalence of hepatitis B and C viral markers in black and white patients with hepatocellular carcinoma in the United States. *J Natl Cancer Inst* 1990;**82**:1038-1041

17. Kew MC, Houghton M, Choo QL, Kuo G. Hepatitis C virus antibodies in Southern African blacks with hepatocellular carcinoma. *Lancet* 1990;**1**:873-874

18. Coursaget P, Bourdil C, Kastally R *et al.* Prevalence of hepatitis C virus infection in Africa: Anti-HCV antibodies in the general population and in patients suffering from cirrhosis or primary liver cancer. *Res Virol* 1990;**141**:449-454

19. Simonetti RG, Cottone M, Craxì A *et al.* Prevalence of antibodies to hepatitis C virus in hepatocellular carcinoma. *Lancet* 1989; **2**:1338

20. Kaklamani E, Trichopoulos D, Tzonou A *et al.* Hepatitis B and C viruses and their interaction in origin of hepatocellular carcinoma. *Jama* 1991;**265**:1974-1976

21. Tanaka S. Type C hepatitis and hepatocellular carcinoma in Japan. In: *International Symposium on Viral Hepatitis and Liver Disease.* (The 8th Triennial Congress). 1993: 60

22. Chuang WL, Chang WY, Lu SN, *et al.* The role of hepatitis B and C viruses in hepatocellular carcinoma in hepatitis B endemic area. *Cancer* 1992;**69**:2052-2054

23. Colombo M, Romeo R. Human primary liver cancer and hepatitis C virus in Western countries and Africa. In: *Etiological and progression factors of human hepatocellular carcinoma.* Brechot C (ed). CRC Press Inc. London, 1994, 49-56

24. Naito M, Hayashi N, Moribe T *et al.* Hepatitis C viral quasispecies in hepatitis C virus carriers with normal liver enzymes and patients with type C chronic liver disease. *Hepatology* 1995; **22**: 407-412

25. Takano S, Yokosuka O, Imazeki F, Tagawa M, Omata M. Incidence of hepatocellular carcinoma in chronic hepatitis B and C: A predictive study of 251 patients. *Hepatology* 1995; **21**: 650-655

26. Nousbaum JP, Pol S, Nalpas B *et al.* Hepatitis C virus type 1, (II) infection in France and Italy. *Ann Intern Med* 1995; **122**: 161-8

27. Colombo M, de Franchis R, Del Ninno E *et al.* Hepatocellular carcinoma in Italian patients with cirrhosis. *N Engl J Med* 1991; **325**:675-680.

28. Sato Y, Nakata K, Kato Y *et al.* Early recognition of hepatocellular carcinoma based on altered profiles of alpha-fetoprotein. *N Engl J Med* 1993; **328:** 1802-1806

29. Cottone M, Turri M, Caltagirone M ***et al.*** Screening for hepatocellular carcinoma in patients with Child's A cirrhosis: a 8 year prospective study by Ultrasound and Alfafetoprotein. *J Hepatol* 1994; **21**: 1029-34

30. Borzio M, Bruno S, Roncalli M *et al.* Liver cell dysplasia is major risk factor for hepatocellular carcinoma in cirrhosis: A prospective study. *Gastroenterology* 1995; **108**: 812-817

31. Tsukuma H, Hiyama T, Tanaka S *et al.* Risk factors for hepatocellular carcinoma among patients with chronic liver disease. *N Engl J Med* 1993; **328**: 1797-1801

32. Simon IW. Membranous obstruction of the inferior vena cava and hepatocellular carcinoma in South Africa. *Gastroenterology* 1982; **82**: 171-178

33. Sell S, Hunt JM, Dunsdorf HA, Chisari FV. Synergy between hepatitis B virus expression and chemical hepatocarcinogens in transgenic mice. *Cancer Res* 1991; **51**: 1278-1285

34. Ozturk M, Bressac B, Puisieux A, *et al.* p53 mutation in hepatocellular carcinoma after aflatoxin exposure. *Lancet* 1991; **338**:1356-1359

35. Yu H, Harris RE, Kabat GC, Wynder EL. Cigarette smoking, alcohol consumption and primary liver cancer: A case-control study in the USA. *Int J Cancer* 1988; **42**: 325-328

36. Pagliaro L, Simonetti RG, Craxì A, *et al.* Alcohol and HBV infection as risk factors for hepatocellular carcinoma in Italy: a multicenter controlled study. *Hepato-gastroenterology* 1983; **30**: 48-50

37. Yamauchi M, Nakahara M, Maezawa Y *et al.* Prevalence of hepatocellular carcinoma in patietns with alcoholic cirrhosis and prior exposure to hepatitis C. *Am J Gastroenterol* 1993; **88**: 39-43

38. Benvegnù L, Fattovich G, Noventa F *et al.* Concurrent hepatitis B and C virus infection and risk of hepatocellular carcinoma in cirrhosis. A prospective study. *Cancer* 1994; **74**: 2442-2448

39. Ohnishi K, Iida S, Iwama S *et al.* The effect of chronic habitual alcohol intake on the development of liver cirrhosis and hepatocellular carcinoma: Relation to hepatitis B surface antigen carriage. *Cancer* 1982; **49**: 672-677

40. Brechot C, Nalpas B, Couroué AM *et al.* Evidence that hepatitis B virus has a role in liver-cell carcinoma in alcoholic liver disease. *N Engl J Med* 1982; **306**: 1387-1387

41. Doll R, Peto R. The causes of cancer: Quantitative estimates of aviodable risk of cancer in the United States today. *J Natl Cancer Inst* 1981; **66**: 1191-1308

42. Yu MW, Hsieh HH, Pan WH, Yang CS, Chen CJ. Vegetable consumption, serum retino level, and risk of hepatocellular carcinoma. *Cancer Res* 1995; **55**: 1301-1305

43. La Vecchia C, Negri E, Decarli A, D'Avanzo B, Franceschi S. Risk factors for hepatocellular carcinoma in northern Italy. *Int Cancer* 1988; **42**: 872-876

44. Nagasue N, Kohno H. Hepatocellular carcinoma and sex hormones. *HPB-Surg* 1992; **6**: 1-6

45. Yu MW, Chen CJ. Elevated serum testosterone levels and risk of hepatocellular carcinoma. *Cancer Res* 1993; **53**: 790-794

46. Austin H. The role of tobacco use and alcohol consumption in the etiology of hepatocellular carcinoma. In: Tabor E, Di Bisceglie AM, Purcell RH, eds. *Etiology, Pathology and Treatment of Hepatocellular Carcinoma in North America.* Houston: Gulf Publishing Company 1991, 57-76

47. Ames B. Dietary carcinogens and anticarcinogens. *Science* 1983; **221**: 1256-1264

48. Von Kaick G, Wesch H. Follow-up study. In: Von Kaick G, Muth A, Kaul A, eds. *The German Thorotrst Study.* Luxembourg: Commission of the Europe on Communities, 1984: 190-211

49. Shun-Zang Y. Drinking water and primary liver cancer. In: Tang ZY, Wo MC, Yia SS, eds. *Primary Liver Cancer.* Springer-Verlag Berlin. Heidelberg, 1990, 30-37

50. Cordier S, Le TB, Verger P *et al.* Viral infections and chemical exposure as risk factors for hepatocellular carcinoma in Vietnam. *Int J Cancer* 1993, **55**: 196-201

3

Molecular basis

M Levrero, P Chirillo, C Balsano and G Natoli

GENETIC AND ACQUIRED FACTORS IN HEPATOCELLULAR CARCINOMA

Carcinogenesis is a multifactorial and multistep process. Although only 1% of total cancer patients inherit their tumors, genetic factors are considered to play a pivotal role.[1-3] Genetic abnormalities - including chromosomal aberrations,[4] activation of oncogenes,[5] abnormalities in growth factors and their receptors,[6] inactivation of tumor suppressor genes[7] and other less characterized predisposing changes such as genomic instability,[8] have been demonstrated in all types of cancer.

Hepatocellular carcinoma (HCC) is a major disease in many parts of the world and ranks eighth in the world's top 10 list of tumors, with an annual incidence of 250,000 cases.[9,10] A number of risk factors are now well recognized and some of the steps involved in the molecular pathogenesis of HCC have been elucidated. Indeed, most HCCs are late complications of HBV and HCV related chronic hepatitis and cirrhosis.[10] Additional environmental factors, such as aflatoxin B1 exposure, contribute and appear to determine the geographic clustering of the disease.[11,12] However, our under-standing of how the multiple factors involved in hepatic carcinogenesis operate and interact at the molecular level is far from complete.[13] Indeed, hepatocyte transformation may occur irrespective of the etiologic agent in the context of the increased cellular turnover induced by chronic liver injury and regeneration, with genetic mutations being a common phenomenon prior to the development of HCC, and the risk of hepatocellular carcinoma is increased several fold in patients with liver cirrhosis, regardless of its etiology. Whether the hepatitis viruses are directly oncogenic or merely participate in the transformation process by inducing chronic cellular injury and regeneration is not entirely clear. This review focuses on the progress that has been made in our understanding of liver cell growth and death regulation, of the role of viral and environmental factors in the molecular pathogenesis of hepatocyte transformation and of the molecular and genetic changes involved in HCC development.

REGULATION OF LIVER CELL GROWTH

The liver has an optimal functional mass relative to body size and when this equilibrium is disturbed, either by functional liver deficit (partial hepatectomy, *small for size* transplants, toxic or viral injury) or excess capacity (*large for size* transplants, drug induced liver hyperplasia, some cases of heterotopic transplantation), the appropriate liver weight/body weight ratio is rapidly restored by either hepatic growth or a reduction in size through programmed cell death (apoptosis), respectively.

Most of the understanding of the mechanisms of hepatocyte replication derives from studies of the compensatory hyperplasia, commonly termed liver regeneration, which takes place after partial hepatectomy (PH). The replicative response of quiescent hepatocytes after PH involves multiple steps, each requiring different sets of controls and circuits.[14] Hepatocyte need to be *primed* to become competent to proliferate in response to mitogenic stimuli. Hepatocytes *priming* involves the post-translational modification and increased binding to DNA of at least three *nuclear transcription factors (NFkB* – nuclear factor kappa B; *STAT3* – signal transducer and activator of transcription; and *AP1* – the c-fos/c-jun heterodimers),[14-16] which in turn regulate the expression of a set of proto-oncogenes (c-fos, c-jun, c-myc) and other proliferation related genes, collectively termed *immediate early genes*. Both extracellular signals, such as TNF-α, and intracellular signals, involving the generation of reactive oxygen intermediates, contribute to the initiation of liver regeneration by activating both NFkB and AP1.[14,17] The most important factors which drive competent hepatocytes from quiescence (GO) into the G1 phase of the cell cycle are the Transforming Growth Factor Alpha (TGF-α) and the Hepatocyte Growth Factor (HGF).[14] On the other hand, TGF-β and activin, which are potent inhibitors of hepatocyte proliferation, contribute to keeping hepatocytes in a non-proliferative state. TGF-β1 has also been shown to induce apoptosis in primary hepatocyte cultures and hepatoma cells in vitro as well as in the regressing liver.[18,19] When cells enter G1 a critical regulatory event for cell cycle progression involves the sequential expression of cyclins, which regulate the activity of their associated kinases (Cdks) and phosphatases.[20,21] Phoshorylation of pRb (retinoblastoma) in G1 by cyclins/Cdks complexes leads to its inactivation, resulting in the release of free active forms of the E2F transcription factor, needed for the sequential activation of many genes involved in DNA replication.[20] Recent evidence indicates that cyclin E may be rate limiting for G1 progression and that the formation of cyclin E-Cdk2 complexes may be the target for the inhibitory effect of TGF-β on hepatocyte DNA replication.[14] A cascade-like expression of cyclin mRNAs in the regenerating liver occurs, in which cyclins E and D mRNAs appear at around 12 hours after the operation prior to the entry into the S phase, while cyclin A and B1 mRNAs are elevated at 24 hours[22]. The mRNA for the tumor suppressor gene p53 peaks between 8 and 16 hours after PH, corresponding to the middle of the G1 phase for hepatocytes undergoing the first round of replication. Its expression in the regenerating liver is related to its function of "genome guardian" involved in slowing down the cell cycle progression to permit repair of genomic injury.[14,23] As a part of the late response, the Ras family genes are expressed 18-24 hours after the operation, in conjunction with the peak of DNA synthesis and the mitotic period.[14] The relative difficulty of eliciting growth responses from hepatocytes in intact livers indicates that hepatocyte quiescence is under stringent control. Although after PH both TGF-β and activin mRNA levels increase, the balance between stimulators (TGF-α and HGF) and inhibitors (TGF-β and activin) of DNA synthesis during liver regeneration favors hepatocyte proliferation during the first 24 hours, this gradually shifts towards inhibition in subsequent days.

APOPTOSIS AND LIVER CANCER

Several lines of evidence suggest that cancer might be the result of defects in the regulation of apoptosis,[24,25] an active process of cellular self-destruction with distinctive morphological and biochemical features.[26] The founder cells of cancers might be those in which DNA damage inflicted by carcinogens does not trigger apoptosis.[24] Chronic HBV and HCV viral hepatitis and cirrhosis, all predisposing factors for HCC development, are characterized by mononuclear cell infiltration of the parenchyma at the margins of liver lobules and "disappearance" of contiguous hepatocytes due to apoptosis.[26] Failure of apoptosis could allow the survival of hepatocytes that are prone to undergo genetic damage as a consequence of both exposure to reactive oxygen intermediates, increased proliferative rate and, in the case of HBV infection, direct integration of the HBV-DNA. An important role in the regulation of hepatocyte apoptosis in the context of chronic viral infections is played by Fas (APO-1 or CD95), a 43 kD cell surface glycoprotein belonging to the tumor necrosis factor (TNF) receptor superfamily.[27] Fas is expressed in normal mouse and human liver and during chronic hepatitis the expression of Fas is upregulated in the hepatocytes nearby the infiltrating lymphocytes. Hepatocyte susceptibility to apoptotic stimuli provided by infiltrating lymphocytes, could represent a critical restraint to hepatocellular transformation and it has been recently demonstrated that resistance to anti-Fas mediated apoptosis is a common phenotype of transformed liver cells.[28]

HEPATITIS VIRUSES

Although epidemiologic studies have convincingly shown that HCC is closely associated with chronic HBV infection,[29] the mechanisms responsible for malignant transformation in HBV-related HCCs are incompletely defined.[30] Integration of viral DNA sequences into the cellular DNA of HCC and chronic hepatitis tissues is frequently found and has been associated with chromosomal deletions and translocations.[31] However, the analysis of the integrated viral and flanking sequences of several hepatomas revealed in a few cases only that integration has occurred in the vicinity of genes associated with growth control and differentiation (myc,[32] retinoic acid receptor,[33] cyclin A[34]), suggesting that *insertional mutagenesis* cannot be regarded as a general mechanism of transformation in human HCC. A different situation occurs in the HCC arising with very high frequency in woodchucks infected by the HBV-related woodchuck hepatitis virus (WHV), in which the viral DNA is almost invariably integrated within or in the proximity of the c-myc and N-myc family genes.[35] Interestingly, HCC also occurred in a proportion of woodchucks that had serologically recovered from WHV infection and WHV DNA has been found in these tumors.[36]

Similarly, HBV-DNA sequences and HBV transcripts - mainly the HBV-X mRNA, have been detected in a high proportion of HCCs from HBsAg negative patients.[37]

An additional mechanism by which viruses can cause tumors involves the activation and/or the repression of the expression of genes crucial for cell growth regulation, thus leading to the development of the neoplastic phenotype. The product of the HBV X gene, pX, has been shown to function as a promiscous *transactivator* of many viral and cellular RNA polymerase II as well as RNA polymerase III promoters, including those of genes involved in cell growth regulation such as c-fos, c-myc, c-jun and the epidermal growth factor (EGF) receptor.[38-40] A second class of HBV transactivators, the preS/S^{tr} proteins, are frequently generated by truncation of the envelope genes in the process of viral DNA integration into the host genome,[41,42] but their properties are much less well characterized. pX exerts its transactivating activity through the modulation of intracellular signalling pathways that control the activity of multiple nuclear transcription factors (including AP1 and NFkB, both involved in the control of hepatocyte proliferation in the regenerating liver).[43-46] pX expression also alters the growth properties of mouse immortalized fibroblasts and induces quiescent cells to progress from the G0/G1 phase into the S phase of the cell cycle and proliferate.[47] However, the relative potency of pX in the transformation of mouse fibroblasts in standard *in vitro* assays is quite low and it is clearly enhanced in the presence of the entire HBV genome.[48] Thus, although pX clearly upregulates cellular signalling pathways involved in the control of cell proliferation and has a direct effect on cell cycle regulation, it is still controversial whether pX transactivating activity alone is relevant for HBV-associated liver carcinogenesis or other HBV functions have to be considered.

Whether HCV directly contributes to hepatocyte transformation is even more controversial.[49] HCV, a single stranded RNA virus with similarities to the Flavi and Pestiviruses, is not an integrating virus; it has no reverse transcriptase and cDNA copies of the virus have never been found in the livers of either infected chimpanzees or HCC patients.[49] Nevertheless, viral genomes and replication have been detected in neoplastic liver cells[50] and it has recently been demonstrated that mouse fibroblasts become transformed upon transfection with a cDNA encoding the aminoterminal portion of HCV NS3, a non structural protein with a serine proteinase function, and form tumors in nude mice.[51] In addition, the structural core protein, in its shorter version of 16 kD, has also been described to enter into the nucleus[52] and to enhance NFkB regulated transcription.[53] The core protein has also been shown to bind members of the TNFR family, suggesting that it may modulate susceptibility of cells to TNF or Fas modulated apoptosis, thus interferring with the immune elimination of infected hepatocytes.[54]

In conclusion, several lines of evidence indicate a direct carcinogenic role for HBV while HCV, alcohol, metabolic liver diseases and certain environmental factors may act predominantly through a pathway of chronic liver injury, that eventually leads to cirrhosis.

GROWTH FACTORS, ONCOGENES AND TUMOR SUPPRESSOR GENES IN HCC DEVELOPMENT

Several studies indicate that TGF-α, besides its role in liver development and regeneration, may also contribute to neoplastic transformation. In fact, blockade of TGF-α activity by antisense oligonucleotides results in inhibition of tumor development from hepatocellular carcinoma progenitor cells[55] and overexpression of TGF-α in transgenic mice leads to hepatocyte hyperplasia and up to 90% of the animals finally develop liver tumors.[56] Interestingly, TGF-α expression is upregulated in the HBV replicating hepatoma cell line 2.2.15, as compared to the parental HepG2 cells,[57] and the HBV transactivator pX enhances the expression of the EGF receptor, which is shared by TGF-α, on cells of hepatic lineage.[40] These findings provide a molecular link between the viral infection and the autocrine regulation of liver regeneration in HBV chronically infected livers. TGF-α overexpression has been frequently detected in HCCs and in the adjacent nontumorous liver,[58] mostly in patients with HBV-related HCCs from different geographical areas. Insulin-like growth factor II (IGF-II) expression is also elevated in a number of human HCCs,[59] but its relation with HBV or HCV infection is less clear.[13]

The frequency of *oncogene activation* by mutation or amplification in HCCs appears to be low, while overexpression of N-ras, c-myc and c-fos has been described in a variable percentage of HCC cases.[13,60] Loss and/or mutation of tumor suppressor genes seems to play a more important role in the development of HCC.[61] Deletion of one allele of a tumor suppressor gene through various mechanisms results in a loss of heterozygosity for that genetic locus and can be detected by restriction fragment length polymorphisms (RFLPs) using the appropriate probe. In HCCs allele losses have been frequently documented on chromosomes 1, 4, 5, 8, 10, 11, 13, 16, 17, and 22, irrespective of HBV status, but none of these losses has led so far to the identification of a tumor suppressor gene specific for HCC.[61]

Mutations and allelic deletions of the p53 gene are the most common genetic alterations found in human tumors.[62,63] p53 is a sequence specific DNA-binding phosphoprotein that can regulate transcription (both activation of growth suppressor genes and repression of growth promotion genes) and inhibits DNA replication causing either growth arrest or apoptosis.[23] Indeed, part of the tumor suppression function of p53 stems from its crucial role in the execution of some forms of programmed cell death, including the apoptosis in response to DNA injury and or when unwarranted activation of cell cycle occurs.[23] p53 activities appear to be modulated by phosphorylation, binding with cellular (mdm2) as well as viral (SV4O TAg) proteins, degradation rate via ubiquitination (HPV E6 protein and its associated protein E6-AP) and mutations.[62] Abnormalities of the structure and expression of the p53 gene have been observed in several continuous HCC cell lines.[13] An association between a specific p53 mutation, a G to T transversion in the third nucleotide of codon 249, resulting in an arginine to serine substitution, has been described in HCCs from two regions of the world, the Quidong region of China and Mozambique, with high exposure to aflatoxins and endemic HBV infection.[64,65] Subsequent larger studies indicated that mutations in codon 249 of p53 are restricted to aflatoxin B1 contamination of food in both duck and human HCCs.[66] Moreover, aflatoxin B1 induces the same G to T mutation of p53 codon 249 in cultured cells.[67] This mutation is present in apparently normal livers and predates the development of HCC in individuals with high exposure to aflatoxin,[68] suggesting that this genetic alteration occurs early during hepatocarcinogenesis. Whether this mutation is sufficient to explain the carcinogenic effect of aflatoxin B1 is less clear. p53Ser249, like most mutated p53 proteins isolated from human tumors, has lost its growth suppression properties and transforms fibroblasts in culture but appears to retain the apoptotic effect of the wild type p53 in hepatoma cells.[69] Recently, a direct interaction between p53 and pX has been reported.[70] pX binding to p53 results in the inactivation of p53 effects on transcription[71,72] but does not impair p53 functions involved in induction of apoptosis.[73] Indeed, pX, is both able to directly induce apoptosis as well as to prompt cells to programmed cell death after exposure to DNA damaging drugs and requires a functional p53 for this effect.[73] This observation provides an explanation for a number of apparent paradoxes on pX, i.e. efficient induction of cell cycle progression, binding to p53 and inactivation of its transactivating function[70-72] vs. an unexpectedly low potency in the transformation of mouse fibroblasts in *in vitro* assays[48] and equivocal results in transgenic mice.[74] Indeed, the demonstration of pX ability to sensitize cells to DNA damage-induced apoptosis, links the expression of the viral protein to the pathogenesis of liver inflammatory damage in the context of chronic HBV hepatitis. In addition, the finding that this activity of pX is dependent on some p53 function and that pX fully exerts its effects on cell growth only when p53 is lost, provides a new key to understanding the molecular basis of HBV-related hepatocellular carcinoma and the role of viral products. It will be important in the future to focus investigations on the events that can lead to a disturbance of the balance between cell growth and apoptosis in the context of chronic inflammation in infected livers (changes in the bcl-2 family of apoptosis regulators, naturally occurring viral mutations selectively affecting the ability of pX to induce apoptosis, coexistence of pX expression and the presence of p53 mutations able to abrogate the execution of the cell apoptotic program).

REFERENCES

1. Bishop JM. The molecular genetics of cancer. *Science* 1987; **235**: 315-315
2. Lasko D, Cavanee W, Nordenskjold M. Loss of constitutional heterozygosity in human cancer. *Annu Rev Genet* 1991; **25**: 281-314
3. Mulvihill JJ. Genetic repertory of human neoplasia. In: Mulvihill JJ, Miller RW, Fraumeni JJ, eds. *Genetics of human cancer.* New York: Raven, 1977; 137-142
4. Solomon E, Borrow J, Goddard AD. Chromosome aberrations and cancer. *Science* 1991; **254**: 1153-1160
5. Bishop JM Molecular themes in oncogenesis. *Cell* 1991; **64**: 235- 248
6. Aaronson SA. Growth factors and cancer. *Science* 1991; **254**: 1146-1153
7. Weinberg RA. Tumor suppressor genes. *Science* 1991; **254**: 1138-46
8. Volpe J. Genetic stability and instability in tumors. In: Sluyser M, ed. *Molecular Biology of Cancer Genes*. New York: Ellis Horwood, 1990; 9-23
9. Pisani P, Parkin DM, Ferlay J. Estimates of the worldwide mortality from eigtheen major cancers in 1985. Implications for prevention and projections of future burden. *Int J Cancer* 1993; **55**: 891-903
10. Tabor E, Kobayashi K. Hepatitis viruses as a cause of hepatocellular carcinoma. *J Natl Cancer Institute* 1992; **84**: 86-90
11. IARC. IARC monographs on the evaluation of carcinogenic risks to humans. Some naturally occuring substances: food items and constituents, heterocyclic aromatic amines and mycotoxins. Vol 56 Lyon, France: IARC, 1993: 245-345
12. IARC. IARC monographs on the evaluation of carcinogenic risks to humans. Hepatitis viruses. Vol 59. Lyon, France: IARC, 1994
13. Tabor E. Tumor suppressor genes, growth factor genes and oncogenes in hepatitis B virus-associated hepatocellular carcinoma. *J Med Virol* 1994; **42**: 357-65
14. Fausto N, Laird AD, Webber EM. Role of growth factor and cytokines in hepatic regeneration. *Faseb J* 1995; **9**:1527-1536
15. FitzGerald M, Webber E, Donovan J, Fausto N. Rapid DNA binding by nuclear factor kB in hepatocytes at the start of liver regeneration. *Cell Growth Diff* 1994;**14:** 217-427
16. Tewari M. Dobrzanski P, Mohn KL, Cressman DE, Hsu JC, Bravo R, Taub R. Rapid induction in regenerating liver of RL/IF-1 (an IkB that inhibits NFkB, RelB-p50, and c-Rel-p50) and PHF, a novel kB site binding complex. *Mol Cell Biol* 1990; **12**: 2898-2908
17. Dieh A, Yin M, Fleckenstein J, Yang S, Lin H, Brenner D, Westwick J, Bagby G, Nelson S. Tumor necrosis factor-α induces c-jun during the regenerative response to liver injury. *Am J Physiol* 1994; **267**: 552-561
18. Patel T, Gores GJ. Apoptosis and hepatobiliary disease. *Hepatology* 1995; **21**: 1725-1741
19. Oberhammer FA, Pavelka M, Sharma S, Tiefenbacher R, Purchio A, Bursch W, Shulte-Hermann R. Induction of apoptosis in cultured hepatocytes and in regressing liver by transforming growth factor β1. *Proc Natl Acad Sci* USA 1992; **89**: 5408-5412
20. Weinberg RA. The retinoblastoma protein and cell cycle control. *Cell* 1995; **81**: 323-330
21. Loyer P, Glaise D, Cariou S, Baffet G, Meijer L, Guguen-Guillozo C. Expression and activation of cdks (1and 2) and cyclins in the cell progression during liver regeneration *J Biol Chem* 1991; **269**: 2491-2500
22. Lu X, Koch K, Lew D, Dulic V, Pines J, Reed S, Hunter T, Leffert H. Induction of cyclin mRNA and cyclin-associated histone H1 during liver regeneration. *J Biol Chem* 1992; **267**: 2841-2844
23. Haffner R, Oren M. Biochemical properties and biological effects of p53. *Curr Opin Gen Dev* 1995; **5**: 84-90
24. Raff MC. Social controls on cell survival and cell death. *Nature* 1992; **356**: 397-398
25. Korsmeyer SJ. Bcl-2 initiates a new category of oncogenes: regulators of cell death. *Blood* 1992; **80**: 879-85
26. Kerr JFR, Wyllie AH., Currie AR. Apoptosis: a basic biological phenomenon with wide ranging implications in tissue kinetics. *Br J Cancer* 1972; **26**: 239-44
27. Nagata S, Goldstein P. The Fas death factor. *Science* 1995; **267**: 1449-1456
28. Natoli G, Ianni A, Costanzo A, De Petrillo G, Ilari I, Chirillo P, Balsano C, Levrero M. Resistance to Fas-mediated apoptosis in human hepatoma cells. *Oncogene* 1995; **11**: 1157-1164
29. Beasley RP, Hwang LY, Lin CC, Chien CS. Hepatocellular carcinoma and hepatitis B virus: a prospective study of 22,707 men in Taiwan. *Lancet* 1981; **ii**: 1129-1133
30. Ganem D, Varmus HE. The molecular biology of hepatitis B viruses. *Ann Rev Biochem* 1987; **56**: 651-693
31. Matsubara K, Tokino T. Integration of hepatitis B virus DNA and its implications for hepatocarcinogenesis. *Mol Biol Med* 1990; **7**: 243-260
32. Moroy T, Marchio A, Etiemble J *et al.* Rearrangement and enhanced expression of c-myc in hepatocellular carcinoma of hepatitis virus infected woodchucks. *Nature* 1986; **324**: 276-279
33. Dejean A, Bougueleret L, Grzeschik KH. *et al.* Hepatitis B virus DNA integration in a sequence homologous to v-erb-A and steroid receptor genes in a hepatocellular carcinoma. *Nature* 1986; **322**: 70-72
34. Wang J, Chenivesse X, Henglein B, Brechot C. Hepatitis B virus integration in a cyclin A gene in a hepatocellular carcinoma. *Nature* 1990; **343**: 555-557
35. Fourel G, Trepo C, Bougueleret L. *et al.* Frequent activation of N-Myc genes by hepadnavirus insertion in woodchuck liver tumors. *Nature* 1990; **347**: 294-298
36. Korba BE, Wells FV, Baldwin B *et al.* Hepatocellular carcinoma in woodchuck hepatitis virus infected woodchucks: presence of viral DNA in tumor tissue from chronic carriers and animals serologically recovered from acute infection. *Hepatology* 1989; **9**: 461-470
37. Paterlini P, Puossin K, Kew M, Franco D, Brechot C. Selective accumulation of the X transcript of hepatitis B virus in patients negative for hepatitis B surface antigen with hepatocellular carcinoma. *Hepatology* 1995; **21**: 313-321
38. Balsano C, Avantaggiati ML, Natoli G *et al.* Full-length and truncated versions of the hepatitis B virus X protein transactivate the c-myc protooncogene at the transcriptional level. *Biochem Biophys Res Commun* 1991; **176**: 985-992
39. Avantaggiati ML, Natoli G, Balsano C. *et al.* The hepatitis B virus pX transactivates the c-fos promoter through multiple cis acting elements. *Oncogene* 1993; **8**: 1567-74

40. Menzo S, Clementi M, Alfani E *et al*. Trans-activation of epidermal growth factor receptor by the hepatitis B virus X gene product. *Virology* 1993; **196**: 878-882

41. Kekulé AS, Lauer U, Meyer M, Caselmann WH, Hofschneider PH, Koshy R. The preS/S region of integrated hepatitis B virus DNA encodes a transcriptional transactivator. *Nature* 1990; **343**: 457-461

42. Natoli G, Avantaggiati ML, Balsano C *et al*. Characterization of the Hepatitis B Virus preS/S region encoded transcriptional transactivator. *Virology* 1992; **18**: 663-670

43. Natoli G, Avantaggiati ML, Chirillo P *et al*. Induction of the c-Jun/c-Fos heterodimers DNA binding activity by the hepatitis B virus transactivator pX. *Mol Cell Biol* 1994; **14**: 989-998

44. Natoli G, Avantaggiati ML, Chirillo P *et al*. Ras- and Raf-dependent induction of c-Jun transcriptional activity by the Hepatitis B Virus transactivator pX. *Oncogene* 1994; **9**: 2837-2843

45. Natoli G, Avantaggiati ML, Chirillo P *et al*. Modulation of intracellular signal transduction pathways by the hepatitis B virus transactivator pX.*J Hepatol* 1994; **21**: 144-52

46. Chirillo P, Falco M, Puri PL *et al*. Hepatitis B virus pX activates NFkB dependent transcription through a Raf-independent pathway. *J Virol* 1996; **70**: 254-261

47. Koike K, Moriya K, Yotsuyanagi H, Iino S, Kurokawa K. Induction of cell cycle progression by Hepatitis B Virus HBx gene expression in quiescent mouse fibroblasts. *J Clin Invest* 1994; **94**: 44-49

48. Seifer M, Hohne M, Shaefer S, Gerlich WH. In vitro tumorigenicity of hepatitis B Virus DNA and HBx protein. *J Hepatol* 1991; **13**: 61-65

49. Tabor E., Kobayashi K. Current Issues in Hepatocellular carcinoma: Hepatitis B virus, Hepatitis C Virus and the p53 Tumor suppressor gene. In: *Viral hepatitis and liver disease*. Nishioka K., Suzuki H., Mishiro S., Oda T. (Eds.) Springer Verlag, Tokyo 1994

50. Kobayashi K, Hayashi H, Itoh Y, Asano T, Isono K. Detection of minus strand hepatitis C virus RNA in tumor tissues of hepatocellular carcinoma. *Cancer* 1994; **73**: 48-52

51. Sakamuro D, Furukawa T, Takegami T. Hepatitic C virus non-structural protein NS3 transforms NIH 3T3 cells. *J Virol* 1995; **69**: 3893-3896

52. Ravaggi A, Natoli G, Primi D *et al*. Intracellular localization of full-length and truncated Hepatitis C Virus core protein expressed in mammalian cells. *J Hepatol* 1994; **20**: 225-232

53. Ou J. Personal communication, 1995

54. Lai M. Personal communication, 1995

55. Laird AD, Brown PI, Fausto N. Inhibition of tumor growth in liver epithelial cells transfected with a transforming growth factor alpha antisense gene. *Cancer Res* 1994; **54**: 4424-4432

56. Jhappan C, Stahle C, Harkins RN, Fausto N, Smith GH, Merlino GT. TGF-α overexpression in transgenic mice induces liver neoplasia and abnormal development of the mammary gland and pancreas. *Cell* 1990; **61**: 1369-1371

57. Tabor E, Farshid M, Di Bisceglie AM, Hsia CC. Increased expression of transforming growth factor α after transfection of a human hepatoblastoma cell line with the hepatitis B virus. *J Med Virol* 1992; **37**: 271-273

58. Hsia CC, Axiotis CA, Di Bisceglie AM, Tabor E. Transforming growth factor-alpha in human hepatocellular carcinoma and coexpression with hepatitis B surface antigen in adjacent liver. *Cancer* 1992; **70**: 1049-1056

59. Cariani E, Lasserre C, Seurin D. *et al*. Differential expression of insulin-like growth factorr II mRNA in human primary liver cancer, benign liver tumors and liver cirrhosis. *Cancer Res* 1988; **48**: 6844-6849

60. Zhang X, Huang D, Qiu D. *et al*. The expression of c-myc and N-Ras in human cirrhotic livers, hepatocellular carcinomas and liver tissue surrounding the tumors. *Oncogene* 1990; **5**, 909-14

61. Ding SF, Habib NA. Loss of heterozygosity in liver tumors. *J Hepatol* 1995; **22**: 230-238

62. Levine AJ. The p53 tumor suppressor gene. *N Engl J Med*. 1992; **326**: 1350-1352

63. Harris CC, Hollstein M. Clinical implications of the p53 tumor suppressor gene. *N Eng J Med* 1993; **230**: 319-322

64. Hsu IC, Metcalf RA, Sun T *et al*. Mutational hotspot in the p53 gene in human hepatocellar carcinoma. *Nature* 1991; **350**: 427-428

65. Bressac B, Kew M, Wands J *et al*. Selective G to T mutations of p53 gene in hepatocellular carcinoma from Southern Africa. *Nature* 1991; **350**: 429-431

66. Unsal H, Yakicier C, Marcais C et al. Genetic heterogeneity of hepatocellular carcinoma. *Proc Natl Acad Sci USA* 1994; **91**: 822-826

67. Aguilar F, Hussain SP, Cerutti P. Aflatoxin B1 induces the transversion of G to T codon 249 of the p53 tumor suppressor gene in human hepatocytes. *Proc Natl Acad Sci USA* 1993; **90**: 8586-8590

68. Aguilar F, Harris CC, Sun T, Hollstein M, Cerutti P. Geographic variation of p53 mutational profile in non-malignant human liver. *Science* 1994; **264**: 1317-1319

69. Ponchel F, Puisieux A, Tabone E *et al*. Hepatocarcinoma specific mutant p53-249Ser induces mitotic activity but has no effect on transforming growth factor-b1 mediated apoptosis. *Cancer Res* 1994; **54**: 2064-2068

70. Feitelson MA, Zhu M, Duan XL, London WT. Hepatitis B x antigen and p53 are associated *in vitro* and in liver tissues from patients with primary hepatocellular carcinoma. *Oncogene* 1993; **8**: 1109-1117

71. Wang XW, Forrester K, Yeh H, Feitelson M.A, Gu J.-R, Harris CC. Hepatitis B virus X protein inhibits p53 sequence-specific DNA binding, trascriptional activity, and association with trascription factor ERCC3. *Proc Natl Acad Sci USA* 1994; **91**: 2230-2234

72. Truant R, Antunovic J, Greenblatt J, Prives C, Cromlish JA. Direct interaction of the Hepatitis B Virus HBx protein with p53 leads to inhibition by HBx of p53 response element-directed trasactivation *J Virol* 1995; **69**: 1851-1859

73. Chirillo P, Natoli G, Puri PL, Burgio VL, Balsano C, Levrero M. The hepatitis B virus pX protein induces p53 mediated programmed cell death. 1996; submitted for publication

74. Kim CM, Koike K, Saito I *et al*. HBx gene of hepatitis B virus induces liver cancer in transgenic mice. *Nature* 1991; **351**: 317-320

4

Pathology

M Kojiro

FROM EARLY TO ADVANCED STAGE

Recent dramatic progress in various diagnostic imaging techniques realized much easier detection of small nodular lesions in the liver. Specifically, the introduction and popularization of ultrasound-guided fine needle biopsy allowed histologic diagnosis of minute hepatocellular carcinoma (HCC) at the early stage. Along with such technological progress, various new information on the pathomorphologic characteristics and developmental process of early HCC have been obtained through the histologic examinations of resected HCC tissues of various sizes and of biopsy specimens of minute tumors.[1-4] The most valuable information is that the majority of HCCs first appear as well differentiated cancer and they proliferate with gradual dedifferentiation. In addition, it has been elucidated that a certain proportion of HCC, which is associated with liver cirrhosis, develops from hyperplastic nodular lesions, such as adenomatous hyperplasia.[5,6]

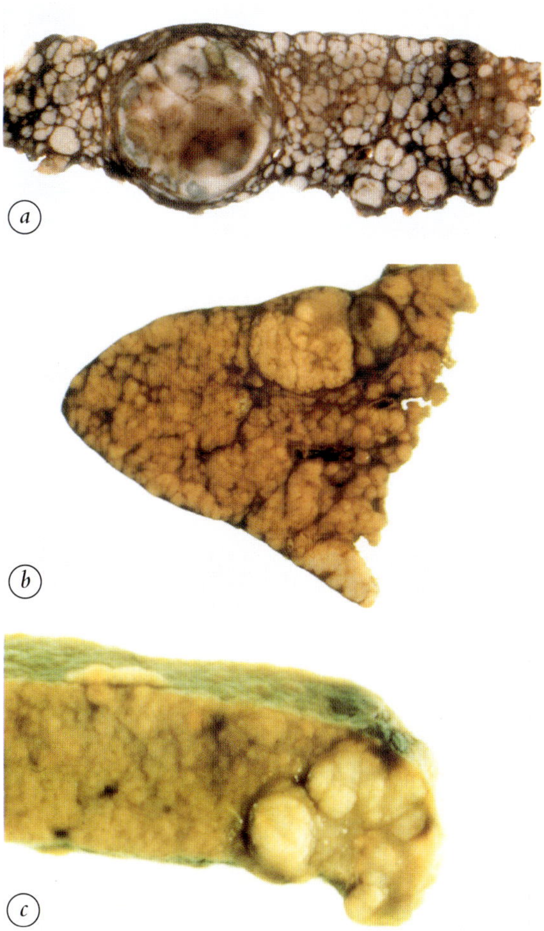

Figure 4.1 – Small HCC with a distinct margin.

a) Single nodular type. Cancer nodule, 2.3 cm in diameter, is encapsulated by a thin-fibrous band.

b) Single nodular type with perinodular growth. Cancer nodule, 2.0 cm in diameter, has perinodular tumor growth.

c) Multinodular confluent type. Tumor, 1.5 cm in diameter, consists of a confluence of minute tumor nodules.

EARLY MORPHOLOGY OF HEPATOCELLULAR CARCINOMA

Gross findings

Small HCC less than 2 cm in diameter can be categorized either into distinct nodular type HCC or indistinct nodular type small HCC.[1] Many resected small HCCs are the distinct nodular type, which presents a clear nodule and, often, a fibrous capsule or septum. This type can be subclassified into single nodular type, single nodular type with perinodular growth, and multinodular confluent type (Fig. 4.1). Most small HCCs seen clinically can be classified into one of these 3 subcategories.

On the other hand, indistinct nodular type small HCCs are about 1-1.5 cm in diameter, and most tumors in this category can be clearly depicted either as a hypoechoic or hyperechoic nodular lesion in ultrasound examinations. However, in gross observations of surgically obtained specimens, their cancerous nodules are usually obscure, or their tumor lesions are difficult to distinguish from non-cancerous areas (Fig. 4.2). These findings are considered to be the morphologic characteristics of the earliest clinically detectable HCC nodule. Cancer lesions of indistinct small HCCs are composed of uniformly proliferated well-differentiated cancerous tissue, and, within the cancerous tissue, there remain many portal tracts as well as fibrous septa of regenerative nodules of liver cirrhosis of varying degrees (Fig. 4.3). Cancer cells of indistinct nodular small HCC do not present an expansive growth pattern, but show "replacing growth pattern," where the cancer cells proliferate along with the adjacent liver cell cord and replace normal hepatocytes; and there is no capsule formation

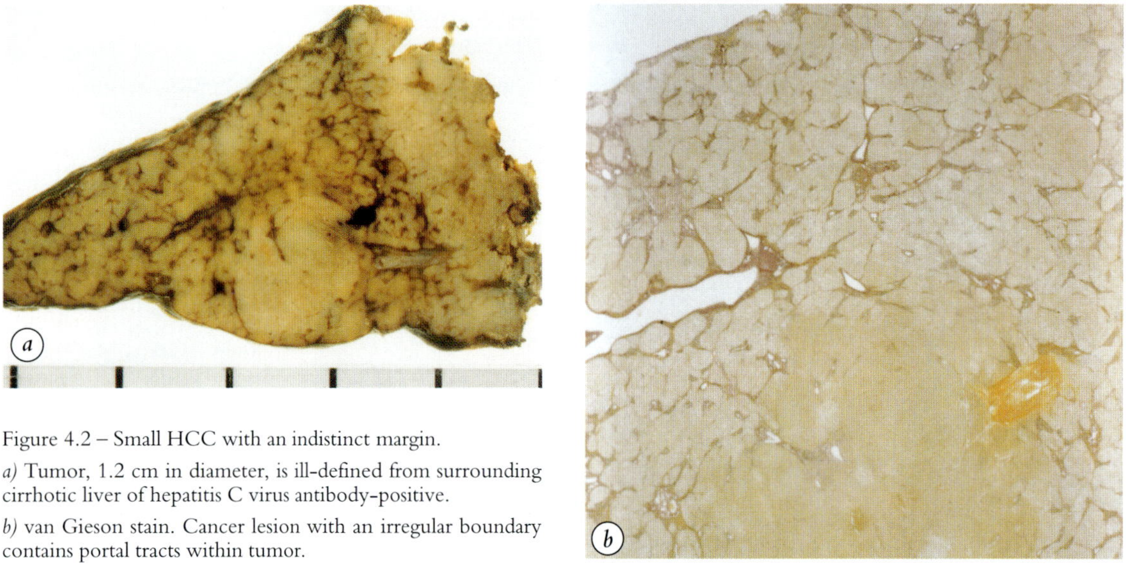

Figure 4.2 – Small HCC with an indistinct margin.

a) Tumor, 1.2 cm in diameter, is ill-defined from surrounding cirrhotic liver of hepatitis C virus antibody-positive.

b) van Gieson stain. Cancer lesion with an irregular boundary contains portal tracts within tumor.

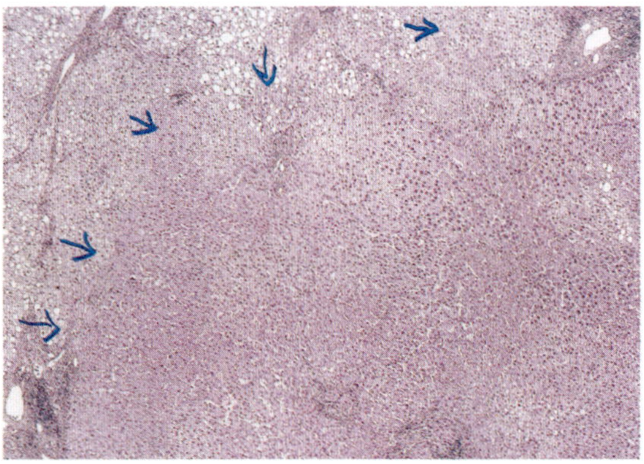

Figure 4.3 – Histologic finding of the tumor of Figure 4.2. The tumor consists uniformly of well-differentiated cancerous tissue with indistinct margins (arrows)(HE stain)

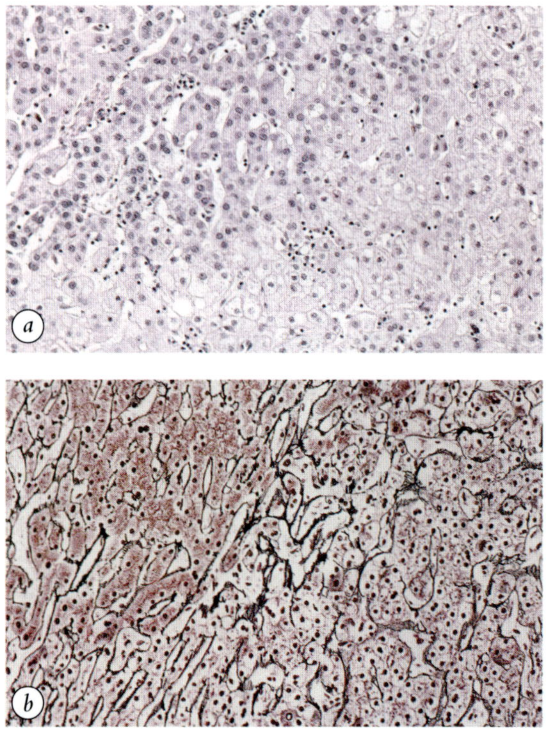

Figure 4.4 – Replacing growth of the cancer cells at the boundary.

a) The well-differentiated cancer cells with a thin-trabecular pattern are proliferating as if they are replacing the hepatocytes along the liver cell cords (HE stain).

b) Reticulin frame-work of the cancerous tissue looks to be contiguous to that of non-cancerous tissue (Reticulin stain)

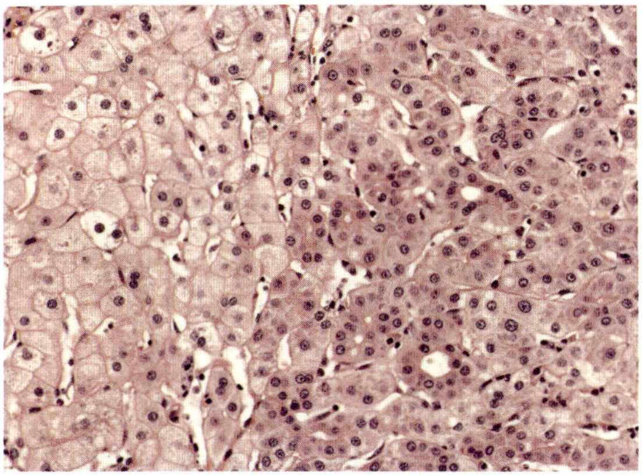

Figure 4.5 – Well-differentiated hepatocellular carcinoma (right half) is characterized by increase of cellularity, irregular thin-trabecular pattern with occasional pseudoglandular structure, and increase of staining affinity. Cancer cells are proliferating in a replacing fashion at the boundary.

at the boundary (Fig. 4.4). When the diameter of indistinct nodular small HCC reaches 1-1.5 cm and the lesion starts to grow expansively, a fibrous capsule is formed at the tumor boundary, and a fibrous septum, within the nodule. When the tumor diameter reaches approximately 2 cm, fibrous capsule and septum can be seen in more than 70% of small HCC, and this percentage is equivalent to that in advanced HCC. Based on these gross findings, it can be considered that morphologic and biologic changes occur on an HCC nodule when it reaches 1-2 cm in diameter, and specifically about 1.5 cm.

Histologic findings

The most important histologic characteristic of early HCC is that the majority of tumors consist of well-differentiated cancerous tissues which present little cellular and structural atypia.[1-4] Histologically, an early HCC lesion presents the following 5 characteristics to varying degrees: (i) increased cell density associated with an increase in nuclear/cytoplasmic (N/C) ratio, (ii) increased eosinophilic staining affinity, (iii) irregular thin-trabecular pattern, (iv) acinar- and/or pseudoglandular pattern, and (v) fatty changes and/or clear changes of cells (Figs. 4.5, 4.6). Among these characteristics, fatty changes of varying degrees are observed in approximately 40% of cancer nodules smaller than 2 cm in diameter, and this makes the other characteristic changes (e.g. increased cell density and appearance of irregular thin-trabecular pattern) indistinguishable, and consequently histologic diagnosis, specifically biopsy diagnosis, difficult.

Tumor dedifferentiation and proliferation

Since the true nature of minute well-differentiated HCC at the early stage was elucidated, much new information on the developmental process from early to advanced HCC has been obtained. The most important is that well-differentiated HCC proliferates along with its dedifferentiation. This suggests that dedifferentiation of cancer cells is closely related to their proliferation.

HCC is known to present various histologic pictures. From the view point of histologic grade, cancer nodules of less than 1 cm in diameter consist of uniform well-differentiated cancerous tissues, with the exception of a few aberrant cases, whereas approximately 40% of cancer nodules of 2-3 cm in diameter consist of cancerous tissues at varying differentiation levels. Within such a nodule, moderately or poorly differentiated cancerous tissues always locate to the inside, and well-differentiated ones to the outside (Fig. 4.7). The most typical case is often clearly depicted as a "nodule in nodule" appearance where moderately or poorly differentiated cancerous tissues without fatty changes are surrounded by well-differentiated ones with fatty changes, and there is a clear boundary between them (Fig. 4.8). Generally, when moderately differentiated cancer tissues without fatty changes are present within a well-differentiated cancerous nodule with fatty changes, the former are surmised to be a newer development

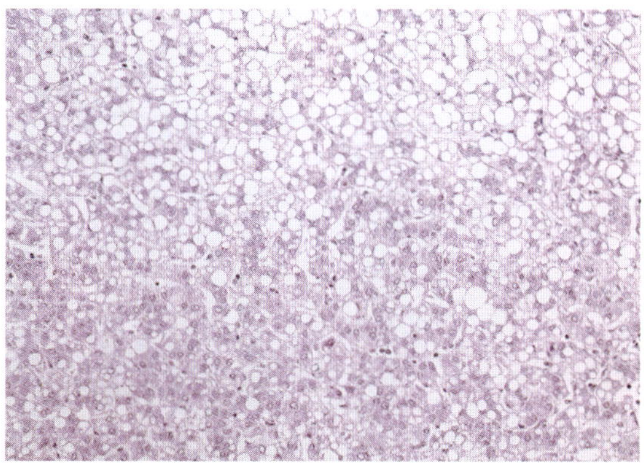

Figure 4.6 – Well-differentiated HCC with diffuse fatty change.

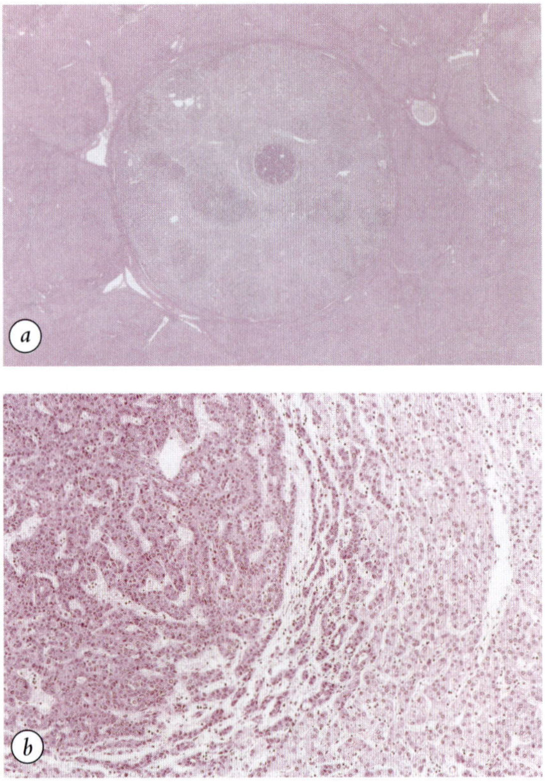

Figure 4.7 – De-differentiation in well-differentiated cancer nodule.

a) A distinct nodule is observed in a well-differentiated hepatocellular carcinoma with 1.6 cm of diameter.

b) A close-up view of the inner nodule. The inner nodule consists of moderately differentiated cancerous tissue with a classical trabecular pattern and is expansively proliferating in a well-differentiated cancerous tissue with a thin-trabecular pattern.

in clinical observations using ultrasonography. An hyperechoic small cancerous nodule appears either as a hypoechoic or isoechoic area within the hyperechoic nodule, gradually increases its area while the hyperechoic area becomes smaller, and then starts to grow. This suggests that the progress of dedifferentiation of the tumor is closely related to tumor proliferation. On the other hand, very slowly growing cancerous nodules (slow growing hepatoma), which usually remain as well-differentiated cancers, start to grow when dedifferentiation has progressed.

The authors studied surgically obtained HCC tissues which consisted of more than 2 cancerous tissues of different histologic grades, and demonstrated that the area of well-differentiated cancer diminishes in size along with an increase in the tumor size. Such a change is caused by the replacement of well-differentiated cancerous tissues with cancerous tissues of lower grade.[7] Based on these findings, growth of early HCC is considered to be related closely to the dedifferentiation of the nodule, i.e., well-differentiated tissues are replaced by newly generated, less well- differentiated tissues having more aggressive proliferative activity.

We also compared histologic pictures of ultrasound-guided fine needle biopsy specimens obtained from 12 HCCs less than 3 cm in diameter and their autopsy specimens 7-26 months after the biopsy. For 10 of 12 HCCs composed of well-differentiated cancer at biopsy, extensively spread cancer lesions in the liver were composed of either moderately or poorly differentiated cells, and no well-differentiated cancerous tissues were found in biopsy specimens. This confirms

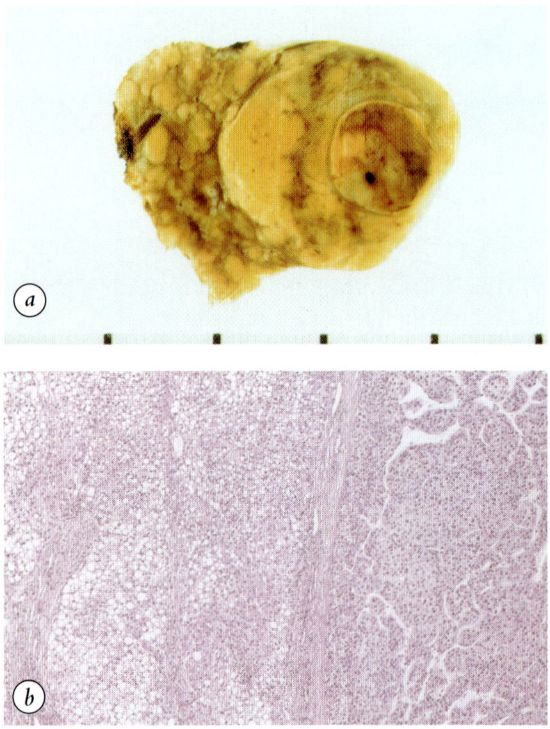

Figure 4.8 – HCC with a typical "nodule in nodule" appearance.

a) Cancer nodule with 2.3 cm of diameter contains a distinct nodule inside.

b) Histologically, the outer nodule consists of well-differentiated cancerous tissue with diffuse fatty change and the inner nodule is composed of a classical hepatocellular carcinoma, moderately differentiated.

the dedifferentiation of early well-differentiated cancerous tissues in individual cases.[8]

Clonal dedifferentiation of HCC cells in a single tumor nodule

We have established a well-differentiated HCC cell line (HAK-lA) and a poorly differentiated HCC cell line (HAK-lB) from a surgically obtained HCC nodule, which was 2.7 x 2.2 cm in size and presented a "nodule in nodule" appearance with a clear boundary between well-differentiated and moderately/poorly differentiated cancer tissues[9] (Fig. 4.9). These 2 cell lines show morphologically and biologically different characteristics: doubling time of HAK-1A is approximately 3 times longer than HAK-1B; DNA ploidy pattern is diploid in HAK-1A but aneuploid in HAK-1B; and HAK-1B is easily transplantable to nude mice but HAK-1A is not, because of its weak proliferative activity. However, these 2 cell lines possess identical structural abnormalities on chromosomes 2 and 17, and an identical point mutation on codon 242 of tumor suppresser gene p53. These findings suggest that the 2 cell lines have the same clonal origin, and that the HAK-1B, which is poorly differentiated, was developed from dedifferentiation of HAK-1A, the well-differentiated cells. Therefore, if HCC consists of cancerous tissues of varying histologic grades, cancer cells at lower differentiation levels would be generated via the dedifferentiation of well-differentiated cells due to certain causes, such as accumulation of p53 mutatuion and some other genomic abnormalities.

Consequently, the following developmental process can be postulated: human HCC develops as a well-differentiated cancer in a hyperplastic nodular lesion, such as adenomatous hyperplasia (AH) or *de novo*; when the tumor grows to 1-1.5 cm in diameter, de-differentiation of well-differentiated cancer cells occurs; cancer tissues at lower histologic grades proliferate within the well-differentiated cancerous nodule; these moderately and/or poorly differentiated cancerous tissues replace the well-differentiated tissues with weak proliferative activity; and they start to grow expansively and develop into advanced HCC (Fig. 4.9).

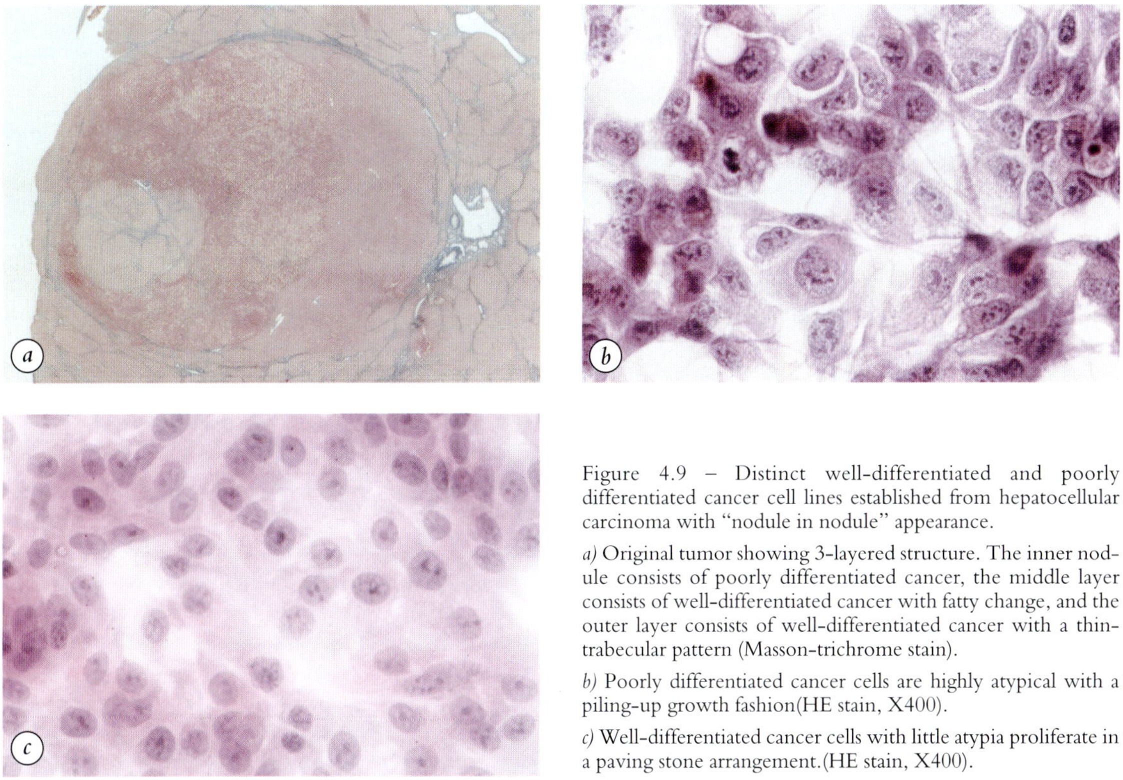

Figure 4.9 – Distinct well-differentiated and poorly differentiated cancer cell lines established from hepatocellular carcinoma with "nodule in nodule" appearance.

a) Original tumor showing 3-layered structure. The inner nodule consists of poorly differentiated cancer, the middle layer consists of well-differentiated cancer with fatty change, and the outer layer consists of well-differentiated cancer with a thin-trabecular pattern (Masson-trichrome stain).

b) Poorly differentiated cancer cells are highly atypical with a piling-up growth fashion(HE stain, X400).

c) Well-differentiated cancer cells with little atypia proliferate in a paving stone arrangement.(HE stain, X400).

MALIGNANT TRANSFORMATION OF ADENOMATOUS HYPERPLASIA

Hyperplastic nodules are frequently observed in liver cirrhosis. They can be divided into two categories; large regenerative nodules and adenomatous hyperplasia (AH). The former is found as distinct nodular lesions of around 1 cm in diameter grossly, but histologically are not significantly different from the surrounding regenerative nodules, and have not been considered to be closely related to the development of HCC.[10] Meanwhile, it has been considered based on clinical follow-up study[11] and the presence of AH containing cancerous foci that AH may be a precancerous lesion.[5,6,12] AH can also be distinguished as a clear nodule approximately 1 cm in diameter from its surrounding regenerative nodule of cirrhotic liver (Fig. 4.10a). Histologically, the cell density is moderately increased in comparison with the surrounding tissue, however no evident structural abnormalities are present. Due to the slight decrease of amount of cytoplasm, the nuclear/cytoplasmic ratio is slightly increased. Also, there is often heterogeneity of nuclear size. The cord structure often appears more prominent than that of the surrounding tissue[13] (Fig. 4.10b). Such hyperplastic nodules are observed in the vicinity of the tumor nodule in approximately 15% of surgically resected HCCs less than 3 cm in diameter and associated with liver cirrhosis.[14] Some AHs are difficult to evaluate as either cancer or benign lesions, because, even though there is no clear structural atypia, they show marked increase of cell density, or they have mild structural atypia. These AH lesions are called "atypical adenomatous hyperplasia (AAH)".[15,16] AAH is the so-called borderline lesion, which cannot be histologically distinguished as

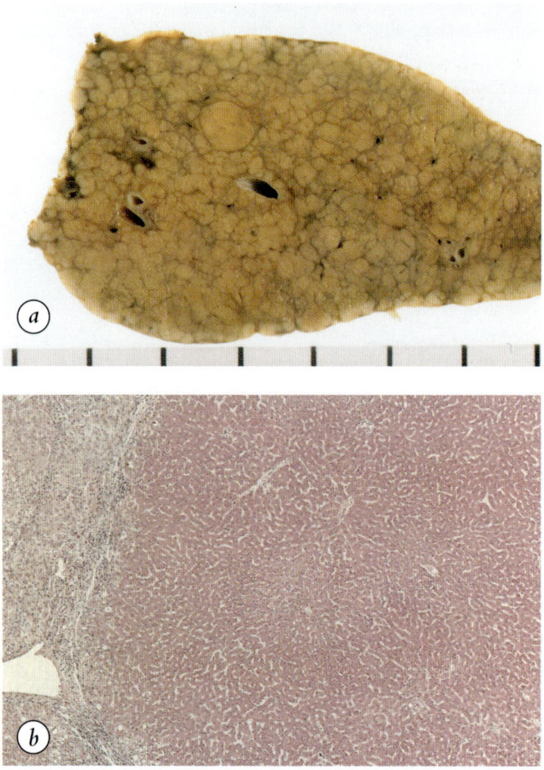

Figure 4.10 – Adenomatous hyperplasia.

a) Distinct tumor nodule with 1.0 cm of diameter is observed in liver cirrhosis of hepatitis C virus antibody-positive.

b) Histologically, tumor nodule shows a mild increase of cellularity, distinct trabecular pattern, and increase of staining affinity.

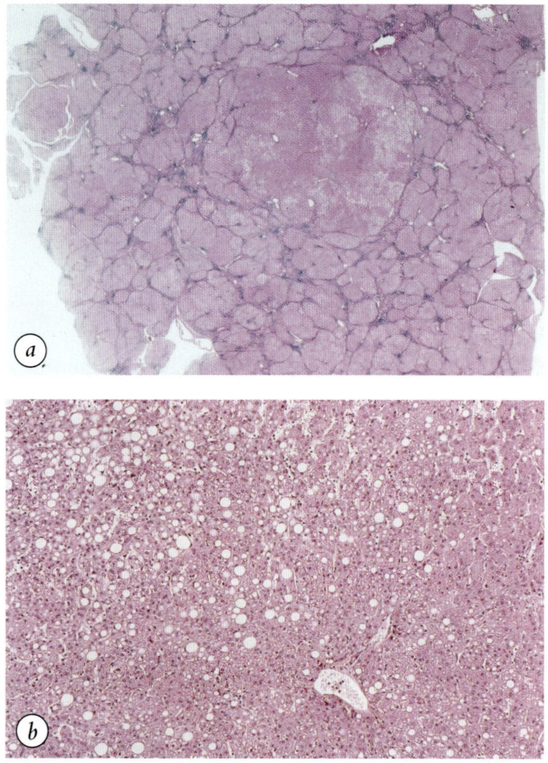

Figure 4.11 – Atypical adenomatous hyperplasia.

a) Tumor nodule, 1.2 cm in diameter, shows an increase of cellularity and staining affinity, and fatty change. Tumor contains portal tracts inside.

b) Histologically, the equivocal areas (left side), which mimic well-differentiated cancer, are observed in the nodule with fatty change.

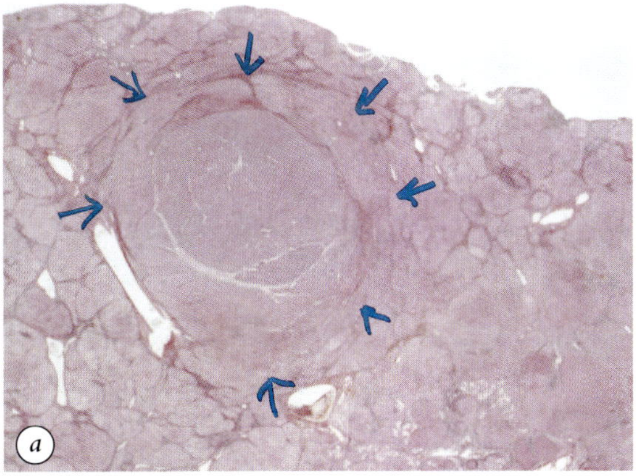

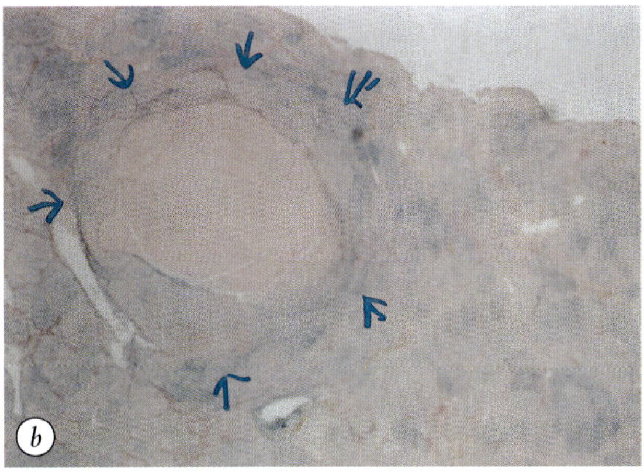

Figure 4.12 – Adenomatous hyperplasia containing cancer nodule.

a) Adenomatous hyperplaisa with 1.4 cm of diameter (arrows) contains well-demarcated cancerous tissue.

b) Adenomatous hyperplasia and cirrhotic liver tissue show prominent iron deposits, but cancer nodule inside adenomatous hyperplasia lacks iron deposits (Berlin blue stain).

either well-differentiated tumor or benign hyperplastic lesion, and such a lesion could be diagnosed differently in different institutions, e.g. as well-differentiated tumor, AAH, or benign hyperplastic lesion (Fig. 4.11).

Some AH nodules contain cancerous foci, and these are called "AH containing cancerous foci".[18,19] The contained cancerous tissue is always well-differentiated cancer. In such a case and if iron deposit is observed in the AH, the contained well-differentiated cancer usually does not show iron deposits (Fig. 4.12).

If the foci is moderately differentiated cancer showing classical trabecular pattern, the nodule should be considered a well-differentiated cancer nodule containing moderately differentiated cancer. A common and interesting finding on AAH and "AH containing cancerous foci" is a frequent association with fatty changes of varying degrees. We presume that many AAHs, specifically those associated with fatty changes, are most probably well-differentiated cancer.

To conclude it can be said that most morphologic features of early HCC have been elucidated. It is important to detect and treat HCC at the early stage while the tumor is well differentiated and has a weak proliferative activity in order to achieve better therapeutic effect and prognosis. However, histologic interpretations of borderline lesions, such as AH or AAH, have been a source of controversy. To reach a consensus, larger numbers of cases should be examined and more objective information including from molecular-oriented study should be obtained.

ADVANCED STAGE

Although increasing numbers of small HCC have been detected along with remarkable advance in various diagnostic modalities, the majority of HCCs are still only detected at the advanced stage. It is also important to understand the morphologic characteristics of advanced HCCs as well as those of small HCCs at the early stage.

FEATURES OF ADVANCED HCC

In general, it is well known that advanced HCCs present a variety of gross appearances according to the histologic heterogeneity, necrosis, hemorrhage, tumor thrombi of the intrahepatic portal veins, intrahepatic metastasis, and associated liver cirrhosis.[17]

Gross classification

Eggel's gross classification[18] continues to be widely used. He classified HCC into nodular, massive and diffuse (Fig. 4.13 a-c). Nodular type is characterized by a single nodular tumor or varying numbers of nodular tumors of different sizes. Massive type consists of a large single tumor occupying almost the

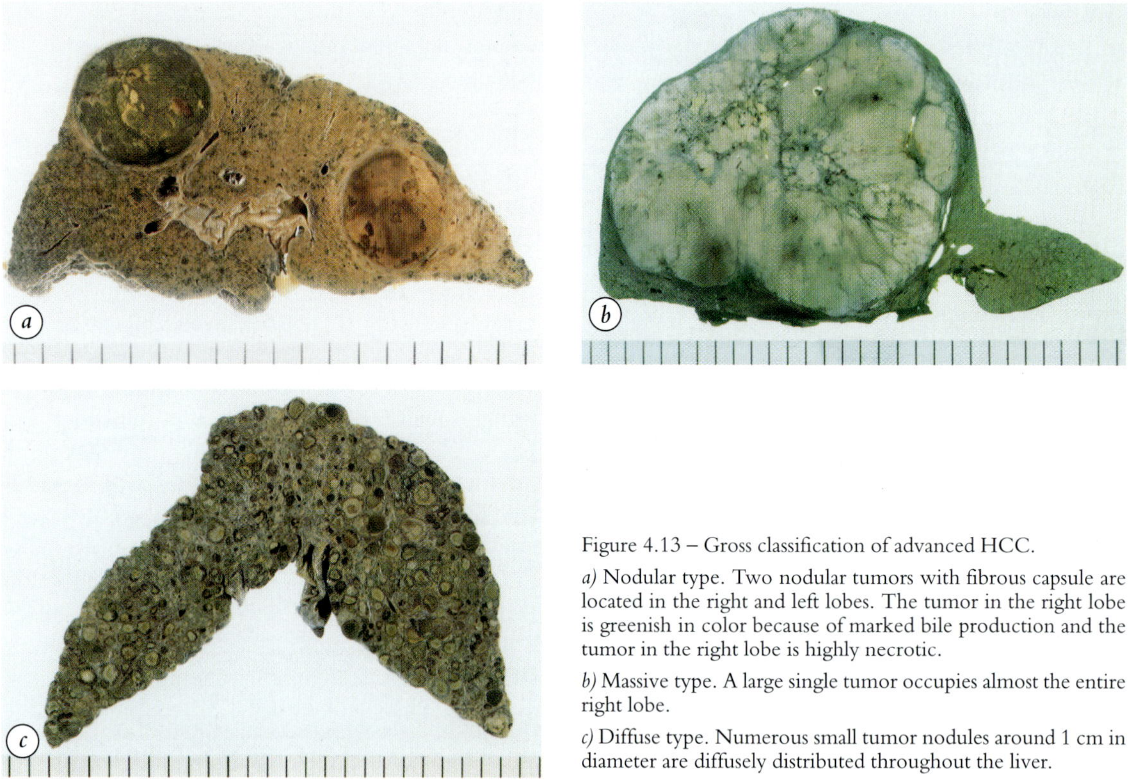

Figure 4.13 – Gross classification of advanced HCC.

a) Nodular type. Two nodular tumors with fibrous capsule are located in the right and left lobes. The tumor in the right lobe is greenish in color because of marked bile production and the tumor in the right lobe is highly necrotic.

b) Massive type. A large single tumor occupies almost the entire right lobe.

c) Diffuse type. Numerous small tumor nodules around 1 cm in diameter are diffusely distributed throughout the liver.

entire lobe. Diffuse type is characterized by diffuse distribution of numerous small tumor nodules throughout the liver.

Histologic features

HCC is one of the neoplasms which show marked histologic heterogeneity, even from the early stage as described above. The basic structure of HCC is generally composed of the tumor parenchyma consisting of cancer cells and stroma comprising sinusoid-like blood spaces lined by a single layer of endothelial cells, and represents a trabecular pattern of varying thickness depending on histologic grade.

Histologic classification

HCC is classified into well-differentiated, moderately differentiated, poorly differentiated, and undifferentiated types by histologic grade.

a) well-differentiated HCC (See above, and Figs. 4. 3-6.)

b) moderately differentiated HCC

This carcinoma is characterized by a trabecular pattern in which tumor cells are arranged in several layers. A pseudoglandular pattern is frequently observed. Cancer cells have abundant eosinophilic cytoplasm and round nuclei with distinct nucleoli. N/C ratio is almost equal to that of the hepatocyte (Fig. 4.14a).

c) poorly differentiated HCC

Cancer cells show a vaguely trabecular or compact (solid) growth pattern. In tumors with a solid growth pattern, a slit-like blood vessel is sparsely observed. Cancer cells show an increased N/C ratio and varying degrees of pleomorphism including mono- and/or multinucleated giant cells (Fig.4.14b).

d) undifferentiated carcinoma

Cancer cells have scant cytoplasm with short spindle-shaped and/or round nuclei, and proliferate in a medullary pattern. The diagnosis of HCC is often difficult from histologic findings only (Fig. 4.14c).

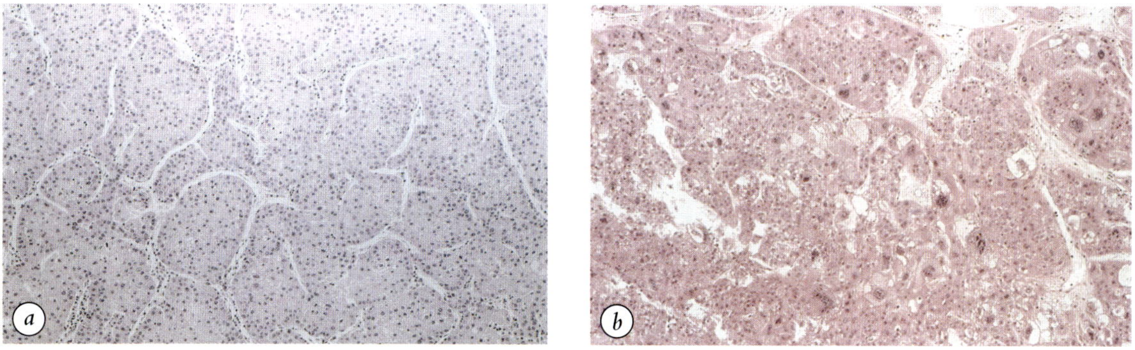

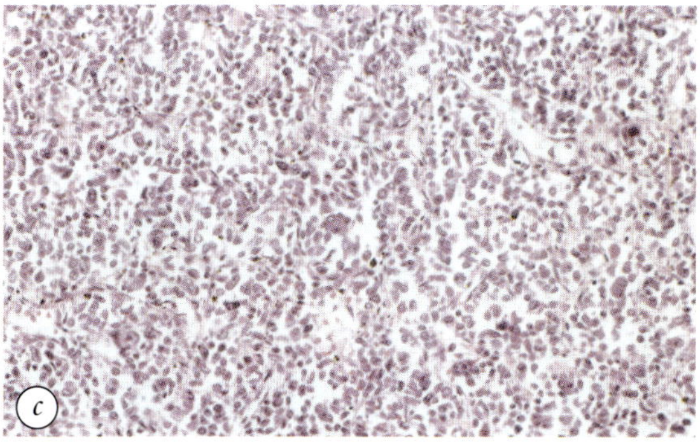

Figure 4.14 – Histologic classification by histologic grade.

a) Moderately differentiated HCC. Cancer cells are arranged in a trabecular pattern and each trabeculae are covered with a single layer of endothelial cells.

b) Poorly differentiated HCC. Tumor consists of pleomophic cancer cells including many bizarre giant cells and shows a vague trabecular arrangement. This carcinoma is also called as giant cell HCC.

c) Undifferentiated HCC. Tumor consists of short-spindle shaped cancer cells with a solid growth pattern. It is difficult to diagnose this tumor as HCC only from histologic features.

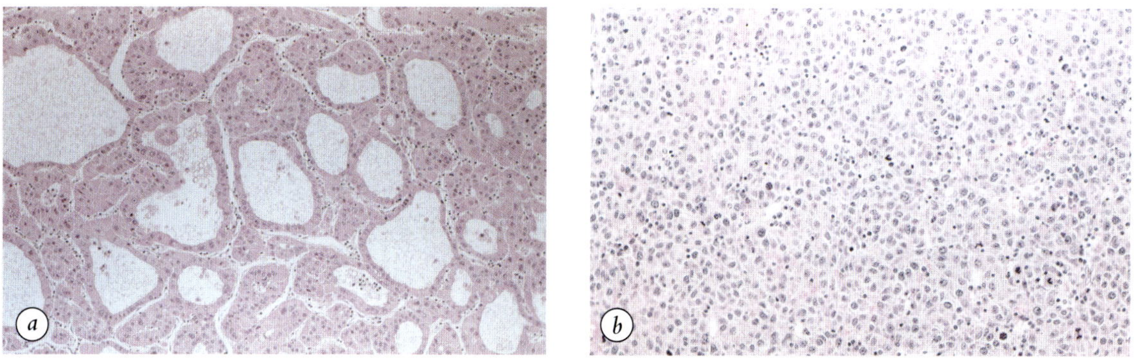

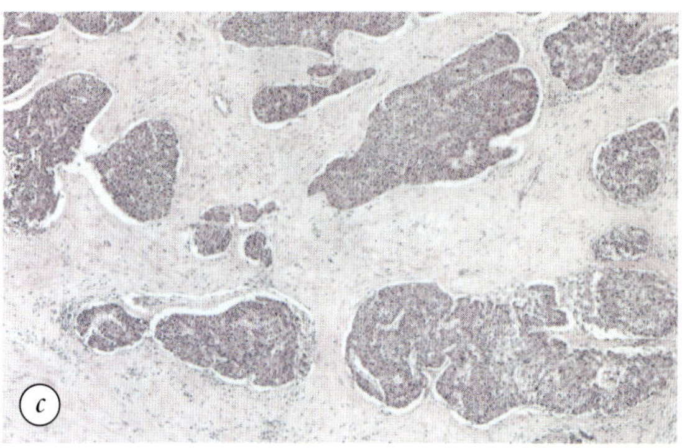

Figure 4.15 – Structural variation in HCC.

a) Pseudoglandular pattern. Cancer cells form varying sized pseudoglands which contain Proteinaceous substances with few cell debri.

b) Compact (solid) pattern. Cancer cells show a solid growth pattern with a few blood vessels. This carcinoma is poorly differentiated.

c) Scirrhous pattern. Blood spaces of the tumor are almost replaced by dense fibrous connective tissue, and tumor nests are atrophic.

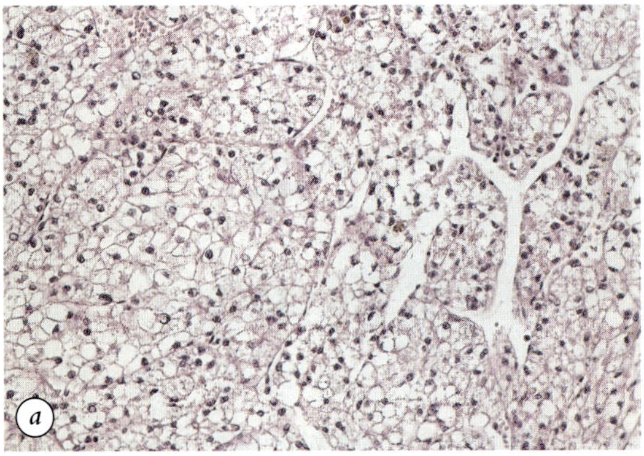

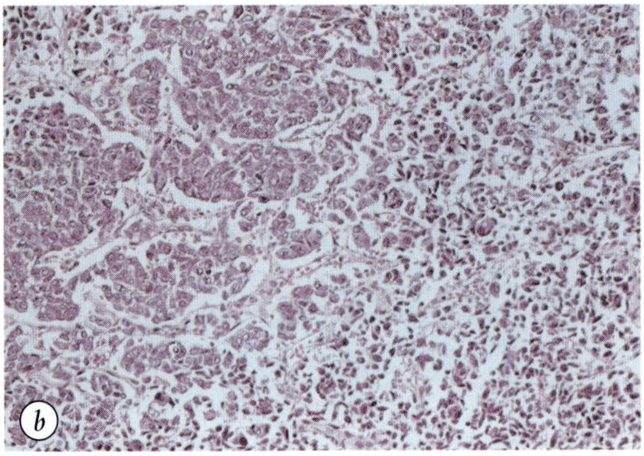

Figure 4.16 – Cytological variation in HCC.

a) Clear cell HCC. The cytoplasms of the cancer cells are watery clear due to abundant glycogen accumulation.

b) HCC with sarcomatous change. Transitional features are observed between trabecular HCC and sarcomatous tumor cells.

Variation in histologic pattern

i) Pseudoglandular/acinar pattern

Pseudoglandular/acinar pattern is as common as a trabecular pattern (Fig. 4.15a), and pseudoglands contain proteinaceous fluid or bile with cell debris.

ii) Compact (solid) pattern

Compact growth pattern is common in poorly differentiated HCC, and HCC with compact growth pattern is often composed of pleomorphic cancer cells with few blood vessels (Fig. 4.15b).

iii) Scirrhous pattern

Marked proliferation of fibrous connective tissue in the tumor is sometimes observed (Fig. 4.15c). It is most often seen after irradiation therapy, chemotherapy, or infarction. It is also found in HCCs without any specific etiologic factors. In our institute, scirrhous HCC accounts for approximately 4% of surgical cases without preoperative anticancer therapies. Such scirrhous appearance should be distinguished from cholangiocarcinoma and fibrolamellar HCC.

Cytologic variation in HCC

Pleomorphism, clear cell change, and spindle cell (pseudosarcomatous or sarcomatoid) changes are noted in HCC. [19]

i) Giant cell HCC

Bizarre pleomorphic cells as shown in Fig. 4.14b are common in poorly differentiated HCCs.

ii) Clear cell HCC

Clear cell HCC is characterized by tumor cells with a watery-clear cytoplasm due to abundant glycogen (Fig. 4.16a). Clear cell HCC resembles some metastatic carcinomas, including renal cell carcinoma, adrenal carcinoma, and clear cell adenocarcinoma of the ovary. Although it was reported that HCC of clear cell variant has a favorable prognosis compared with that of usual HCC,[20] the authors did not find a significant difference in prognosis in a study of 20 cases of clear cell HCC among 215 consecutively resected HCCs. [21]

iii) Sarcomatoid HCC

Occasionally, sarcomatoid HCCs consisting of spindle-shaped or pleomorphic anaplastic tumor cells are found in part of the tumor or almost the entire tumor with or without transitional features between trabecular HCC and the sarcomatoid area (Fig. 4.16b).[22,23]

The author presumes that the majority of sarcomatoid HCCs could be the sarcomatous change of HCC rather than the combination of true sarcoma and HCC. Among more than 62 surgically resected HCCs less than 2 cm in diameter seen in the author's institution, there has been no case with sarcomatoid appearance, and it is found in about 4% of advanced HCCs. Accordingly, sarcomatoid change of HCC seems to be caused by phenotypic changes of cancer cells due to factors including anti-cancer chemotherapy. We have clarified that the incidence of a sarcomatoid HCC is significantly higher among HCC cases with repeated transcatheter arterial chemoembolization therapy compared with non-treated cases. [24]

iv) Intracytoplasmic inclusions in HCC

In HCC, various hyalin inclusions are observed.

a) Reticular hyalins (Mallory bodies) (Fig. 4.17a)

Reticular hyalins are also called Mallory bodies and are commonly seen in alcoholic hepatitis. They are irregular in shape and acidophilic, and are not stained by periodic acid-schiff stain (PAS). Ultrastructurally, they are composed of an accumulation of intermediate filaments. [25]

b) Globular hyalins (Fig. 4.17b)

Globular hyalins are brightly stained with eosin and round to ovoid in shape. Most globular hyalins are diastase-resistant PAS positive.

c) Pale bodies (Fig. 4.17c)

Pale bodies are round to ovoid in shape and eosinophilic. They are immunohistochemically positive to anti-fibrinogen antibody, and are ultrastructurally observed as the accumulation of fibrils (fibrinogen) in dilated endoplasmic reticula.[26,27] Pale bodies are found in about 4% of HCCs and frequently in fibrolamellar HCCs.

Extrahepatic metastasis

Extrahepatic metastasis occurs at a relatively late stage in HCC. The reported incidence of extrahepatic metastasis ranges from around 50% to 70% in Western countries.[28,29] Among 660 consecutive autopsy cases of HCC at the author's institute, extrahepatic metastasis was found in 503 cases (76.2%). The incidence of extrahepatic metastasis tends to be slightly higher in HCC without cirrhosis than HCC with cirrhosis. Peters[29] reported extrahepatic metastases in 67.0% and 46.2% of HCCs without and with cirrhosis, respectively. The authors[30] found the corresponding figures of 74.2% and 58.4%, respectively.

In general, hematogeneous metastases are much more common than lymphatic ones in HCC; the incidence

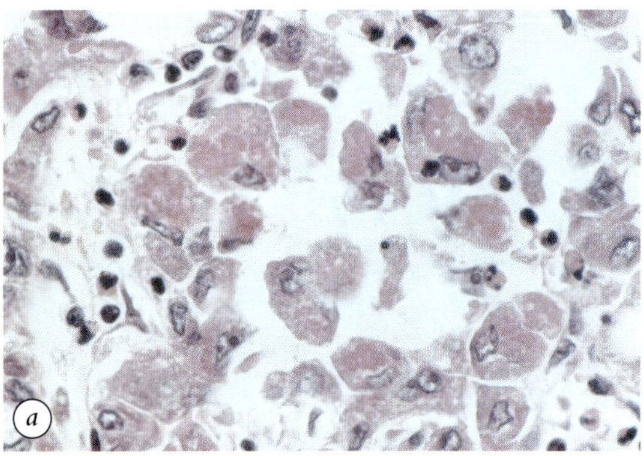

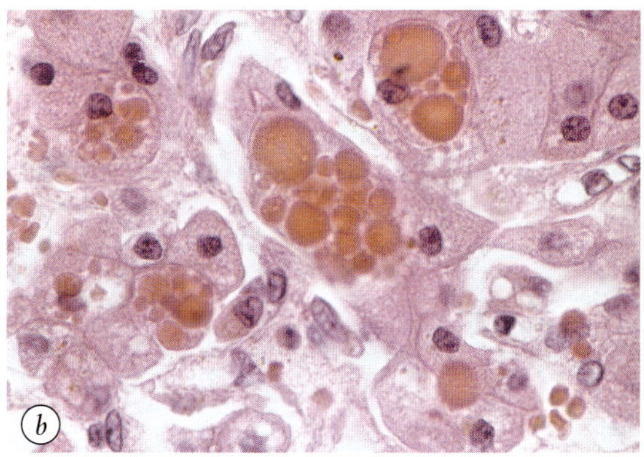

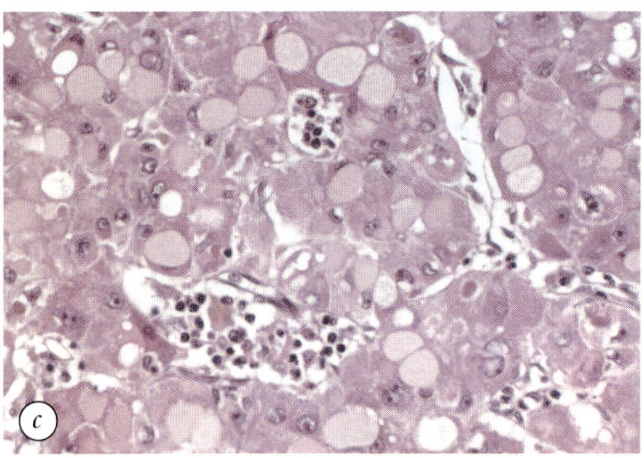

Figure 4.17 – Hyaline inclusions in HCC.

a) Reticular hyalins. Tumor cells contain acidophic inclusions which are irregular in shape.

b) Globular hyalins. Varying sized globular hyalins are brightly stained with eosin.

c) Pale bodies. Tumor cells contain ground-glass-like hyalin inclusions.

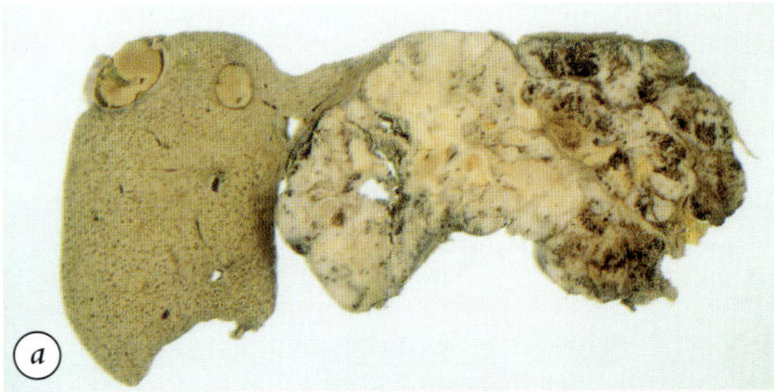

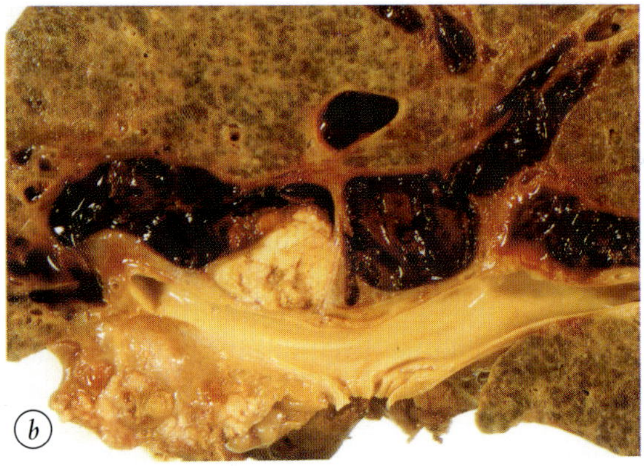

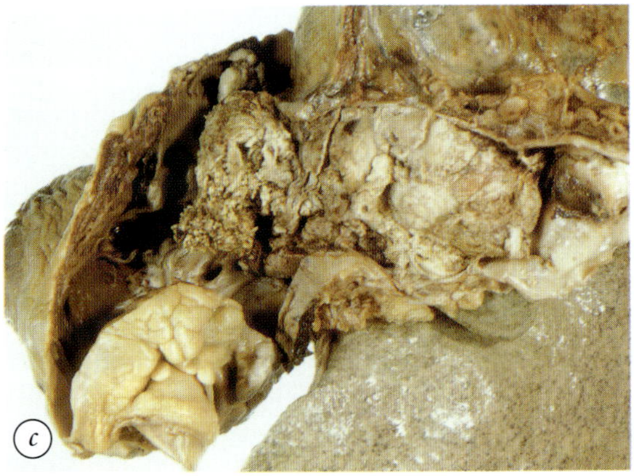

Figure 4.18 – Unusual tumor growth in HCC.

a) Pedunculated HCC. Massive tumor occurring in the left lobe proliferates extrahepatically with a few intrahepatic metastases.

b) Massive hemobilia due to intra-bile duct tumor growth. The tumor proliferates into the bifurcation of the hepatic duct and the patient died of massive hemobilia.

c) Tumor growth in the right atrium. The inferior vena cava and the right atrium were filled with massive tumor casts, but the patient presented no significant cardio-vascular symptoms.

of hematogeneous and lymphatic metastases were 50.8% and 23.5% in our series, respectively. Hematogeneous metastasis is noted in lung (47.6%), adrenal glands (8.3%), bone (5.6%), gastrointestinal tract (4.7%), gall bladder (3.5%) and pancreas (3.0%). Lymphatic metastasis is the most common in the hepatic hilar lymph nodes (58.3%), then peripancreatic nodes (54.2%), perigastric nodes (45.8%), periaortic nodes (33.3%), and superficial lymph nodes such as cervical nodes (about 10%).[30]

Unusual tumor growth

Pedunculated tumor growth, intra-bile duct tumor growth, and intra-atrial tumor growth through the inferior vena cava are sometimes encountered in HCC.

1) Pedunculated HCC

An extrahepatic tumor growth with little tumor proliferation in the liver is occasionally found in HCC. Most pedunculated HCCs occur in the subcapsular portion of the liver and grow extrahepatically with or without a pedicle (Fig. 4.18a). Among pedunculated HCCs, there are rare cases suggestive of tumor development in an accessory lobe.

2) Intra-bile duct tumor growth

Tumor invasion into the hepatic duct and/or common bile duct is not a rare event in HCCs and it accounts for about 6% of autopsy cases of HCC.[31] In most of the cases presenting with tumor invasion into the hepatic duct and/or common bile duct, progressive obstructive jaundice is one of the major clinical signs. Patients with HCC growing into the bile duct have a significantly shorter survival after the time of diagnosis than usual HCC cases. Massive hemorrhage in the bile duct (hemobilia) due to tumor invasion into the bile duct is occasionally encountered and it is often fatal (Fig. 4.18b).

3) Intra-atrial tumor growth

It is not uncommon to find massive tumor growth into the right atrium with or without tumor extension into the right ventricle through the inferior vena cava (IVC) in HCC.[32] Among 439 autopsy cases of HCC in the past 2 decades in our institute, tumor extended into the IVC in 48 (10.9%) cases, and into the right atrium in 18 (4.8%) cases (Fig. 4.18c). A tumor bolus crossed the tricuspid valves and entered the ventricle in 5 of the 18 cases and direct tumor invasion into the myocardium was found in 2 cases. Despite massive tumor casts in the right atrium through the IVC, serious cardiovascular symptoms among the patients were uncommon. Only diuretic-resistant edema in the lower extremities and/or marked venous dilatation in the abdominal wall were observed. The serious clinical problems in the patients with an intra-atrial tumor growth were sudden cardiac arrest or severe dyspnea due to obstruction of tricuspid valves by ball-shaped tumor thrombus. Only 1 case died of sudden cardiac arrest due to tricuspid obstruction among 18 autopsy cases of HCC patients with right atrial tumor growth.

REFERENCES

1. Nakashima O, Sugihara S, Kage M, *et al*: Pathomorphologic characteristics of small hepatocellular carcinoma: A special reference to small hepatocellular carcinoma with indistinct margins.*Hepatology,* 1995; **22**:101-105,
2. Kojiro M, Sugihara S, Nakashima O: Pathomorphologic characteristics of early hepatocellular carcinoma. In:Okuda K, Tobe T, Kitagawa T (eds), Early detection and treatment of liver cancer. *Gann monograph on cancer research No.38*, Japan Scientific Societies Press, Tokyo, 1991, p29-38
3. Kondo F, Wada K, Nagato,Y, *et al*: Biopsy diagnosis of well-differentiated hepatocellular carcinoma based on new morphologic criteria. *Hepatology*,1989; **9**: 751-755
4. Kondo Y, Niwa Y, Akikusa B, *et al*: A histopathologic study of early hepatocellular carcinoma. *Cancer,* 1983; **52**: 687-692
5. Ohno Y, Shiga J, Machinami R: A histopathological analysis of five cases of adenomatous hyperplasia containing minute hepatocellular carcinoma. *Acta Pathol Jpn*, 1990; **40**:267-278,
6. Arakawa M, Kage M, Sugihara S, *et al*: Emergence of malignant lesions within an adenomatous hyperplastic nodule in a cirrhotic liver. Observations in five cases. *Gastroenterology*, 1986; **91**:198-208
7. Kennmochi K, Sugihara S, Kojiro M, *et al.*:Relationship of histologic grade of hepatocellular carcinoma (HCC) to tumor size, and demonstration of tumor cells of multiple different grade in single HCC. *Liver,*1987; **7**:18-26
8. Sugihara S, Nakashima O, Kojiro M, *et al*: The morphologic transition in hepatocellular carcinoma -A comparison of the individual histological features disclosed by ultrasound-guided fine-needle biopsy with at autopsy. *Cancer,* 1992; **70**: 1488-1492,
9. Yano H, Iemura A, Fukuda K, *et al* : Establishment of two distinct human hepatocellular carcinoma cell lines from a single nodule showing clonal dedifferentiation of cancer cells. *Hepatology*, 1993; **18**: 320-327
10. Kondo F, Ebara M, Sugiura N, *et al*: Histological features and clinical course of large regenerative nodules: Evaluation of their precancerous potentiality. *Hepatology*, 1990; **12**:529-598
11. Takayama T, Makuuchi M, Hirohashi S, *et al.*: Malignant transformation of adenomatous hyperplasia to hepatocellular carcinoma. *Lancet*, 1990; **336**:1150-1153
12. Terada T, Kadoya M, Nakanuma Y, *et al*: Iron-accumulating adenomatous hyperplastic nodule with malignant foci in the cirrhotic liver. *Cancer*, 1990; **65**:1994-2000
13. Liver Cancer Study Group of Japan: *The general rules for the clinical and pathological study of primary liver cancer*, 3rd ed., Kanehara Shuppan, Tokyo, 1992
14. Eguchi A, Nakashima O, Okudaira S, *et al*: Adenomatous hyperplasia in the vicinity of small hepatocellular carcinoma. *Hepatology*, 1992; **20**:843-848
15. Sakurai M, Wakasa K, Monden M, *et al*: Hepatocellular carcinoma in adenomatous hyperplasia of the liver. *Cancer Chemother Pharmacol*, 1989; **23**(Suppl):110-113
16. Kaji K, Terada T, Nakanuma Y: Frequent occurrence of hepatocellular carcinoma in cirrhotic livers after surgical resection of atypical adenomatous hyperplasia (borderline hepatocellular lesion): a follow-up study. *Am J Gastroenterol* , 1994; **89**:903-908
17. Nakashima T, Kojiro M: *Hepatocellular carcinoma - An atlas of its pathology.* Tokyo, Springer-Verlag, 1987
18. Eggel H: Uber das primare Carcinom der Leber. Beitr Pathol *Anat Allg Pathol* , 1901; **30**:506
19. Ishak KG, Anthony PP, Sobin LH: *Histological typing of tumours of the liver*, 2nd ed.,WHO international histological classification of tumours. Berlin, Springer-Verlag, 1994, p20
20. Lai CL, Wu PC, Lam KC, Lok ASF: Histologic prognostic indicators in hepatocellular carcinoma. *Cancer*, 1979; **44**: 1677-1683
21. Yang SH, Watanabe J, Nakashima O, Kojiro M: Clinicopathologic study on clear cell hepatocellular carcinoma. *Pathol Intern* 1996;**46**:505-509
22. Kakizoe S, Kojiro M, Nakashima T: Hepatocellular carcinoma with sarcomatous change. Clinicopathologic and immunohistochemical studies of 14 autopsy cases. *Cancer,* 1987; **59**:310-316
23. Maeda T, Adachi E, Kajiyama K, Takenaka K, Sugimachi K, Tsuneyoshi M: Spindle cell hepatocellular carcinoma. A clinicopathologic and immunohistochemical analysis of 15 cases. *Cancer*, 1995; **77**:51-57
24. Kojiro M, Sugihara S, Kakizoe S, Nakashima O, Kiyomatsu K: :Hepatocellular carcinoma with sarcomatous change: a special reference to the relationship with anticancer therapy. *Cancer Chemother Pharmacol* , 1989; **23**(Suppl):4-8
25. Nakanuma Y, Ohta G: Is Mallory body formation a preneoplastic change? A study of 181 cases of liver bearing hepatocellular carcinoma and 82 cases of cirrhosis. *Cancer*, 1984; **55**:2400-2404
26. Stromeyer FW, Ishak KG, Gerber MA, Mathew T: Ground-glass cells in hepatocellular carcinoma. *Am J Clin Pathol*, 1980; **74**:254-258
27. Nakashima O, Sugihara S, Eguchi A, Taguchi J, Watanabe J, Kojiro M: Pathomorphologic study of pale bodies in hepatocellular carcinoma. *Acta Pathol Jpn*, 1992; **42**:414-417
28. MacDonald RA: Primary carcinoma of the liver. *Arch Intern Med*, 1957; **99**:266-279
28. MacSween RNM: A clinicopathological review of 100 cases of primary malignant tumors of the liver. *J Clin Pathol*, 1974; **27**:669-682

29. Peters RL: Pathology of hepatocellular carcinoma. In: Okuda K, Peters RL, eds. *Hepatocellular carcinoma*. New York, Wiley, 1976, p107-168

30. Watanabe J, Nakashima O, Kojiro M: Clinicopathologic study on lymph node metastasis of hepatocellular carcinoma: A retrospective study of 660 consecutive autopsy cases. *Jpn J Clin Oncol*, 1994; **24**:37-41

31. Kojiro M, Kawabata K, Kawano Y, Shirai F, Takemoto N, Nakashima T: Hepatocellular carcinoma presenting as intrabile duct tumor growth: a clinicopathologic study of 24 cases. *Cancer*, 1982; **49**:2144-2124

32. Kojiro M, Nakahara H, Sugihara S, Murakami T, Nakashima T, Kawasaki H: Hepatocellular carcinoma with intraatrial tumor growth: a clinicopathologic study of 18 autopsy cases. *Arch Pathol Lab Med*, 1984; **108**:989-992

PART II

CLINICAL ASPECTS

5

Clinical presentation

J Bruix, JM Llovet, C Bru and J Rodés

A decade ago most patients with HCC were diagnosed at an advanced stage with the clinical pattern of a neoplasic patient exhibiting constitutional syndrome (weight loss, malaise and anorexia) associated with clinical signs of severe hepatic disease, such as jaundice, encephalopathy, ascites and gastrointestinal bleeding due to ruptured esophageal varices. Nowadays, the diagnosis of HCC is achieved at earlier stages and thus the clinical pattern of these patients varies from the completely asymptomatic individual to the "classical" picture of an end-stage terminally ill case. Furthermore, it has to be taken into account that in most parts of the world liver cirrhosis underlies HCC in the vast majority of the patients[1] and thus, some of the symptoms at diagnosis will reflect the functional status of the liver rather than the evolutionary stage of the tumor. By contrast, in the minor proportion of patients in which the HCC develops in an otherwise normal liver (as seen in half of black patients in South Africa[2]), the clinical presentation is related exclusively to the development of the tumor.

ETIOLOGY OF THE UNDERLYING LIVER DISEASE

HCC has been described in patients with all etiologic types of liver cirrhosis.[2] Obviously, the most frequent etiologies of chronic liver disease are those that are more frequently reported in patients without HCC and the geographic discrepancies that appear when comparing series of patients from different geographic areas, reflect the heterogeneous prevalence of the etiologic agents in the world.[3] Thus, most of the patients are diagnosed with HCC on cirrhosis related to alcohol and/or HBV antibody or HCV viruses.[4] In fact, in western countries the prevalence of anti-HCV in patients with HCC is as high as 75%.[5] There is no evidence that a different etiology of the underlying liver disease would promote a special characteristic in the clinical presentation. The only exception would be the age at diagnosis which has been repeatedly shown to be lower in those cases with HBV related HCC.

CLINICAL CHARACTERISTISTICS

Age

The median age at the time of diagnosis is usually between the 5th and 6th decade of life. This moderately advanced age may be the consequence of the time needed to first develop liver cirrhosis and then generate the HCC. However, as previously commented, patients with HCC related to HBV infection are younger, probably reflecting the acquisition of the infection during delivery or early after birth. Therefore, it has been shown that most cases diagnosed during childhood and adolescence may be attributed to HBV[6] and when dividing the patients according to the etiology of the disease, the HBV-positive patients appear to be younger. [7]

Sex

HCC has a male predominance with the male to female ratio varying between series.[3] However, this male preponderance is tempered at advanced age,[8] thus suggesting that androgenic hormones favor the development of the tumor, while estrogens, are to some extent, protective.

Physical examination

Most of the features reported in patients with HCC are those of chronic liver disease. If patients are diagnosed at an advanced stage it will be easier to detect a palpable abdominal mass on which it may be possible to auscultate an arterial bruit reflecting arterio-venous fistulae. The palpation of an hepatic mass is more frequent in patients with an underlying normal liver since the non affected liver mantains a normal function until advanced stages, thus precluding early recognition of the disease. A minor proportion of patients present fever at the time of diagnosis and, in very infrequent cases, the distinction between HCC and liver abscess may be difficult.[9] The development of an HCC is sometimes associated with the appearance/increase of vascular spiders.

Symptoms

A decade ago only a minor proportion of HCC patients were diagnosed at an asymptomatic phase, but in recent years almost 40% of our patients are diagnosed while having no symptoms. This sharp increase has not only been due to the engagement of early detection programs in patients with cirrhosis (we include in the HCC early detection plan all the cirrhotic patients), but also to the fact that all the patients referred to our unit for evaluation of a liver disease and/or a clinical or biochemical abnormality related to a potential liver disease are explored by ultrasonography. This has allowed the recognition of solitary small asymptomatic HCC that otherwise would only have been diagnosed when the tumoral disease was far more advanced.

The clinical picture of those patients classified as symptomatic covers a wide spectrum of manifestations either alone or in combination. In patients diagnosed at an intermediate stage it is possible to register only one of the potential symptoms summarized below, but in advanced cases or as the disease progresses the clinical pattern may be more complex.

Pain

This is one of the most frequent manifestations in HCC patients. It appears mostly at advanced stages and/or when the tumor affects the liver capsule. Pain is located in the right upper quadrant and its intensity varies largely from mild pain that is easily controllable to severe pain requiring powerful analgesics. Since its appearance is usually associated with an advanced stage, pain may have prognostic implication. Acute onset pain may reflect bleeding into the peritoneal cavity due to the rupture of the tumor, and represents in a minority of patients (5%) the first symptom of the disease. In this circumstance, the abdominal pain is diffuse and if the bleeding is not controlled, the patients deteriorate rapidly because of hypovolemic shock. Therefore, this complication is life threatening and frequently leads to death.

Constitutional syndrome

This is characterized by malaise, weight loss and anorexia and its presence reflects advanced disease, which may also be recognized by other clinical classifications such as the Performance Status Test[10] or the Karnofsky scale.[11]

Since in most patients HCC develops on a cirrhotic liver, a large proportion will present signs and symptoms of chronic liver disease either at diagnosis or during follow-up, and it may be impossible to determine to what extent the appearance of liver decompensation is due to the appearance of the tumor or to the evolution of the underlying liver disease itself. Jaundice, encephalopathy and ascites are not specific features of HCC patients.

Jaundice

In some subjects, the infiltration of the biliary tree prompts obstruction due to the tumor or to blood clots and this may induce obstructive jaundice. However, the development of jaundice is usually due to the functional impairment of the non-tumoral liver.

Hemorrhagic ascites

This symptom may be suggestive of HCC reflecting minor or major tumoral bleeding. In necropsic series up to 50% of patients are found to have hemorrhagic ascites, but it has to be stressed that cirrhotic patients, although very seldom, may also present this feature.

Variceal bleeding

A significant proportion of patients present with variceal bleeding. Up to 15% of patients admitted to hospital because of variceal bleeding may be diagnosed with HCC if properly explored.[12] Variceal bleeding is not unequivocally associated with the existence of portal vein thrombosis due to tumoral invasion. However, it has been suggested that the development of an HCC induces a further increase in a previously hypertensive portal vein and that this may favor bleeding not only from esophageal varices, but also from hypertensive gastropathy associated with portal hypertension. Furthermore, HCC development has been suggested to be an important factor in determining the failure of pharmacologic treatment in preventing new episodes of variceal bleeding in cirrhotic patients who first bled when free of HCC.[13] This suggested increase in portal pressure could also explain some of the hepatorenal syndromes observed in HCC patients, but obviously this may be the case in advanced stages only, while in non-terminal cases the most important cause of renal failure is the administration of non steroidal anti-inflammatory agents. These drugs are frequently used for controlling pain but in cirrhotic patients they may prompt irreversible functional renal failure due to renal prostaglandin inhibition[14] and thus should be avoided.

Spontaneous bacterial peritonitis

Both cirrhosis and HCC decrease systemic immunity and this favors the development of infections. We have recently shown that up to 20% of the patients with this complication present underlying HCC.

Metastases

HCC is considered to be a neoplasm with a highly metastatic potential. Recent studies have shown that it is possible to detect circulating malignant cells even at early stages of the disease,[15] whose ultimate development into clinically recognizable metastases depends on several additional parameters, such as immunologic factors and attachment-invasion capability of these cells.[16] In addition to these cellular mechanisms, the patients should survive long enough to allow the microscopic nests to grow until reaching a sufficient volume to be clinicallly relevant and/or detectable by imaging techniques or at necropsy. The most frequently affected sites are hilar nodes, bone, lung and adrenal glands. As expected, the rate of dissemination runs parallel to the stage of the tumor, but in a minority of patients the symptoms due to the metastatic spread may be the first symptom of the disease.[17]

Most of these cases exhibit bone metastases with pathologic fractures, but in a few cases lung metastases may prompt repeated episodes of dyspnea due to the appearance of tumoral emboli in the pulmonary vascular bed, and these episodes are the sole clinical manifestation of the HCC. Finally, in some patients the first manifestation of the disease is the infiltration of the surrounding organs such as the stomach and duodenum, giving rise to bleeding and/or perforation.[18]

Paraneoplasic syndromes

Systemic manifestations secondary to the development of the tumor are present in less than 25% of cases at the time of diagnosis and are rarely recognized as the first manifestation of the disease. The most frequent of these is diarrhea, which can be registered in more than 50% of cases in the 3 months prior to diagnosis.[19] The mechanism of this frequent clinical manifestation is not known, but it is probably related to the production of several vasoactive substances (vasoactive intestinal peptide (VIP), gastrin, prostaglandins) by the tumor. Erythrocytosis can be present in 10% of cases but may be difficult to recognize due to the fact that the increased red blood cell mass may be hidden by the expanded plasma volume of cirrhotic patients, thus resulting in a normal hematocrit value. Hypoglycemia is more common with large tumors and it has been divided into type A, which appears in patients with fast growing tumors and is apparent only at a preterminal stage, and type B, which is not a terminal event that appears quickly after fasting and is very difficult to control.[20]

Hypercalcemia, sexual precocity, gonadotrophin production, cryofibrinogenemia, dysfibrinogenemia and carcinoid syndrome are very infrequent.

BIOCHEMICAL PROFILE

Once again the degree of the analytical abnormalities will depend on the stage of the tumor and the functional capability of the underlying liver disease. Patients with HCC who are detected early may present minor hypertransaminasemia with the other liver function tests remaining almost within normal values. By contrast, decompensated cirrhotic patients in whom HCC detection was prompted by tumoral symptoms, exhibit a more abnormal profile with increased alkaline phosphatase and gamma-glutamyl-transpeptidase associated with hyperbilirubinemia, hypoalbuminemia, hypergammaglobulinemia and reduced prothrombin ratio.

Alpha-fetoprotein (AFP) is the sole tumoral marker with a proven clinical value (see Chapter 7). However, most patients with a small HCC exhibit a normal concentration.[21] In fact, less than 10% of patients with uninodular HCC smaller than 5 cm shown AFP levels above 100 ng/dl. Thus, the detection of increased AFP should raise the suspicion of advanced disease.

REFERENCES

1. Johnson PJ, Williams R. Cirrhosis and the etiology of hepatocellular carcinoma. *J Hepatol* 1987; **4**: 140-147.
2. Kew MC. Hepatocellular carcinoma with and without cirrhosis. A comparison in southern African blacks. *Gastroenterology* 1989; **97**: 136-139.
3. Bruix J, Castells A, Bru C. Caracteristicas clinicas y pronostico del carcinoma hepatocelular. Existen diferencias geograficas? *Gastroenterol Hepatol* 1991; **14**: 520-524.

4. Okuda K. Hepatocellular carcinoma: recent progress. *Hepatology* 1992; **15** : 948-963.

5. Bruix J, Calvet X, Costa J, Ventura M, Bruguera M, Castillo R, Barrera JM, Ercilla G, Sanchez Tapias JM, Vall M, Bru C, Rodés J. Prevalence of antibodies to hepatitis C virus in Spanish patients with hepatocellular carcinoma and hepatic cirrhosis. *Lancet* 1989;II:1004-1006.

6. Chang MH, Chen PJ, Chen JY, Lai MY, Hsu HC, Lian DC, Liu YG *et al.* Hepatitis B virus integration in hepatitis B virus related hepatocellular carcinoma in childhood. *Hepatology* 1991; **13**: 316-320.

7. Lee SD, Lee FY, Wu JC, Hwang SJ, Wang SS, Lo KJ. The prevalence of antihepatitis C virus among Chinese patients with hepatocellular carcinoma.*Cancer* 1992; **69**: 342-345.

8. Nomura F, Ohnishi K, Honda M, Satomura Y, Nakai T, Okuda K. Clinical features of hepatocellular carcinoma in the elderly: a study of 91 patients older than 70 years. *Br J Cancer* 1994; **70**:690-693.

9. Okuda K, Kondo Y, Nakano M, Kage M, Arakawa M, Kojiro M, Ohtsuki T *et al.* Hepatocellular carcinoma presenting with pyrexia and leukocytosis: report of five cases. *Hepatology* 1991; **13**:695-700.

10. Sorensen JB, Klee M, Palshof T, Hansen HH. Performance status assessment in cancer patients. An interobserver variability study. *Br J Cancer* 1993; **67**:773-775.

11. Karnofsky DA, Adelmann WH, Craver LF, Burchenal JH. The use of nitrogen mustards in the palliative treatment of carcinoma. *Cancer* 1948; **1**:634-656.

12. Llach J, Teres J, Garcia-Pagan JC, Calvet X, Saperas E, Rodes J. Hipertransaminasemia en el curso de una hemorragia digestiva alta por varices esofagicas en pacientes cirroticos. Su asociacion con el carcinoma hepatocellular. *Gastroenterol Hepatol* 1988; **11**: 273-275.

13. Lebrec D. Long term management of variceal bleeding: the place of pharmacotherapy. *World J Surg* 1994; **18**:229-232

14. Arroyo V, Gines P, Rimola A, Gaya J. Renal function abnormalities, prostaglandins, and effects of nonsteroidal anti-inflammatory drugs in cirrhosis with ascites. An overview with emphasis on pathogenesis. *Am J Med* 1986; **81**:104-122

15. Hillaire S, Barbu V, Boucher E, Moukhtar M, Poupon R. Albumin messenger RNA as a marker of circulating hepatocytes in hepatocellular carcinoma. *Gastroenterology* 1994; **106**:239-242

16. Kohn EC, Liotta L. Molecular insights into cancer invasion: strategies for prevention and intervention. *Cancer Res* 1995; **55**: 1856-1862.

17. Liaw CC, Ng KT, Chen TJ, Liaw YF. Hepatocellular carcinoma presenting as bone metastasis. *Cancer* 1989; **64**: 1753-1757.

18. Humbert P, Sarmiento J, Boix J, Planas R, Quintero E, Franquet T, Villagrasa M. Hepatocellular carcinoma presenting with bleeding due to duodenal perforation by the tumor. *Endoscopy* 1987; **19:** 37-38.

19. Bruix J, Castells A, Calvet X, Feu F, Bru C, Sole M, Bruguera M *et al.* Diarrhoea as a presenting syndrome of hepatocellular carcinoma. *Dig Dis Sci* 1990; **35**:681-685

20. Shapiro ET, Bell GI, Polonsky KS, Rubenstein AH, Kew MC, Tager HS. Tumor hypoglycemia: a relationship to high molecular weight insulin-like growth factor-II. *J Clin Invest* 1990;**85**:1672-1679.

21. Calvet X, Bruix J, Bru C, Gines P, Vilana R, Sole M, Ayuso MC, Bruguera M, Rodes J. Natural history of hepatocellular carcinoma in Spain. Five year experience in 249 cases. *J Hepatol* 1990; **10**:311-317

6

Natural history

L Bolondi and G Zironi

Hepatocellular carcinoma (HCC) is one of the commonest tumors worldwide and epidemiologic data show a significant increasing trend in HCC incidence in many countries.[1-3] Usually HCC is associated with chronic liver disease and cirrhosis in particular. As viral hepatitis represents the leading cause of chronic liver disease and considering the wide spread of hepatitis, a reduction in the incidence of HCC is unlikely in the near future.

MORPHOGENESIS OF HCC

The advances in imaging techniques allowing the investigation of large series of patients with liver disease and the increasing number of liver transplantations and resections have made possible the study of this neoplasm at an early stage, both from a clinical and a pathologic perspective, and therefore the analysis of the natural course of human hepatocarcinogenesis.

Pathologic studies show that the nodular lesions detectable in chronic liver disease may have different evolutions: it is possible to identify preneoplastic lesions which have been named regenerative nodules, adenomatous hyperplasia and atypical adenomatous hyperplasia.[4] Histopathologic criteria defining different types of nodular lesions in cirrhotic and non cirrhotic livers and distinguishing macroregenerative nodules from dysplastic nodules have been recently reported[5] and consider both cellular and stromal characteristics. However separation of macroregenerative nodules from low-grade and high-grade dysplastic nodules is sometimes impossible, mainly when the entire lesion is not available for study as in the case of echo-guided biopsy.

Clinical studies underlined the precancerous nature of some of these lesions;[6,7] nodule-in-nodule lesions, i.e. the peripheral area of early, well differentiated HCC with a central area of less differentiated HCC, were also described. The pathologic distinction between these different lesions lies in the detection of morphometric changes, cellular density and atypia, cytoplasmic eosinophilia or basophilia, nuclear crowding, and structural abnormalities such as small acinar structures or abnormal cord structures. Nevertheless the differentiation between dysplastic nodules and early HCC can be difficult[8]. Therefore other methods, such as the evaluation of DNA synthesis, cellular ploidy and proliferation-related cellular antigens (e.g. Ki67, PCNA etc), have been proposed. We have found a reduction of binuclear hepatocytes within an increased poliploid compartment, an increased AgNOR protein quantity and abnormalities in the activity and distribution of dipeptydil-peptidase IV in regenerative nodules with subsequent malignant transformation.[9] These alterations have also been described in cirrhotic livers without HCC and in livers that subsequently developed HCC,[10-12] thus suggesting their possible prognostic relevance.

HEPATITIS VIRUSES AND OTHER RISK FACTORS

Research suggests a strong epidemiologic relationship between HBV infection and HCC: a strict association has been described between the HBsAg carrier rate and the incidence rate of HCC.[13] The HBsAg positivity rate is higher in HCC patients than in control groups or in patients without HCC; HBsAg carriers show higher risk of developing HCC; the relative risk was greater than 100 in a study of 22,707 men in Taiwan.[14] Beside the epidemiologic considerations, many experimental studies strongly support the carcinogenic role of HBV. A malignant transformation of transgenic hepatocytes transfected with HBV DNA has been described.[15] Furthermore HBV belongs to the hepadnaviruses, which are retrovirus-like agents; integrated viral HBV DNA sequences have been found in the DNA of HCC cells.[16] Obviously the HBV-DNA integration plays an important role in the development of HCC, but several observations suggest that this is only an initiator of hepatocarcinogenesis and does not have a specific role. It is demonstrated that the viral DNA is also integrated in non-tumor hepatocytes from HCC patients and in livers of HBV infected patients without HCC[17,18] and that the cellular site of HBV integration is random. It is hypothesized that the gene mutations, translocations and rearrangements that follow viral DNA integration[19-21] represent a first step in a cascade of events that lead to cancer. Again, some viruses possess viral oncogenes (v-onc) but this is not the case with HBV. Nevertheless the HBV X gene product displays transactivating properties[22] like the pre-S2 region of integrated HBV DNA,[23] while the HBV DNA polymerase displays a reverse transcriptase activity.[24]

Studies regarding tumor suppressing genes found a loss of heterozygosity in advanced HCC, mainly on chromosomes 16 and 17 [25, 26] and the most common mutation involves the p53 gene at codon 249.[27,28] Interestingly, the mutation in the p53 gene was also observed in HCC after aflatoxin exposure:[29] in experimental studies, chemical carcinogens can induce cirrhosis and HCC, but in humans there is no evidence that aflatoxin directly induces HCC. The increased risk of HCC among people exposed to aflatoxin seems to be mainly related to chronic HBV infection in the same population.[30]

In Japan the observation that in the last 15 years the incidence of HCC has increased, while the rate of HBsAg positive HCC patients has decreased, suggested a role for factors other than HBV infection in hepatocarcinogenesis: an increased number of HCC patients positive for hepatitis C virus antibody (anti-HCV) were found. Similar results were also described in Europe[31, 32]. Kiyosawa *et al.* found a prevalence of patients positive for anti-HCV in 89% of chronic hepatitis, in 86% of liver cirrhosis and in 94% of HCC while, in the same study group, HBV was present in 6%, 17% and 34%, respectively.[33] The clinical course of patients infected by HCV after blood transfusion suggests a mean time interval of 10 years for the diagnosis of active chronic hepatitis, of 21.2 years for the diagnosis of cirrhosis and of 29 years for the diagnosis of HCC.[33] The evolution from HCV hepatitis to HCC seems to imply different mechanisms from those of HBV: HCV is a single positive strand RNA virus and, as reverse transcription for its replication has not been proved, it is unlikely that the HCV genome can integrate into cellular DNA. HCV probably plays a role in hepatocarcinogenesis only in the presence of other risk factors: in HCC patients with cirrhosis and a history of alcohol abuse and in those who were HBsAg positive Farinati *et al* found a high prevalence of anti-HCV[34]. Furthermore anti-HCV is more frequent among HBsAg positive patients with HCC than without HCC and the same result was found in alcoholic cirrhotics. Ikeda *et al*[35] showed that alcohol abuse and elevated values of α-fetoprotein (AFP) are related to a higher incidence of HCC in anti-HCV positive patients, but not in HBV positive ones.

A direct hepatocarcinogenetic role for HCV is therefore suspected, but it is more likely that HCV plays a co-carcinogenic role which is augmented by chronic inflammation, cirrhosis and cell regeneration, which take place in the infected liver. Other experimental studies emphasize the role of necrosis and hepatocyte regeneration in hepatocarcinogenesis. In the model of transgenic mice proposed by Chisari *et al* [36] the severity of hepatitis and necrosis correlates with the development of HCC.

The observation of iron-free foci in livers of patients with genetic hemochromatosis suggests a clonal origin of HCC in humans. Hemochromatosis has been estimated to increase the risk of HCC 200-fold above that of the general population while HCV, HBV, alcohol and cigarette smoking act as co-factors for the development of HCC in these patients. In about 7.6% of cirrhosis due to genetic hemochromatosis, iron-free nodules were described[37] and the follow-up showed a higher incidence of HCC in patients with iron-free nodules. Moreover hepatocellular dysplasia was generally noted in these nodules and proliferative cell nuclear antigen staining was greater in iron-free nodules. It has been hypothesized that the hepatocytes of these nodules represent a group of younger clonal cells; other observations seem to further support the hypothesis of clonality of HCC[38]. This hypothesis is not inconsistent with the multicentric genesis of HCC as the same carcinogenetic events could occur in different areas of the same liver.

INCIDENCE OF HCC IN LIVER CIRRHOSIS

Data regarding the evolution of HCC emerge from prospective and retrospective studies of cirrhotic populations. Colombo *et al* found a 3% incidence of HCC/year[39] and the risk of developing HCC was higher in patients with persistently high levels of AFP regardless of the etiology and severity of cirrhosis. Patients older than 60 years were also at higher risk than patients under 40. In another prospective study of cirrhotic patients[35] on the cumulative incidence of HCC, the rate was 19.4% after 5 years, 44.3% after 10 years and 58.2% after 15 years, with higher risk in anti-HCV than in HBsAg positive patients. A possible explanation for the lower incidence of HCC in HBV infected patients could be the reduction of necrosis and inflammation after the HBeAg/HBeAb seroconversion or the higher mortality rate for liver disease before the development of HCC.

Tsukuma *et al*[40] found a cumulative risk of developing HCC after 3 years of 12.5% in cirrhosis and of 3.8% in chronic active hepatitis; the severity of the liver disease represented an independent risk factor. Furthermore alcohol and cigarette smoking were related with an higher risk only in cirrhotic and not in chronic hepatitis patients.

Our screening program for the early detection of liver lesions and the evaluation of risk factors was based on a group of 324 cirrhotic patients: each patient was submitted to a liver ultrasonographic examination, AFP and liver biochemical tests every 6 months. After a mean follow-up of 33 months we found an overall incidence of HCC of 11.7% (38 cases: unifocal at ultrasonography in 31 cases) with an incidence of 4.3% per year of follow-up. The multivariate analysis with Cox proportional hazard model identified AFP, Child-Pugh classes B and C and male sex as independent risk factors for developing HCC. Among the 38 HCC detected during the follow-up only 22 (58%) were treated by surgery, OLT or local therapy and in only 9 (23%) was the treatment successful (stable disease after 12 months). These results show that at present extensive survey programs for cirrhotic patients do not have a great clinical efficacy and their cost-effectiveness will be improved only when better risk factors are identified or other more efficacious treatments are available.

GROWTH PATTERN AND CLINICAL PRESENTATION

Studies regarding the growth rate of HCC appeared in the literature at the beginning of the 80's[41] mainly due to the use of ultrasonography as an imaging technique for the early detection and diagnosis of HCC. Further studies demonstrated that the growth rate of HCC, evaluated as tumor volume doubling time, differs greatly, ranging from 1 to 19 months with a median of 6 months.[42-46] This wide growth rate variability is detectable among and within patients:[46,47] some HCC show no growth or very slow growth at the beginning, whereas others grow quickly at first and then enter a steady period or a slower growth

Table 6.1 – Frequency of symptoms at the time of HCC detection in 439 HCC cirrhotic patients.

General malaise	54%
Anorexia	48%
Abdominal pain	45%
Weight loss	37%
Abdominal mass	18%
Ascites	18%
Fever	15%
Jaundice	8%
Nausea/vomiting	7%
Gastrointestinal bleeding	4%

period, while others show a constant growth rate. This finding has important implications: firstly it contributes to the heterogeneity of clinical presentation of the tumor. In the past, when a tumor was discovered in advanced stages, symptoms were directly related to the size of the tumor, like abdominal pain, sensation of abdominal fullness and palpable mass in the abdomen, or to the decompensation of cirrhosis (jaundice and ascites). At present, the diagnosis of HCC is often made when the tumor is still asymptomatic: nevertheless anorexia, general malaise and fever could be the first clinical signs (Table 6.1). It must be outlined, however, that clinical signs in patients affected by HCC overlap with those of the underlying liver cirrhosis. The different growth rates justify the detection of relatively advanced HCCs also in patients submitted to strict sonographic follow-up.

The spontaneous rupture of HCC into the peritoneal cavity may occur, but represents a rare complication that seems to be more frequent in African and Oriental patients than in Caucasians. It occurs suddenly and abdominal pain, anemia, shock and hemoperitomeum are the usual findings: superficial, large and hypervascularized nodules are at higher risk of spontaneous rupture and this may also be the consequence of a guided puncture.

Apart from the growth rate, different growth patterns have been described: the replacing growth pattern is characterized by a replacement of tumoral cells along the liver cell cords while in the sinusoidal type the tumor cells grow in an infiltrating fashion. Geographic variability in growth pattern was described: the infiltrative pattern is more common in South African patients while the other modality prevails in

Oriental, French and Italian populations. The growth pattern also influences the incidence of extrahepatic metastasis, as demonstrated by the higher incidence of metastasis in infiltrating HCC;[48] hematogenic metastasis to lungs, bone and adrenal glands are generally the most common. The invasion of hepatic vessels by tumor cells, as well as the extracapsular microscopic invasion of surrounding liver tissue, are related to tumor size: larger HCC generally show some kind of invasion and, as a consequence, 61% of patients with a 3-5 cm HCC had multiple tumors.[49] Tumor size is also related to histologic features: nodules larger than 3 cm in diameter usually consist of moderately, or poorly-differentiated HCC, while small HCC (less than 2 cm) are generally well differentiated.[50] The presence of single or multiple nodules and their location obviously influence the decision to treat and the results of therapy. Furthermore multiple nodules can be related both to an intrahepatic spread of a single HCC or more probably to a multifocal origin of the tumor. The need for correct staging has become mandatory particularly since a recent study showed that sonography and computed tomography were not sensitive enough to diagnose all HCC nodules in the same liver.[39]

SURVIVAL

As previously reported HCC is generally associated with chronic liver disease and therefore any prognostic consideration is influenced by the severity of the underlying liver disease. In the past, due to the impossibility of an early diagnosis, the life expectancy for HCC patients was very low: the tumor was generally discovered in an advanced stage and in the presence of advanced cirrhosis.

Several studies analyzed the prognostic significance for survival of a wide number of characteristics: age, laboratory findings, tumor size, histologic features, surgical factors, presence of metastasis, alcohol intake etc.[44-46, 50-58] Clinical features were closely analyzed (Table 6.2): Okuda *et al*[45] in a retrospective analysis, staging patients on the basis of tumor size, ascites, serum bilirubin and serum albumin, found that the median survival of HCC patients in stage III (severe disease) was 0.7 months while in stage I it was 8.3 months. Calvet *et al*[55] proposed a prognostic index

Table 6.2 – Clinical prognostic factors in HCC cirrhotic patients

Clinical prognostic factors
Male sex[46,51,52]
Older age[51,53,55]
Increased bilirubin[45,53-55]
Disease symptoms[51]
Encephalopathy[54]
Ascites[45,46,55]
Serum albumin[45]
Tumor size[45,46,55]
Alcohol intake[46]
g-GT[46,55]
Prothrombin time[46]
HBsAg[46]
Child-Pugh class[46]
Blood urea nitrogen[55]
Serum sodium[55]
Tumor metastasis[55]

based on clinical and laboratory findings for the stratification of HCC patients. A more recent paper[46] found a cumulative estimated survival rate comparable with that of other authors,[43,44] but a longer 3-year survival probability resulted when only the Child-Pugh A class of patient was considered. Furthermore the statistical differences among survival rate in the three Child-Pugh classes were significant, thus emphasizing the critical prognostic role of liver functional impairment. This observation, in part, further confirms the previous findings[45, 55]. The bulk of information regarding the survival predictors can also be applied to the differentiation of HCC patients into groups characterized by a similar life expectancy. This stratification could be of particular interest when the efficacy of different treatment modalities is compared: a recent paper demonstrates the efficacy of surgical resection and percutaneous ethanol injection in improving survival of HCC patients with single, small HCC (≤ 5cm in diameter) stratified according to the Child-Pugh classes.[59] This study comprised 116 untreated patients, 73 of Child-Pugh class A and 43 of class B, with 1, 2, 3, 5 year survival rates of 86, 51, 26, 11% and 65, 22, 13, 0% respectively; of the 73 Child-Pugh class A patients 43 were deemed potentially operable and the survival rates in this group were 89, 51, and 30% at 1, 2 and 3 years, respectively.

REFERENCES

1. Manderson WG, Patrick RS, Peters EE. Incidence of primary carcinoma of the liver in the west of Scotland between 1949 and 1965. *Gut* 1968; **9**: 480-484
2. Bartoloni ST, Omer F, Giannini A, Napoli P. Hepatocellular carcinoma and cirrhosis: a review of their relative incidence in a 25-year period in the Florence area. *Hepatogastroenterology* 1984; **31**: 215-217
3. Okuda K, Fujimoto I, Hanai A, Urano Y. Changing incidence of hepatocellular carcinoma in Japan. *Cancer Res* 1987; **47**: 4967-4972
4. Sakamoto M, Hirohashi S, Shimosato Y. Early stages of multistep hepatocarcinogenesis: adenomatous hyperplasia and early hepatocellular carcinoma. *Hum Pathol* 1991; **22**: 172-178
5. International Working Party. Terminology of nodular hepatocellular lesions. *Hepatology* 1995; **22**: 983-993
6. Takayama T, Makuuchi M, Hirohashi S, Sakamoto M, Okazaki N, Takayasu K, Kosuge T, Motoo Y, Yamazaki S, Hasegawa H. Malignant transformation of adenomatous hyperplasia to hepatocellular carcinoma. *Lancet* 1990; **336**: 1150-1153
7. Arakawa M, Kage M, Sugihara S, Nakashima T, Suenaga M, Okuda K. Emergence of malignant lesions within an adenomatous hyperplastic nodule in a cirrhotic liver. Observation in five cases. *Gastroenterology* 1986; **91**: 198-208
8. Wada K, Kondo F, Kondo Y. Large regenerative nodules and dysplastic nodules in cirrhotic livers: a histopathologic study. *Hepatology* 1988; **8**: 1684-1688
9. Bolondi L, Gramantieri G, Chieco P, Melchiorri C, Trere D, Stecca B, Derenzini M, *et al.* Enzymatic cytochemistry, DNA ploidy and AgNOR quantitation in hepatocellular nodules of uncertain malignant potential in liver cirrhosis. *Dig Dis Science*, 1996; **41**: 800-808
10. Tarao K, Shimizu A, Harada M, Kuni Y, Ito Y, Tamai S, Iimori K, *et al.* Difference in the in vitro uptake of bromodeoxyuridine between liver cirrhosis with and without hepatocellular carcinoma. *Cancer* 1989; **64**: 104-109
11. Tarao K, Shimizu A, Ohkawa S, Harada M, Ito Y, Tamai S, Kuni Y, *et al.* Development of hepatocellular carcinoma associated with increase in DNA synthesis in the surrounding cirrhosis. *Gastroenterology* 1992; **103**: 595-600
12. Derenzini M, Treré D, Oliveri F, David E, Colombatto P, Bonino F, Brunetto MR. Is high AgNOR quantity in hepatocytes associated with increased risk of hepatocellular carcinoma in cirrhotic liver disease? *J Clin Pathol* 1993;**46**: 727-729
13. Szmuness W. Hepatocellular carcinoma and the hepatitis B virus: evidence for a causal association. *Prog Med Virol* 1978; **24**: 40-69
14. Beasley RP, Hwang L-Y, Lin C-C, Chien C-S. Hepatocelluar carcinoma and hepatitis B virus - a prospective study of 22,707 men in Taiwan. *Lancet* 1981; **2**: 1129-1133
15. Hohne M, Schafer S, Seifer M, Feitelson MA, Paul D, Gerlich WH. Malignant transformation of immortalized transgenic hepatocytes after transfection with hepatitis B virus DNA. *EMBO J* 1990; **9**: 1137-1145
16. Brechot C, Pourcel C, Louise A, Rain B, Tiollais P. Presence of integrated hepatitis B virus DNA sequences in cellular DNA of human hepatocellular carcinoma. *Nature* 1980; **286**: 533-535
17. Shafrits DA, Shouval D, Sherman M. Integration of hepatitis B DNA into the genome of liver cells in chronic liver disease and hepatocellular carcinoma. *N Engl J Med* 1981; **305**: 1067-1073
18. Kam W, Rall LB, Smuckler EA, Schmid R, Rutter WJ. Hepatitis B viral DNA in liver and serum of asymptomatic carriers. *Proc Natl Acad Sci USA* 1982; **79**: 7522-7526
19. Tokino T, Fukushige S, Nakamura T, *et al.* Chromosomal translocation and inverted duplication associated with integrated hepatitis B virus in hepatocellular carcinomas. *J Virol* 1987; **61**: 3848-3854;
20. Zhou Y-Z, Slagle BL, Donehower LA, *et al.* Structural analysis of a hepatitis B virus genome integrated into chromosome 17p of a human hepatocellular carcinoma. *J Virol* 1988; **62**: 4224-4231
21. Meyer M, Wiedorn KH, Hofschneider PH, *et al.* A chromosome 17:7 translocation is associated with a hepatitis B virus DNA integration in human hepatocellular carcinoma. *Hepatology* 1992; **15**: 665-671
22. Two JS, Schloemer RH. Transcriptional trans-activating function of hepatitis B virus. *J Virol* 1987; **61**: 3448-3453
23. Kekule AS, Lauer U, Meyer M, *et al.* The pre2/s region of integrated hepatitis B virus DNA encodes a transcriptional transactivator. *Nature* 1990; **343**: 457-461
24. Summers J, Manson WS. Replication of the genome of a hepatitis B-like virus by reverse transcription of a RNA intermediate. *Cell* 1982; **29**: 403-415
25. Nishida N, Fukuda Y, Kokuryu H, *et al.* Accumulation of allelic loss on arms of chromosomes 16q and 17 p in the advanced stages of human hepatocellular carcinoma. *Cancer Res* 1992; **52**: 6358-6364
26. Nose H, Imazeki F, Ohto M, Omata M. p53 gene mutations and 17p allelic deletions in hepatocellular carcinoma from Japan. *Cancer* 1993; **72**: 355-360
27. Bressac B, Galvin KM, Liang TJ, *et al.* Abnormal structure and expression of p53 gene in human hepatocellular carcinoma. *Proc Natl Acad Sci* USA 1990; **87**: 1973-1977
28. Scorsone K, Zhou Y, Butel J, Slage BL. p53 mutations cluster at codon 249 in hepatits B virus-positive hepatocellular carcinomas from China. *Cancer Res* 1992; **52**: 1635-1638
29. Osturk M. p53 mutation in hepatocellular carcinoma after aflatoxin exposure. *Lancet* 1991; **338**: 1356-1359
30. Yeh F-S, Yu MC, Mo C-C, *et al.* Hepatitis B virus, aflatoxins, and hepatocellular carcinoma in Southern Guanxi, China. *Cancer Res* 1989; **49**: 2506-2509
31. Bruix J, Barrera JM, Calvet X, *et al.* Prevalence of antibodies to hepatitis C virus in Spanish patients with hepatocellular carcinoma and hepatic cirrhosis. *Lancet* 1989; **ii**: 1004-1006
32. Colombo M, Kuo G, Choo QL, *et al.* Prevalence of antibodies to hepatitis C virus in Italian patients with hepatocellular carcinoma. *Lancet* 1989; **ii**: 1006-1008
33. Kiyosawa K, Sodeyama T, Tanaka E, Gibo Y, Yoshizawa K, Nakano Y, Furuta S, Akhane Y, Nishioka K, Purcell RH, Alter HJ. Interrelationship of blood transfusion, non-A, non-B hepatitis and hepatocellular carcinoma: analysis by detection of antibody to hepatitis C virus. *Hepatology* 1990; **12**: 671-675
34. Farinati F, Fagiuoli S, De Maria N, Chiaramonte N, Aneloni V, Ongaro S, Salvagnini M, Naccarato R. Anti-HCV positive hepatocellular carcinoma in cirrhosis. Prevalence, risk factors and clinical features. *J Hepatol* 1992; **14**: 183-187

35. Ikeda K, Saitoh S, Koida I, Arase Y, Tsubota , Chayama K, Kumada H, Kawanihi M. A multivariate analysis of risk factors for hepatocellular carcinogenesis: a prospective observation of 795 patients with viral and alcoholic cirrhosis. *Hepatology* 1993; **18**: 47-53

36. Chisari FV, Klopchin K, Moriyama T, *et al.* Molecular pathogenesis of hepatocellular carcinoma in hepatitis B virus transgenic mice. *Cell* 1989; **59**: 1145-1156

37. Deugnier YM, Guyader D, Crantock L, *et al.* Primary liver cancer in genetic hemochromatosis: a clinical, pathological and pathogenetic study of 54 cases. *Gastroenterology* 1993; **104**: 228-234

38. Hsu H, Chiou T, Chen J, *et al.* Clonality and clonal evolution of hepatocellular carcinoma with multiple nodules. *Hepatology* 1991; **13**: 923-928

39. Colombo M, De Franchis R, Del Ninno E, *et al.* Hepatocellular carcinoma in Italian patients with cirrhosis. *N Engl J Med* 1991; **325**: 675-680

40. Tsukuma H, Hiyama T, Tanaka S, Nakao M, Yabuuchi T, Kitamura T, Nakanishi K, Fujimoto I, Inoue A, Yamazaki H, Kawashima T. Risk factors for hepatocellular carcinoma among patients with chronic liver disease. *N Engl J Med* 1993; **328**: 1797-1801

41. Chen DS, Sheu JC, Sung JL, Lay MY, Lee CS, Su CT, Tsang YM, *et al.* Small hepatocellular carcinoma. A clinicopathological study in thirteen patients. *Gastroenterology* 1982; **83**: 1109-1119

42. Okazaki N, Yoshino M, Yoshida T, Suzuki M, Moriyama N, Takayasu K, Makuuchi M, *et al.* Evaluation of the prognosis for small hepatocellular carcinoma based on tumor volume doubling time. *Cancer* 1989; **63**: 2207-2210

43. Ebara M, Ohto M, Shinagawa T, Sugiura N, Kimura K, Matsutani S, Morita M, *et al.* Natural history of minute hepatocellular carcinoma smaller than 3 centimeters complicating cirrhosis. *Gastroenterology* 1986; **90**: 289-298

44. Cottone M, Virdone R, Fusco G, Orlando A, Turri M, Caltagirone M, Maringhini A, *et al.* Asymptomatic hepatocellular carcinoma in Child's A cirrhosis. *Gastroenterology* 1989; **96**: 1566-1571

45. Okuda K, Ohtsuky T, Obata H, Tomimatsu M, Okazaky N, Hasegawa H, Nakajima Y, *et al.* Natural history of hepatocellular carcinoma and prognosis in relation to treatment. Study of 850 patients. *Cancer* 1985; **56**: 918-928

46. Barbara L, Benzi G, Gaiani S, Fusconi F, Zironi G, Siringo S, Rigamonti A, *et al.* Natural history of small untreated hepatocellular carcinoma in cirrhosis: a multivariate analysis of prognostic factors of tumor growth rate and patient survival. *Hepatology* 1992; **16**: 132-137

47. Sheu JC, Sung JL, Chen DS, Yang PM, Lai MY, Lee CS, Hsu HC, *et al.* Growth rate of asymptomatic hepatocellular carcinoma and its clinical implications. *Gastroenterology* 1985; **89**: 259-266

48. Kojiro M. Pathomorphology of advanced hepatocellular carcinoma. In: Tobe T, Kaneda H, Okudaira M, Ohto M, Endo Y, Mito M, Okamoto E, Tarika K, Koijro M (eds) *Primary liver cancer in Japan*. Springer-Verlag Tokyo, 1992; 31-37

49. Ohto M, Kondo F, Ebara M. Pathology, diagnosis, and treatment for small liver cancer. In: Tobe T, Kaneda H, Okudaira M, Ohto M, Endo Y, Mito M, Okamoto E, Tarika K, Koijro M (eds) *Primary liver cancer in Japan*. Springer-Verlag Tokyo, 1992; 365-373

50. Oka H, Kurioka N, Kim K, Kanno T, Kuroky T, Mizoguchi Y, Kobayashi K. Prospective study of early detection of hepatocellular carcinoma in patients with liver cirrhosis. *Hepatology* 1990; **12**: 680-687

51. Falkson G, Cnaan A, Schutt AJ, Ryan LM, Falkson CH. Prognostic factors for survival in hepatocellular carcinoma. *Cancer Res* 1988; **48**: 7314-7318

52. Sutton FM, Russell NC, Guinee VF, Alpert E. Factors affecting the prognosis of primary liver carcinoma. *J Clin Oncol* 1988; **6**: 321-328

53. Clebowski R, Tong M, Weissman J, Block JB, Ramming KP, Weiner JM, Bateman JR, *et al.* Hepatocellular carcinoma - Diagnostic and prognostic features in North American patients. *Cancer* 1984; **53**: 2701-2706

54. Attali P, Prod'Homme S, Pelletier G, Papoz L, Ink O, Bufet C, Etienne JP. Prognostic factors in patients with hepatocellular carcinoma. Attempts for selection of patients with prolonged survival. *Cancer* 1987; **45**: 2108-2111

55. Calvet X, Bruix J, Gines P, Bru C, Vilana R, Rodes J. Prognostic factors of hepatocellular carcinoma in the West. A multivariate analysis in 206 patients. *Hepatology* 1990; **12**: 753-760

56. Lai CL, Wu PC, Lam KC, Todd D. Histologic prognostic indicators in hepatocellular carcinoma. *Cancer* 1979; **44**: 1677-1683

57. Lee CS, Hwang LY, Beasley RP, Hsu HC, Lee HS, Lin TY. Prognostic significance of histologic findings in resected small hepatocellular carcinoma. Acta Chir Scand 1988; **154**: 199-203

58. Hsu HC, Wu TT, Wu MZ, Sheu JC, Lee CS, Chen DS. Tumor invasiveness and prognosis in resected hepatocellular carcinoma. *Cancer* 1988; **61**: 2095-2099

59. Livraghi T, Bolondi L, Buscarini L, Cottone M, Mazziotti A, Morabito A, Torzilli G, *et al.* No treatment, resection and ethanol injection in hepatocellular carcinoma: a retrospective analysis of survival in 391 patients with cirrhosis. *J Hepatol* 1995; **22**: 522-526

7

Early detection and serum markers

M Cottone and A D'Antoni

PROCEDURES FOR EARLY DIAGNOSIS

Before the introduction of ultrasound (US) in the follow-up of cirrhosis, α-fetoprotein (AFP) was considered the only marker useful for the early diagnosis of HCC. However, because of the low sensitivity of AFP most cases of HCC were diagnosed only when symptomatic. US has been a big step forward in the early diagnosis of HCC and it is now adopted as a screening tool worldwide. Despite the major role of US, AFP and other markers (fucosydase AFP, des-gamma-carboxy prothrombin, serum α-L-fucosidase) continue to be used as screening tools in clinical practice. Their use is complementary to US and has limited indications which will be discussed.

α-FETOPROTEIN

AFP is a serum protein normally synthesized by fetal liver cells, by yolk-sac cells and in trace amounts by the fetal gastrointestinal tract. Its production is increased in pregnant women in the second and third trimesters and in fetal and neonatal life, while it declines gradually after birth. The simple standard approach for the detection of AFP is usually a radio-immunoassay technique.[1]

The increase in serum AFP is not specific to HCC because it can be seen in a variety of non malignant conditions such as chronic hepatitis, fulminant hepatic failure or cirrhosis.[1-3] These conditions are all characterized by hepatic necrosis and/or inflammation of the hepatic parenchyma. So the increase may reflect selective transcriptional activation of the AFP gene which is induced by the hepatic damage *per se* rather than by simple regeneration as may be seen after hepatic resection.[4] In most patients with a non malignant cause of AFP elevation, the elevation is mild and transient: however 26% of the elevations exceed 200 ng/ml and 9% persist for a long time.

The degree of tumor differentiation and tumor size appears to be important in determining the level of AFP produced. Most well differentiated HCCs are smaller than 2 cm, hence AFP levels in these tumors are often normal[4] and the sensitivity of the test is blunted. Nonetheless it appears that the major determinant of AFP levels is the degree of tumor differentiation,[1] which explains why a certain percentage of

Table 7.1 – Characteristics of AFP in five screening studies

Author (reference)	Sensitivity (%)	Specificity (%)	PPV
Colombo[14] (a)	79	NR	NR
Cottone[15] (b)	30	89	43
Oka[16] (c)	39	76	32
Pateron[17] (d)	50	86	33
Imberti[18] (e)	39	NR	NR

PPV = Predictive Positive Value; cut off values used:
(a) 20-400 ng/ml (either fluctuating or persistent values);
(b) > 50-400 ng/ml;
(c) < 20 ng/ml;
(d) 15 ng/ml;
(e) 20-200 ng/ml
NR = Not reported

small HCCs are AFP positive in spite of their small dimension. A relationship between AFP levels and HBsAg positivity has been observed in some studies[6] though this is not supported by other workers:[7,8]the reason for this correlation is unclear.

The level of AFP which has been considered specific to HCC is above 400 ng/ml: if this value is chosen the sensitivity of AFP, in asymptomatic HCC as compared to US, varies from 0 to 20 %. In fact levels of AFP are frequently normal (below 20 ng/ml), particularly in the case of small HCC and they often rise above normal levels when lesions become larger and are sometimes unresectable. For small HCCs (<3 cm) the sensitivity at two cut-off levels of 20 ng/ml and 200 ng/ml are low, varying from 33% to 65% and from 9.1% to 26% respectively.[9-13] In five screening studies cirrhotic patients were monitored to evaluate the development of HCC using different cut-off levels: specificity was high ranging from 76% to 89%, while sensitivity ranged from 30 to 79 %[14-18] (Table 7.1). Therefore in these studies the levels of AFP above 20-50 ng/ml were predictive of the development of HCC. So it is generally agreed that patients with initial, persistent AFP levels of >20 ng/ml should be followed up carefully and monitored with US every 3 months.

The role of AFP in screening programs is far from clear, so that at present it cannot be recommended as the sole screening tool, taking into account also the cost effectiveness of this test. Therefore more useful and reliable tumor markers should be sought in order to detect HCCs at an early, treatable stage. At present the role of AFP is limited to: a) the identification of patients with higher risk of developing HCC from values between 20 ng/ml and 400 ng/ml; and b) the diagnosis of HCC from values above 400 ng/ml.

FUCOSYLATED AFP

Human AFP exhibits associated sugar chain heterogeneity and new methods for quantitative AFP measurement using lectin-affinity electrophoresis have been developed. A study in 1981 described the lectin-dependent fractionation of AFP using chromatography and electrophoresis.[19] Several investigators have since shown that HCC is associated with an increased specific proportion of AFP L3 and AFP P4+P5 when analyzed with Lens Culinaris agglutinin A (LCA-A) and with erythroagglutinating phytohemagglutinin (E-PHA).[20] In 1988 Aoyagy *et al.*[21] utilized the fucosylation index (the percentage of lectin-reactive species of AFP in total AFP) to differentiate benign liver disease from HCC. They found that sensitivity was 69%, and specificity 96%. These figures were affected by a minimum AFP level (which was above 100 ng/ml) needed to perform an analysis of fucosylation and by the fact that the lesions were larger than 2 cm.

A modest improvement, at a cut-off level of 15-18%, in sensitivity and specificity (73% and 100% respectively) was obtained by Sato *et al.*,[22] who modified this technique by coupling lectin-affinity electrophoresis with antibody-affinity blotting which enabled them to achieve test performance at an AFP level of over 30 ng/ml.

A recent study[23] found a sensitivity of 61% and specificity of 90%, using a cut-off level of 15%. In this study a correlation with tumor size was observed and the sensitivity for lesions less than 2 cm in diameter was 48%. An interesting finding was that in 41% of patients the positive lectin reactive AFP was present up to 10 months before the HCC was detected by other diagnostic techniques.

Because of the low sensitivity of fucosylated-AFP for the diagnosis of small HCCs and its high cost, this marker is not easily adaptable to mass screening. Recently Concanavalin A affinity electrophoresis of serum AFP by antibody-affinity electrophoresis and Western blotting has been shown to discriminate HCC from benign chronic liver disease.[24] It is easy, cheap and seems more sensitive and specific than LCA-A and E-PHA methods for detecting HCC. The sensitivity of this marker for small HCC is not very high (48%) so its role in screening programs must be evaluated.

DES-GAMMA-CARBOXY PROTHROMBIN (DCP)

DCP is an abnormal prothrombin which cannot interact with other coagulation enzymes. The enzyme cannot bind calcium ions because of a deficiency in gamma-carboxy glutamic acid content. The mechanism of its production in primary HCC is unclear but it is attributed to synthesis by the tumor itself, resulting from an acquired defect in the vitamin K dependent carboxylase system of the malignant hepatocytes.[25] DCP levels in the plasma may be measured using either the enzyme immunoassay method (ELISA) to determine DCP antigen levels or the staphilocoagulase method (SC) to assay the DCP activities.

In 1984 Liebman *et al.*[26] first reported that 67% of patients with HCC had abnormally high levels of DCP (at levels above 300 ng/ml). Plasma DCP does not correlate with AFP levels as was shown from comparisons between the two assays;[17,25] combined use of DCP and AFP raises sensitivity values but this is not true for small HCC. DCP has been used in combination with AFP measurements as a marker of response to therapy; it seems that the serum DCP concentration normalizes after surgical treatment or transcatheter embolization while it increases with the recurrence of the disease.[27] In Table 7.2 the main clinical studies of DCP in HCC are summarized.[26-36] These studies show a sensitivity varying between 35% and 91%, but differences in the assay methods used to measure DCP must be considered. Sensitivity for small HCC (<3 cm) ranged between 19% and 48%.

More recently Saitoh *et al.*[37] have proposed a quantitative assay of serum DCP concentration in patients with HCC smaller than 20 mm in maximum diameter using an Avidin Biotin Complex (ABC) method to increase the sensitivity. They reported a sensitivity of 39%, a specificity of 89% and a predictive

Table 7.2 – Clinical studies of DCP in HCC

Author (reference)	Assay	Total number of HCCs	DCP-positive (%)	DCP-positive (%) in HCC <3 cm
Liebman[26]	RIA	76	69 (91)	NR
Soulier[27]	SC	70	51 (74)	NR
Soulier[28]	SC	75	53 (71)	NR
Okuda[30]	EIA	52	30 (58)	6/24 (25)
Fujiyama[29]	EIA-C	120	76 (64)	0/12 (0)
Tanabe[31]	EIA	31	11 (35)	0/5 (0)
Deyashiki[32]	EIA-C	70	54 (77)	NR
Ono[36]	EIA-C	29	16 (55)	NR
Tsai[33]	EIA-C	107	59 (55)	4/21 (19)
	SC		69 (63) ⋆	10/21 (48)
Nakao[34]	EIA-C	91	42 (46)	3/9 (33)
Nakao[35]	EIA-C	39	37 (95)	NR
Total		*750*	*498 (66)*	*23/71 (32)*

NR = not reported; RIA = polyclonal anti-DCP RIA; SC = Staphylococcus coagulase activity assay; EIA = monoclonal antibody competitive ELISA; EIA-C = antigen capture, monoclonal ELISA.
⋆ Not calculated in total sum Modified from Weitz & Liebman[25]

positive value of 61.6%. Nevertheless it still remains a test that is not sensitive enough to be proposed for early diagnosis or the screening of small HCC.

SERUM α-L-FUCOSIDASE

This marker is a lysosomal enzyme present in all mammalian cells and is involved in the catabolism of fucose-containing glycoconjugates. It has been recently proposed as a useful marker in the diagnosis of HCC. Giardina *et al.*[38] reported a sensitivity of 76% and specificity of 90.9% when 443 nmol/ml/h was taken as the cut-off value and they described this test as complementary to AFP and US. However, their study does not report the size and the stage of the 21 HCCs evaluated with this marker: therefore it is difficult to infer its role as a screening marker.

In conclusion all the above mentioned serum markers have failed so far as screening tools in asymptomatic patients with cirrhosis. They have a minor role in comparison with US and may be used for research purposes.

ULTRASONOGRAPHY

US fits quite well the description of a screening technique. It is cheap, widely accessible, easy and quick to perform, safe, sensitive and reproducible. US equipment has a limited cost and is widely used, as today virtually every hospital has its own instrument. The cost of a single examination is quite modest, so it can be serially repeated at an acceptable cost per year, and in the hands of experienced examiners the hepatobiliary system may be thoroughly studied.

Sonographic characteristics of hepatic nodular lesions

For screening purposes it is important to detect small lesions because they are potentially treatable (by surgery, PEI and OLT). Small hepatic lesions are defined in the most recent literature as nodules of less than 3 cm in diameter.[39] In an attempt to standardize the terminology applied to nodular hepatic lesions, at the World Congress of Gastroenterology 1994 an International Working Party suggested a new terminology and definitions of all mass lesions of the liver.[40,41] They have been histologically classified as regenerative lesions and dysplastic or neoplastic lesions. In practical terms a distinction can be made between benign, precancerous and malignant lesions (see Table 7.3). In cirrhotic patients differential diagnosis is usually restricted to regenerative nodules, adenomatous hyperplasia and small HCC.

Ultrasonographic features common to all nodular

Table 7.3 – Ultrasonographic characteristics of small hepatic nodules

Benign	Regenerative nodules	Hypo- or isoechoic
Precancerous	Adenomatous hyperplasia	Hypo- or hyperechoic
Malignant	Small HCC	Hypo-, iso- or hyperechoic

lesions are: a hypoechoic or isoechoic pattern, a round or oval shape and well defined margins with respect to the surrounding parenchyma. Less frequently small lesions can be hyperechoic. Differential diagnosis is not always possible on ultrasonographic grounds. In fact regenerative nodules can be either hypo- or isoechoic; adenomatous hyperplasia shows a hypo- or hyperechoic pattern, while small HCC may be hypo-, iso- or hyperechoic (see Table 7.3). Nevertheless there are some features which can help in differentiating between lesions:

Regenerative nodules: They are usually 0.3-1.0 cm in diameter.[42] Their presence is frequently suggested by nodularity of the hepatic contour. The multiple closely spaced nodules and their thin connective tissue borders produce a cobblestone appearence and are recognized because of their thin, slightly more echogenic borders, which correspond pathologically to fibrous and fatty connective tissue surrounding and separating the nodules.[43]

Adenomatous hyperplasia shows a hypoechoic pattern with features similar to those of regenerating nodules and HCC; they lack peculiar ultrasonographic characteristics which may help in establishing a diagnosis.

Small HCC: this tumor is most commonly hypo- (77%) or isoechoic (6.4%), but may be hyperechoic (16.1%); the presence of a thin, peripheral hypoechoic halo is seen most often in small HCCs.[44] This halo, which corresponds to a fibrous capsule in resected specimens, is a characteristic finding in small HCCs[45] and can be found in 88% of hypo- or hyperechoic small HCCs.[46] It has been reported as being quite specific (86%).

Recently Kitamura *et al*[47] observed that the small diffuse hypoechoic pattern is associated with a higher risk of hepatocellular carcinoma (14.0 relative risk). They found that this type of pattern was present in 50% of patients with cirrhosis but this observation needs be confirmed by other studies.

Useful clues to differential diagnosis can be obtained with color Doppler ultrasonography. HCCs are most often hypervascular with an arterial flow; they are more commonly deficient in portal or hepatic vein supply and show an enhanced arterial vasculature. Several characteristic patterns are recognized:[48] a basket pattern is the most usual one (75%); but other patterns described are a spot pattern, a detouring pattern and a single arterial vessel in tumor. The reported sensitivity for the presence of a pulsatile arterial flow is 53-76%, with a specificity of 69-100%.[49]

It is important to underline that the gold standard for the evaluation of accuracy in techniques for diagnosis of HCC is the histologic examination of explanted liver. So far most of the studies on accuracy of US have been carried out without this gold standard and therefore are biased. Nevertheless prospective studies of surveillance by US and AFP, despite the fact that sensitivity was calculated with respect to lesions detected by other means, are a useful source of information because of the long follow-up. In these studies the sensitivity of US for the diagnosis of small HCC ranged from 78% to 100%,[14-18] and specificity was high (93-100%).

Dodd *et al.*[50] prospectively interpreted 200 preoperative sonograms from 200 patients with cirrhosis who underwent hepatic transplantation. These were cor-related with specimens of freshly resected whole livers. Pathologic examination showed 80 malignant lesions in 34 patients (28 with HCC). US correctly showed 36 of the 80 malignant lesions, with a lesion sensitivity of 45% and a specificity of 98%. Of the 44 missed lesions 24 were 1 cm or less, 12 were between 1 and 3 cm, and 8 were more than 3 cm in diameter. These data show that sensitivity is dependent upon the size of lesions (74% of the missed lesions were less than 3 cm in diameter). Others factors which can determine the low sensitivity of US are: the lesion can lie in a site difficult to visualize, intra-observer variability, the coarse appearence of the liver parenchyma, the isoechogenicity of small lesions with respect to surrounding parenchyma, and the inability of the patient to collaborate in the examination.

Although imaging techniques like US and CT allow an high resolution of hepatic focal lesions, none can yield an accurate diagnosis of the nature of the lesion. Differentiation between benign and malignant lesions is mandatory; therefore US-guided biopsy is necessary if a final diagnosis is to be obtained. Ultrasound-guided fine needle biopsy (FNB) is an accurate diagnostic invasive tool for hepatic tumors with a sensitivity ranging in different series between 80% and 95%, a specificity of 100% and an accuracy of 90.1%.[51]

SCREENING

We have shown that US is highly sensitive in the early diagnosis of HCC. This technique is not invasive or very expensive and is therefore an ideal tool in the screening of HCC. The crucial point is whether screening is worthwhile. For the evaluation of a screening program the following points need to be considered: selection of population (general population? high risk population?), validity, cost acceptance. The benefits of screening are improved prognosis for some cases, less radical treatment, and reassurance for those with negative results, whereas disadvantages are cost, longer morbidity, overtreatment of borderline lesions and false positives.

SELECTION OF POPULATION

General population (mass screening): studies of this kind carried out in South Africa and China (high risk populations) using AFP as a screening tool have produced discordant results.[52-53] Whereas in South Africa no asymptomatic patient with cancer was found in a large population (9000), in China 800 HCCs (44% asymptomatic) were picked up among 1,967,511 persons screened over 5 years. This discrepancy could be due to a different behavior pattern of HCC (being more aggressive in South Africa). However despite the encouraging results obtained in China the high cost of the screening and the lack of a control population do not allow this method of screening to be considered effective.

Population at risk: Discordant results have so far been published on the risk of HBsAg carriers. Whereas in 1394 Alaskan natives infected with hepatitis B virus, Heyward *et al.* found 9 HCCs during a 26 month screening period,[54] De Franchis *et al.*, in a cohort of 92 HBsAg carriers, followed-up for 130 months, did not detect any patient with HCC.[55] This discrepancy does not support the introduction of screening programs in this group of patients. It is not clear if the condition of HCV carrier exists and therefore no prospective studies have been carried out on the risk of HCV carriers. In Japan and China a higher incidence of HCC has been shown in HBsAg and antiHCV positive chronic active hepatitis.[56-58] This high rate has not been confirmed in other countries.[14,59] Differences in clinical outcomes among different countries may explain these results and suggest that in anti-HCV and HBsAg positive chronic active hepatitis the evaluation of effectiveness of screening programs needs to be limited to high risk areas.

HCC almost always occurs in patients with cirrhosis[60-62] and the cumulative incidence is high. Therefore it is worthwhile carrying out screening studies in this class of patients. Figure 7.1 shows the cumulative incidence of cancer in carriers, chronic hepatitis and cirrhosis, calculated by the mean annual incidence reported in five studies[14-18] for cirrhosis, in three studies for chronic active hepatitis[56,58] and in two studies for HBsAg carriers.[54,55]

Studies of early detection have been performed in cirrhosis whatever the etiologic risk factor and the results show that the incidence of HCC is quite comparable in all the different risk groups. This observation suggests that the risk of cancer is related to the presence of cirrhosis *per se*: therefore no selection among patients with different risk factors should be performed in planning screening programs. Men and older patients have been shown to have higher risk of HCC[63-65] but not all studies have identified these demographic characteristics as risk factors.[58,66] Dysplasia has been shown to be associated with a higher risk of HCC: Borzio *et al*[67] observed at enrolment 75 patients with dysplasia (according to the criteria of Anthony[81]) in a cohort of 307 consecutive cirrhotic patients. These patients had a 3.8 independent relative risk of HCC in comparison to other cirrhotic patients. According to these results patients with dysplasia should be strictly monitored. However the definition of dysplasia has been disputed by other authors.[68]

In conclusion screening studies should be performed in all patients with cirrhosis regardless of risk factors. It is likely that dysplasia and an hypoechoic diffuse pattern identify patients at higher risk, who should be monitored more frequently.

VALIDITY

The basic measurement of screening benefit is its effect on the population mortality rate. A comparison of survival rates involving screening detected cases is unreliable because of lead time and length bias.[69] Lead time bias occurs when survival appears to be lengthened because the diagnosis was made earlier rather than the death delayed. Length bias refers to the tendency of screening to generate favorable outcomes by preferentially detecting slow growing indolent tumors. A longer survival of untreated HCC, detected at an early stage, has been shown in many studies.[9,70,71] In order to evaluate the effectiveness of a screening procedure a randomized trial is the correct method as it removes the necessity for considering confounders and bias. No randomized studies exist which show that patients with cirrhosis who are regularly screened survive longer than patients who are not regularly screened. Such a study seems impossible to carry out for various reasons:

a) US in patients with cirrhosis is performed for other reasons: portal hypertension, biliary problems or detection of ascites. Therefore it is impossibile to have a true control population which does not undergo US.

b) mortality from cirrhosis is high so that a large number of patients would have to be evaluated in order to show any difference in survival between screened and unscreened patients.

c) although no controlled evidence exists of the therapeutic measures, surgery, transplantation (OLT) and ethanol injection (PEI) have been introduced into clinical practice and it is unlikely that patients would accept to be randomized for a screening study. Two studies[57,72] have evaluated the difference in survival between people undergoing periodic US and AFP examination and people who are not screened. The authors showed a significantly longer survival time in patients receiving periodic examination than in those without periodic examination. However the studies are retrospective, not randomized and the criteria for selection are not reported. Despite this lack of evidence for the effectiveness of screening many studies have been performed in different parts of the world. These studies have given relevant information on the real incidence of HCC, on the best screening methods, on the survival rate of patients who receive treatment. Unfortunately, they do not prove that the screening approach is effective.

Incidence of cancer

Before the introduction of US as a screening tool in the follow-up of cirrhosis the cumulative incidence of HCC was underestimated because patients with HCC died from complications of cirrhosis before cancer could be searched for.[73] Prospective screening studies have shown that the incidence of HCC is higher than previously reported[14-17,74] All the prospective studies performed have shown only small differences in the incidence of cancer in cirrhosis. The yearly incidence seems to be 3-6% independently of

Table 7.4 – Prospective screening studies for early detection of HCC

Author	Number of patients	Mean age (years)	Follow up (months)	Cumulative incidence* (%)	Number of lesions detected	Unifocal lesions (%)	Treated patients (%)
Oka[16]	140	57	41	52	40	88	82
Colombo[14]	417	55	33	24	29	58	14
Cottone[15]	147	58	65	31	30	88	30
Pateron[17]	118	55	35	46	14	32	7
Imberti[18]	200	60	44	41	38	66	24
Mean value		*57*	*43.6*	*39*		*66*	*31*
Total	*1022*				*151*		

* calculated after 8 years by the mean annual incidence reported in the study

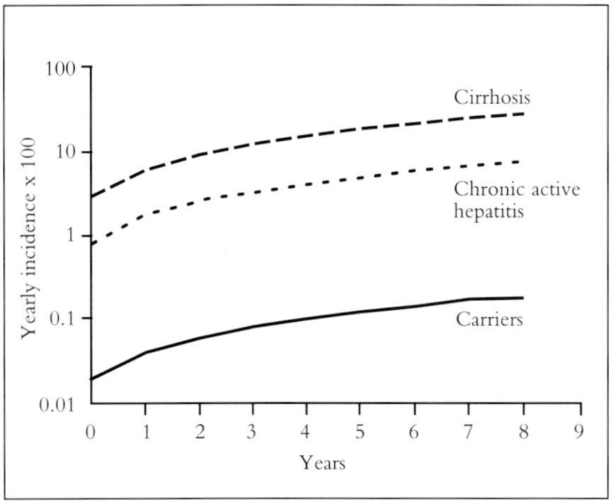

Figure 7.1 – Incidence of HCC in carriers, chronic active hepatitis and cirrhosis

risk factors. The 8 year cumulative incidence varies from 24 to 52 % in the different studies. In Table 7.4 the main prospective studies are presented. A higher incidence was observed in Japan (52%): this discrepancy may be due to the different protocol adopted (in Oka's study[16] screening was carried out by US every 3 months, whereas in Colombo's study[14] it was performed every year except on patients with an intermediate value of AFP) or to a real difference in incidence in the various geographical areas.

Screening modality

In all these studies screening was carried out using US and AFP but the time interval chosen was different (from 3 months to 1 year). The minimum interval seems to be 3 months on the basis of growth rate studies.[75] Sheu *et al.*[75] have shown that the mean doubling time of HCC is 110 days. However there is great variability in the pattern of growth. Three patterns of growth have been described worldwide:[71, 76,70]

a) tumors with a long period of no growth;

b) tumors with a declining growth rate over time;

c) tumors with an almost constant growth rate.

These differences may justify an approach tailored to the modality of growth: however no variable has been shown to be related to the pattern of growth. The presence of high AFP values has been advocated as a possible predictor: intermediate values (>20 and <400 ng/ml) have been associated with an higher risk of HCC even if a relationship between AFP level and growth rate has never been demonstrated. It is sound policy to screen patients with these values every 3 months. On the basis of the studies on growth rate and on AFP as a predictor of subsequent HCC development two methods of screening may be proposed:

a) US every 3 months without AFP

b) US and AFP every 6 months with 3-month controls in cases with AFP > 20 ng/ml, with dysplasia and with an hypoechoic diffuse nodular pattern.

Since these two modalities are almost economically equivalent, the choice may be based on practical reasons alone.

Survival rate of treated patients

In the absence of any randomized control studies on screening, indirect evidence of its effectiveness comes from the demonstration that therapy prolongs survival of patients with small HCC. Therefore the survival rate of treated patients in a screening study is an important measure if compared to a control population.

The rate of treatment was discordant in the different screening studies. It ranged from 7 % to 83% (Table 7.3). The reasons for these differences are:

1) not all modalities of treatment (PEI, transplantation, chemoembolization) were available in every center;

2) the protocol of screening adopted (US every 3 months,[16] every 6 months,[15,17,18] every year[14]);

3) the stage of the cirrhosis at which the screening is performed; patients with more advanced cirrhosis seeming to have a higher risk of HCC;[16,66]

4) the rate of unicity of lesions detected (varies from 88% to 32%); this discrepancy being due either to the protocol adopted or to the different selection of the patients;

5) geographic differences in the behavior of the HCC.

The conclusions are discordant: Colombo *et al.*[14] and Pateron *et al.*[17] state that on the basis of their experience screening is not worthwhile, whereas Oka *et al.*[16] state that screening allows the mortality for HCC to be reduced. This discordant view reflects different attitudes toward the role of treament. To date the studies on the therapy of HCC, despite the absence of randomized trials, seem to show that:

A) in Child's A cirrhotic patients with small HCC below 65 years, surgery, PEI and OLT prolong survival;[77-79]

B) in Child's B patients below 65 years only OLT may have a role;

C) above age 65 only PEI in Child's A class patients has a role in prolonging survival.[80] It has not been clearly shown that PEI has a role in prolonging survival in Child's B patients.

On the basis of these statements and because of the impossibility of carrying out randomized studies on the role of screening it is sound to propose screening studies on Child's A and B patients under 65 and on Child's A patients above 65 years.

Multicenter prospective screening studies from different geographical areas, which include cost-benefit analysis, adopting the same protocol, should be carried out in order to give an answer to the open question on what is the real incidence of unifocal lesions and consequently what is the treatment rate.

The lack of evidence that early detection translates into improved clinical outcome strengthens the concept that the primary goal in the battle against HCC should focus on the prevention of cirrhosis by vaccinating against hepatitis, by minimizing the risk of hepatitis C and by decreasing the incidence of alcoholism.

REFERENCES

1. Taketa K. α-Fetoprotein: reevaluation in hepatology. *Hepatology* 1990; **12**:1420-1432.
2. Lok A, Lai CL. AFP monitoring in Chinese patients with chronic hepatitis B virus infection:role of early detection of hepatocellular carcinoma. *Hepatology* 1989; **9**:110-115
3. Di Bisceglie AM, Hoffnagle JH. Elevations in serum alpha-fetoprotein levels in patients with chronic hepatitis B. *Cancer* 1989; **64**:2117-2120
4. Alpert E, Feller E. Alpha-fetoprotein (AFP) in benign liver disease: evidence that normal liver regeneration does not induce. AFP synthesis. *Gastroenterology* 1978; **74**:856-858
5. Kondo F, Wada K, Nagato Y, Nakajima T, Kondo Y, Hirooka N, Ebara M, *et al*. Biopsy diagnosis of well-differentiated hepatocellular carcinoma based on new morphologic criteria. *Hepatology* 1989; **9**:751-755.
6. Kashala LO, Conne B, Kapanci Y *et al*. Hepatitis B virus, alphafetoprotein synthesis and hepatocellular carcinoma. *Liver* 1992; **12**:330-340
7. Silver HKB, Denault J, Gold P, Thompson WG, Shuster J, Friedman SO. The detection of alphafetoprotein in patients with viral hepatits. *Cancer Res*. 1974; **34**:244-47.
8. Chen DS, Sung JL. Relation of hepatits B surface antigen to serum alphafetoprotein in non malignant disease of the liver. *Cancer* 1979; **44**:984-992.
9. Ebara M, Ohto M, Shinagawa T, Sugiura N, Kimura K, Matsutani S, Morita M,*et al*. Natural history of minute hepatocellular carcinoma smaller than three centimeters complicating cirrhosis: a study in 22 patients. *Gastroenterology* 1986; **90**:289-298
10. Chen DS, Sung JL, Sheu JC, Lai MY, How SW, Hsu HC, Lee CS *et al*. Serum alpha-fetoprotein in the early stage of human hepatocellular carcinoma. *Gastroenterology* 1984; **86**:1404-1409.
11. Shinagawa T, Ohtho M, Kimura K, Tsunetomi S, Morita M, Saisho H, Tsuchiya Y *et al*. Diagnosis and clinical features of small hepatocellular carcinoma with emphasis on the utility of real time ultrasonography: a study in 55 patients. *Gastroenterology* 1984; **86**:495-502.
12. Sonoda K, Shirabe K K, Takenaka K, Kanematsu T, Yasumori K, Sugimachi K. Angiographically undetected small hepatocellular carcinoma: clinicopathological characteristics, follow-up and treatment. *Hepatology* 1989; **10**:1003-1007.
13. Okuda K. Early recognition of hepatocellular carcinoma. *Hepatology* 1986; **6**:729-738.
14. Colombo M, De Franchis R, Del Ninno E. Hepatocellular carcinoma in Italian patients with cirrhosis. *New Engl J Med* 1991; **325**:675-680.
15. Cottone M, Turri M, Caltagirone M *et al*. Screening for hepatocellular carcinoma in patients with Child's A cirrhosis: an 8-year prospective study by ultrasound and alphafetoprotein. *J Hepatology* 1994, **21**:1029-1034.
16. Oka H, Tamori A, Kuroki T, Kabayashi K, Yamamoto S. Prospective study of alfafetoprotein in cirrhotic patients monitored for devolpment of hepatocellular carcinoma. *Hepatology* 1994; **19**:61-66.
17. Pateron D, Ganne N, Trinchet JC *et al*. Prospective study of screening for hepatocellular carcinoma in Caucasian patients with cirrhosis. *J Hepatology* 1994; **20**:65-71.
18. Imberti D, Fornari F, Sbolli G, Buscarini E, Squassante L, Buscarini L. Hepatocellular carcinoma in liver cirrhosis. A prospective study. *Scand J Gastroenterol* 1993; **28**:540-544.
19. Breborowicz J, Mackiewicz A, Breborowicz D. Microheterogeneity of alpha-fetoprotein in patient serum as demonstrated by lectin affino-electrophoresis. *Scand J Immunol* 1981; **14**:15-20.
20. Taketa K, Sekiya C, Namili M, Akamatsu K, Ohta Y, Endo Y, Kosaka K. Lectin-reactive profiles of alpha-fetoprotein characterizing hepatocellular carcinoma and related conditions. *Gastroenterology* 1990; **99**:508-518.
21. Aoyagi Y, Suzuki Y, Isemura M, Nomoto M, Sekine C, Igarashi K, Ichida F. The fucosylation index of alpha-fetoprotein and its usefulness in the early diagnosis of hepatocellular carcinoma. *Cancer* 1988; **61**:769-774.
22. Sato Y, Nakata K, Shima M. Early recognition of hepatocellular carcinoma based on alterd profiles of alpha-fetoprotein. *N*

Engl J Med 1993; **328**:1802-1806.

23. Shiraki K, Takase K, Tameda Y, Hmada M, Kosaka Y, Nakano T. A clinical study of alpha-fetoprotein as an early indicator of hepatocellular carcinoma in the follow-up of cirrhotic patients. *Hepatology* 1995; **22**:802-807.
24. Saitoh A, Ikeda K, Koida I *et al*. Diagnosis of hepatocellular carcinoma by concanavallin A affinity electrophoresis of serum AFP. *Cancer* 1995; **76**:1139-44.
25. Weitz IC, Liebman HA. Des-gamma-carboxy (abnormal) prothrombin and hepatocellular carcinoma: a critical review. *Hepatology* 1993; **18**:990-997.
26. Liebman HA, Furie BC, Tong M, Blanchard RA, Lo JK, Lee SD, Coleman MS,*et al*. Des-gamma-carboxy (abnormal) prothrombin as a serum marker of primary hepatocellular carcinoma. *N Engl J Med* 1984; **310**:1427-1431.
27. Soulier JP, Lefrere JJ, Gozin D. Le dosage de la decarboxyprothrombin: son intérpetet dans le diagnostic des carcinomes hepatocellulaires. *Ann Med Interne* 1988; **139**:7-11
28. Soulier JP, Gozin D, Lefrere JJ. A new method to assay des-g-carboxyprothrombin. *Gastroenterology* 1986; **91**:1258-1262
29. Fujiyama S, Morishita T, Sato T, Sagawa K, Motohara K, Matsuda I. Clinical evaluation of plasma abnormal prothrombin in patients with hepatocellular carcinoma. *Hepatogastroenterology* 1986; **33**:201-205
30. Okuda H, Obata H, Nakanishi T, Furukawa R, Hashimoto R. Production of abnormal prothrombin (des-gamma-carboxyprothrombin) by hepatocellular carcinoma:a clinical and experimental study. *J Hepatol* 1987; **4**:357-363.
31. Tanabe Y, Oshinishi K, Nomura F, Iida S. Plasma abnormal prothrombin levels inpatients with small hepatocellular carcinoma. *Am J Gastroenterol* 1988; **83**:1386-1389.
32. Deyashiki Y, Nishioka Y, Takahashi K, Kosaka Y, Suzuchi K. Evaluation of des-gamma-carboxyprothrombin as a marker protein of hepatocellularcarcinoma. *Cancer* 1989; **64**:2546-2551.
33. Tsai SL, Huang GT, Yang PM, Sheu JC, Sung JL, Chen DS. Plasma desgammacarboxy-protrombin in the ealry stage of hepatocellular carcinoma. *Hepatology* 1990; **11**:481-487
34. Nakao A, Vsuziki Y, Isshiki K, Kimura Y, Takeda S, Kishimoto W, Nonami T *et al*. Clinical evaluation of plasma abnormal prothrombin (des-gamma-carboxy prothrombin) in hepatobiliary malignancies and other diseases. *Am J Gastroenterol* 1991; **86**:62-66.
35. Nakao A, Virji A, Carr B, Iwatsuki S, Starzel E. Abnormal prothrombin (des-gamma-carboxy prothrombin) in hepatocellular carcinoma. *Hepatogastroenterology* 1991; **38**:450-453.
36 Ono M, Ohta H, Ohira M, Sekiya C, Namiki M, Measurements of immunoreactive prothrombin, des-gamma-carboxy prothrombin, and vitamin K in human liver tissues:overproduction of immunoreactive prothrombin in hepatocellular carcinoma. *Am J Gastroenterol* 1990; **85**:1149-54.
37. Saitoh S, Ikeda K, Koida I, Tsobota A, Arase Y, Chayama K, Kumada H. Serum des-gamma-carboxyprothrombin concentration determined by the avidin-biotin complex method in small hepatocellular carcinomas. *Cancer* 1994; **74**:2918-2923.
38. Giardina MG, Matarazzo M, Varriale A, Morante R, Napoli A, Martino R. Serum Alpha-L-Fucosidase. A useful marker in the diagnosis of hepatocellular carcinoma.*Cancer* 1992; **70**:1044-48
39. Choi BI, Takayasu K, Han MC. Small hepatocellular carcinomas and associated nodular lesion of the liver: pathology, pathogenesis and imaging findings *AJR* 1993; **160**:1177-1187;
40. International working party. Terminology of nodular hepatocellular lesions. *Hepatology* 1995; **22**: 983-933
41. Ludwig L *et al*. Terminology of chronic hepatitis, hepatic allograft rejection, and nodular lesions of the liver: summary of recommendation developed by an International Working Party, supported by the World Congresses of Gastroenterology, Los Angeles, 1994. *Am J Gastroenterol* 1994; **89**:S177-181
42. Kondo F, Wada K, Nagato Y. *et al*. Biopsy diagnosis of well-differentiated hepatocellular carcinoma based on new morphologic criteria.*Hepatology* 1989; **9**:751-755.
43. Freeman MP, Vick CW, Taylor KJW, Carither RL, Brewer WH. Regenerating nodules in cirrhosis: sonographic appearance with anatomic correlations. *AJR* 1986; **146**:533-536.
44. Sheu JC, Sung LJ, Chen DS. Ultrasonography of small hepatic tumors using high-resolution linear-array real-time instruments.*Radiology* 1984; **150**:797-802.
45. Okuda K, Musha H, Nakajima Y. *et al*. Clinicopathologic features of encapsulated hepatocellular carcinoma: a study of 26 cases.*Cancer* 1977; **40**:1240-1245
46. Wernecke K, Vassallo P, Bick U, Diederich S, Peters PE. The distinction between benign and malignant liver tumors on sonography: value of a hypoecoic halo.*AJR* 1992; **159**: 1005-1009.
47. Kitamura S, Iishi S, Tatsuta M, *et al*: Liver with Hypoechoic nodular pattern as a risk factor for hepatocellular carcinoma.*Gastroenterology* 1995; **108**:1778-1784.
48. Tanaka S, Kitamura T, Fujita M, Nakanishi K, Okuda S. Color doppler flow imaging of liver tumors.*AJR* 1990; **154**:509-514.
49. Nino-Murcia M, Ralls PW, Brooke, Jeffrey R, Johnson M. Color flow doppler characterization of focal hepatic lesions.*AJR* 1992; **159**:1195-1197.
50. Dodd GD, Miller WJ, Baron RL, Skolnick M, Campbell WL. Detection of malignant tumors in end-stage cirrhotic livers: efficacy of sonography as a screening technique.*AJR* 1992; **159**:727-733.
51. Fornari F, Filice C, Rappaccini G *et al*. Small (<3cm) hepatic lesions. Results of sonographically guided biopsy in 386 patients.*Dig Dis Sci* 1994; **39** :2267-2275.
52. Purves LR. Alphafetoprotein and the diagnosis of liver cancer in: Cameron HM, Linsell DA, Warwick GP, eds *Liver cell cancer*.Amsterdam Holland Elsevier, 1976; 61-79.
53. Tang ZY, Yu Ex, Wu CE *et al*. Diagnosis and treatment of hepatocellular carcinoma in early stage. Report of 134 cases.*Chin Med J* 1979; **92**:801-806.
54. Heyward W, Lanier A, McMahon B, Fitzgerald MA, Kilkenny S, Paprocki. TR Early detection of primary hepatocellular carcinoma. *JAMA* 1985; **254**:3052-3054
55. De Franchis R, Meucci G, Vecchi M *et al*. The natural history of asymptomatic Hepatitis B surface antigen carriers. *Ann Int Med* 1993; **118**:191-194
56. Liaw YF, Tai DI, Chu CM *et al*. Early detection of HCC in patients with Chronic Type B hepatitis. A prospective study. *Gastroenterology* 1986; **90**:263-267
57. Tanaka S, Kiyamura T, Nakanishi K, Okuda S, Yamazaky H, Hiyama T, Fujimoto I. Effectiveness of periodic checkup by ultrasonography for early diagnosis of hepatocellular carcinoma. *Cancer* 1990; **66**:2210-2214.

58. Tsukuma H, Hiyama T, Tanaka S *et al*. Risk factors for HCC among patients with chronic liver disease. *N Engl J Med* 1993; **328**:1797-1801

59. Seef L, Buskell-Basel Z, Wright EC *et al*. Long term mortality after transfusion associated non A-non B hepatitis. *N Engl J Med* 1992; **327**:1906-1911

60. Eggel H. Ueber das primary carcinoma der Leber. *Beitr Pathol Anat Allg Pathol* 1901; **30**:506-604

61. Edmonson HA, Steiner PE. Primary carcinoma of the liver. A study of 100 cases among 48900 necropsies. *Cancer* 1954; **7**:462-503

62. Miyaji T. Association of hepatocellular carcinoma with cirrhosis among autopsy cases in Japan during 14 years from 1958 to 1971. *Gann.Monogr Cancer Res*. 1976;**18**:129-49.

63. Simonetti RG, Cammà C, Fiorello F, Politi F, D'Amico G, and Pagliaro L. Hepatocellular carcinoma. A worldwide problem and the major risk factors.*Dig Dis Sci* 1991; **7** suppl:962-72

64. Zaman SN, Melia WM, Johnson RD, Portman BC, Johnson PJ, Willimas R: Risk factors in development of hepatocellular carcinoma in cirrhosis; prospective study of 613 patients. *Lancet* 1985:1357-1360

65. Benvegnù L, Fattovich G, Noventa F *et al*. Concurrent hepatitis B and C virus infection and risk of hepatocellular carcinoma in cirrhosis. *Cancer* 1994; **74** :2442-2448

66. Mandelli C, Fraquelli M, Fargion S,*et al*. Comparable frequency of hepatocellular carcinoma in cirrhosis of different etiology. *Eur J Gastroenterol Hepatol* 1994; **6**:1129-1134.

67. Borzio M, Bruno S, Roncalli M *et al*. Liver cell dysplasia is a major risk for hepatocellular carcinoma in cirrhosis: a prospective study. *Gastroenterology* 1995; **108**: 812-817

68. Henmi A, Uchida T, and Shikata T. Karjometric analysis of liver cell dysplasia and hepatocellular carcinoma. Evidence against precancerous nature of liver cell dysplasia.*Cancer* 1985; **55**:2594-2599

69. Sackett D, Haynes B, Guyatt G, Tugwell P. *Clinical Epidemiology. A basic science to clinical medicine*. 1991 Little Brown and Company, Boston

70. Barbara L, Benzi G, Gaiani S *et al*:Natural history of small untreated hepatocellular carcinoma in cirrhosis:a multivariate analysis of prognostic factors of tumor growth rate and patients survival. *Hepatology* 1992; **16**:132-137

71. Cottone M, Virdone R, Fusco G *et al*.Asymptomatic Hepatocellular carcinoma in Child's A cirrhosis. A comparison of natural hystory and surgical treatment. *Gastroenterology* 1989; **96**:1566-1571.

72. Unoura M, Kaneko S, Matsushita *et al*. High risk groups and screening strategies for early detection of hepatocellular carcinoma in patients with chronic liver disease. *Hepatogastroenterology* 1993; **40**:305-310.

73. D'Amico G, Morabito A, Pagliaro L, Marubini E, The Liver Study Group of V Cervello Hospital. Survival and prognostic indicators in compensated and decompensated cirrhosis. *Dig Dis Sci* 1986; **31**:468-475.

74. Oka H, Kurioka N, Kim K,*et al*. Prospective study for early detection of hepatocellular carcinoma in patients with cirrhosis. *Hepatology* 1990; **12**:680-687.

75. Sheu JC, Sung JL, Chen DS *et al*. Growth rate of asymptomatic hepatocellular carcinoma and its clinical implications *Gastroenterology* 1985; **89**:259-266.

76. Okuda K, Ohtsuki T, Obata H *et al*. Natural history of hepatocellular carcinoma and prognosis in relation to treatment: study of 850 patients. *Cancer* 1985; **56**: 918-928.

77. Koneru B, Cassavilla A, Bowman J, Iwatsuki S, Starzl. Liver transplantation for malignant tumors. *Gastroenterol Clin North Am* 1988; **17**:277-93

78. Bismuth H, Chiche L, Adam R, Castaing D. Surgical treatment of hepatocellular carcinoma in cirrhosis: liver resection or transplantation? *Transplant Proc* 1993; **25**:1066-1067

79. Livraghi T, Bolondi L, Buscarini L *et al*. No treatment, resection, and ethanol injection in hepatocellular carcinoma: a retrospective analysis of survival of 391 patients with cirrhosis. *J Hepatol*. 1995; **22**:522-526.

80. Lencioni R, Bartolozzi C, Caramella D *et al*. Treatment of small hepatocellular carcinoma with PEI. *Cancer* 1995; **75**:1737-1746

81. Anthony PP, Vogel CL, Barker LF. Liver cell dysplasia: a premalignant condition. *J Clin Pathol* 1973;**26**:217-223

PART III
DIAGNOSIS

8

Ultrasonography: Conventional

L Buscarini and T Livraghi

In the management of patients with hepatocellular carcinoma (HCC) or in those at risk, ultrasonography plays many roles: detection, characterization, differential diagnosis, pathologic diagnosis, staging, guide for locoregional therapies and follow-up.

a) Detection is the identification of a mass lesion in the liver, its location, size and number. Beside the mass forming HCC (unique or multiple) there is a diffuse very infrequent type, which can be misinterpreted as advanced cirrhosis.

b) Characterization establishes if the mass lesion has the characteristics associated with HCC.

c) Differential diagnosis involves HCC and other primary malignant liver tumors; HCC and metastatic tumors; HCC and benign liver tumors or pseudotumors.

d) Pathologic diagnosis can be achieved by US-guided biopsy.

e) Staging determines if the tumor is unique or multiple; with or without portal vein and/or hepatic vein and/or biliary tree involvement; with or without extrahepatic spread, obviously only in sites where US examination is possible.

f) locoregional therapies include US-guided percutaneous alcohol injection, radiofrequency interstitial thermal ablation or interstitial laser photocoagulation obtained by inserting under US guidance a needle electrode or a laser fiber.

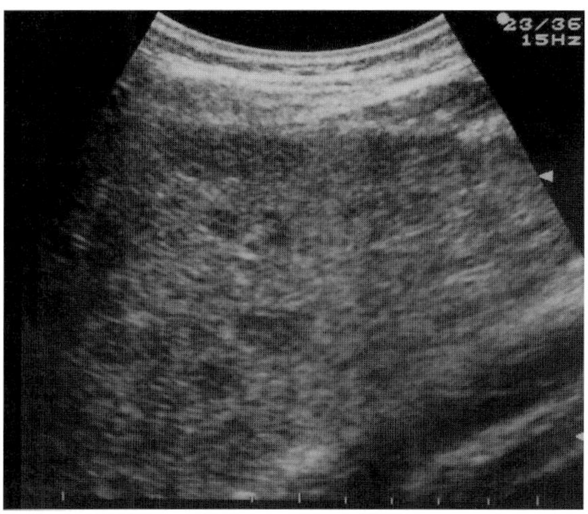

Figure 8.1 – Diffuse alteration of the liver echostructure because of multiple hypoechoic areas simulating diffuse HCC.

g) follow-up of patients at risk of developing HCC, namely patients with cirrhosis or patients already treated for HCC, is supported by US combined with measurement of serum AFP levels.

US-guided biopsy and locoregional therapies will be described in chapters 19, 25 and 26.

For the indications cited in points a–e above, other imaging techniques, particularly CT can be used in addition to US; the high risk patient follow-up is typically supported by US, as the technique is easily repeated, cheap (in comparison with other methods) and without any X-ray exposure.

DETECTION

The first rule in identifying a liver mass lesion is to find the corresponding image in two orthogonal sections; if its echotexture shows a marked difference from that of surrounding liver parenchyma, diagnosis of the mass is definitive. If the mass is superficially located it bulges through the liver surface; if the lesion is near to a venous structure, the vessels can be compressed, dislocated, infiltrated or encased; if it is near to the gallbladder its wall can be clearly compressed. US specificity in detecting a liver mass lesion is high but some pitfalls are possible: the most common are induced by nodular steatosis, presence of spared areas in fatty liver; alterations of echogenicity and liver margins due to the cirrhosis (Fig. 8.1).

Detection rate with US is increasing with improvements in existing technology and with operator experience. Today it is possible to identify a mass with a diameter of about 0.5 cm. This improved detectability has induced a change in the definition of small HCC based on its dimensions. Currently small HCC is a single tumor less than 2 cm; however other investigators[1] define small as a tumor less than 5 cm.

Detection rates depend on the dimensions of the tumor, its location, and its echostructure, as well as the experience and involvement of the operator. The first three characteristics counteract each other; for example, a tumor of 0.5 cm in diameter can be visualized if it is deeply located; the same tumor located on the surface can easily be missed. However the detection rate of US for HCC has been satisfactory even for tumors of small dimensions (Table 8.1).

Table 8.1 – Detection rate of HCC in relation to the size of the tumor

Author	Number of tumor detected/ total number of tumors (%)		
	Size HCC		
	1–2 cm	2-3 cm	3-5 cm
Sheu *et al* [2]	18/19 (94.7%)	13/14 (92.8%)	
Choi *et al* [3]	14/27 (52%)	17/20 (85%)	22/26 (85%)
	<1 cm	1-3 cm	
Takayasu *et al* [4s]	7/19 (37%)	101/110 (92%)	
	<2 cm	2-3 cm	3-4cm
Matsui & Itai[5s]	51/109 (46.7%)*	27/33 (82%)	20/20 (100%)

s= surgical control

*= 14 nodules were <0.5 cm (detection rate 0%); 31 nodules were 0.5–1 cm (detection rate 13%); 34 were 1–1.5 cm (detection rate 68%); 30 were 1.5–2 cm (detection rate 80%).

The detection rate with US was found to be 100% in a group of tumors ranging between 1.2 and 9.5 cm: 10 lesions were smaller than 3 cm[6]; it was 98% in a series of 174 patients: the tumor appeared as a single nodule of < 5 cm in 53 cases.[7]

HCC is more frequently located in the right lobe (about 65% of the cases) than in the left lobe and very uncommonly in the caudate lobe (Fig. 8.2).[8] Detection rate is influenced by tumor location: for tumors situated in anterior segments of the right lobe it is

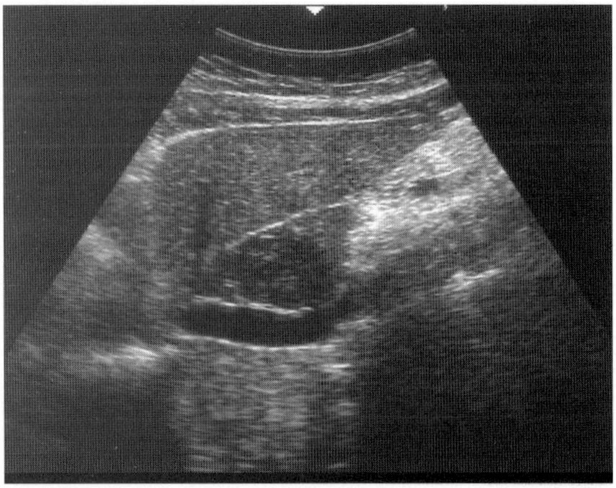

Figure 8.2 – Hypoechoic round-shaped HCC located in the caudate lobe.

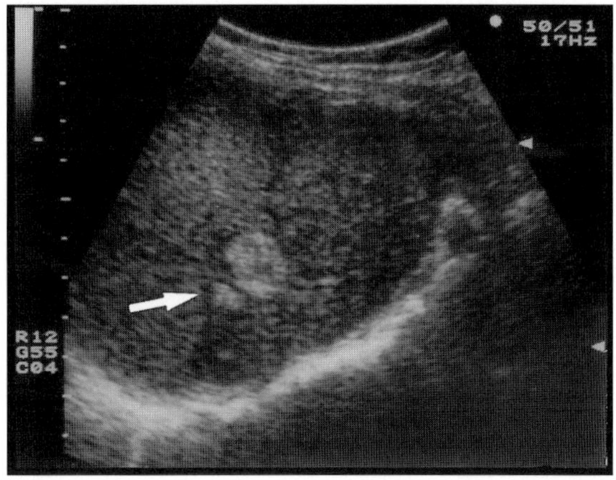

Figure 8.3 – Hyperechoic HCC with a minute daughter nodule (arrow); also hyperechoic.

80.3%; in posterior segments, 73%; in the medial part of the left lobe, 68%; in the lateral part, 77%. Overall no differences in detection rates have been found between the two lobes.[9]

Location of a tumor in a specific segment (according to Couinaud nomenclature[10]) is not always easy and is somewhat dependent on the operator's expertise; for this reason it is difficult to obtain by US the detailed information useful for surgery.[11]

When the echostructure is not dissimilar to that of the surrounding liver only indirect signs of the mass lesion are found: compression of the vessels, bulging of the surface or, as an early indirect sign, isolated dilation of a small biliary capillary. In contrast, even minute nodules that are clearly hyperechoic are easily detectable (Fig. 8.3).

Sensitivity of US is strongly influenced by the experience and attentiveness of the operator. Detection rates of 80% were found in a group of 50 HCCs smaller than 5 cm; this increased to 92% in a second more accurate examination.[1]

The number of tumors is not easily established from US (as with other imaging techniques) and frequently multiple nodules are missed at examination, particularly in end-stage cirrhotic livers, as shown by histologic studies of resected HCCs, or comparing the US results before transplantation and the results of pathologic examination of explanted livers; moreover US in many instances fails to detect the presence of tumoral satellites.[12-15] However US seems to be

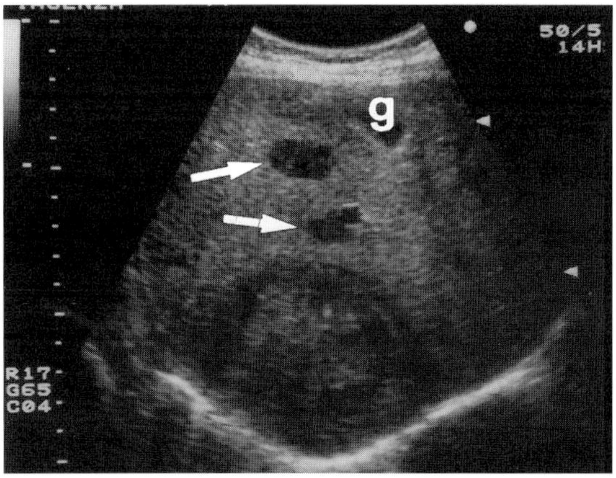

Figure 8.4 – Intrahepatic metastases (arrows) of the main HCC deeply located; g = gallbladder.

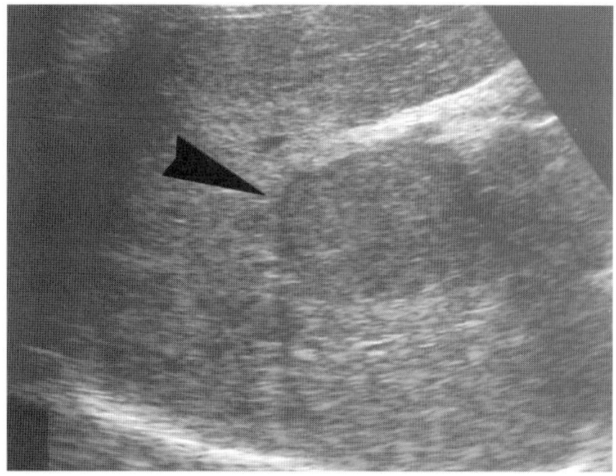

Figure 8.5 – Oval-shaped HCC (arrow) with well defined boundary; the tumor exhibits posterior enhancement and lateral shadows.

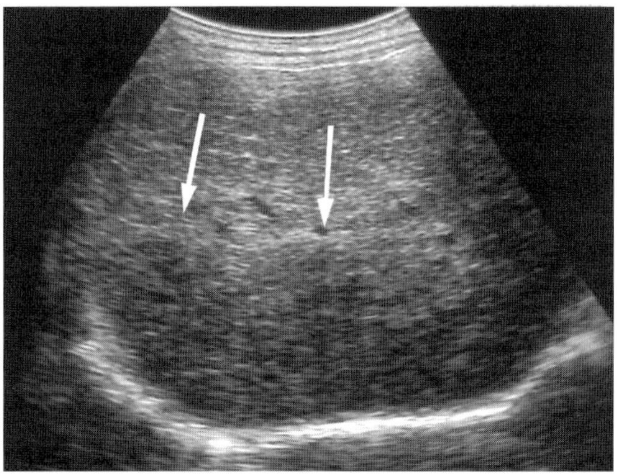

Figure 8.6 – Hypoechoic infiltrative HCC not clearly demarcated from the surrounding liver (arrows).

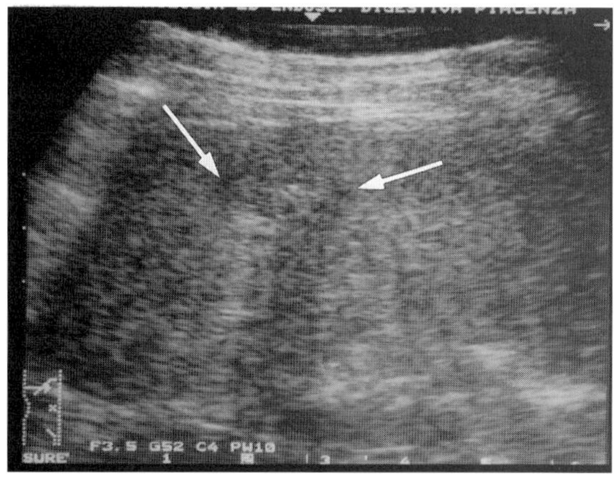

Figure 8.7 – Isoechoic HCC (arrows) with posterior shadow.

highly specific; therefore any lesion sonographically identified in a cirrhotic liver should be considered malignant until the contrary is proved.[14]

CHARACTERIZATION

In Western and far Eastern countries, HCC arises for the most part in patients with chronic liver disease: ancillary signs useful in characterizing the disease are therefore represented by US patterns of cirrhosis (caudate lobe hypertrophy; margin deformation; coarse echotexture; splenomegaly; signs of portal hypertension).

The number of tumors detected in the liver can suggest the correct diagnosis: in cases of HCC, the number of nodules is generally less than 5.[16] Minute nodules located in the same segment or in an adjacent segment of the main tumor can be considered as daughter nodules. Plural nodules in both lobes are considered multicentric tumors, when none is large enough to be regarded as the main mass and the remainder are considered intrahepatic metastases (Fig. 8.4).[17]

The shape of nodular HCC is generally round or oval and the boundary between the mass and surrounding liver is well defined (Fig. 8.5). In the infiltrative type, however, the border is not clearly visible (Fig. 8.6). An important element in reaching a diagnosis is the internal echo pattern, which can be classified into 4 types: isoechoic (Fig. 8.7), hyperechoic (Fig. 8.3),

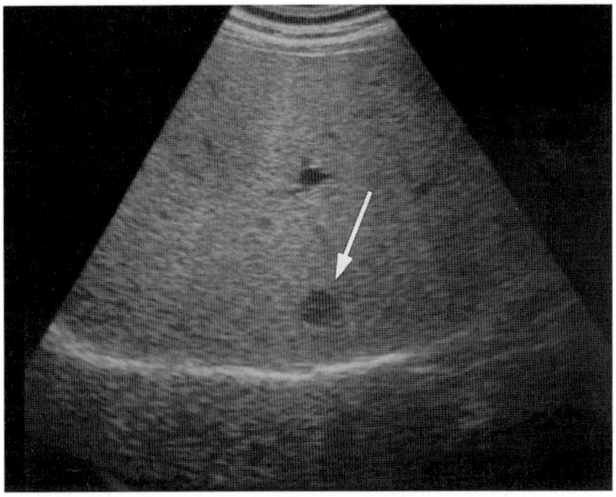

Figure 8.8 – Minute hypoechoic HCC (arrow).

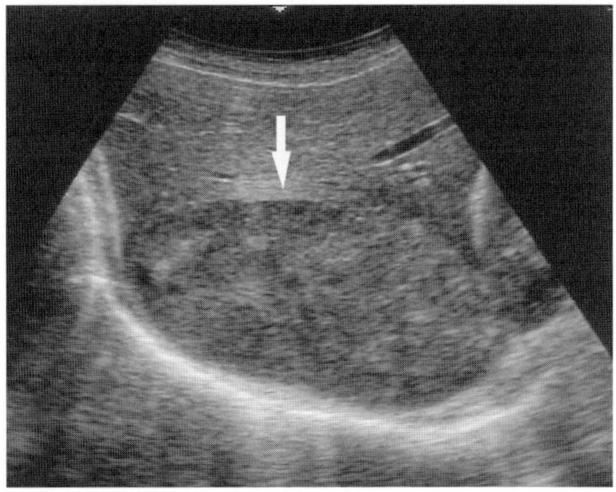

Figure 8.9 – Large potato-shaped HCC (arrow) with mixed echo pattern.

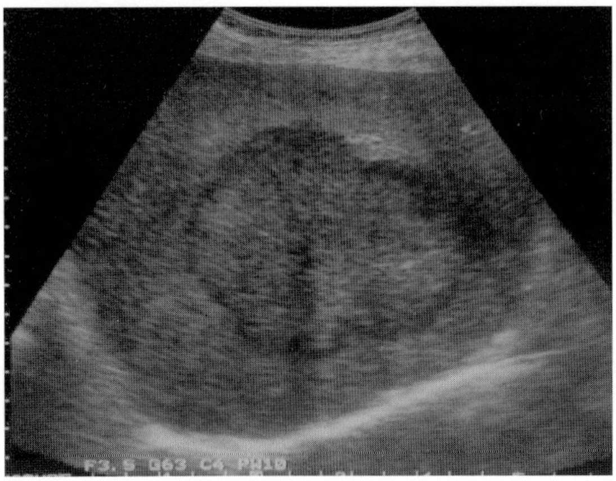

Figure 8.10 – Large isoechoic HCC with peripheral hypoechoic halo.

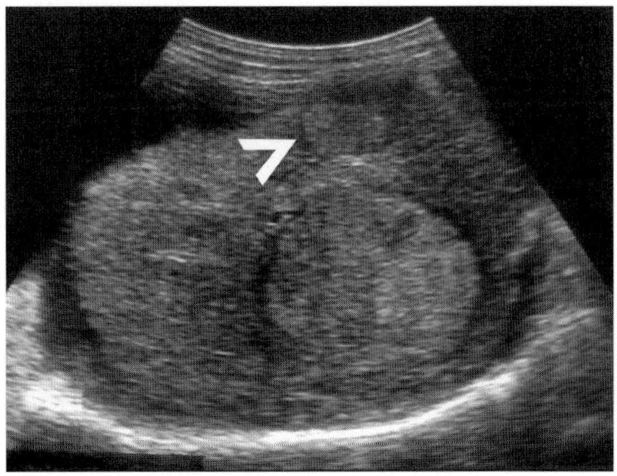

Figure 8.11 – Round-shaped HCC with mixed echo pattern with hypoechoic halo; a daughter nodule is also visible (arrow); the liver is surrounded by ascites.

Table 8.2 – Ultrasound pattern of small HCC

	Number of patients with characterized tumor/ total number of patients (%)			
Author	**Hypoechoic**	**Hyperechoic**	**Isoechoic**	**Mixed**
		Size ≤3 cm		
Sheu *et al* [2]	24/31 (77.4)	5/31 (16.1)	2/31 (6.5)	
Yoshida *et al* [18]	10/13 (76.9)			
Choi *et al* [19]	14/29 (48.3)	13./29 (44.9)	1/29 (3.4)	1/29 (3.4)
		Size ≤ 5 cm		
Buscarini *et al* [7]	21/53 (39.6)			

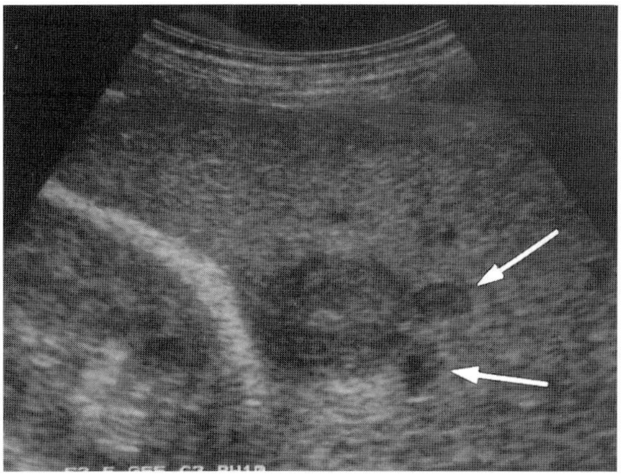

Figure 8.12 – Hypoechoic HCC with two sites of extranodular growth (arrows).

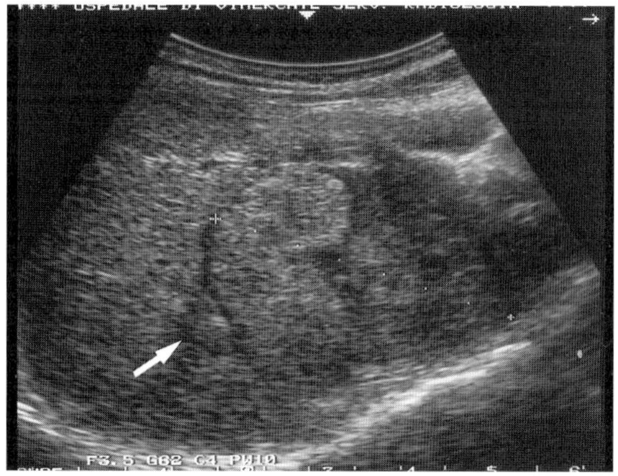

Figure 8.13 – A small nodule (arrow) is detectable close to the hypoechoic halo of the large HCC indicated by the markers.

hypoechoic (Fig. 8.8) or mixed (Fig. 8.9) in relation to the aspect of the echogenicity of the surrounding liver parenchyma. The so called low-periphery echopattern indicates a mass demarcated by a hypoechoic rim, being internal iso, hyper, or mixed echoes (Fig. 8.10). Echopattern is highly dependent on the tumor dimensions (Table 8.2). Tumors less than 3 cm in diameter are generally hypoechoic. This is due to the presence of a pure cellular mass, without sinusoidal dilation, fatty metamorphosis, hemorrhage, necrosis.

However an hyperechoic presentation is not unusual in small tumors. In a group of 34 HCCs less than 2 cm, 6 tumors appeared as hyperechoic, 7 as mixed (that is coexistence of hyperechoic and hypoechoic areas), while 18 patients had hypoechoic tumors and only 3 isoechoic ones. The hyperechoic characteristic was related to cancer cells with fat droplets, without necrosis, with poor development of sinusoids: the tumoral cells had mild nuclear atypia with rare mitoses; in hypoechoic areas, cancer cells did not show fat droplets and appeared well differentiated but slightly less differentiated than cancer cells with fatty metamorphosis.[20] The occurrence of hyperechoic aspect has been found very infrequently (less than 2%) in other series.[21]

In about half of small HCCs, it is possible to see a hypoechoic halo, which is a thin hypoechoic band around the tumor (Fig. 8.11).[19] The thickness of this band is smaller than 10% of the tumor diameter. Hypoechoic halos in resected specimens correspond to a fibrous capsule or a peritumoral liver cell compression (pseudocapsule).[22, 23] This feature is more often found in small HCCs but it can be visualized in larger tumors. The encapsulated type of HCC is a well differentiated tumor with an expansive growth. A careful examination of capsular structure is necessary to identify its eventual disruption with an extranodular growth (Figs. 8.12, 13). Occasionally a hyperechoic rim borders the tumor, tentatively attributed to local fatty metamorphosis (Fig. 8.14).[24]

In some cases lateral shadows are visible, that is an acoustic shadows behind the edges of the tumor, said to correspond to the capsule. More probably this phenomenon is not unique to HCC and depends on the incidence of the US beam on the lateral profile of a round mass acting as a refracting lens. In small tumors (more frequently than in large ones) a posterior acoustic enhancement is visible due to a local

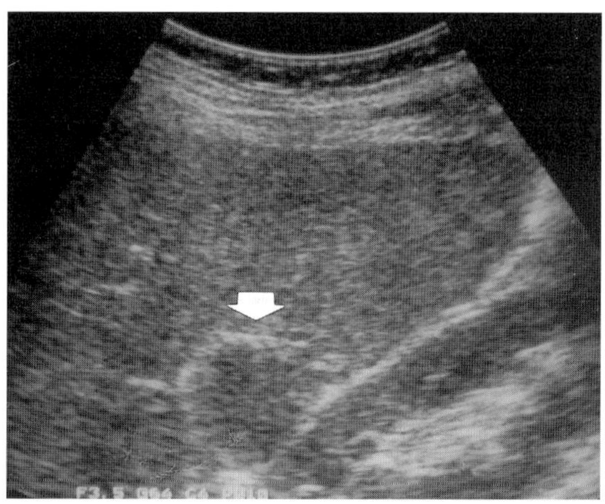

Figure 8.14 – HCC with hyperechoic ring (arrow).

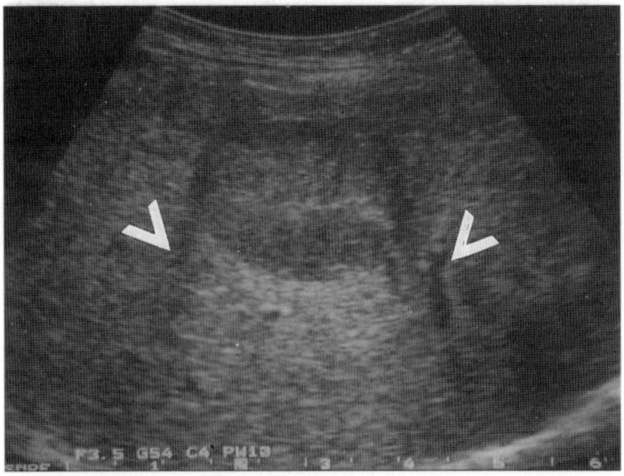

Figure 8.15 – HCC with lateral shadows (arrows) and posterior enhancement.

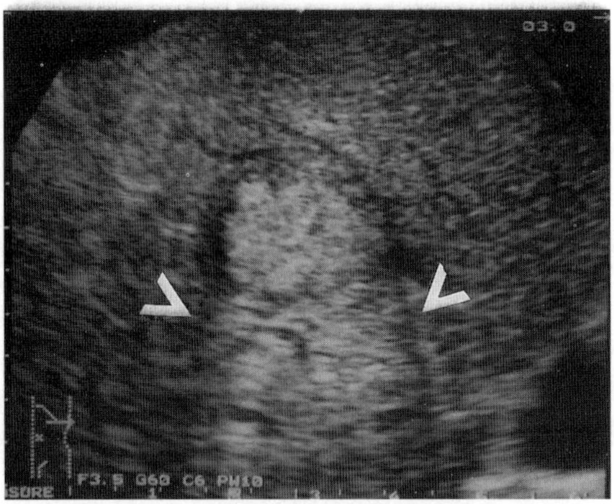

Figure 8.16 – HCC with lateral shadows (arrows) and posterior enhancement.

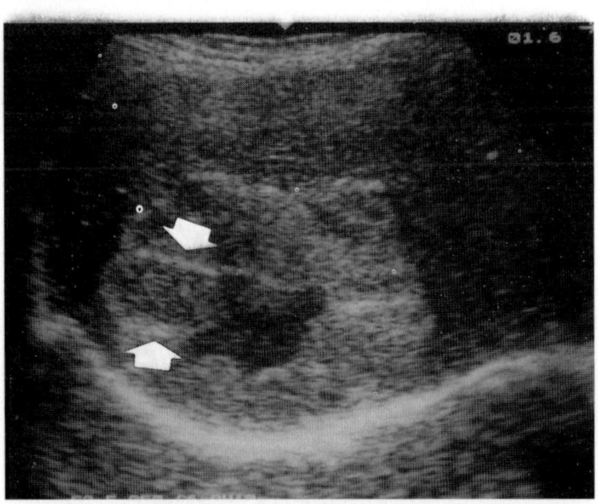

Figure 8.17 – Large HCC with mosaic pattern, in which internal septa are clearly visible (arrows).

Table 8.3 – Three conditions for US diagnosis of HCC[16]

I)	Tumor has at least one of the following features:
	a) peripheral halo
	b) mosaic pattern
	c) hypoechoic lesion
II)	Number of nodules is less than 5
III)	Findings suggesting chronic liver diseases

increase of echogenicity behind the tumor. Posterior enhancement corresponds to facilitated transmission of ultrasonic waves through the tumor, probably because of structural characteristics which, however, have not been identified (Figs. 8.5, 15, 16).[19]

In larger tumors the presence of internal septa can be visualized. This feature, defined as a mixed or mosaic pattern (Fig. 8.17), is more common in tumors larger than 3 cm representing a model of tumoral growth. The tumor is composed of small areas with different or the same echogenicity, being separated from each other by an echoic rim representing a fibrous septum: it could depend on the coexistence of different clones of cancer cells generating fibrous septa as a boundary or on the association of two encapsulated tumors with infiltration beyond the capsule. Detection of a capsule or septa by US is easier in larger tumors, but the sensitivity of US is less than that of other imaging techniques such as CT or MR.[6]

Obviously in determining the mosaic pattern, other factors can play a role, such as changes in vascular features, presence of necrosis phenomena, fatty metamorphosis.

For diagnosis of HCC sensitivity was 58.9% and specificity was 99.9% by following the three US parameters detailed in Table 8.3.[16] Sensitivity improved to 68.6% in a successive study. [25]

Posterior echo enhancement, lateral shadow and mosaic pattern have been regarded as quite specific features of HCC in comparison with liver metastases (Table 8.4).

In large tumors involvement of hepatic vessels is very common, while biliary tree invasion is less frequent. The tumor partially or completely fills the lumen of the vessel, which appears either less or more echogenic than normal liver parenchyma.[26] In some

Table 8.4 – Efficacy of different US characteristics in diagnosis of HCC[18]

	Number of cases*	Sensitivity %	Specificity %
Mosaic pattern	151	65.6 (42/64)	96.6 (84/87)
Posterior echo enhancement	151	53.1 (34/64)	90.8 (79/87)
Lateral shadow	151	32.8 (21/64)	98.9 (86/87)

*= The series included 64 patients with HCC and 87 patients with metastatic liver tumors. True positive and false negatives are cases of HCC (according to the presence or the absence of the recalled US characteristics), while true negatives and false positives are cases of metastatic liver tumor (according to the absence or the presence of the same characteristics).

cases HCC can be only represented by portal vein thrombosis;[27] in this case thrombus biopsy is mandatory (Fig 8.18). [28]

A diffuse type of HCC is characterized by multiple minute nodules, with altered hepatic texture shown by the presence of scattered foci within the parenchyma (Figs. 8.19, 20). Diffuse tumors are difficult to identify and characterize because the diffuse and faint parenchyma alteration can be misinterpreted as due to cirrhosis.

Finally, in infiltrative type HCC the tumor boundaries are irregular and difficult to distinguish from the non tumor tissue (Fig. 8.21).

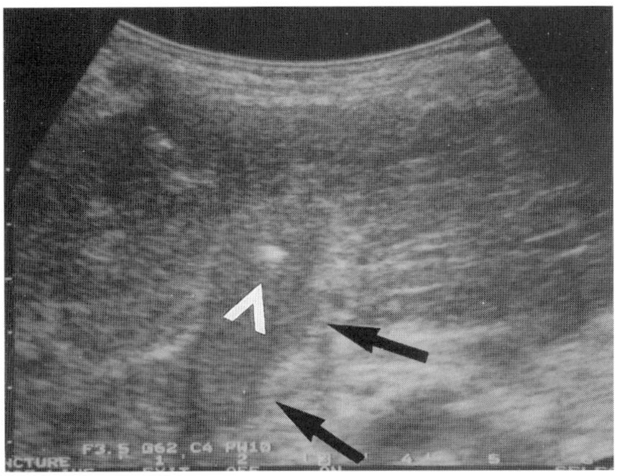

Figure 8.18 – Complete portal thrombosis (arrows) in a patient with suspected HCC: the biopsy of the thrombus (arrowhead) demonstrates the neoplastic growth within the vessel.

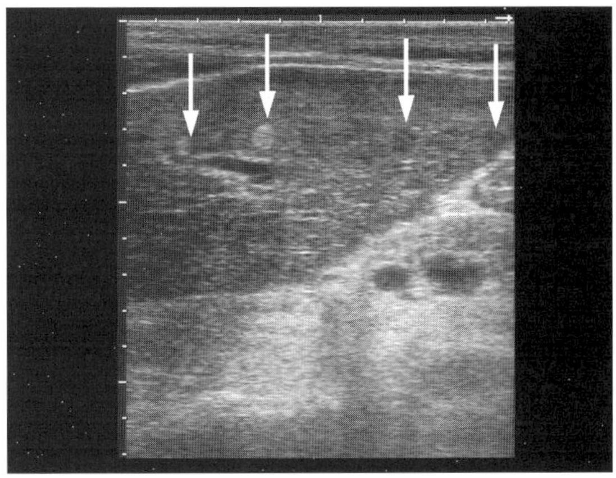

Figure 8.19 – Diffuse HCC with hyper and hypoechoic (arrows) nodules.

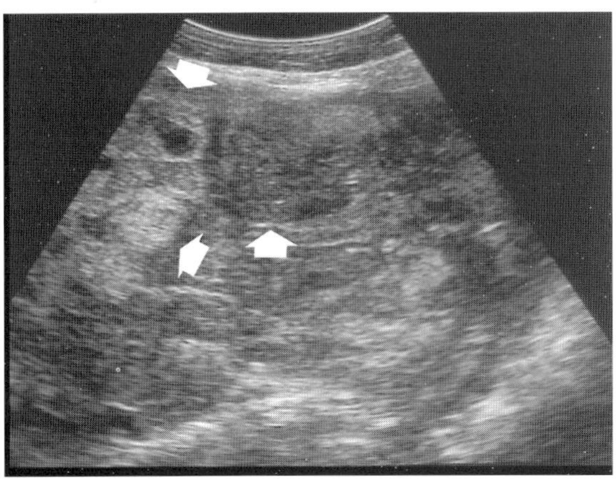

Figure 8.20 Diffuse HCC with multiple and confluent nodules hypo, hyperechoic and mixed (arrows).

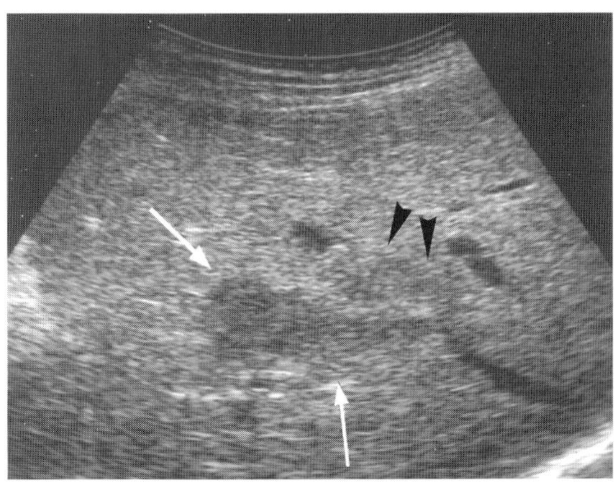

Figure 8.21 – Infiltrative HCC presenting as hypoechoic area not well demarcated (arrows), invading the hepatic vein (arrowheads).

NATURAL HISTORY OF HCC

US allows, in untreated cases, modifications in the tumor to be easily followed over time, as well as the modality of growth and calculation of the doubling time of the tumor (Figs. 8.22a-c).

A tumor less than 2 cm generally appears as an hypoechoic lesion; by increasing in volume it becomes isoechoic with an hypoechoic halo. This step lasts about 11 months. The successive changes lead the tumor to appear hyperechoic with a halo and then with the so-called mixed pattern, described above. The end stage is a form of massive tumor. The time for evolution from isoechoic with halo to a massive form is quite variable: from several months to about 2 years. [29]

Follow-up of hyperechoic HCCs showed that hypoechoic areas emerged at the periphery or within the tumor, increasing in volume and compressing the pre-existing hyperechoic zones (Figs. 8.23a-b).[20]

The nature of tumoral growth varies: constant growth, late growth, declining growth rate with possible volume reduction, or progressive increase of volume with sudden enlargement or cessation in growth.[29, 30] In some patients no growth has been observed for a period longer than 1 year.[31] The small hypoechoic tumors tend to have a slow growth whereas those that are isoechoic with a halo tend to grow faster. For the most part tumor doubling time ranged from 5 to 6.5 months.[29, 30]

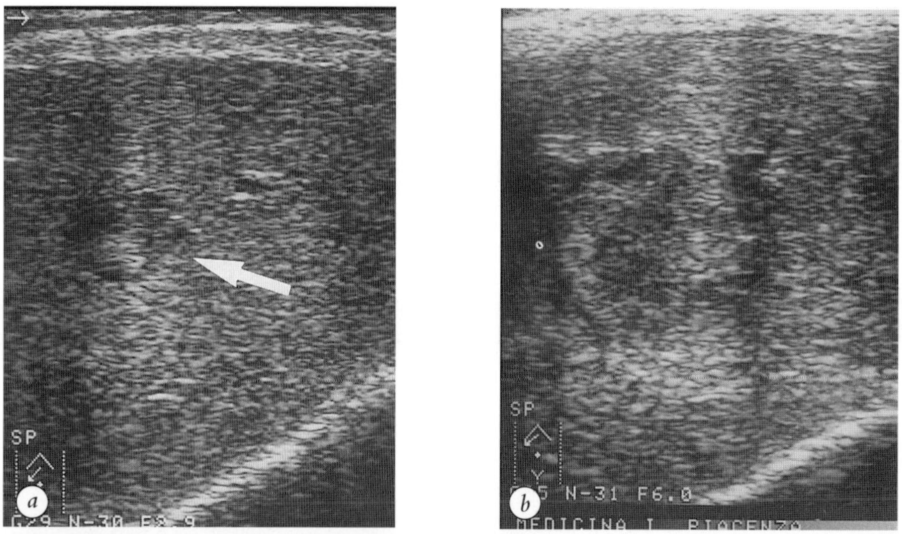

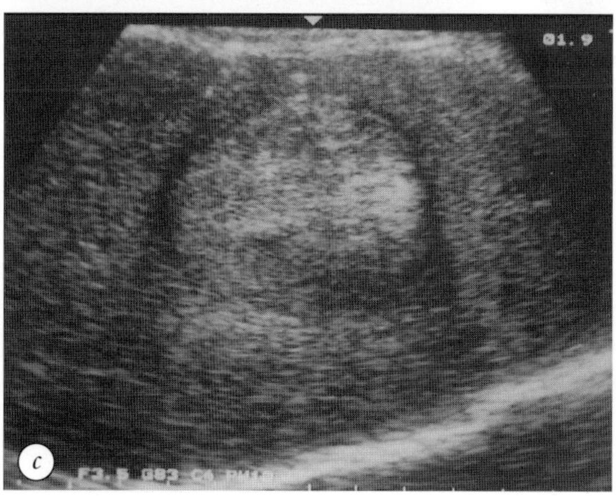

Figure 8. 22 –

a) Natural history of HCC presenting as 2.8 cm mixed nodule (arrow).

b) After 25 months the nodule measures 5.2 cm, and it has posterior enhancement and lateral shadows.

c) After 30 months the HCC becomes predominantly hyperechoic with hypoechoic halo, lateral shadows and posterior enhancement. The diameter is 6 cm long.

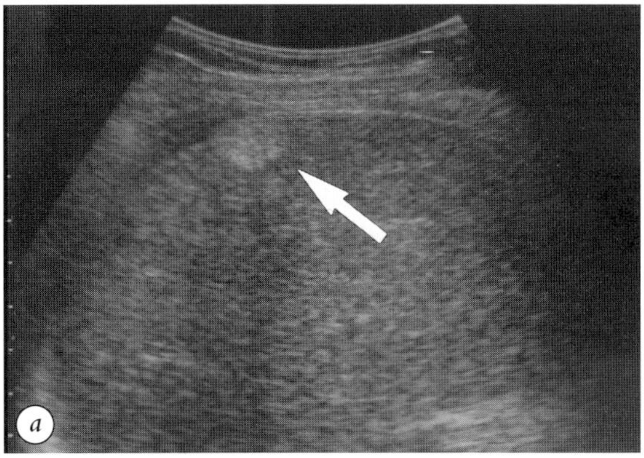

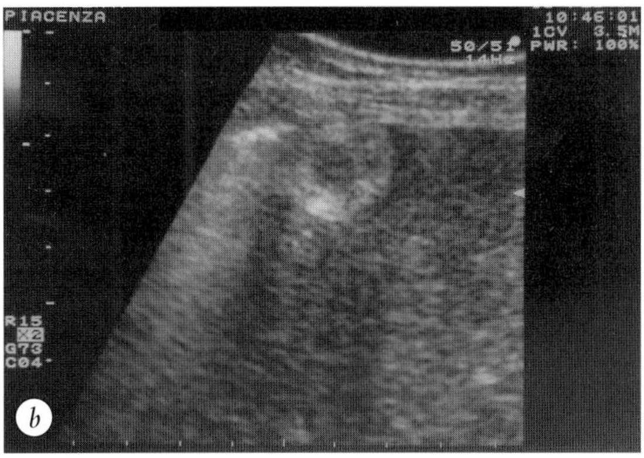

Figure 8.23 –

a) Small HCC detected as hyperechoic oval nodule (arrow) (1.2 x 2 cm).

b) After 10 months the nodule becomes round with hypoechoic center (2 cms in diameter).

DIFFERENTIAL DIAGNOSIS

Many nodular pathologies of the liver can present with a characteristic US picture: abscess, echinococcal cyst, small angioma, HCC itself, various kinds of metastases. Also, all nodular liver pathologies can manifest an anomalous picture. Therefore, US differential diagnosis can be difficult and it has to be supported by other clinical and laboratory data; often it involves other imaging techniques or indicates the need for a biopsy.

Some simple general rules to approach the problems of differential diagnosis of US images in the field of liver nodular pathology can be summarized as follows.

HCC in Western and far Eastern countries arises generally in cirrhotic livers; therefore the search for related ancillary signs is very important. For HCC developing in non cirrhotic liver, it is important to remember that in normal liver a mass lesion less than 15 mm in diameter has a very high probability of being a benign tumor, even in patients with oncologic history.[32] Moreover, the diagnosis of HCC in normal liver is generally made in advanced stage, when the tumor is large.

An increase in serum AFP over 400-500 ng/ml can be considered a sure index of HCC (recently the AFP diagnostic cut-off has been lowered to values of 200 ng/ml). A possible exception is represented by extra-hepatic tumors with liver metastasis, producing AFP.

In cirrhotic livers, the occurrence of metastatic tumors is significantly less than that of HCC.[33] Focal nodular hyperplasia (FNH) is absent in cirrhotic liver.

Nevertheless some situations, either benign or malignant, can be difficult to differentiate from HCC. Pathologies which have practical relevance in this sense are represented by some benign mass lesions (atypical hemangioma, focal nodular hyperplasia, adenoma); another primary liver malignancy (cholangio-carcinoma (CC)); eventually liver metastases, and by liver lymphomatous involvement.

Atypical hemangioma, for instance cavernous hemangioma, has large dimensions, irregular borders without a capsule, and a complex echostructure. It can be found also in middle-advanced age and in cirrhotic liver. In these cases the correct diagnosis requires other imaging techniques (Tc labeled red cells scintigraphy; angio CT; MR). In cirrhotic livers, a typical hemangioma can be difficult to differentiate from a form of hyperechoic small HCC and requires other imaging techniques and often biopsy.[34]

FNH has a non specific echopattern (isoechoic with halo; hyperechoic; mixed pattern). It can present many of the same characteristics as the fibrolamellar variant of HCC: clinical signs, such as age, female sex, absence of cirrhosis or ultrasonographic signs such as the presence inside the tumor of a central scar. In this case even a complete series of imaging techniques (Tc scintigraphy; CT; MR) can fail to make a correct diagnosis, thus compelling the use of biopsy.[35] Fine cutting needle echoguided biopsy performed either on the lesion and on the normal parenchyma can easily allow the diagnosis.[36]

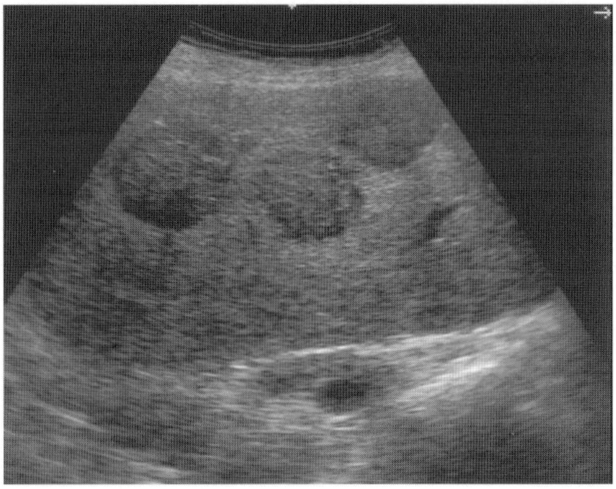

Figure 8.24 – Peripheral nodular form of CC presenting with three hypoechoic nodules.

Liver cell adenoma is generally restricted to females, with the history of prolonged intake of estro-progestational hormones. The US picture is not characteristic, the lesion being round or oval without any capsule, appearing isoechoic, hypoechoic or hyperechoic, perhaps with a hypoechoic center or a central scar bound to previous hemorrhages. A formal diagnosis can be performed only on the basis of biopsy, preferably under laparoscopic control if the lesion is superficially located.[37]

Among other primary malignant tumors, cholangiocarcinoma (CC) (even if its prevalence is only about 1% of HCC cases) has to be differentiated from HCC. CC generally arises in non cirrhotic liver, and AFP values are normal. The peripheral nodular form is usually located in the right lobe (Fig. 8.24); intrahepatic bile ducts irradiating from the tumor are dilated (Fig. 8.25),[38] the small tumors are generally hypoechoic, while lesions larger than 3 cm are more frequently hyperechoic. A hypoechoic halo is present in one third of cases. Diagnosis can be performed only by biopsy. As a rule, unlike HCC, no portal vein thromboses occur.[39] In many instances, CC arises in the larger bile ducts: scans of the involved segments reveal intraluminal soft-tissue echoes with the presence, in some cases, of extraductal masses.[40-42]

Metastatic tumors generally arise in non cirrhotic livers and more often the primary tumor is known. Sometimes the correct characterization can be very difficult. Metastases are frequently multiple: many nodules of similar size located in both liver lobes suggest a metastatic nature. Liver metastases have potato or cauliflower shape and irregular boundaries. Metastases present various echopatterns which can coexist in the same liver; the target aspect is frequently observed (and frequently bound to a colon cancer); a rapid growth can import an insufficient arterial blood supply with necrosis phenomena and appearance of hypoechoic areas. Portal vein thrombosis, which was considered rare in liver metastases, is detectable in some;[43] however its presence is more indicative of HCC.

Hematologic liver malignancies are, from a practical point of view, represented by Hodgkin and non Hodgkin lymphomas (NHL). The primary lymphomatous involvement of the liver is very rare. Lymphomatous involvement is generally in nodular form. The mass lesions are hypoechoic of various dimension and shape. It has been pointed out that tumors of B lymphocytes (namely NHL) is the second tumor most frequently associated with HCC, either as previous, synchronous or metachronous tumor.[44] Even if this case is not frequent, it is important to remember that in cases of lymphoma already diagnosed, a new lesion in the liver is not necessarily of lymphomatous origin but could be HCC; on the other hand, a new lesion during follow up of treated HCC, is not necessarily a recurrence but could be a lymphoma. Finally, a recent report has described the coexistence of lymphoma and HCC in the same liver.[45] Ignorance of these possibilities can be a serious drawback to the correct management of the patient.

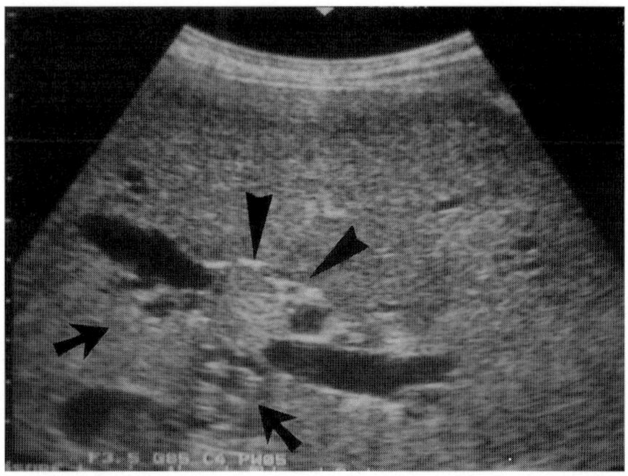

Figure 8.25 – Hyperechoic CC (arrowheads) inducing focal dilatation of bile ducts (arrows).

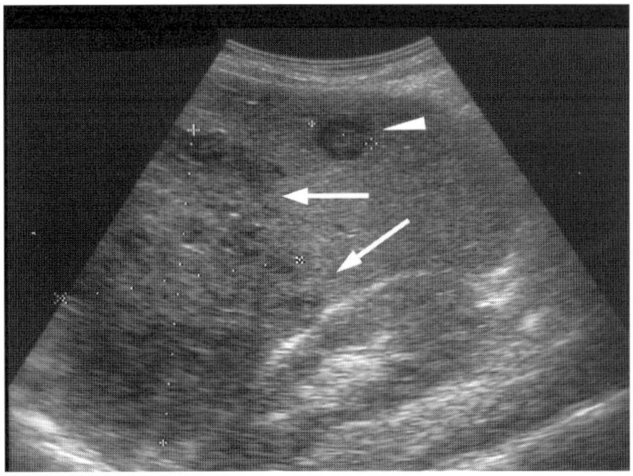

Figure 8.26 – Large HCC with no distinct boundary (arrows) and a small daughter nodule (arrowhead).

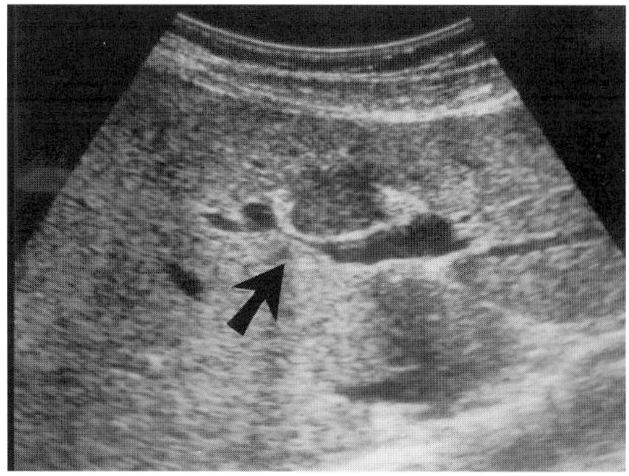

Figure 8.27 – Hypoechoic HCC compressing the portal vein (arrow)

Non malignant nodules in cirrhotic livers identified as dysplastic nodules (according to a recent classification[46]) are a difficult diagnostic problem. In fact, the US picture is indistinguishable from that of small HCC.[47] The only US characteristic of malignancy is the appearance of a hypoechoic area (the so-called nodule in nodule) inside the tumor. The inner nodule represents the advanced tumoral component while the peripheral mantel is regarded as the early component; the form is defined as early advanced HCC.[48] The increase of volume is another element suggesting the transformation of a dysplastic nodule in HCC, but, in some cases, even the nodule growth is not accompanied by the emergence of an overt HCC. Multiple US guided biopsies can fail to reach a correct diagnosis, either because the sampling involves a very limited part of the nodule, or because of the intrinsic difficulties of pathologic judgment. Useful approaches to distinguish a dysplastic nodule from an overt HCC can be the study of vascularization or MRI tissue characterization.[49]

STAGING

US examination can identify the number of nodules, but easily underestimates it;[13,50] distinguish daughter nodules (small nodules contiguous to the main tumor) or intrahepatic metastases (Fig. 8.26);

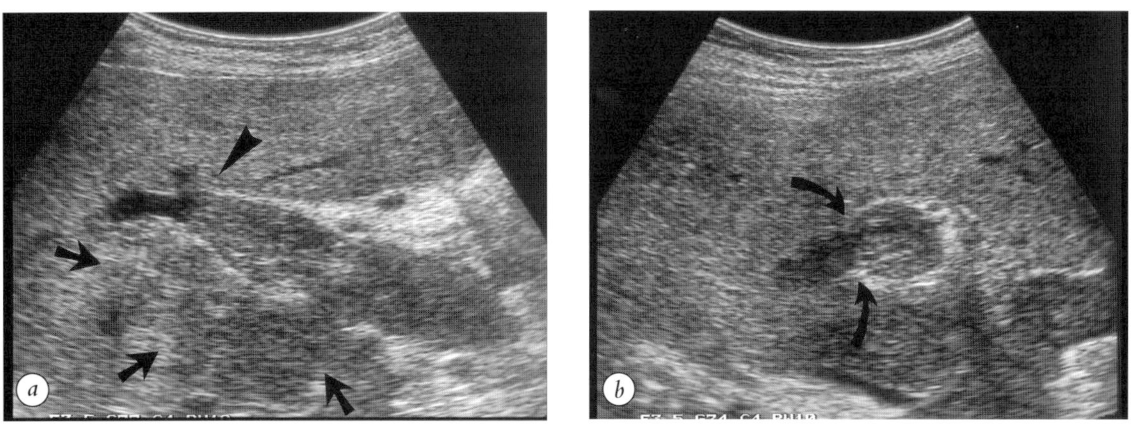

Figure 8.28 –

a) Hypoechoic HCC (arrows) invades the portal vein: in oblique scan the neoplastic thrombus is clearly visible up to the right bifurcation of the main trunk (arrowhead);

b) it is possible to see in sagittal scan the tumor disrupting the vessel wall (arrows)

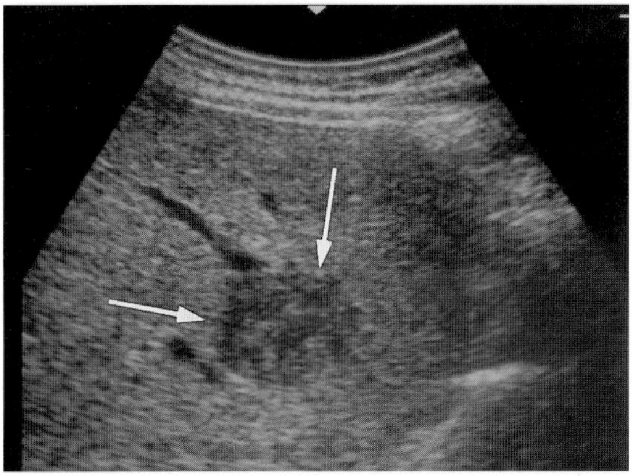

Figure 8.29 – HCC invading an hepatic vein (arrows).

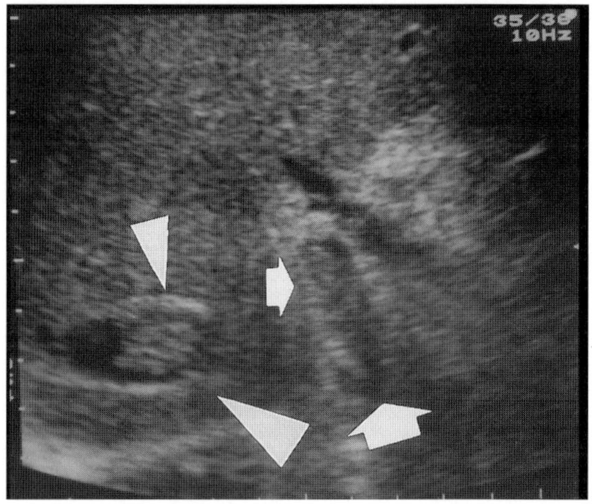

Figure 8.30 – Thrombosis of both vena cava (arrowheads) and portal vein (arrows) caused by HCC.

portal/hepatic vein or biliary tumoral involvement, locoregional node involvement, and abdominal extrahepatic spread. According to autopsy studies either intrahepatic and extrahepatic spread is found more frequently in tumors larger than 5 cm than in smaller tumors.[51]

HCC tends to invade the portal vein (Figs. 8.27, 28) and, to a lesser extent, the hepatic veins (Fig. 8.29): tumor emboli in the portal vein were found in 459/838 of autopsied cases (62.2%); in the hepatic veins, emboli were found in 164/725 autopsied cases (26.2%).[52] Sonography is reliable for detection of hepatic vein invasion even if the underlying cirrhosis does not always allow correct visualization. [53]

Sonography is useful in detecting portal vein thrombosis, which correlates with tumor size (Table 8.5).

In a recent paper portal/caval vein thrombosis was found, at diagnosis, in 56/407 patients, 14% (Fig. 8.30).[55] As patients with cirrhosis are at a high risk of developing portal vein thrombosis, this phenomenon cannot be immediately related to the presence of HCC. In rare situations portal vein thrombosis is the unique detectable localization of the tumor. Multiple papers have been published about the possibilities of differentiating benign from malignant portal vein thrombus on the basis of imaging appearance, without practical results; this aim, crucial for the management of the patient, is partially acquirable by Doppler sonography.[56]

Invasion of the right atrium is rare, even in cases of large tumors.[57] Paradoxically the hepatic component remains undetectable at US, while intra-atrial tumor is visible.[58]

Table 8.5 – Prevalence of portal vein thrombosis in a series of patients with HCC, identified by US at the time of tumor diagnosis[54]

Tumor size	Number of patients	%	Number of patients with portal thrombosis	%
Uninodular ≤5 cm	41	17.2	4	9.8
Uninodular >5 cm	53	22.2	13	25.5
Multinodular	47	1.7	15	31.7
Diffuse	98	41.0	63	64.7
Total	239		95	39.7

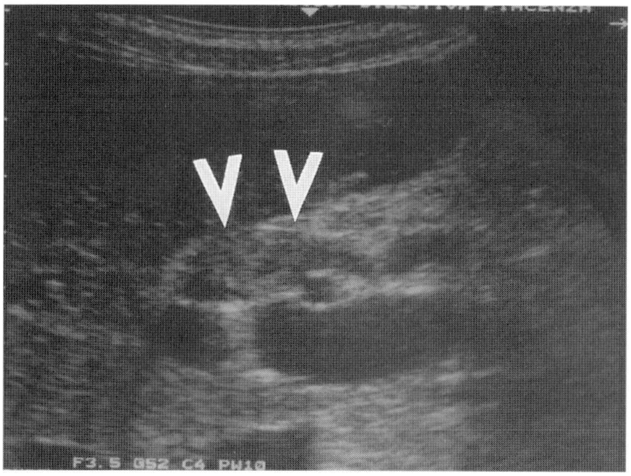

Figure 8.31 – HCC invades the common bile duct (arrows).

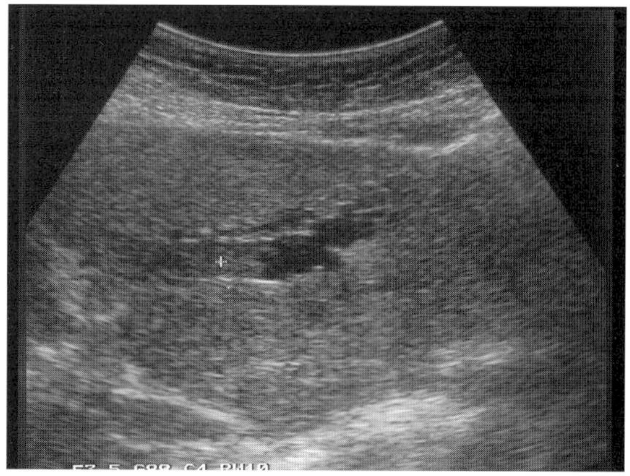

Figure 8.32 – HCC proliferating into the left bile duct (+).

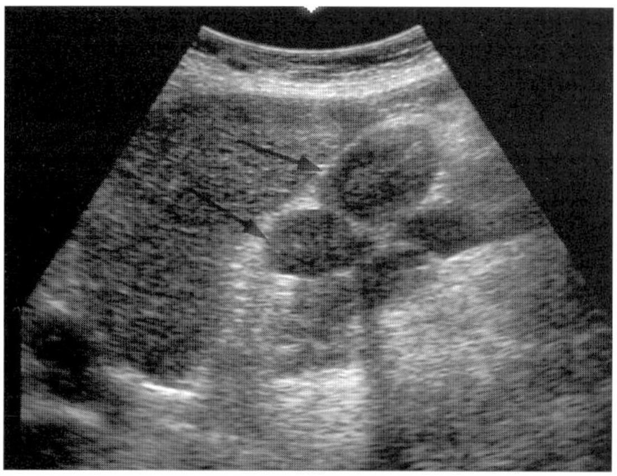

Figure 8.33 – Large hypoechoic lymph nodes (arrows) involved in metastatic spread of HCC, below the liver margin.

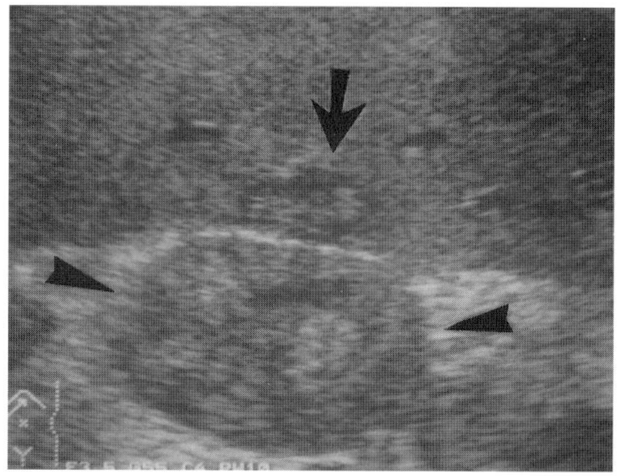

Figure 8.34 – Small HCC (arrow) with large adrenal metastasis (arrowheads).

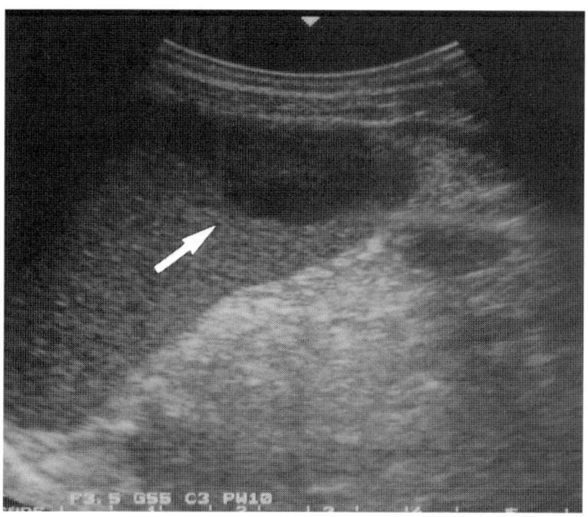

Figure 8.35 – Hypoechoic metastasis of HCC (arrow) to the spleen.

Biliary tree involvement is rare and not easily detectable. The incidence was 9% in a series of 238 autopsies and 21 surgical cases, this subgroup usually having infiltrative or mixed (nodular and infiltrative) type of HCC.[59] Tumor invasion into the biliary system can induce a mechanical obstruction of the main duct due to continuous tumoral growth (Fig. 8.31) or to migration of tumoral thrombi or to hemobilia. US can identify the presence of a dilated biliary system and tumor tissues in the major bile ducts (Fig. 8.32) and/or common bile duct.[60]

Metastases, in clinical studies, have been found in about 14% of patients[7,54] being located in 2/3 in bone and lung; metastases involving abdominal tissues or organs (lymph-nodes Fig. 8.33, peritoneum, adrenal glands Fig. 8.34, spleen, Fig. 8.35) can be detected by US.

FOLLOW-UP OF PATIENTS AT RISK OF DEVELOPING HCC

The most important series of patients at risk of developing HCC are those with cirrhosis or with HCC in cirrhosis who have undergone an effective treatment. In fact, cirrhotic patients show an incidence of HCC ranging between 5-11%;[61] 3%,[62] 5.1%;[63] 5.8% year.[64] The risk of developing HCC during follow-up is higher among patients who at recruitment had elevated AFP values (but obviously lower than values considered diagnostic for HCC) than among patients with normal AFP levels.[62, 63] Sensitivity and specificity of US in detecting HCC during follow-up of cirrhotic patients have been found to be 78% and 93% respectively.[64]

US examination is suggested every 6 months[62] or 3 months[61,63] together with serum AFP measurement. Only in patients with increased AFP values should the follow-up timing be shortened (perhaps every two months). The real impact of this policy has been refuted as the percentage of patients eligible for effective treatment remains low;[62] however, comparing two consecutive series of patients, one in a cross-section study, the second in a prospective study of cirrhotic patients, the number of small tumors detected was significantly higher in this second series even if the percentage of patients with multiple-diffuse HCC was the same in the two series. This fact probably reflects the clinical expression of two forms of HCC: the unicentric and the multicentric. In any case the increased number of small HCCs allowed a higher percentage of patients to undergo a potentially curative treatment,[65] confirming previous data.[66]

A similar policy concerns patients who undergo a treatment with curative intent and with an effective result. The percentage of HCC recurrence of patients surgically treated or receiving percutaneous treatment such as percutaneous alcohol injection or radiofrequency thermal ablation ranges between 80% and 100% at five years.[67, 68]

CONCLUSION

The diagnostic accuracy of US for hepatocellular carcinoma can be considered very high; the exam is useful for early detection of the tumor, and its characterization; it can be easily and efficiently repeated. Obviously the tumor can be biopsied under US guidance. Moreover US is the first step for tumor staging, but in this field other imaging techniques are necessary. Finally, US can be considered the ideal method for prospective study of patients at risk of developing HCC.

REFERENCES

1. Kudo M, Hirasa M, Takakuwa H *et al.* Small hepatocellular carcinomas in chronic liver disease: detection with SPECT. *Radiology* 1986; **159**: 697-703
2. Sheu JC, Sung JL, Chen DS *et al.* Ultrasonography of small hepatic tumors using high-resolution linear-array real-time instruments. *Radiology* 1984; **150**: 797-802
3. Choi BI, Park JH, Kim BH, Kim SH, Han MC, Kim CW. Small hepatocellular carcinoma: detection with sonography, computed tomography (CT), angiography and lipiodol-CT. *Br J Radiol* 1989; **62**: 897-903.
4. Takayasu K, Moriyama N, Muramatsu Y *et al.* The diagnosis of small hepatocellular carcinomas: efficacy of various imaging procedures in 100 patients. *AJR* 1990; **155**: 49-54
5. Matsui O, Itai Y. Diagnosis of primary liver cancer by computed tomography. In Tobe T, Kameda H, Okudaira M *et al*, eds. *Primary liver cancer in Japan*. Tokyo : Springer-Verlag, 1992: p 132
6. Honda H, Onitsuka H, Murakami J *et al.* Characteristic findings of hepatocellular carcinoma: an evaluation with comparative study of US, CT, and MRI. *Gastrointest Radiol* 1992; **17**: 245-249
7. Buscarini L, Fornari F, Canaletti R *et al.* Diagnostic aspects and follow-up of 174 cases of hepatocellular carcinoma: second report. *Oncology* 1991; **48**: 26-30
8. Ricca Rosellini S, Arienti V, Nanni O *et al.* Hepatocellular carcinoma. Prognostic factors and survival analysis in 135 Italian patients. *J Hepatol* 1992; **16**: 66-72
9. Clarke MP, Kane RA, Steele G *et al.* Prospective comparison of preoperative imaging and intraoperative ultrasonography in the detection of liver tumors. *Surgery* 1989; **106**: 849-855
10. Lafortune M, Madore F, Patriquin H, Breton G. Segmental anatomy of the liver: a sonographic approach to the Couinaud nomenclature. *Radiology* 1991; **181**: 443-448
11. Scott Gazelle G, Haaga JR. Hepatic neoplasms: surgically relevant segmental anatomy and imaging techniques. *AJR* 1992; **158**: 1015-1018
12. Utsonomiya T, Matsumata T, Adachi E, Honda H, Sugimachi K. Limitations of current preoperative liver imaging techniques for intrahepatic metastatic nodules of hepatocellular carcinoma. *Hepatology* 1992; **16**: 694-701
13. Miller WJ, Federle MP, Campbell WL. Diagnosis and staging of hepatocellular carcinoma: comparison of CT and sonography in 36 liver transplanted patients. *AJR* 1991; **157**: 303-306
14. Dodd III GD, Miller WJ, Baron RL, Skoinick ML, Campbell WL. Detection of malignant tumors in end-stage cirrhotic livers: efficacy of sonography as a screening technique. *AJR* 1992; **159**: 727-733

15. Rizzi PM, Kane PA, Ryder SD *et al.* Accuracy of radiology in detection of hepatocellular carcinoma before liver transplantation. *Gastroenterology* 1994; **107**: 1425-1429

16. Tanaka S, Kitamura T, Ahshima A *et al.* Diagnostic accuracy of ultrasonography for hepatocellular carcinoma. *Cancer* 1986; **58**: 344-347

17. Nagasue N, Yukaya H, Ogawa Y, Sasaki Y, Chang YC, Niimi K. Clinical experience with 118 hepatic resections for hepatocellular carcinoma. *Surgery* 1986; **99**: 694-702

18. Yoshida T, Matsue H, Okazaki MD, Yoshino M. Ultrasonographic differentiation of hepatocellular carcinoma from metastatic liver cancer. *J Clin Ultrasound* 1987; **15**: 431-437

19. Choi BI, Kim CW, Han MC *et al.* Sonographic characteristics of small hepatocellular carcinoma. *Gastrointest Radiol* 1989; **14**: 255-261

20. Kanno T, Kurioka N, Kim S *et al.* Implications of hypoechoic lesions in small hepatocellular carcinoma. *Gastroenterol Jpn* 1989; **24**: 528-534

21. Yoshikawa J, Matsui O, Takashima T *et al.* Fatty metamorphosis in hepatocellular carcinoma: radiologic features in 10 cases. *AJR* 1988; **151**: 717-720

22. Tanaka S, Kitamura T, Imaoka S, Sasaki Y, Taniguchi H, Ishiguro S. Hepatocellular carcinoma: sonographic and histologic correlation. *AJR* 1983; **140**: 701-707

23. Ros PR, Murphy BJ, Buck JL, Olmedilla G, Goodman Z. Encapsulated hepatocellular carcinoma: radiologic findings and pathologic correlation. *Gastrointest Radiol* 1990; **15**: 233-237

24. Sakaguchi S, Tohara K, Oka Y. Ultrasonographic diagnosis of hepatocellular carcinoma. In Tobe T, Kameda H, Okudaira M *et al*, eds. *Primary liver cancer in Japan*. Tokyo: Springer-Verlag, 1992: p 115

25. Tanaka S, Kitamura T, Nakanishi K, Okuda S, Kojima J, Fujimoto I. Recent advances in ultrasonographic diagnosis of hepatocellular carcinoma. *Cancer* 1989; **63**: 1313-1317

26. Subramanyam BR, Balthazar EJ, Hilton S, Lefleur RS, Horii SC, Raghavendra BN. Hepatocellular carcinoma with venous invasion. Sonographic-angiographic correlation. *Radiology* 1984; **150**: 793-796

27. Lim JH, Auh YH. Hepatocellular carcinoma presenting only as portal venous tumour thrombosis: CT demonstration. *J Comput Assist Tomogr* 1992; **16**: 103-106

28. Dodd III GD, Carr BI. Percutaneous biopsy of portal vein thrombus: a new staging technique for hepatocellular carcinoma. *AJR* 1993; **161**: 229-233

29. Ebara M, Ohto M, Shinagawa T *et al.* Natural history of minute hepatocellular carcinoma smaller than three centimeters complicating cirrhosis. A study in 22 patients. *Gastroenterology* 1986; **90**: 289-298

30. Sheu JC, Sung JL, Chen DS *et al.* Growth rate of asymptomatic hepatocellular carcinoma and its clinical implications. *Gastroenterology* 1985; **89**: 259-266

31. Cottone M, Virdone R, Fusco G *et al.* Asymptomatic hepatocellular carcinoma in Child's A cirrhosis. A comparison of natural history and surgical treatment. *Gastroenterology* 1989; **96**: 1566-1571

32. Jones EC, Chezmar JL, Nelson RC, Bernardino ME. The frequency and significance of small (<15 mm) hepatic lesions detected by CT. *AJR* 1992; **158**: 535-539

33. Melato M, Laurino L, Mucli E, Valente M, Okuda K. Relationship between cirrhosis, liver cancer, and hepatic metastases. An autopsy study. *Cancer* 1989; **64**: 455-459

34. Ikeda K, Saitoh S, Koida I *et al.* Imaging diagnosis of small hepatocellular carcinoma. *Hepatology* 1994; **20**: 82-87

35. Di Stasi M, Caturelli E, De Sio I, Salmi A, Buscarini E, Buscarini L. Natural history of focal nodular hyperplasia of the liver: an ultrasound study. *J Clin Ultrasound* 1996;**24**:345-350

36. Livraghi T, Belli P, Garavaglia GM, Matricardi L, Torzilli G, Vettori C. Focal nodular hyperplasia of the liver: diagnostic role of smear cytology vs microhistology following ultrasound-guided fine needle biopsy. *J Intervent Radiol* 1993; **8**: 155-158.

37. Buscarini L, Fornari F, Civardi G, Di Stasi M, Buscarini E, Cavanna L. Laparoscopy integrates ultrasound and ultrasound guided biopsy for diagnosis of benign liver tumors. *Acta Endoscop* 1993; **23**: 27-36

38. Cherqui D, Tantawi B, Alon R *et al.* Intrahepatic cholangiocarcinoma. Results of aggressive surgical management. *Arch Surg* 1995; **130**: 1073-1078.

39. Soyer P, Bluemke DA, Reichle R *et al.* Imaging of intrahepatic cholangiocarcinoma: 1. Peripheral cholangiocarcinoma. *AJR* 1995; **165**: 1427-1431.

40. Subramanyam BR, Raghavendra N, Blthazar EJ *et al.* Ultrasonic features of cholangiocarcinoma. *J Ultrasound Med* 1984; **3**: 405-408

41. Choi BI, Lee JH, Han MC, Kim SH, Yi JG, Kim CW. Hilar cholangiocarcinoma: comparative study with sonography and CT. *Radiology* 1989; **172**: 689-692

42. Wibulpolprasert B, Dhiensiri T. Peripheral cholangiocarcinoma: sonographic evaluation. *J Clin Ultrasound* 1992;**20**: 303-314

43. Araki T, Suda K, Sekikawa T, Ishii Y, Hihara T, Kachi K. Portal venous tumour thrombosis associated with gastric adenocarcinoma. *Radiology* 1990; **174**: 811-814

44. Di Stasi M, Sbolli G, Fornari F *et al.* Extrahepatic primary malignant neoplasms associated with hepatocellular carcinoma: high occurrence of B cell tumors. *Oncology* 1994; **51**: 459-464

45. Cavanna L, Civardi G, Fornari F *et al.* Simultaneous relapse of liver cell carcinoma and non-Hodgkin's lymphoma in the liver. Report of a case with diagnosis by ultrasonically guided aspiration biopsy. *Acta Cytol* 1994; **38**: 451-454.

46. Summary of recommendations developed by an international working party, supported by the World Congress of Gastroenterology, Los Angeles, 1994. Terminology of chronic hepatitis, hepatic allograft rejection, and nodular lesions of the liver. *Am J Gastroenterol* 1994; **89**: S177-S181

47. Arakawa M, Kage M, Sugihara S, Nakashima T, Suenaga M, Okuda K. Emergence of malignant lesions within an adenomatous hyperplastic nodule in a cirrhotic liver. Observations in five cases. *Gastroenterology* 1986; **91**: 198-208.

48. Winter III TC, Takayasu K, Muramatsu Y *et al.* Early advanced hepatocellular carcinoma: evaluation of CT and MR appearance with pathologic correlation. *Radiology* 1994; **192**: 379-387

49. Matsui O, Kadoya M, Kameyama T *et al.* Adenomatous hyperplastic nodules in the cirrhotic liver: differentiation from hepatocellular carcinoma with MRI imaging. *Radiology* 1989; **173**: 123-126

50. Garbagnati F, Spreafico C, Marchiano' A, Salvetti M, Segura C, Piragine G. Staging of hepatocellular carcinoma by ultrasonography, computed tomography, and angiography: the role of CT combined with arterial portography. *Gastrointest Radiol* 1991; **16**: 225-228

51. Yuki K, Hirohashi S, Sakamoto M, Kanai T, Shimosato Y. Growth and spread of hepatocellular carcinoma. A review of 240 consecutive autopsy cases. *Cancer* 1990; **66**: 2174-2179

52. The Liver Cancer Study Group of Japan. Primary liver cancer in Japan. Clinicopathologic features and results of surgical treatment. *Ann Surg* 1990; **211**: 277-287

53. Mathieu D, Guinet C, Bouklia-Hassane A, Vasile N. Hepatic vein involvement in hepatocellular carcinoma. *Gastrointest Radiol* 1988; **13**: 55-60

54. Calvet X, Bruix J, Brù C *et al*. Natural history of hepatocellular carcinoma in Spain. Five year's experience in 249 cases. *J Hepatol* 1990; **10**: 311-317

55. Trevisani F, D'Intino PE, Caraceni P *et al*. Etiologic factors and clinical presentation of hepatocellular carcinoma. Differences between cirrhotic and noncirrhotic Italian patients. *Cancer* 1995; **75**: 2220-2232

56. Dodd III GD, Memel DS, Baron RL, Eichner L, Santiguida LA. Portal vein thrombosis in patients with cirrhosis: does sonographic detection of intrathrombus flow allow differentiation of benign and malignant thrombus? *AJR* 1995; **165**: 573-577

57. Chua SO, Chiang CW, Lee YS, Liaw YF, Chang CH, Hung JS. Echocardiographic findings of mobile atrial hepatocellular carcinoma. Report of five cases. *J Ultrasound Med* 1989; **8**: 347-352

58. Morimoto K, Matsui K, Hashimoto T *et al*. Intraatrial extension of hepatocellular carcinoma detected with ultrasound. *J Clin Ultrasound* 1986; **14**: 466-469

59. Kojiro M, Kawabata K, Kawano Y, Shirai F, Takemoto N, Nakashima T. Hepatocellular carcinoma presenting as intrabile duct tumour growth. A clinicopathologic study of 24 cases. *Cancer* 1982; **49**: 2144-2147.

60. Chen MF, Jan YY, Jeng LB, Hwang TL, Wang CS, Chen SC. Obstructive jaundice secondary to ruptured hepatocellular carcinoma into the common bile duct. Surgical experiences of 20 cases. *Cancer* 1994; **73**: 1335-1340

61. Oka H, Kurioka N, Kim K *et al*. Prospective study of early detection of hepatocellular carcinoma in patients with cirrhosis. *Hepatology* 1990; **12**: 680-687.

62. Colombo M, De Franchis R, Del Ninno E *et al*. Hepatocellular carcinoma in Italian patients with cirrhosis. *N Engl J Med* 1991; **325**: 675-680

63. Imberti D, Fornari F, Sbolli G, Squassante L, Buscarini L. Hepatocellular carcinoma in liver cirrhosis. A prospective study. *Scand J Gastroenterol* 1993; **28**: 540-544

64. Pateron D, Ganne N, Trinchet JC *et al*. Prospective study of screening for hepatocellular carcinoma in Caucasian patients with cirrhosis. *J Hepatol* 1994; **20**: 65-71

65. Buscarini L. Di Stasi M, Buscarini E *et al*. Clinical presentation, diagnostic work-up and therapeutic choices in two consecutive series of patients with hepatocellular carcinoma. *Oncology* 1996 ;**53**:204-209

66. Tanaka S, Kitamura T, Nakanishi K *et al*. Effectiveness of periodic checkup by ultrasonography for the early diagnosis of hepatocellular carcinoma. *Cancer* 1990; **66**: 2210-2214

67. Livraghi T, Giorgio A, Marin G *et al*. Hepatocellular carcinoma and cirrhosis in 746 patients: long-term results of percutaneous ethanol injection *Radiology* 1995; **197**: 101-108.

68. Rossi S, Di Stasi M, Buscarini E *et al*. Percutaneous radiofrequency interstitial thermal ablation in the treatment of liver cancer, *AJR* 1996;**167**:759-768

9

Ultrasonography: Doppler

S Tanaka

Thanks to recent improvements in the Doppler equipment, color Doppler US now provides useful information for the differential diagnosis of liver tumors.

The Doppler signal from the tumor blood flow was first detected for breast cancer by the duplex Doppler method.[1] Regarding liver tumors, Taylor *et al*. reported that a Doppler shift of more than 5 kHz, associated with a large pressure gradient due to arteriovenous shunting, was observed in HCC but not in other liver tumors.[2] However, detection of the shunting site by the duplex Doppler method was very difficult, because with this method the course of the blood stream cannot be visualized on the B-mode image.

The color Doppler flow imaging technique was developed by Namekawa *et al*,[3], and it was first applied to HCC by Sukigara *et al*.[4] More recently, owing to advances in the color Doppler equipment, many reports have been published concerning color Doppler diagnosis of liver tumors.[5-10]

EQUIPMENT AND TECHNIQUE

Color Doppler US is a noninvasive method for examining hemodynamic characteristics under physiologic conditions. It was initially employed in hemodynamic studies of the heart and systemic circulation. Recently, technical improvements have permitted the color display of even a relatively slow blood flow. As a result, color Doppler US has been widely utilized in the study of the abdominal organs and tumor characterization. Unlike angiography, in which a viscous contrast medium is injected directly into the blood vessel concerned, color Doppler flow imaging has the outstanding feature of being able to depict the blood flow in the physiologic state. Furthermore, since the procedure is completely noninvasive, it can be repeated, permitting frequent follow-up observations.

According to a histopathologic study,[11] tumor vessels in HCC smaller than 3 cm do not exceed 200 μm in diameter. Under favorable conditions, tumor vessels of even less than 200 μm in size can be adequately visualized by color Doppler flow imaging. However, color Doppler US has many limitations, such as low sensitivity for fine and slow blood flows, noise caused by tissue movement, and so on. Some countermeasures have been attempted. For example, the attenuation in deep areas has been reported to be com-pensated for by intravenous contrast agents,[12,13] and the sensitivity for blood flow perpendicular to the direction of the ultrasonic beam has been increased by use of power mode imaging.[14,15]

COLOR DOPPLER FLOW IMAGING

Velocity mode

Blood flows are visualized in color on the ordinary US. The direction and the velocity of the blood flow are indicated by differences in the color. For example, the blood flow approaching the probe is shown in red to yellow, while the blood flow going away from the probe is depicted in blue to light blue, depending on the range of the Doppler shift.

Power mode

Blood flows are visualized in color on the ordinary US, the same as with the velocity mode. Compared with the velocity mode, slower and finer blood flows can be depicted in color and even blood flows which cross the ultrasound beam vertically can be visualized[14]. However, the direction of the blood flow cannot be distinguished, and the noise caused by tissue movement is greater than with the velocity mode.

Turbulence mode

The turbulent flow is indicated by differences in color. This mode is used mainly for the diagnosis of cardiovascular diseases.

Spectral Doppler analysis

The flow velocity pattern of a blood flow can be observed to adjust the cursor to the blood flow concerned, depicted in color, and fitting the angle bar to the direction of the blood flow.

Based on the flow velocity pattern, arterial pulsating flow, venous pulsating flow and constant flow can be differentiated. Some indices of the hemodynamics, such as the maximum velocity (V max.), pulsatility index (PI)(= maximum/mean velocity), resistive index (RI)(= maximum/minimum velocity), and acceleration index (AI), can be calculated, and there have been attempts to use these indices for the differential diagnosis of various tumors.[16,17]

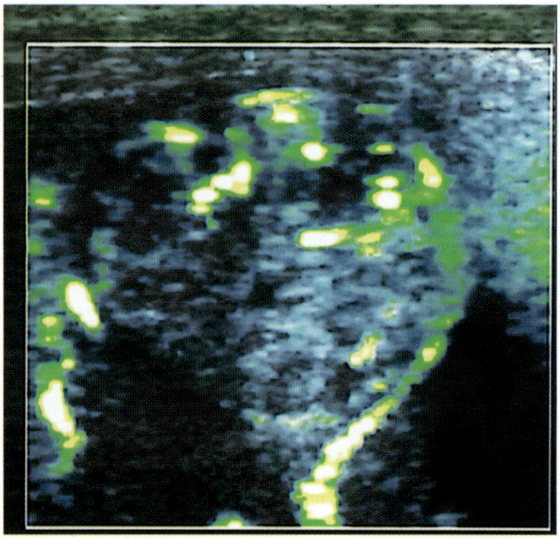

Figure 9.1 – Basket pattern of HCC. A vascular rich lesion of 25 mm in diameter is shown by the power mode imaging. The tumor area is colorfully visualized with abundant tumor vessels clinging along the periphery of the nodule and developing branches within it.

Contrast enhancement

Intravenous contrast agents for use in US are being developed. Some of them are reported to be effective in enhancing the sensitivity of color Doppler US for fine, slow blood flows and deeply-located blood flows.[12,13]

IMAGE FINDINGS

HCC is generally nourished by the hepatic artery, and hypervascularity is its characteristic finding on hepatic angiography. In color Doppler flow imaging as well, HCC is displayed as a vascular-rich region in comparison with the surrounding liver tissue. A basket pattern, which is a fine blood-flow network surrounding the tumor nodule (Fig. 9.1), and tumor vessels flowing into the tumor and branching within it (Fig. 9.2) are the characteristic findings of color Doppler flow imaging. These findings were reported to be observed in 16 (80%) of 20 HCCs, but not in any other liver tumors.[6] Nino-Murcia *et al.*[7] reported that, when taking internal vascularity as a positive finding for HCC, the sensitivity was high enough at 76%. However, this finding was also observed in one-third of metastatic liver tumors, so the specificity was only 69%.

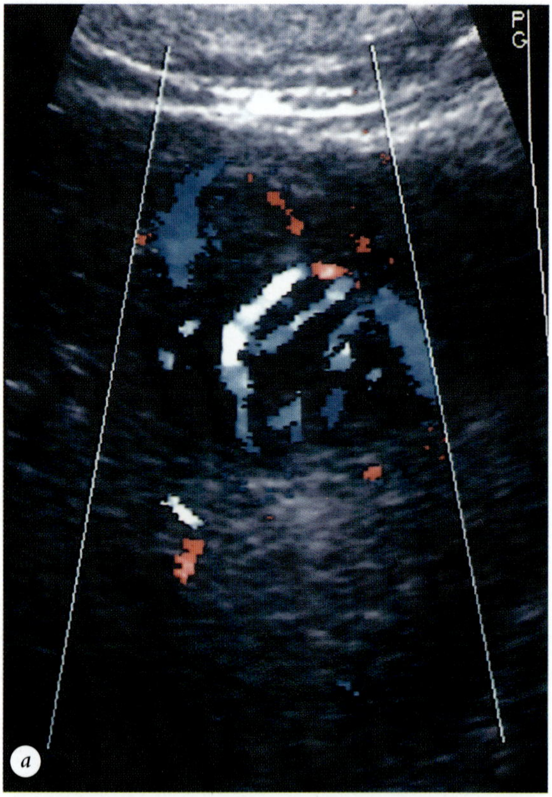

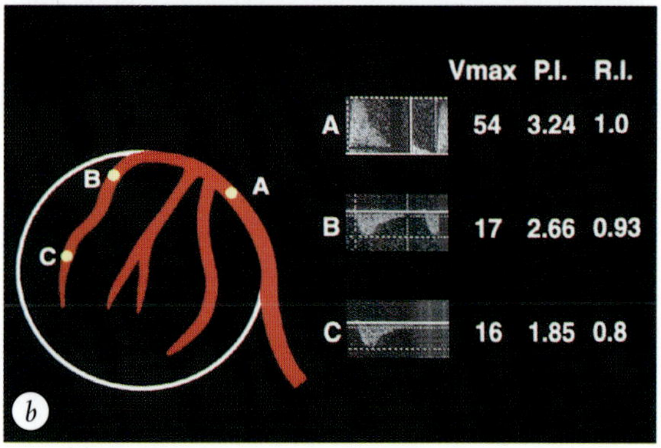

Figure 9.2 – Feeding artery of HCC.

a) A feeding artery, running into the nodule of 20 mm in diameter and branching, is shown in blue color by the velocity mode imaging.

b) The flow velocity pattern of this feeding artery shows the arterial pulsating flow pattern, and all the parameters, maximum velocity, pulsatility index and resistive index are decreasing after running into the nodule.

There have been reports of spectral Doppler analysis. Reinhold *et al.*[16] reported that, when employing Doppler shifts of 4.5 kHz or more as a positive finding for HCC, the specificity was as high as 95%. In their series, the sensitivity was also rather high at 70%, but the majority of the lesions were large HCCs (mean diameter 7.7 cm). Yasuhara *et al.*[17] reported that the distribution of histogram of the flow velocity pattern reflected the turbulent flow caused by the tumor involvement, and they found it to be useful for the differential diagnosis of liver tumors.

In general, typical HCC, especially when larger than 3 cm in diameter, is vascular-rich compared with the surrounding liver tissue, and is visualized as a colorful area with abundant tumor blood flows. Also, the decrease in the tumor vascularity which occurs after treatment of HCC can be used to evaluate the effectiveness of the therapy.

DIFFERENTIAL DIAGNOSIS

Small HCC and adenomatous hyperplastic nodule (AHN)

AHN is thought to be a precancerous lesion and it is the most confusing type of liver mass to differentiate from small HCC. It develops as a complication of liver cirrhosis, like HCC, and its sonographic appearance, a hypo-echoic ellipse without a halo or mosaic pattern, closely resembles that of small HCC. Accordingly the differentiation of small HCC from benign AHN is very important.

There is a report describing the differential diagnosis of these two kinds of lesion by color Doppler US. According to the report, the existence of a feeding artery (Fig. 9.2) and/or a draining portal vein (Fig. 9.3) was a positive finding for small HCC to be differentiated from AHN, and the accuracy of it was high, with 79% sensitivity and 100% specificity [8]. A draining portal vein is a low velocity constant-flow efferent tumor vessel continuing to the portal branch. On the basis of continuity, it is considered to be a branch of the portal vein, but it flows toward the liver hylus, the opposite direction to the normal portal flow. This finding indicates a pathological phenomenon and it is observed in cases without arterio-portal shunt. It is speculated that the outflow route from the sinusoid space to the hepatic venous system is blocked by some cause related to the tumor, thereby producing overflow into the portal system.[8]

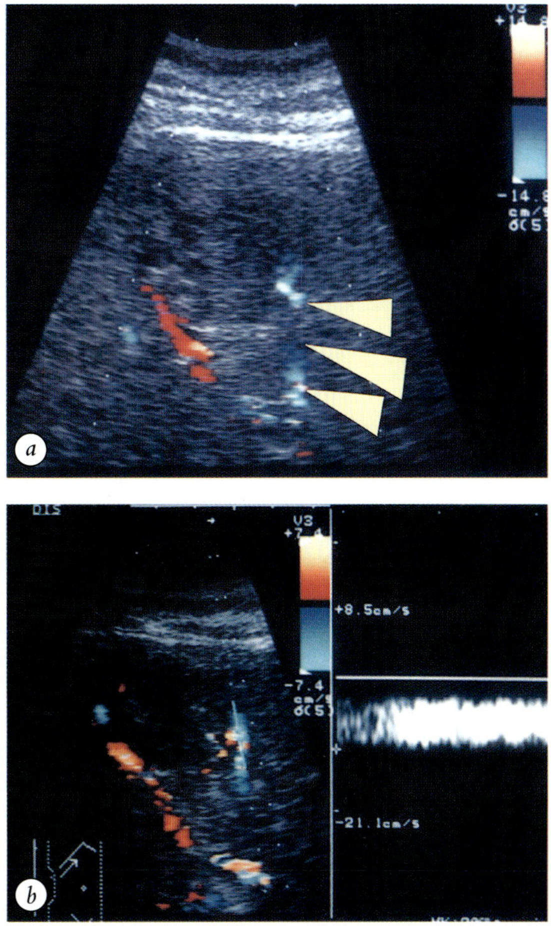

Figure 9. 3 – Draining portal vein of HCC.

a) Blood flow running out of the nodule of 25 mm in diameter, and flowing into a branch of right anterior portal vein is visualized with blue color (arrow heads) by the velocity mode imaging.

b) The flow velocity pattern of this blood flow shows a constant flow pattern .

Tumors located deep below the abdominal surface were excluded from that study. For the diagnosis of deeply-located HCC by color Doppler US, contrast enhancement is reported to be effective (Fig. 9.4) in increasing the sensitivity.[13]

There is always the risk that AHN may become cancerous, even when malignancy is initially ruled out by angiography and biopsy. Therefore, close follow-up observation by a non-invasive modality is

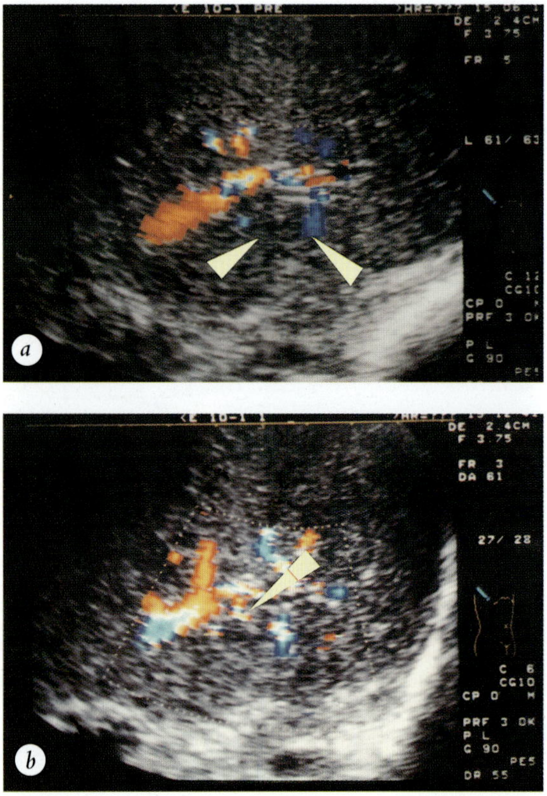

Figure 9.4 – Contrast enhancement of HCC. Pre-enhancement *a)*, blood flows are observed only the periphery of the 15 mm hypoechoic lesion (arrowheads). After injection of Levovist through cubital vein *b)*, a draining portal vein (arrowhead) flowing out of the tumor and flowing into the right posterior superior branch of the portal vein appeared.

necessary (Fig. 9.5). Detection of newly-developed arterial tumor vessels by close observation with color Doppler US provides useful information for the early diagnosis of HCC.[8]

Hemangioma

The tumor blood flow observed in hepatic hemangiomas is not as abundant as that in HCC. In almost half of hemangiomas, color Doppler flow imaging shows a spot pattern, that is, dots or patches in the central region of the tumor nodule (Fig. 9.6). This finding is detected mainly in cases showing extensive pooling in the central region of the tumor on hepatic angiography.[6] However, another report[7] described tumor vascularity in only one of 12 hemangiomas. A high-velocity blood flow or high-degree Doppler shift are reported to be rare in hemangioma.[10, 16]

Metastatic liver tumor

When a large number of metastatic cancer foci are scattered in the liver, the intrahepatic portal branches are generally dilated and meander around the tumor nodule without branching within tumor nodules (Fig. 9.6). This is referred to as a detouring pattern.[6] Metastatic liver tumors are not as vascular-rich as HCCs in general. However, depending on the properties of the original tumor, some of them show internal vascularity on the peripheral area of the nodule in color Doppler US (Fig. 9.7). Nino-Murcia *et al.*[7] reported that intra-tumoral blood flow was detected in one-third of metastatic liver tumor cases.

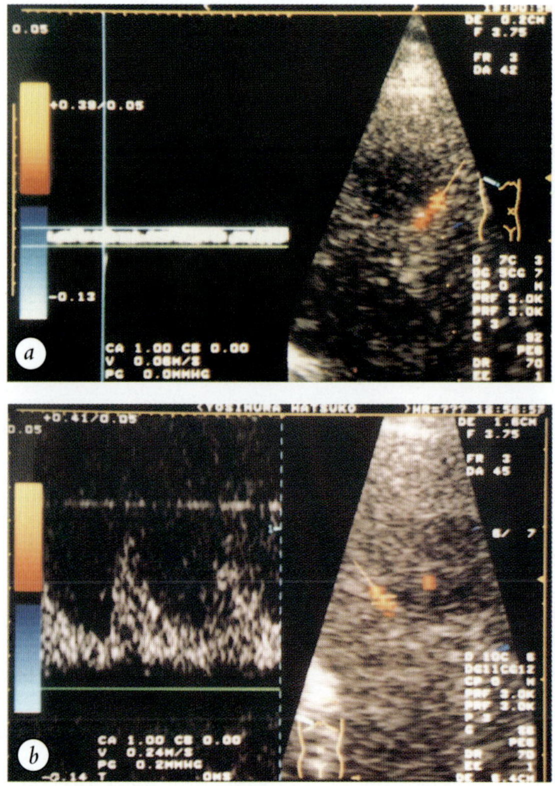

Figure 9.5 – Follow-up by color Doppler US.

a) Only constant flows were shown at the periphery of the 13 mm hypoechoic nodule, when the nodule was first detected on the cirrhotic liver. Hepatic angiography reveals no focal lesion and the FNB shows no malignancy.

b) 13 months later, the size of the nodule showed no change by ordinal US, though a feeding vessel flowing into the nodule appeared and the blood flow at the periphery of the tumor changed from constant flow to arterial pulsating flow. Detailed examination was performed again and an early HCC within AHN was surgically resected.

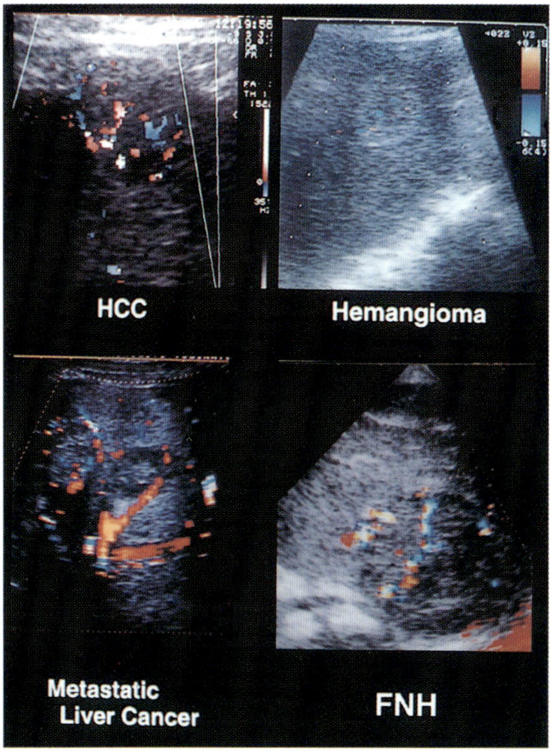

Figure 9.6 – Characteristic color Doppler findings of liver tumors HCC: Vascular-rich lesion compared with the surrounding. liver, Hemangioma: Spot pattern, Multiple metastases: Detouring pattern and FNH: Spoke wheel pattern.

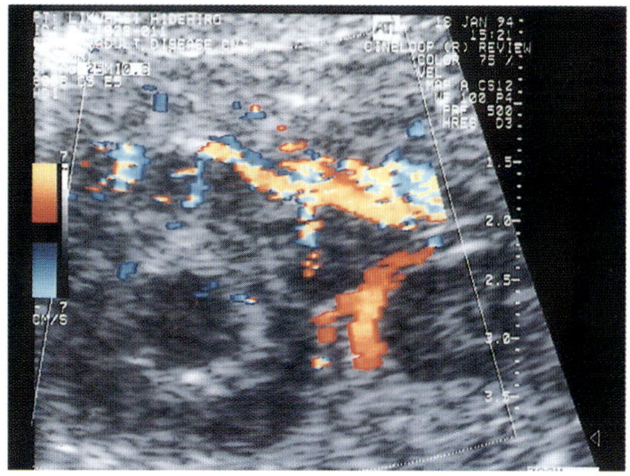

Figure 9.7 – Metastatic liver tumor from stomach. A 25 mm tumor nodule with central liquefactive necrosis is observed. Tumor vessels are distributed to the peripheral area of the nodule.

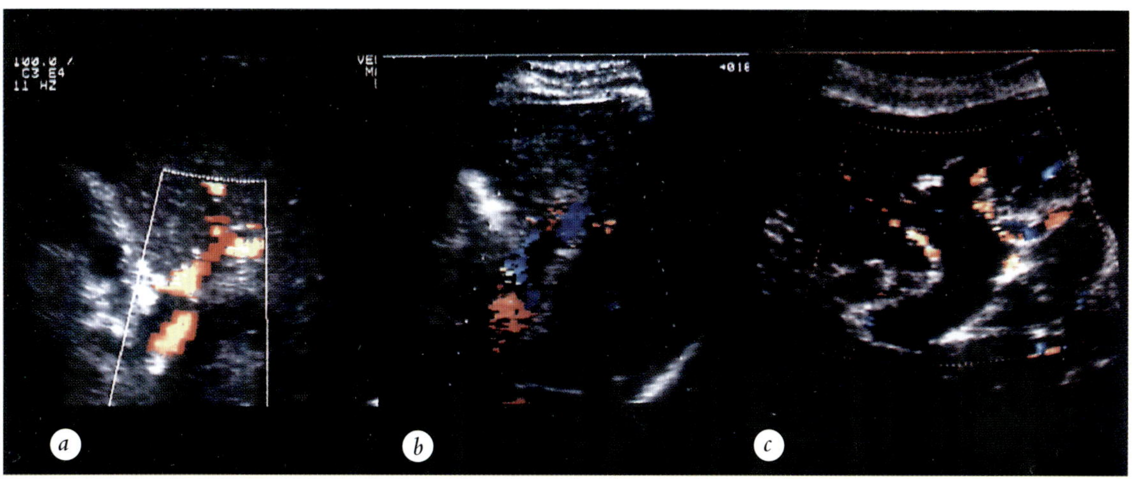

Figure 9.8 – Staging of portal tumor embolus accompanied HCC. Along with the stage of the tumor involvement, findings of *a)* a simple color defect area with normal flow direction, *b)* a turbulent flow due to the portal flow disturbance, *c)* complete obstruction of portal flow with the enhancement of the hepatic arterial flow along the portal vein, are shown.

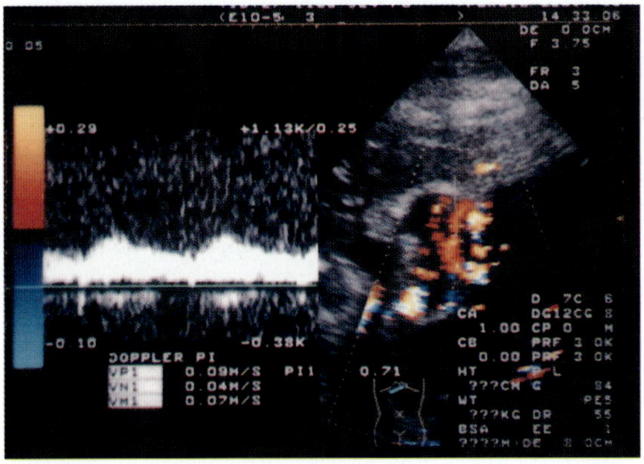

Figure 9.9 – Arterial pulsating flow within portal tumor embolus. The low velocity arterial flow is observed within the embolus (with contrast enhancement). This finding, comparable to the thread and streaks sign shown on the hepatic angiography is a specific finding for malignant embolus.

Using power mode imaging, internal vascularity was expected to be visualized more often.

Focal nodular hyperplasia (FNH)

FNH is characterized by a spoke wheel pattern with blood vessels running radially and rather straight from the center to the periphery of the tumor (Fig. 9.6). Kudo *et al.* reported a case in which this particular pattern was observed.[18] Golli *et al.* reported central spots with pulsating flow in 13 of 19 FNHs.[19]

Portal tumor embolism and benign thrombosis

Portal tumor embolism often accompanies advanced HCC. The characteristic color Doppler findings of portal tumor thrombus are as follows. In the early stage (Fig. 9.8a), the diameter of the portal vein increases to maintain the blood flow. At this stage, tumor embolus appears as a defect area of color with the portal flow in normal direction. With the growth of the tumor thrombus (Fig. 9.8b), the portal flow becomes impaired and turbulence appears. With further growth (Fig. 9.8c), the portal flow is completely obstructed, and the arterial flow along the portal vein accentuated. Also the slow and fine arterial flow indicating the thread and streaks sign seen in hepatic angiography appeared within tumor embolus (Fig.9.9). This finding of arterial flow within embolus suggests a diagnosis of malignant thrombus, not a benign one, accompanied by inflammation or bleeding[20, 21].

Accurate evaluation of impairment of the portal blood flow makes it possible to conduct effective therapy for HCC.

When the disturbance of the portal blood flow continues, collateral routes toward the liver are usually formed besides the original portal vein. When extensive collateral blood flow routes are formed, there is a characteristic image of cavernous transformation, as if the strings were knitted together along the obstructed portal vein.

REFERENCES

1. Burns PN, Halliwell M, Webb AJ, Wells PNT. Ultrasonic Doppler studies of the breast. *Ultrasound Med Biol* 1982; **8**: 127-143
2. Taylor KJW, Ramos I, Morses SS, Fortune KL, Hammers L, Taylor CR. Focal liver masses: differential diagnosis with pulsed Doppler US. *Radiology* 1987; **164**: 643-647
3. Namekawa K, Kasai C, Tsukamoto M, Koyano A. Imaging of blood flow using auto correlation. *Ultrasound Med Biol* 1982; **8** [suppl 1]: 138
4. Sukigara M, Takamoto S, Komazaki T, *et al.* Observation of the hepatoma by the real-time two dimensional echography: its clinical significance and prospect (English abst.). *Acta Hepatol Jpn* 1985; **26**: 747-752
5. Merritt CRB. Doppler color flow imaging. *J Clin Ultrasound* 1987;**15**: 591-597
6. Tanaka S, Kitamra T, Fujita M, Nakanishi K, Okuda S. Color Doppler flow imaging of liver tumors. *AJR* 1990; **154**: 509-514
7. Nino-Murcia M, Ralls PW, Jeffrey RB, Johnson M. Color flow Doppler characterization of focal hepatic lesions. *AJR* 1992; **159**: 1195-1197
8. Tanaka S, Kitamra T, Fujita M, Kasugai H, Inoue A, Ishiguro S. Small hepatocellular carcinoma : differentiation from adenomatous hyper plastic nodule with color Doppler flow imaging. *Radiology* 1992; **182**: 161-165
9. Shimamoto K, Sakuma S, Ishigaki T, Ishiguti T, Itoh S, Fukatsu H. Hepatocellular carcinoma: evaluation with color Doppler US and MR imaging. *Radiology* 1992; **182**:149-153
10. Numata K, Tanaka K, Mitsui K Morimoti M, Inoue S, Yonezawa H. Flow characteristics of hepatic tumors at color Doppler sonography: correlation with arteriographic findings. *AJR* 1993; **160**: 515-521
11. Edamitsu O. Pathomorphologic study on tumor vessels of hepatocellular carcinoma (English Abstract). *Acta Hepatologica Jpn* 1992; **33**: 15-20
12. Goldberg BB, Hilpert PL, Burns PN, *et al.* Hepatic tumors : signal enhancement at Doppler US after intravenous injection of a contrast agent. *Radiology* 1990; **177**: 713-717

13. Tanaka S, Kitamra T, Yoshioka F, *et al.* Effectiveness of galactose-based intravenous contrast medium on color Doppler sonography of deeply located hepatocellular carcinoma. *Ultrasound Med Biol* 1995; **21**: 157-160

14. Jain SP, Fan PH, Philpot EF, *et al.* Influence of various instrument settings on the flow information derived from the power mode. *Ultrasound Med Biol.* 1991; **17**: 49-54

15. Rubin JM, Bude RO, Carson PL, Bree RL, Adler RS. Power Doppler US: a potentially useful alternative to mean frequency-based color Doppler US. *Radiology* 1994; **190**: 853-856.

16. Reinhold C, Hammers L, Taylor CR, Quedens-Case CL, Holland CK, Taylor KJW. Characterization of focal hepatic lesions with duplex sonography: findings in 198 patients. *AJR* 1995; **164**: 1131-1135.

17. Yasuhara K, Kimura K, Ohto M, *et al.* Pulsed Doppler in the diagnosis of small liver tumors. *Br J Radiol* 1988; **61**: 898-902.

18. Kudo M, Tomita S, Minowa K, *et al.* Color Doppler flow imaging of hepatic nodular hyperplasia. *J Ultrasound Med* 1992; **11**: 553-557.

19. Golli M, Mathieu D, Anglade MC, Cherqui D, Vasile N, Rahmouni A. Focal nodular hyperplasia of the liver: value of color Doppler US in association with MR imaging. *Radiology* 1993; **187**: 113-117.

20. Tanaka K, Numata K, Okazaki H Nakamura S, Inoue S, Takamura Y. Diagnosis of portal vein thrombosis in patients with hepatocellular carcinoma : efficacy of color Doppler sonography compared with angiography. *AJR* 1993; **160**: 1279-1283.

21. Dodd GD, Memel DS, Baron RL, Eichner L, Santiguida LA. Portal vein thrombosis in patients with cirrhosis. *AJR* 1995; **165**: 573-577.

10

Ultrasonography: Intraoperative

K Kubota and M Makuuchi

In the era when intraoperative ultrasound (IOUS) was not available for hepatic surgery, it was difficult to determine the location of an invisible or impalpable tumor and the extent of resection required during hepatectomy.[1] However, since IOUS was introduced for abdominal surgery, the examination has also been found to yield important information for performing hepatectomy.[2-6] In this chapter, the utility of IOUS when performing hepatectomy for hepatocellular carcinomas (HCCs) is described from the diagnostic and surgical viewpoints.

APPLICATION OF INTRAOPERATIVE ULTRASOUND TO DIAGNOSIS

Liver scanning

Preoperatively, surgeons should scan the liver themselves to determine the number and location of tumors and grasp the three-dimensional vascular structure of the liver; this makes the IOUS findings more comprehensive. We routinely employ a convex finger-grip probe with a 7.5-MHz transducer (Fig. 10.1), which is connected to a real-time scanning system. Scanning of the liver should be performed before dissecting the ligaments, such as the coronary or falciform ligaments, as such dissection occasionally results in air entering the dissection plane, which makes it difficult to observe main tumors, detect small lesions and visualize the portal and hepatic venous branches. First, the liver should be scanned as follows:

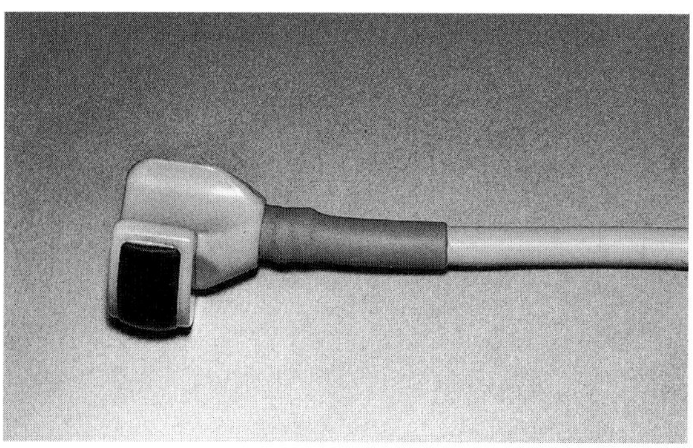

Figure 10.1 – Finger grip intraoperative ultrasound probe with a 7.5-MHz transducer, which is connected to a real-time B-mode scanning system (Aloka SSD 650).

1. Trace the right, middle and left hepatic veins and their tributaries and check them for tumor thrombi.
2. Trace all the intrahepatic portal venous branches and check them for tumor thrombi.
3. Examine the liver parenchyma for a main tumor, intrahepatic metastatic lesions and other primary lesions.
4. Confirm the three-dimensional relationship between the tumor and the portal and hepatic venous branches.

If this scan suggests that hepatectomy is possible, the falciform, bilateral coronary and triangular ligaments, and the bare area should be dissected to mobilize the liver. Then, IOUS should be repeated, paying particular attention to the following points:

1. Check for lesions in the liver, especially in the posterosuperior area.
2. Reconfirm the three-dimensional relationship between the tumor and the portal and hepatic venous branches.
3. Decide the most appropriate extent of hepatectomy in the light of both curability and liver function.

After mobilization of the liver, although the lesions can be observed from the ventral, visceral, dorsal and diaphragmatic surfaces, the correct orientation for IOUS may occasionally be difficult to achieve if the surgeon is inexperienced and/or unskilled.

Determination of tumor location

Although tumor locations can be evaluated preoperatively by diagnostic imaging modalities, such as US, computed tomography (CT), magnetic resonance imaging and angiography, impalpable or invisible tumors cannot always be localized intraoperatively on the basis of preoperative information. IOUS, however, can visualize not only an impalpable or invisible tumor, but also the portal and hepatic venous branches. The location of a tumor can be determined based on the relationship between the tumor and the portal and hepatic venous branches. First, the segment in which a tumor is located should be confirmed by scanning the hepatic veins and next, the portal venous branches should be traced to the tumor. The portal venous branches were mapped by Takayasu *et al.*[7] and have become the landmarks for

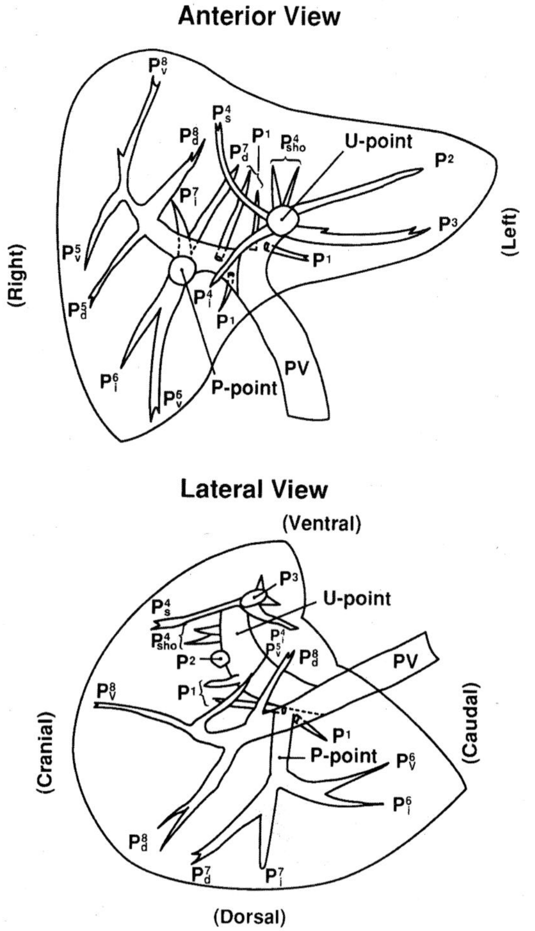

Figure 10.2 – Map of intrahepatic portal venous branches (Modified from ref. 7 with permission from the publisher). *a)* Anterior and *b)* lateral views of the liver. Superscripts refer to the eight Couinaud's subsegments and subscripts to the subsegmental branches named after their major feeding areas in the subsegments: v = ventral, d = dorsal, l = lateral, s = superior, and i = inferior areas, PV = portal vein, U-/P- point = umbilical/posterior point, sho = short branches.

deciding the resection area of the liver (Fig. 10.2). This scanning procedure contributes to determining the Couinaud's segment in which a tumor is located.

Diagnosis of tumors

Characteristic US features of HCCs include a mosaic pattern of internal echoes, posterior echo enhancement, a thin halo and lateral shadows.[8] However, several histological types of small tumor, such as HCCs (Fig. 10.3), cholangiocellular carcinomas, regenerative nodules, adenomatous hyperplasias, hemangiomas, adenomas and metastatic lesions (Fig. 10.4), may be detected by IOUS. When a tumor has a diameter greater than 2 cm, it may show US findings characteristic of a particular histological nature , whereas nodules smaller than this do not show characteristic US features and are usually visualized as hypoechoic lesions. US of 61 HCCs ranging from 2.1 to 5.0 cm in diameter revealed a mosaic pattern, posterior echo enhancement, a halo and lateral shadows in 77, 74, 48 and 23%, respectively, whereas these four US features were observed in 35, 18, 0 and 0%, respectively, of 17 HCCs smaller than 2.0 cm in diameter.[9] Such small tumors are usually detected by IOUS, but cannot always be diagnosed ultrasonographically, in which case, a core-needle biopsy is indicated.

Core-needle biopsy

The histologic nature of small nodules can be evaluated by histological examination of fine-needle aspiration and core-needle biopsy specimens. The latter technique usually yields larger samples for histological examination, helping to make an accurate diagnosis. First, the IOUS probe is placed on the liver surface where a lesion is clearly visualized and there are no major vessels between the surface and the lesion. Then, the lesion is punctured with a core needle using a free-hand technique under IOUS guidance. The needle is visualized clearly as a hyperechoic glittering line and the sampling site of the

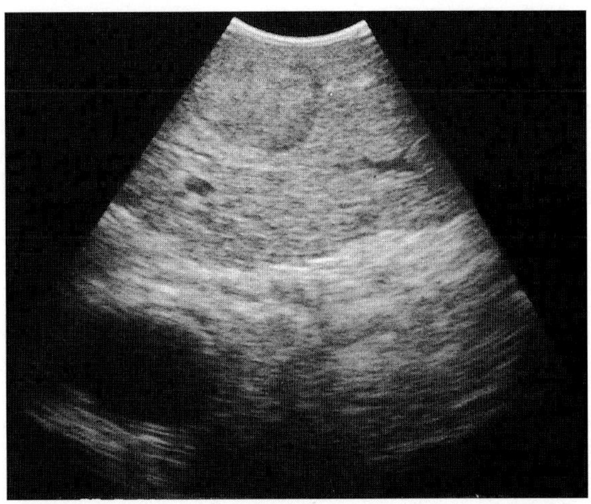

Figure 10.3 – Intraoperative ultrasonographic findings of a hepatocellular carcinoma about 2 cm in diameter. The tumor has a mosaic pattern internal echo with a halo (view from the ventral surface).

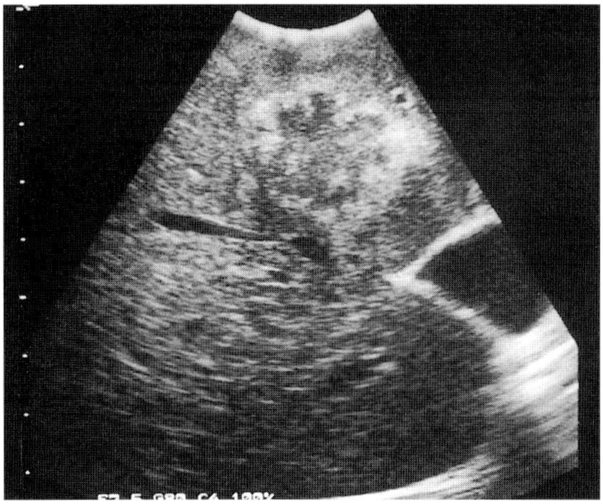

Figure 10.4 – Intraoperative ultrasonographic findings of a metastatic lesion from a colonic cancer. The metastatic lesion is hyperechoic with a bosselated margin (view from the visceral surface).

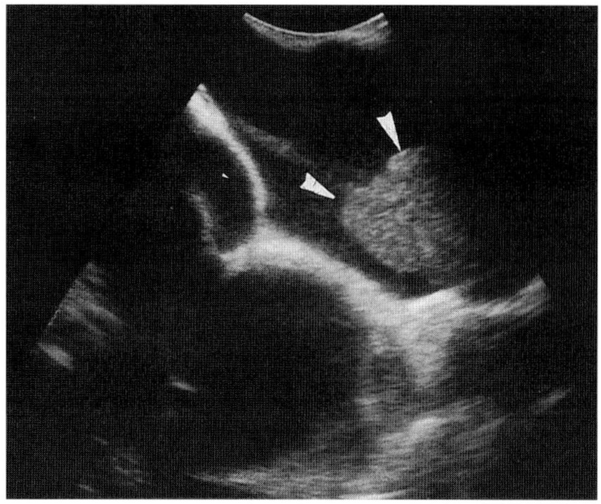

Figure 10.5 – Tumor thrombus in the inferior vena cava budding into the right atrium. The tumor thrombus (white arrows) buds into the lumen of the right atrium (view from the ventral surface).

lesion together with the surrounding liver parenchyma can be confirmed by the echo-free line.

Detection of tumor thrombi

Patients with advanced HCCs may develop tumor thrombi in the portal or hepatic venous branches or in the bile ducts and tumor thrombi in the hepatic venous branches may grow into the inferior vena cava (Fig. 10.5). Information about tumor thrombi is important for deciding operative procedures. Postmortem examinations of 61 patients with HCCs revealed that 56 (92%) had macroscopically detectable tumor thrombi: 33 (54%) had tumor thrombi in the portal venous branches, 22 (36%) had them in both the portal and hepatic venous branches and one (1.6%) had one only in the hepatic vein.[10] These data suggest that when there is no tumor thrombus in the portal vein, it is rare for one to be present in the hepatic vein. Of 188 patients with HCCs who underwent hepatectomies, 27 tumor thrombi were detected in 23 patients: 18 (67%) were detected by IOUS, seven (26%) by preoperative US and nine (33%) angiographically.[9] Furthermore, a tumor thrombus may develop in the bile duct and usually presents as jaundice or stone-like attacks.[11] Such tumor thrombi are usually visualized as isoechoic lesions with the main HCC occupying the lumen and their extent can be confirmed by IOUS. Although small tumor thrombi limited to the region around the tumor are often recognized in resected specimens, at present, IOUS is the best means for detecting them during surgery.

APPLICATION OF INTRA-OPERATIVE ULTRASOUND TO HEPATECTOMY

Extent of hepatectomy

In our department, the maximum extent of hepatectomy is determined preoperatively according to the flow chart shown in Fig. 10.6. However, the actual extent of hepatectomy is finally decided on the basis of the IOUS findings and the pathological diagnoses of small nodules, bearing in mind the patient's liver function. Most patients with HCCs have cirrhotic livers and consequently, limited resection is required, which can be confirmed by employing IOUS.

Orientation of hepatectomy

When hepatectomy was performed on the basis of anatomical knowledge without IOUS, HCCs were not always resected correctly in some situations: for example, a resected liver specimen did not include the tumor or a tumor was exposed on the dissected surface. Lau *et al.*[12] reported that in 8 of 51 patients whose parenchymal dissection lines were determined without IOUS, tumor infiltration was confirmed

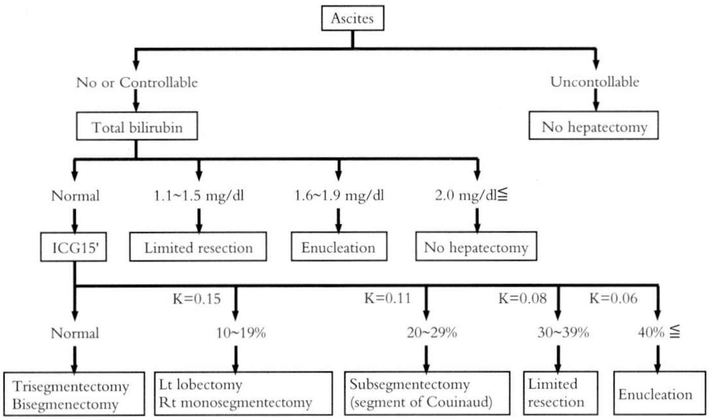

Figure 10.6 – Criteria for selection of operative procedures in patients with impaired liver function. The criteria consist of ascites, the serum total bilirubin value and the indocyanine green disappearance rate.

histologically on the resected margins, compared with none of 25 patients in whom the dissection line was determined using IOUS. Even if the tumor is invisible or impalpable, IOUS enables surgeons to decide the direction of the dissection plane and resect the tumor with adequate margins. However, it is questionable whether hepatectomy only with adequate margins is the optimal surgical procedure. We have developed "systematic subsegmentectomy" which involves limited, but adequate hepatectomy, that is resection of the portal area containing a HCC.[4]

Systematic subsegmentectomy

Intrahepatic spread via the portal vein is characteristic of HCCs. When a tumor thrombus in a portal venous branch grows toward the hepatic hilus, tumor cells are likely to spread to other areas along the portal venous branches (Fig. 10.7). Therefore, total resection of the portal area containing the tumor and tumor thrombus is necessary and can be substantiated using an IOUS-guided operative procedure termed "systematic subsegmentectomy" (Fig. 10.8).[4] First, the portal venous branches feeding the tumor are located by IOUS. Second, the point for ligating the portal venous branch is determined and then the distal point of the branch is punctured under IOUS guidance to enable 3-5 ml indigo carmine to be injected (Figs. 10.9 a and b), which stains the surface of the portal area containing the tumor and the stained area is marked by electrocautery. In order to prevent the dye regurgitating into other portal venous branches which should be preserved, the puncture point in the portal venous branch must be 1 to 2 cm distal from the ligation point and the speed of dye injection should be adjusted by observing the injected dye in the portal venous branch ultrasonographically. If possible, the tip of the needle

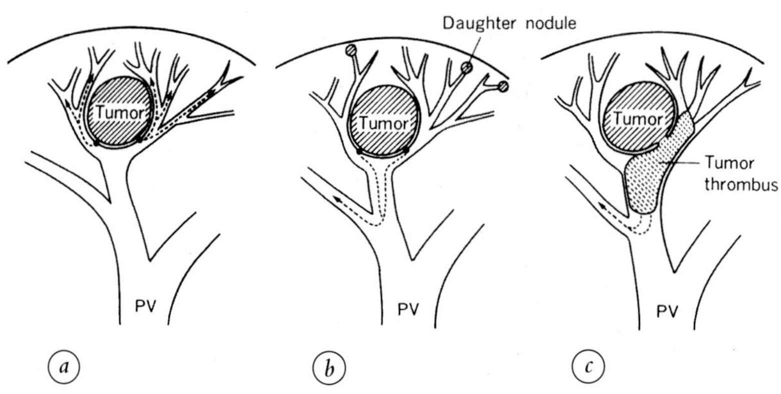

Figure 10.7 – Schema of hypothetical intrahepatic spreading of hepatocellular carcinoma.

a) Hepatocellular carcinoma grows expansively and invades the portal venous branches, PV= portal vein.

b) Intrahepatic metastatic lesions then grow at the distal end of the portal venous branch.

c) Hepatocellular carcinomas occasionally form tumor thrombi in the portal vein. Therefore, the ligation point of the portal vein should be as proximal as liver function permits.

(Reproduced from ref. 4 with permission from the publisher).

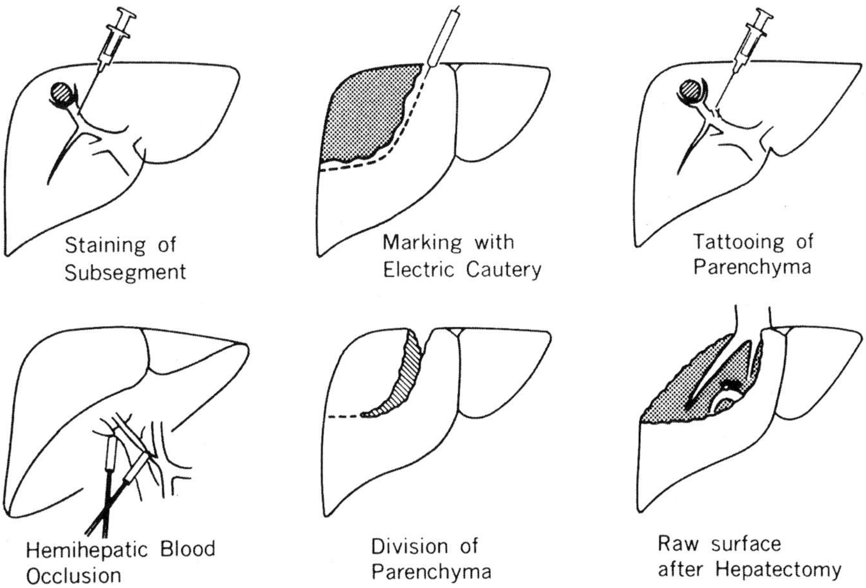

Figure 10.8 – Operative procedure for systematic subsegmentectomy. (Reproduced from ref. 4 with permission from the publisher).

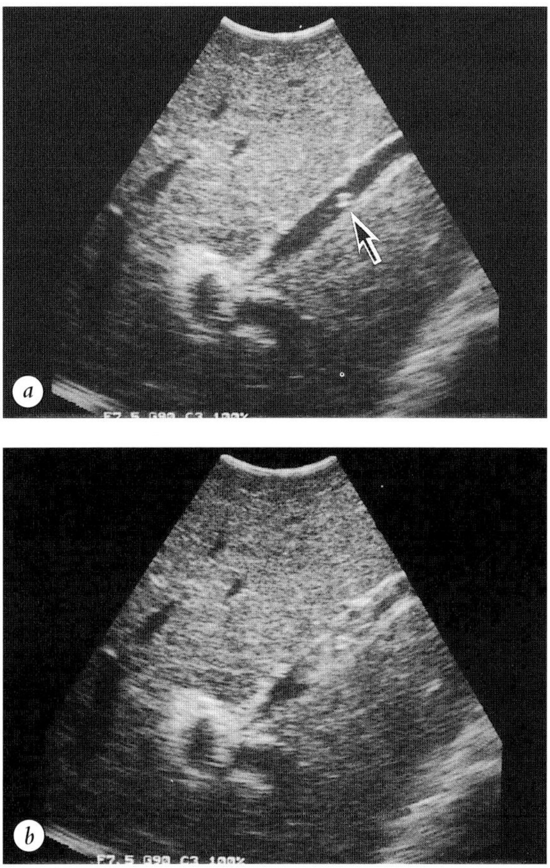

Figure 10.9 – Sonograms recorded from the ventral surface at the time of staining.

a) Puncture of the portal venous branch to the posteroinferior segment. The arrow indicates the tip of the needle.
b) Injection of indigo carmine. The injected dye is visualized as hyperechoic flow.

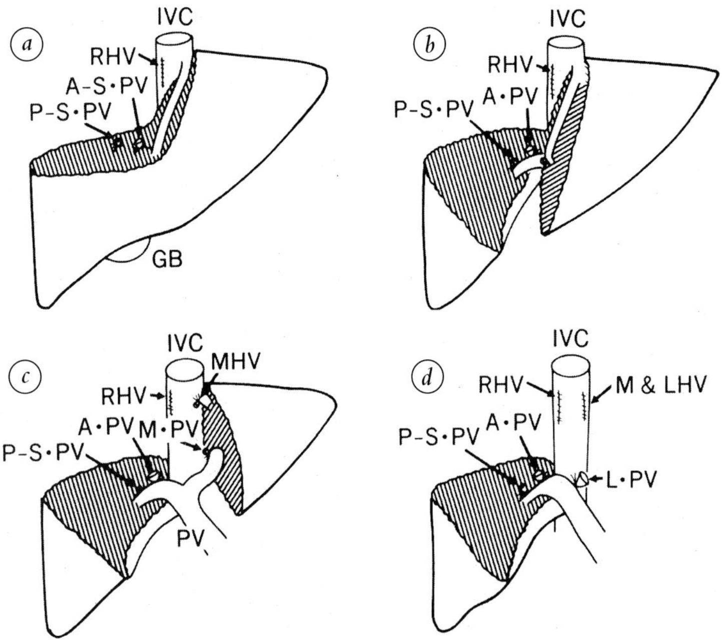

Figure 10.10 – Four types of hepatectomy preserving the inferior right hepatic vein.

a) Resection of the right anterosuperior and posterosuperior areas.

b) Resection of the right anterior segment and right posterosuperior area.

c) Resection of the left medial and right anterior segments and right posterosuperior area.

d) Resection of the left lobe, right anterior segment and right posterosuperior area. (Reproduced from ref. 14 with permission from the publisher).

should be directed toward the distal site in the direction of the portal venous flow. HCCs may be associated with arterio-portal venous shunting, which occasionally interferes with staining of the portal area. In such instances, the portal area can be stained clearly by occluding the hepatic artery at the hepatic hilus or by puncturing the feeding hepatic arterial branch, if it has been revealed by IOUS. Portal venous flow regurgitation caused by arterio-portal venous shunting may promote the spread of cancer cells and, therefore, if the patient's liver function permits, the entire stained area, including that probably stained by regurgitation as a result of arterio-portal venous shunting should be resected. When the portal area containing the tumor is fed by two or more portal venous branches, the deeper or dorsal branch should be punctured first, otherwise small air bubbles may enter the ventral branch and obscure the dorsal branch. Once the resection area and the ligation point have been selected, the parenchymal dissection line is self-evident. When a definite landmark for dissecting the parenchyma is necessary, 1-2 ml patent blue should be injected into the parenchyma just in front of the vessels to be ligated, which can be clearly identified during dissection. This technique is termed "tattooing of the liver parenchyma".[13]

The liver parenchyma is routinely dissected by crushing it using forceps. Parenchymal dissection is begun under vascular occlusion at the hepatoduodenal ligament and crushing the parenchyma leaves only small vessels and bile ducts, which are subsequently ligated and divided. The direction of the dissection plane can be confirmed and corrected using IOUS. The dissection plane, which includes small air bubbles, is usually visualized as a glittering line by US or it can be demonstrated by the surgeon inserting an index finger into it and thus, the root of the portal venous branch is exposed, ligated and divided. Liver parenchyma division is continued in this manner until the scheduled hepatectomy is completed. In Japan, this operative procedure is now accepted as the standard technique for hepatectomy.

Hepatectomy preserving the inferior right hepatic vein

Resection of a HCC which is localized in the posterosuperior area and invades the right hepatic vein requires entire posterior segmentectomy. However, when a thick inferior right hepatic vein is present, resection of the posterosuperior area with preservation of the posteroinferior area is possible.[14]

Anatomically, the inferior right hepatic vein has been reported to exist in 20-24% of specimens[15] and it can usually be identified preoperatively by US or CT. At present, there are four types of hepatectomy that preserve the inferior right hepatic vein: extended central bisegmentectomy, which includes resection of the left medial and right anterior segments and the posterosuperior area; resection of the right anterior segment and posterosuperior area; resection of the right anterosuperior and postero- superior areas and extended left lobectomy, which preserves only the posteroinferior area (Fig. 10.10). However, since preoperative portal embolization was introduced,[16] the safety of major hepatectomy has improved and therefore, the number of ideal candidates for these four techniques may now be small.

CONCLUSION

IOUS is useful for confirming the location of a HCC, detecting and diagnosing other lesions, deciding the extent of hepatectomy and correcting the direction of the dissection plane. Furthermore, IOUS has contributed to establishing new surgical procedures, such as systematic subsegmentectomy and hepatectomy with preservation of the inferior right hepatic vein. Surgeons should note the fact that adequate hepatectomy is only possible using IOUS.

REFERENCES

1. Shanghai Coordinating Group for Research on Liver Cancer. Diagnosis and treatment of primary hepatocellular carcinoma: Efficacy of various imaging procedures in 100 patients. *AJR* 1979; **92**: 801-810
2. Makuuchi M, Yamazaki S, Hasegawa H, *et al.* Ultrasonically guided liver surgery. *Jpn J Ultrasonics Med* 1980; **7**: 45-49
3. Makuuchi M, Hasegawa H, Yamazaki S: Intraoperative ultrasonic examination for hepatectomy. *Jpn J Clin Oncol* 1981; **11**: 367-390
4. Makuuchi M, Hasegawa H, Yamazaki S: Ultrasonically guided systematic subsegmentectomy. *Surg Gynecol Obstet* 1985; **161**: 346-350
5. Makuuchi M, Hasegawa H, Yamazaki S, *et al.* The use of operative ultrasound as an aid to liver resection in patients with hepatocellular carcinoma. *World J Surg* 1987; **11**: 615-621
6. Makuuchi M, Takayama T, Kosuge T, *et al.* The value of ultrasonography for hepatic surgery. *Hepato-Gastroenterol* 1991; **38**: 64-70
7. Takayasu K, Moriyama N, Muramatsu Y, *et al.* Intrahepatic portal vein branches studied by percutaneous transhepatic portography. *Radiology* 1985; **154**: 31-36
8. Makuuchi M, Hasegawa H, Yamazaki S, *et al.* Ultrasonic characteristics of the small hepatocellular carcinoma less than five centimeters in diameter, mosaic pattern of internal echoes and posterior echo enhancement. *Acta Hepatol Jpn* 1981; **22**: 1740.
9. Makuuchi M: *Abdominal Intraoperative Ultrasonography*. Tokyo, New York, Igaku-Shoin, 1987, p1-159.
10. Kuwao S. Pathomorphological study on primary liver cancer. *Acta Hepatol Jpn* 1979; **20**: 828-838
11. Lau WY, Leung JWC, Li AKC: Management of hepatocellular carcinoma presenting as obstructive jaundice. *Am J Surg* 1990; **160**: 280-282
12. Lau WY, Leung KL, Lee TW, *et al.* Ultrasonography during liver resection for hepatocellular carcinoma. *Br J Surg* 1993; **80**: 493-494
13. Takayama T, Makuuchi M, Watanabe K, *et al.* A new method for mapping hepatic subsegment: counterstaining identification technique. *Surgery* 1991; **109**: 226-229
14. Makuuchi M, Hasegawa H, Yamazaki S: Four new hepatectomy procedures for resection of the right hepatic vein and preservation of the inferior right hepatic vein. *Surg Gynecol Obstet* 1987; **164**: 68-72
15. Nakamura S, Tsuzuki T: Surgical anatomy of the hepatic veins and the inferior vena cava. *Surg Gynecol Obstet* 1981;**152**:43-50
16. Makuuchi M, Thai BL, Takayasu K, *et al.* Preoperative portal embolization to increase safety of major hepatectomy for hilar bile duct carcinoma: A preliminary report. *Surgery* 1990; **107**: 521-527

11

Ultrasonography: Contrast agents

C Spreafico, LF Frigerio and F Garbagnati

Diagnostic tests in oncology should detect tumors accurately and at an early stage and offer information about the nature of the lesions.

The use of color Doppler ultrasound in oncology aims to aid differential diagnosis of tumors by its ability to demonstrate small normal and tumor vessels by a non-invasive technique.

In the case of focal hepatic lesions, color Doppler ultrasound attempts to identify the vascularity of a lesion and provide a diagnosis, giving an evaluation that takes account both of morphologic and qualitative criteria and of quantitative assessments of vascular flow. The anatomopathologic assumption, which is also that on which angiographic diagnostic criteria are based, stems from numerous studies conducted on experimentally induced tumors, demonstrating that the vessels of malignant lesions have peculiar characteristics that differ from those of benign lesions: tumor vascular structures are particularly dense at the periphery of nodular lesions, have an irregular pattern and thin walls without a muscular tunica, and they have numerous arteriovenous shunts.[1] The color Doppler image of these vessels correlates closely with their morphology in that the signals are most easily obtained at the periphery, extremely high velocity flow is present at the shunts, and the thin walls give rise to minimal systo-diastolic variation because of the reduced peripheral resistance. For hepatocellular carcinoma (HCC) in particular, numerous patterns of central and peripheral vascularity of tumor nodules have been described and, although there is not complete agreement, the most frequent finding in these neoplasms seems to be the presence of pulsating flow within and around the tumor ("basket pattern" and "vessels within the tumor").[2,3] This type of tumor vascularization differs from that of benign lesions, among which the best known pattern is that of angiomas which, as a result of the extremely slow flow, do not show Doppler signals.

This attempt at tissue characterization through color Doppler ultrasound poses some difficulties due both to the characteristics of the vasculature, which cannot always be evaluated unequivocally, and to the fact that it is often impossible to obtain images of optimum quality: in fact the result depends upon the characteristics of the nodules, such as their site and dimensions, how co-operative the patient is and lastly the poor sensitivity of Doppler systems in detecting the slower neovascular flow within the tumor. The low velocity of flow in smaller vessels results in smaller Doppler frequency differences, to the point of becoming indistinguishable from those produced by normal tissue movement. At the same time the amount of blood in a certain tissue volume decreases and consequently the intensity of the backscattered echo from the blood decreases until a point is reached where the signal is too weak to be picked up by the transducer. Recent technological advances in ultrasound equipment and the use of increasingly high frequencies can reduce these limitations, increasing both the Doppler shift corresponding to a given flow velocity and the intensity of the backscattered echo (the Rayleigh relationship). In clinical practice the increase in the ultrasound frequency used is restricted by tissue penetration. This becomes particularly clear in the study of abdominal organs, especially the liver, where frequencies between 3 and 5 MHz are normally employed.

This explains the rapid development and intense research activity on ultrasound contrast agents. Since it is not possible to modify the velocity of blood flow at the periphery and within the tumor, there is particular interest in the development of substances capable of enhancing the acoustic backscatter of the blood itself, enhancing visualization of small neovascular structures within tumors. Besides increasing the sensitivity of color Doppler examinations, the use of contrast agents can be directed at improving the contrast resolution of conventional ultrasound and thus the ability to distinguish between normal and abnormal tissue. This can be achieved thanks to selective uptake of certain contrast agents by certain tissues or particular lesions, suggesting a diagnosis based on this behavior, as is the case for iodized contrast agents in computerized tomography (CT) and the para-magnetic contrast agent in magnetic resonance (MR).

DEFINITION

The term ultrasound contrast agent is used to describe a substance which, when introduced into the organism, is capable of producing changes in the normal ultrasonic characteristics of the tissues. The most important of these characteristics is acoustic backscatter and the purpose of US contrast agents is the enhancement of this property. This is done by using substances containing extremely small particles which act as additional reflectors and cause an increase in the number and/or intensity of the interfaces.

As far as the ability of the injected particles to increase acoustic backscatter is concerned, three principal characteristics must be considered: their diameter, which must not be too small with respect to the wavelength of the ultrasonic beam employed; the direct proportion between the backscatter and the difference in acoustic impedance between the particles and the tissues being examined; and lastly the number of particles in the contrast agent: the larger the number of particles the greater the acoustic backscatter will be.[4]

The most important requirements of an ultrasound contrast agent, besides modifying the acoustic properties of tissue, are that it should be injectable into the vascular system; it should be stable throughout the duration of the US examination; it should have no or extremely low toxicity; it should be excreted or metabolized in a relatively short time.

CLASSIFICATION

As regards the contrast effect of contrast agents in the liver parenchyma, two groups can be identified on the basis of their principal mechanism of action:

- the first is produced by phagocytosis of the contrast agent by the cells of the reticuloendothelial system present within the liver parenchyma;
- the second mechanism involves the transport of particles of contrast agent with the blood flow as far as the small vessels within the parenchyma and particularly as far as the newly formed tumor vessels.

Colloidal suspensions and emulsions

Colloidal suspensions and emulsions belong to the first group. **Colloidal suspensions** consist of particles of extremely small dimension suspended in a liquid medium. Among the products that have been developed are collagen microspheres and gelatin particles with diameters between 2 and 3 μm and particles of ethyl ester of iodipamide, an iodized contrast agent, with a diameter of 0.5-1 μm.[5,6]

The other possibility is to use chemical substances consisting of carbon atoms and halogens which, being fat soluble, can be introduced into the circulation in **emulsion form**. The most widely used compound is perfluorooctylbromide (PFOB) emulsified in lecithin. This substance can be used both orally and intravenously; the diameter of the particles in the emulsion ranges from 0.1 to 0.2 μm and they remain in the intravascular space for about 6 hours, after which they are removed by evaporation through the lungs and phagocytosis by the reticuloendothelial system. The contrast effect of PFOB is due to the large acoustic impedance difference between its particles and human tissue, estimated to be over 30%. The emulsion also causes an increase in absorption of the ultrasonic beam, so the calculation of the dosage used becomes critical, as absorption can be so high as to prevent the study of the deeper tissues. As a result of the behaviour of the emulsion within the parenchyma, the contrast effect of PFOB is manifested in two stages: first there is an increase in acoustic backscatter from the blood, while the emulsion is in the intravascular space; and then the parenchyma is enhanced, following phagocytosis by the reticuloendothelial system. The use of this contrast agent to detect the presence, number and site of focal hepatic lesions is based on the assumption that the majority of these lesions lack reticuloendothelial cells. Clinical tests in humans, however, have yielded equivocal and often conflicting results, with tumor lesions that have become hyperechoic following administration of PFOB, clearly owing to a greater abundance of macrophages, whilst in other cases the lesions have become less echogenic than the surrounding parenchyma.[5,7-10]

The second group of contrast agents, those which diffuse in the circulation to normal and tumor vessels, comprise two main categories: free gas microbubbles and stabilized gas microbubbles.

Gas bubbles

The first contrast agent used for enhancement of ultrasound images belongs to the category of **free gas microbubbles**. This was normal saline injected into the heart and its contrast effect was due to air micro-bubbles produced by cavitation during injection.[11,12]

The gas bubbles produced have some drawbacks: they are unstable and above all they have a larger diameter than that of the pulmonary capillaries, so the bubbles are destroyed as they pass through the pulmonary circulation. This precludes their use in the systemic arterial circulation and therefore the ultrasound investigation of internal organs.[4]

Much more recently use has been made of CO_2 bubbles injected selectively into the hepatic artery. This method combines selective angiographic catheterization with an ultrasound examination that is made more sensitive by the gas contrast. The CO_2 microbubbles are normally prepared by mixing 10 ml of CO_2 with 10 ml of heparinized normal saline and 5 ml of the patient's own blood. The microbubbles are injected at a rate of 1-2 ml/s for a total of about 10 s. Plain ultrasound examination is always done prior to injection of CO_2. The whole procedure is then divided into three phases: an early phase in which the microbubbles fill the vascular bed of the entire liver parenchyma; a middle phase generally lasting from 10-60 s after the end of injection during which the microbubbles remain in the parenchyma and a late phase, lasting from 1-3 minutes, when CO_2 is washed out from the liver parenchyma. Dynamic ultrasound image observation during these three phases enables the vascularity of nodular hepatic lesions to be evaluated and, on the basis of this vascularity, Kudo *et al.*[13] have suggested that the nodules be classified as hypervascular, isovascular and hypovascular. Within the hypervascular group a further classification into four sub-types has been suggested according to the distribution of the contrast generated by CO_2 within the nodules. More than 90% of HCC are hypervascular in appearance and this is shown by a persistent increased echogenicity of HCC compared with the surrounding liver parenchyma from which the gas has already been washed out (Figs. 11.1a,b). This method can be useful in detecting small deep lesions that are difficult to demonstrate with conventional US, as it can also be used for detection of hypovascular or isovascular HCC nodules which are very difficult to diagnose angiographically or by conventional ultrasound examination. What should also be stressed is that this investigation has virtually no cost and takes little time to perform, adding only 10-15 minutes to a normal angiographic procedure.[13,14] Ultrasound images with CO_2 also have a characteristic appearance in the case of focal nodular hyperplasia (FNH) and hepatic angiomas, whereas metastases have heterogeneous vascular characteristics and differentiation from other tumors is difficult and unreliable, particularly if they are hypervascular and thus hyperechoic after CO_2 injection. The use of CO_2 microbubbles has clearly enhanced the sensitivity of conventional ultrasound in detecting liver nodules. Particularly interesting at present is the use of ultrasound with CO_2 for staging of hepatocellular carcinoma prior to surgical management, by resection or transplantation (OLT), in order to diagnose small, often hypovascular, satellite nodules less than 1 cm in diameter, at deep or peripheral sites, which are difficult to diagnose with other more complex and costly imaging modalities such as computerized tomography during arterial portography and CT after intra-arterial injection of Lipiodol.

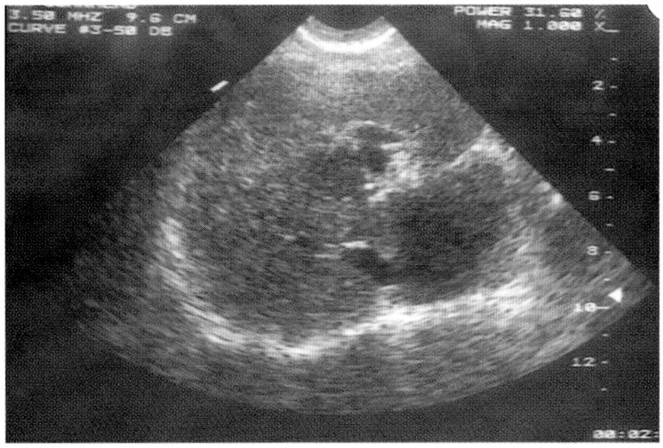

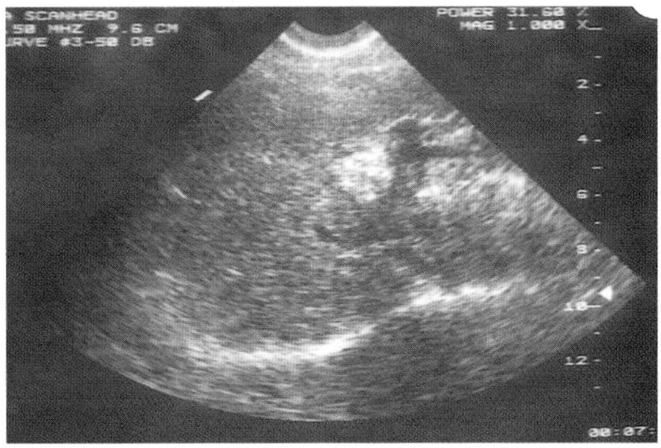

Figure 11.1 –

a) Small hypoechoic HCC nodule in a peri-hilar site, adjacent to the left hepatic vein: baseline study.

b) After CO_2 intra-arterial injection a persistent hypervascularity can be observed inside the nodule in comparison with the remaining parenchyma.

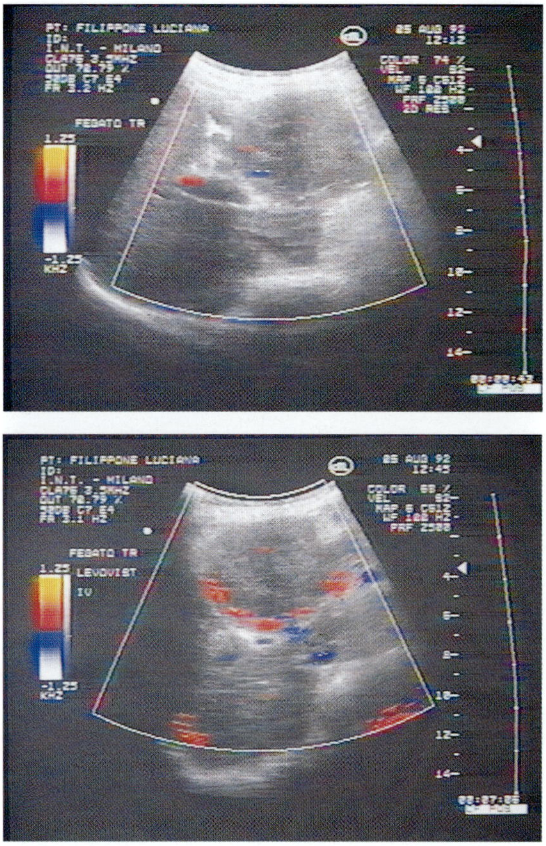

Figure 11.2 –

a) Large HCC nodule in the left lobe of the liver. In this baseline color Doppler study few vascular signals can be seen.

b) After Levovist injection an intense enhancement in color signals is observed with a prevalent distribution at the perifery of the lesion.

Lastly, another suggested use for this method is in the follow-up of loco-regional treatment for HCC, such as chemoembolization, alcoholization and heat therapy, where it could provide a more reliable evaluation of residual tumor tissue.

In an attempt to overcome some of the limitations of free gas bubbles, especially their instability and lack of uniform size, whilst maintaining their echogenic characteristics, many studies have focused on the development of **stabilized gas microbubbles** that are as stable and uniform in size as possible but are small enough to traverse the pulmonary bed and can therefore be used as an intravenous contrast agent for the study of the left cardiac chambers, peripheral arterial circulation and organs.

These bubbles have been prepared by different methods and have given rise to different types of contrast agent, which are currently in the advanced trial stage.

One procedure consists of the formation of so-called "aerosomes", lipid shells inside which gas microbubbles of CO_2 or nitrogen are trapped. The liposomes consist of lecithin, either pure or combined with various percentages of cholesterol. The particles thus obtained are smaller than 0.5 μm in diameter and have increased the echogenicity of the liver when injected intravenously in animal studies.[15]

A second method of preparation is to trap air microbubbles inside a protein shell, as is the case for Albunex, which consists of air-filled albumin microspheres produced by sonication of 5% human serum albumin. The microspheres thus produced are stable, capable of traversing the pulmonary circulation and strongly echogenic, but they have a very short plasma half-life after intravenous injection. Studies with ^{125}iodine radiolabeled albumin microspheres show that the concentration in the blood falls by half in less than 1 minute and at 3 minutes they have virtually disappeared from the vessels.[16-18]

A third type of contrast agent is prepared by making air microbubbles adhere to a sugar molecule. The biochemical principle of this ultrasound contrast agent is the stabilization of gas microbubbles with echogenic properties by enclosing them inside particles of a monosaccharide that can be considered physiologic for the organism: galactose. Two contrast agents based on this principle have been developed: the first of these, Echovist, provided stable homogeneous microbubbles, but did not show sufficient ability to pass through the pulmonary circulation. A second contrast agent, SH U 508 A (Levovist) was therefore prepared, meeting the need for greater chemical stability by using a palmitic acid molecule. The formulation thus obtained is characterized by the presence of structurally and volumetrically stable microbubbles of uniform size, capable of surviving the pulmonary circulation after being injected into a peripheral vein.[19-24] Levovist is supplied in vials ready for extemporaneous preparation with water for injection. The diameter of microparticles in the suspension thus obtained was less than 4 μm in 99% of cases. The plasma half-life of SH U 508 A is about 10-11 minutes in healthy adults and about 7-9 minutes in children.

This contrast agent has undergone extensive clinical trials firstly to establish its complete lack of toxicity and safety in patients, then to evaluate its efficacy in enhancing the color Doppler signal in the left heart, the systemic arterial system and the organs.[25]

We took part in a Phase III multicenter study in which 38 HCC patients with a total of 43 examinable nodular lesions were evaluated.[26] All the nodules had been selected on the basis of a vascular color Doppler signal judged to be sub-optimal at plain examination (Figs. 11.2, 3). For each patient two to four venous injections of Levovist at concentrations of 300-400 mg/ml were used. After contrast agent injection there was significant enhancement of the color Doppler signal in 35 out of 43 nodules (81.4%), with a duration ranging from 40 to 240 seconds. In 8 out of 43 (18.6%) there was no change in the flow signals, a finding related to portal vein thrombosis in two cases, to marked hypovascularity already evident at CT and digital subtraction angiography in four cases, and to the deep site of the nodule in one case; lastly, in one case the lesion had been subjected to trans-arterial chemoembolization (TACE) a few days previously, with complete devascularization, also already demonstrated by angiography. This finding is interesting and again suggests that ultrasound contrast agents are potentially of great value in the follow-up of local therapy for HCC nodules, such as chemoembolization, alcoholization and heat therapy. In the above study another 3 of the 43 lesions examined in addition to that described above had already been subjected to TACE, but in these three cases enhancement of the color Doppler signal could be demonstrated after injection of Levovist, indicating an incomplete therapeutic result that was subsequently confirmed.

Experimental findings also show that SH U 508 A, besides improving detection of vascularization in and around the tumor, is able to enhance visualization of normal venous and arterial vasculature. This can be valuable in the investigation of pathologies at this level (portal vein thrombosis, vascular involvement in tumor processes, etc.). Ultrasound contrast agents are also potentially useful in the study of surgical vascular anastomoses, particularly in follow-up after liver transplantation.

Very recently a new ultrasound method called "harmonic imaging" has been developed. This is

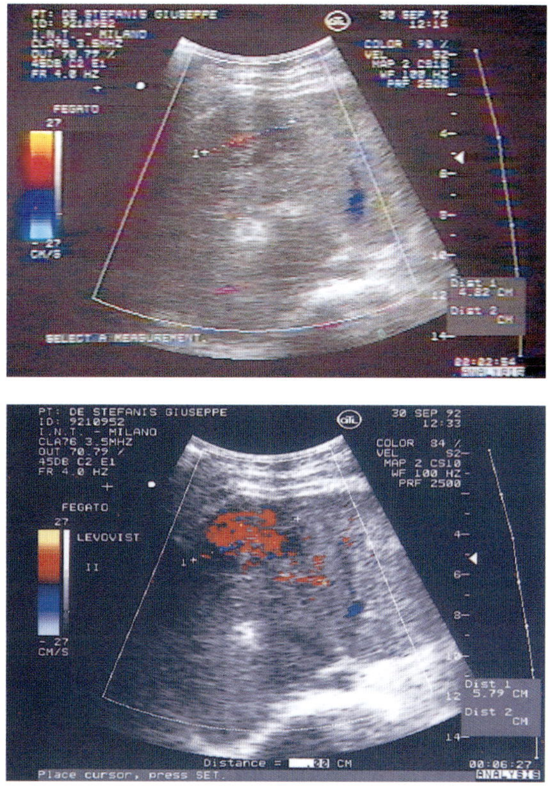

Figure 11.3 –

a) Hypoechoic HCC nodule with some intra-lesional signals at the color Doppler examination.

b) After Levovist injection a very intense enhancement can be demonstrated with vascular signals homogeneously distributed throughout the nodule.

based on the principle of exploiting the non linear generation of harmonics by air microbubbles in contrast agent (Levovist) in an ultrasound field and the broad bandwidth of a commercially available digital ultrasound system (ATL Inc., Seattle, WA, USA). This system was modified so as to transmit at 3-4 MHz and receive at 6-8 MHz. The images thus obtained show a great improvement in the signal-to-noise ratio caused by the Doppler effect in solid tissues. The purpose of harmonic imaging is to allow real-time subtraction imaging of flowing blood, making it possible to detect blood flow in vessels in which it was not otherwise detectable.[27,28]

TOXICITY

As already stated above, the potential toxicity of an ultrasound contrast agent is particularly important and it is essential for clinical use that the substance should be well tolerated and have no adverse effects.

In animals no functional alterations in organs or systems were demonstrated following injection of contrst agent nor were histologic changes encountered in killed animals. No teratogenic or embryotoxic effects have so far been demonstrated.[8,16,22]

Local tolerance at the injection site was always good for all contrast agents, even for hyperosmolar agents like Levovist, for which slight drawbacks were described, mainly a transient localized sensation of warmth. Again for Levovist, the other minimal adverse effects recorded in the course of clinical trials were: dysgeusia, pruritus, rash, headache, and transient paresthesias. There were no significant changes in blood chemistry parameters at the doses used in clinical trials.

The side effects with PFOB were comparatively greater: transient pain, raised temperature, fatigue, allergy and, in some cases, elevated transaminases. The greatest risk is that of pulmonary emphysema, resulting from interstitial damage following pulmonary evaporation of perfluorchemicals; however, sporadic use for diagnostic purposes seems unlikely to cause such an effect.[7,10]

With Albunex, the risk of possible contamination of the albumin must be considered and hence the need for the controls already in force for therapeutic use. In theory there is also the possibility of immune reactions triggered by injection of human albumin.

CONCLUSION

HCC is a neoplasm for which the therapeutic approach is greatly influenced by the early diagnosis and by the staging of the disease, which in the majority of cases consists of multiple nodules in the liver parenchyma. Only in the initial stages can liver transplantation, currently considered the best possible therapy for these patients, be proposed. Alternatively, other well-known loco-regional therapeutic approaches are used, such as percutaneous alcoholization or heat therapy and, in selected cases, chemoembolization, the results of which depend upon tumor spread. The possibility of controlling HCC in the advanced stages is very poor.

Ultrasound plays a major role both in diagnosis and in staging, as it has high sensitivity and specificity and in the majority of cases is the first investigational method used, often within screening programs for patients at risk. Among ultrasound contrast agents, CO_2 is injected intra-arterially as a complement to angiography in order to increase the sensitivity of ultrasound in detecting small HCC satellite nodules that are poorly detectable even with considerably more sophisticated and costly imaging modalities.[13,14] All the other substances proposed and tested as contrast agents are injected intravenously. In the majority of cases these contrast agents act by improving visualization of vascular structures.

HCC being highly vascularized, is one of the tumors most widely studied with Doppler techniques, first with pulsed Doppler[29,30] and then color Doppler,[2,3,31,32] which permits direct imaging of small normal and tumor vessels, whether at the periphery or in the central portion of the lesion. The main difficulties in these studies spring from the relatively poor sensitivity to the low flow velocity in vessels of small size and to the weak signals coming from deep sites, which mean that about 20% of HCC nodules are avascular on color Doppler examination.[33] The use of contrast agents aims to overcome or at least reduce these limitations, thus making it possible to improve the overall diagnostic impact of the method. Further studies will nevertheless be necessary to evaluate the new semeiotics deriving from the use of contrast agents and the clinical value of the information thus acquired in diagnosing and staging tumors.

REFERENCES

1. Folkman J: Tumor angiogenesis. *Adv Cancer Res* 1985; **43**: 175-203
2. Shimamoto K, Sakuma S, Ishigaki T *et al* Hepatocellular carcinoma: evaluation with color Doppler US and MR imaging. *Radiology* 1992; **182**: 149-153
3. Tanaka K, Inoue S, Numata K *et al* Color Doppler sonography of hepatocellular carcinoma before and after treatment by transcatheter arterial embolization. *AJR* 1992; **158**: 541-546
4. Ophir J, Parker KJ: Contrast agents in diagnostic ultrasound. *Ultrasound Med Biol* 1989; **15**: 319-333
5. Parker KJ, Tuthill TA, Lerner RM *et al*. A particulate contrast agent with potential for ultrasound imaging of the liver. *Ultrasound Med Biol* 1987; **13**: 555-666

6. Violante MR, Parker K, Lerner R: Particulate contrast agents for improved ultrasound detection of liver metastases: *Invest Radiol* 1990; **25**: 165-166

7. Behan M, O'Connell DJ, Carney DN *et al.* Perfluorooctylbromide as a US contrast agent for liver metastases: preliminary findings and clinical tolerance. *Radiology* 1989; **173**: (P): 361

8. Mattrey RF: Sonographic enhancement of Doppler signals and perfused tissues with perfluorooctylbromide. *Invest Radiol* 1990; **25**: 158-159

9. Mattrey RF, Leopold GR, van Sonnenberg E *et al.* Perfluorochemicals as liver-and spleen-seeking ultrasound contrast agents. *J Ultrasound Med* 1983; **2**: 173-176

10. Mattrey RF, Strich G, Shelton RE *et al.* Perfluorochemicals as US contrast agents for tumor imaging and hepatosplenography: preliminary clinical results. *Radiology* 1987; **167**: 339-343,

11. Gramiak R, Shah PM: Echocardiography of the aortic root. *Invest Radiol* 1968; **3**: 356-366

12. Gramiak R, Shah PM, Kramer DH: Ultrasound cardiography: contrast studies in anatomy and function. *Radiology* 1969; **92**: 939-947

13. Kudo M, Tomita S, Tochio H *et al.* Specific findings at dynamic contrast-enchanced US with carbon dioxide microbubbles. *Radiology* 1991; **179**: 377-382

14. Matsuda Y, Yabuuchi I: Hepatic tumors: US contrast enhancement with CO_2 microbubbles. *Radiology* 1986;**161**: 701-705

15. Unger EC, Lund P, Fritz T *et al.* "Aerosomes" Liposomes as US contrast agents. *Radiology* 1990; **177** (P): 252,

16. Barnhart J, Levene H, Villapando E *et al.* Characteristic of Albunex: airfilled albumin microspheres for echocardiography contrast enhancement. *Invest Radiol* 1990; **25**: 162-164

17. Goldberg BB, Hilpert PL, Burns PN *et al.* Hepatic tumors: signal enhancement at Doppler US after intravenous injection of a contrast agent. *Radiology* 1990; **177**: 713-717

18. Hilpert PL, Mattrey RG, Mitten RM *et al.* IV injection of airfilled human albumin microspheres to enhance arterial Doppler signal: a preliminary study in rabbits. *AJR* 1989; **153**: 613-616

19. Burns PN: Mezzi di contrasto per ecografia nella diagnostica radiologica. *Radiol Med* 1994; **87**(Suppl.): 71-82

20. Burns PN, Liu JB, Hilpert P *et al.* Intravenous US contrast agent for tumor diagnosis: quantitative studies. *Radiology* 1990; **177** (P): 140

21. Fobbe F, Ohnesorge O, Reichel M: Transpulmonary contrast agent and color-coded duplex sonography; first clinical experience. *Radiology* 1992; **185**(P): 142

22. Fritzsch T, Hillmann J, Kampfe M *et al.* SH U 508, a transpulmonary echocontrast agent: initial experience. *Invest Radiol* 1990; **25**: 160-161

23. Goldberg BB, Liu JB, Burns PN *et al.* Galactose-based intravenous sonographic contrast agent: experimental studies. *J Ultrasound Med* 1993; **12**: 463-470

24. Schlief R: Ultrasound contrast agents: *Curr Opinion Radiol* 1991; **3**: 198-207

25. Derchi LE, Rizzatto G, Solbiati L: I mezzi di contrasto in ecografia. *Radiol Med* 1992; **84**: 208-215

26. Angeli E, Carpanelli R, Crespi G *et al.* Efficacia del SH U 508 A (Levovist) nella valutazione con color-Doppler della vascolarizzazione dell'epatocarcinoma. *Radiol Med* 1994; **87**(Suppl.): 24-31

27. Burns PN, Powers JE, Fritzsch T: Harmonic imaging: a new imaging and Doppler method for contrast enhanced ultrasound. *Radiology* 1992; **185**(P): 142

28. Burns PN, Powers JE, Hope Simpson D *et al.* Harmonic contrast enhanced Doppler as a method for the elimination of clutter. In vivo duplex and color studies. *Radiology* 1993; **189**: 285

29. Taylor KJW, Ramos I, Morse SS *et al.* Focal liver masses: differential diagnosis with pulsed Doppler US. *Radiology* 1987; **164**: 643-647

30. Taylor KJW, Ramos I, Carter D *et al.* Correlation of Doppler US tumor signals with neovascular morphologic features. *Radiology* 1988; **166**: 57-62

31. Numata K, Tanaka K, Mitsui K *et al.* Flow characteristic of hepatic tumors at color Doppler sonography: correlation with arteriographic findings. *AJR* 1993; **160**: 515-521

32. Tomita S: Color-Doppler imaging of hepatic tumors: *Medical Review* 1993; **43**: 28-35

33. Tanaka S, Kitamura T, Fujita M *et al.* Color Doppler flow imaging of liver tumors. *AJR* 1990; **154**: 509-514

12

Angiography

A Roche

During the seventies – the golden age of arteriography – angiography was the spearhead of the exploration of hepatic tumors. Today and generally speaking, it is relegated by non invasive imaging techniques to a position of secondary importance. Nevertheless, among hepatic tumors, HCC is probably the lesion in which exploration – and treatments – still closely depend on angiography. Even if its role in detecting lesions has decreased, it still has value in tumor characterization and staging before surgical resection or locoregional percutaneous treatments. Moreover, its diagnostic place depends more and more on the development of efficient intra-arterial therapeutic methods (such as intra-arterial chemotherapy, chemoembolization or interstitial radiotherapy) and outstanding coupled diagnostic techniques: CT-portography, CT-arteriography, CT following intra-arterial injection of Lipiodol, intra-arterial CO_2 injection for US study improvement. Consequently, although it is an invasive technique, angiography is indicated in HCC more than in any other liver tumor, among other things because it is frequently the first step in intra-arterial therapy.

EQUIPMENT

The advantages of digital subtraction (DSA) upon conventional angiography are well known and widely accepted, and DSA is systematically preferred for HCC study where its advantages have been demonstrated.[1,2] A 14 inch field of view image intensifier is generally sufficient to completely visualize the liver. With smaller fields of view (9 or 10 inches), multiple injections and studies are generally needed and at least one localized on each liver lobe.

A C-arm is recommended since oblique projections may be useful, especially for separating the left lobe parenchyma from spine bone structures .

As already mentioned, sensitivity of CT or US may be improved by intra-arterial injection of conventional contrast media, lipiodol or CO_2,which justify the need of the three imaging modalities to be closely placed in the department.

TECHNIQUE

Comparative study of both arterial and portal opacification of liver vessels and parenchyma is essential to correct interpretation.[3] Separated opacification of the arterial system and portal veins is mandatory, which makes intravenous digital subtraction angiography inappropriate to HCC study. "Pure" portal opacification is of the best quality after superior mesenteric artery injection because this artery generally contributes about 70% of the portal vein blood. When a right hepatic artery originates from the superior mesenteric artery, or in the case of arterial flow reversal in duodenal pancreatic arcades and gastroduodenal artery (due to stenosis of celiac trunk or high arterial flow in the liver), the catheter tip must be advanced beyond the origin of the hepatic feeders to obtain a "pure" portal hepatogram. Intra-arterial administration of 4cg of papaverin, in 30 seconds and immediatly before contrast medium injection, shortens the arterial phase and improves the quality of the venous opacification.

Global opacification of the celiac trunk and superior mesenteric artery maps the hepatic arteries. Arterial hepatic feeders all arise from the common hepatic artery in only about 50% of cases; replaced hepatic arteries may arise from the left gastric, superior mesenteric or gastroduodenal arteries as well as from the aorta; trifurcation of the celiac trunk in the splenic artery and two hepatic arteries is less frequent; in contrast, an accessory gastric artery may originate from the left hepatic artery.

Selective opacification of hepatic arteries allows precise study of the tumoral vascularization. The proper hepatic artery may be occluded after intra-arterial chemotherapy, chemoembolization or surgical ligation; hepatic vascularization is then assumed by collateral circulation to have been explored, ie duodenal pancreatic, inferior diaphragmatic, left gastric, intercostal, lumbar, internal mammary arteries. When exploring a subcapsular and extraperitoneal area of the liver (especially in the dorsal and internal territory of the right lobe), hypervascular tumors may be spontaneously partially vascularized by some posterior parietal pedicles (mainly inferior diaphragmatic artery) and these should be systematically explored. Very occasionally, HCC has been reported as developping into an accessory liver, either pedunculated or ectopic, located in the retroperitoneal space, right intrathoracic space or left diaphragm.[4]

Infusion hepatic arteriography - arteriography with injection of a large amount of contrast medium at a

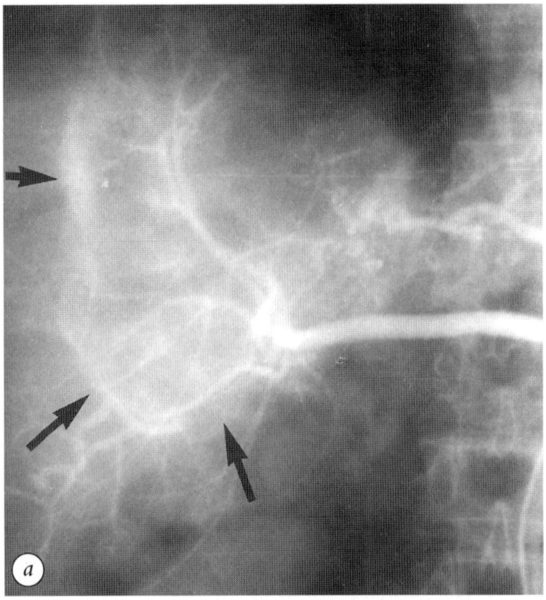

Figure 12.1 – Interest of infusion arteriography technique.

a) selective hepatic artery conventional injection shows the main HCC (arrows).

b) infusion technique clearly demonstrates complementary small daughter nodules (arrows).

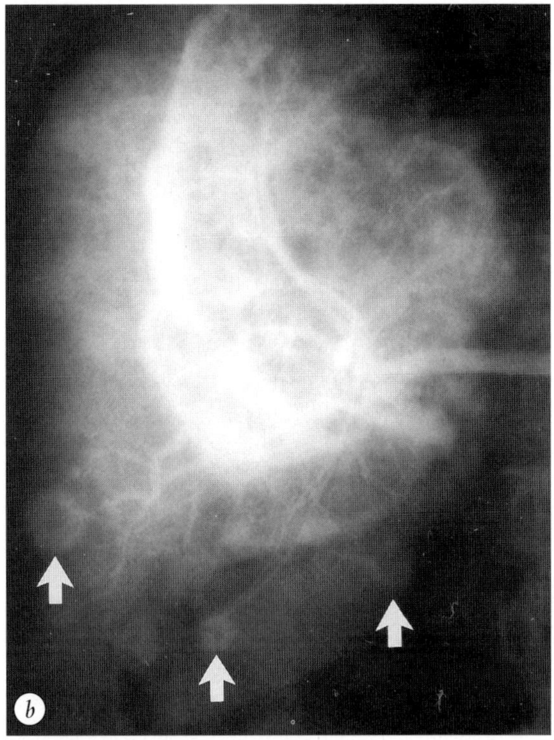

rate of <2 ml/s – has been reported to improve detection of small HCC [5](Fig. 12.1). Combination of infusion and balloon occlusion techniques, with early and delayed films (>1 minute) after contrast medium injection, may also be useful in detecting small lesions.[6] Certain drugs induce vasoconstriction of normal arteries while being almost ineffective against tumoral vascularization; injected into the hepatic artery, adrenalin – 6 to 8 μg injected in 15 seconds immediately prior to the injection of contrast medium – may be used for this purpose and improve tumor detection.

IMAGING FINDINGS

Arteriographic presentation of huge HCC is very characteristic. Most of these forms are very hypervascular, with many dilated neovessels throughout the tumor and increased capillary blush during the venous phases, arteriovenous shunting and sometimes endoportal invasion (Fig. 12.2) ; when this characteristic constellation of arteriographic signs is present, the diagnosis is made easily because no other tumor has this appearence.

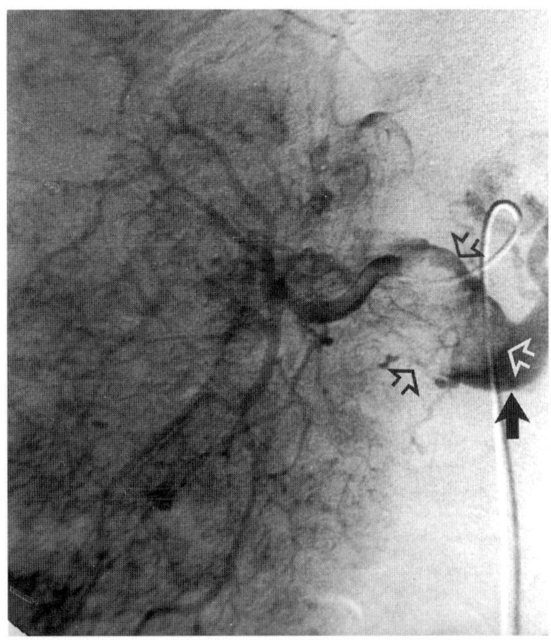

Figure 12.2 – Typical huge infiltrative HCC with intraportal tumor overgrowth (open arrow) and arterioportal shunting (plain arrow). One can note that the tumor cast expands the lumen of the portal trunk.

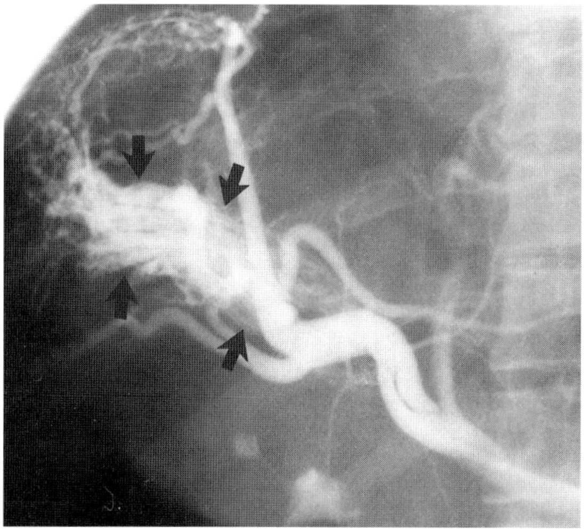

Figure 12.3 – Growing cast of HCC in the right branch of the portal vein showing typical thread and streaks sign (arrows)

Endoluminal portal and/or hepatic vein invasion by a tumor cast is very typical of HCC;[7] it is found by the pathologist in more than 70% and 40% of cases respectively.[8] Arteriography detects intraportal tumor overgrowth in 44%, the thrombus being hypervascular in 63%;[9] nevertheless, Doppler US is actually more reliable at detecting portal thrombosis in patients presenting with HCC.[10] Angiographic demonstration of endoluminal invasion of the hepatic vein is less frequent but also very typical;[11] it is hypervascular in 75% of cases[9] and is found in 4-45% of angiographic studies.[9] In almost all cases the tumor cast leads to an enlargement of the invaded vein. The vascularization of growing casts of HCC in portal or hepatic vein is very typical, described by Okuda *et al.* as the thread and streaks sign[7] (Fig. 12.3). Sometimes, a tumor thrombus partially occluding an intrahepatic portal vein is the only manifestation of HCC on imaging investigations.[12] Progressive retrograde invasion of intrahepatic veins may lead to the complete occlusion of the main portal vein division, then its trunk and even sometimes its infrahepatic tributaries (splenic or mesenteric veins, left gastric vein and esophageal varices). The intraluminal evolution of hepatic vein invasion may be similarly extensive towards the inferior vena cava, the right atrium and even the pulmonary artery[13] (Fig. 12.4).

Angiography identifies arterioportal shunting in 24 to 63% of cases;[9,14,15] arteriovenous shunting with hepatic veins occurs less frequently. These shunts generally directly develop from intravenous tumor thrombus and may result from two main mechanisms: (i) a periportal arterial vessel drains into intraportal vein tumor thrombus neovessels, and then into the portal vein itself, either up- or downstream; (ii) invasion of contiguous periportal arteries by the intraportal vein tumor produces direct communication between these arteries and the vein lumen. Arterioportal shunting may also result from intrahepatic tumor invasion of contiguous arteries and veins.[8]

HCC nodules may be surrounded by a capsule. It is defined as a thin, sharply marginated rim of tissue, with or without contrast enhancement, surrounding

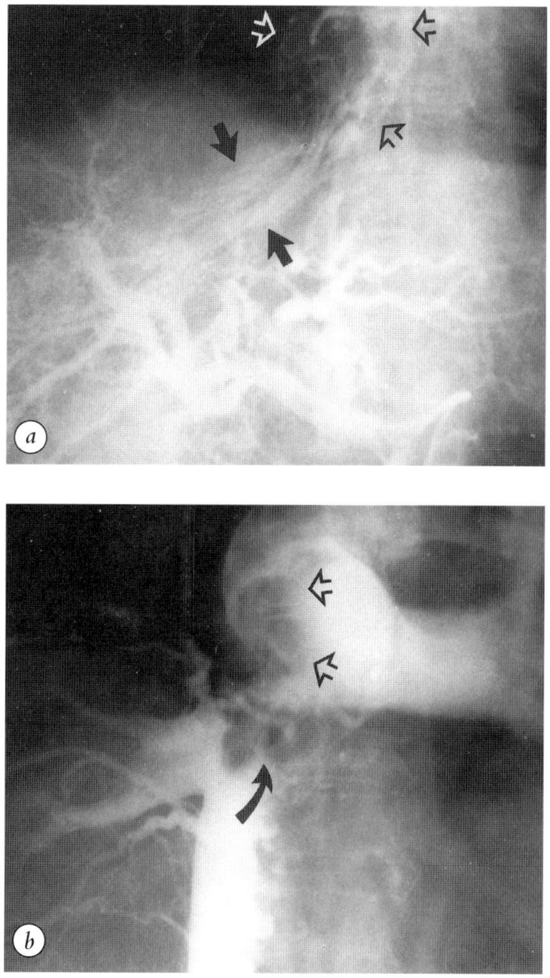

Figure 12.4 – HCC with endovenous overgrowth. Arteriography *a)* and cavography, *b)* show endoluminal invasion of the right hepatic vein (plain arrows), the inferior vena cava (curved arrow) and the right atrium (open arrows).

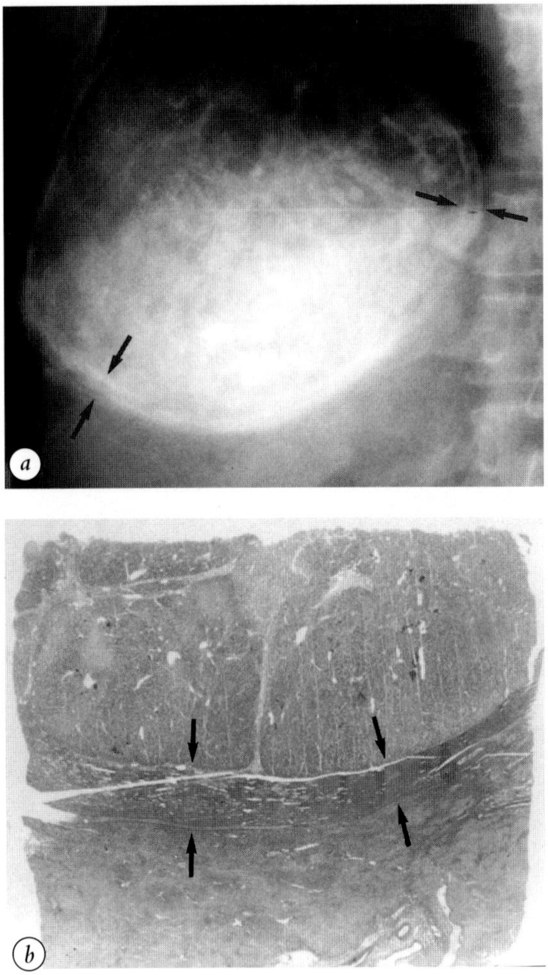

Figure 12.5 – *a)* Nodular HCC surrounded by a capsule (arrows) visible on arteriography and b) histology.

completely or partially a nodule (Fig. 12.5). The capsule has two layers; the inner layer consists of collagen and reticulum fibers; compressed liver parenchyma and peritumoral vessels make up the outer layer. In non-Asian populations, its frequency is estimated to be 15%;[16,17] it is circumferential in 40% and hypervascular in 93%.[9] In Japan, it has been reported in up to 58% of HCC.[18,19]

The gross morphologic structure of HCC is either expansive (uni- or multifocal) or infiltrative (diffuse).[20] Infiltrative forms represent 15% of all HCC.[21] Fibrolamellar HCC is a special type that mostly develops on healthy liver and preferentially affects young women. The tumor is nearly always hypervascular, generally huge when the diagnosis is made (mean diameter 14 cm) and well demarcated.[22] It presents a fibrous septation that leads to compartmentation, and sometimes a fibrous central scar; these two signs may mimick a focal nodular hyperplasia.

Only patients who do not enter a systematic screening program - because they are not identified as belonging to a risk group for HCC - present a huge and symptomatic HCC when the diagnosis is made. In contrast, in those with known chronic liver disease, small HCC may be diagnosed early. Because surgical resection is the most effective treatment, the detection of such small and asymptomatic HCC has become an essential goal.[23] Gross aspects of small HCCs have been classified into four distinctive structural patterns. Type 1 is a single nodular type, presenting as a sharply defined, round expansile nodule, often surrounded by a capsule. Type 2 is a single nodular type with extranodular growth. Type 3 is a contiguous multinodular type that presents as a cluster of small contiguous nodules, each one being surrounded by fibrous connective tissue. Type 4 is a poorly demarcated nodular type in which the border with non cancerous tissue is ambigous. The majority of type 1 tumors are well differentiated whereas types 2 or 3 are moderately or poorly differentiated. The frequency of types 1, 2, 3 and 4 is respectively 21%, 34%, 31% and 2%.[24] Small HCC are usually defined as tumors smaller than 3.0 cm in diameter. These small tumors are rarely as hypervascular as large HCC. In a series of 68 well differentiated HCC (up to 5.0 cm in diameter),[25] 20.5% of all the lesions, and 50% of the tumors smaller than 3.0 cm in diameter, were hypovascular; hypovascular tumors were significantly smaller and better differentiated.

Peritoneal bleeding due to tumor rupture is a severe complication of HCC. It may occur either spontaneously or as a complication of a locoregional treatment. Angiographic diagnosis permits its emergency treatment by arterial embolization. Direct visualization of contrast medium leakage in the peritoneal cavity is a reliable but infrequent angiographic sign (Fig. 12.6). The diagnosis of active bleeding by angiography is based on visualization of contrast medium pooling that appears in the early phase, and persists to the latest phase, but modifies its aspect over time; on a frontal projection it is frequently

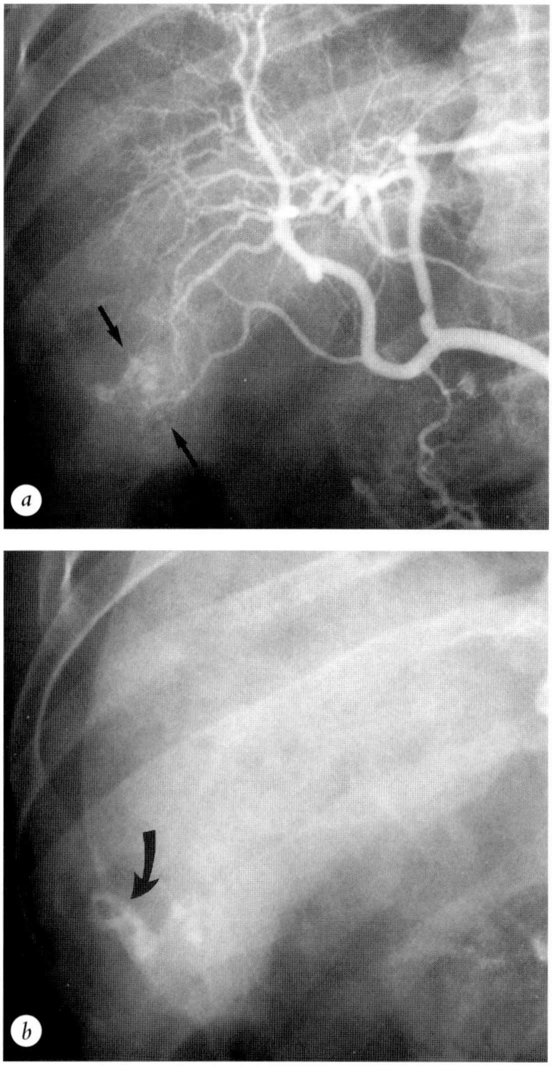

Figure 12.6 – Spontaneous rupture of HCC. *a)* on the early phase of arteriography a small HCC (arrows) can be located in lower segment of the right lobe. *b)* active bleeding in the peritoneal cavity (curved arrow) is visualized on delayed films. Diagnosis and treatment could be achieved by arterial approach.

difficult to differentiate it from low-flow HCC neovascularization.

Angiographic pretherapeutic staging requires systematic analysis of the following data:

i) number of lesions as well as their segmental localization and their location relative to the main portal and hepatic vessels. Preoperative knowledge of anatomical arterial variations is essential, especially the presence of a retro-portal hepatic artery. One can note that diagnosis of the retro-portal course of a replaced hepatic artery arising from the superior mesenteric artery is frequently easy on a frontal projection (Fig. 12.7);

ii) identification of a peritumoral capsule, due to its important prognostic value;

iii) portal staging based on: pattency of intra- and infrahepatic portal branches, signs of portal hypertension, quality of the portal perfusion of the liver parenchyma that must be appreciated before any embolization or chemoembolization;

iv) hepatic vein staging: patency or presence of an endovenous tumor growth that is associated with a higher risk of pulmonary metastasis;

v) diagnosis of locoregional metastatic adenomegalies, present in about 10% of cases, but identified by angiography in very rare hypervascular forms (Fig. 12.8).

Arteriography is also reliable in identifying tumor recurrence or persistance after local treatment by percutaneous tumor ablation or transarterial embolization. Recurrences are generally located in the periphery of the treated lesion and detected as hypervascular tissue.

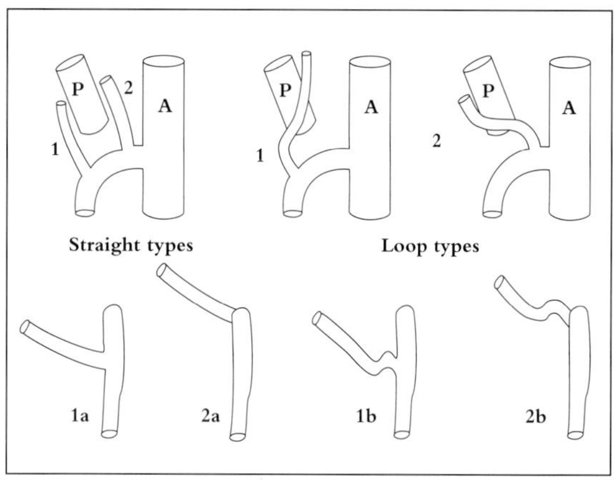

Figure 12.7 – How to recognize pre- and retro-portal accessory hepatic artery arising from superior mesenteric artery on front projection. Absence (a) or presence (b) of a proximal loop, and early origination (2) or not (1) of the replaced artery, are the two key points for correct interpretation. Lateral representation (top row), shows that, on a frontal projection, types 1a and 2b can be diagnosed as retroportal, and types 1b and 2a as pre-portal. (A: Aorta, P: Portal vein)

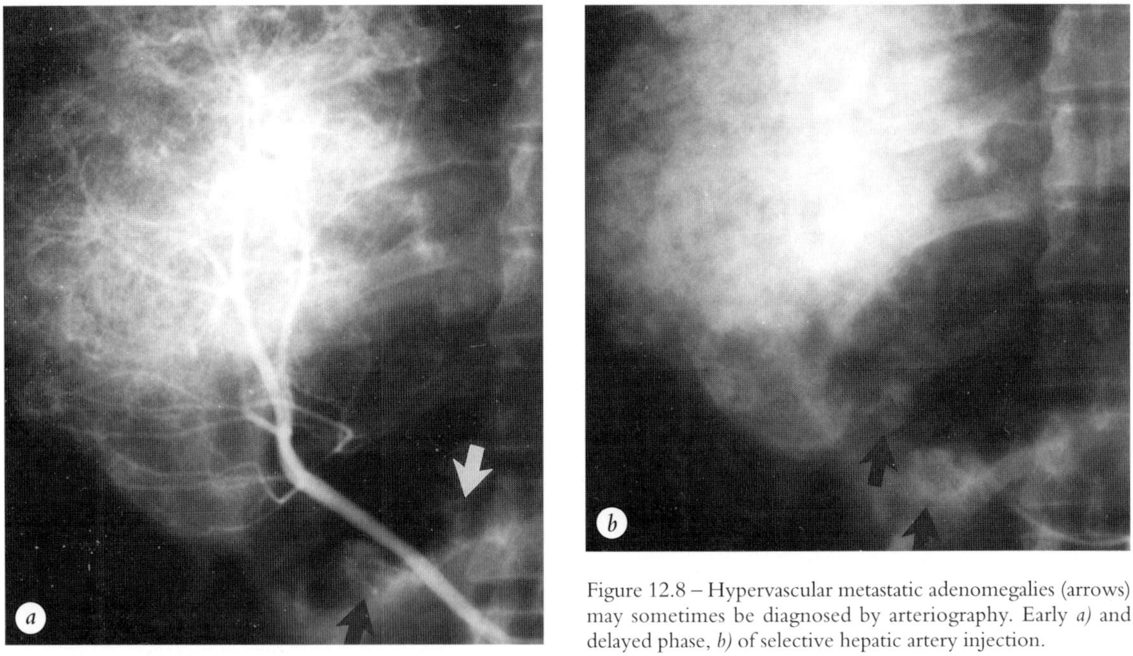

Figure 12.8 – Hypervascular metastatic adenomegalies (arrows) may sometimes be diagnosed by arteriography. Early *a)* and delayed phase, *b)* of selective hepatic artery injection.

DIFFERENTIAL DIAGNOSIS

In the cirrhotic liver, various types of nodular lesions, ranging from benign to malignant, may be present. Nevertheless, very few of these lesions are visible on arteriography except for HCC. Consequently, when a hypervascular tumor is visible on an hepatic arterial injection in a cirrhotic patient – or a patient presenting signs of porto-caval collateral shunting, which means intrahepatic portal hypertension – HCC is almost definitely diagnosed. Moreover, regenerative nodules, that are frequently present in cirrhotic liver, are never vascularized by the arterial system. However, one can rarely find more or less hypervascular masses in cirrhotic liver (adenoma, focal nodular hyperplasia, angioma, abcess, metastases, hyperplastic nodular hyperplasia) as well as HCC developing in a non cirrhotic liver.[26]

Portal study is a key examination in the angiographic exploration of liver tumors. It gives strong indications as to the malignancy, and also distinguishes between HCC and metastases.[3] Portal amputations (distal or proximal) are a feature of large HCC, which contrasts with benign tumors where they are present in only 19%. In late phases of the portal opacification (= portal hepatography), benign tumors show well-defined lacuna in all cases, since HCC leads to ill-defined lacuna in 51%. HCC leads to proximal (portal trunk or its two main branches) amputation three times more frequently than metastases. Portal stenosis is nearly always irregular in HCC, a consequence of its tendency to intraportal tumor overgrowth. Finally, the association of angiographic portocaval collateral circulation (related to portal hypertension) with proximal portal amputation is only noticed in HCC.

Numerous reports, from Asian and non-Asian countries,[17, 27] have described various types of nodular lesions in cirrhotic liver, ranging from regenerative nodules to HCC. These lesions are generally divided into three histologic groups: adenomatous hyperplasia without atypia, HCC, and intermediate lesions represented by adenomatous hyperplasia either atypical or containing malignant foci. In these lesions, intranodular portal blood flow tends to decrease – while at the same time, nodular arterial feeding increases – as the grade of malignancy increases; thus in adenomatous hyperplasia and small HCC, portal feeding is respectively 96% and 6% and arterial flow respectively 4% and 94%.[28] Finally, an isovascular nodule detected on selective arterial injection may correspond to HCC or a regenerative nodule; on the other hand, a hypovascular nodule may be HCC, a regenerative nodule, adenomatous hyperplasia or an inadvertent lesion such as metastases, lymphoma or granuloma.

Arterioportal shunting is frequent in HCC, but it carries poor specificity[29] since it may also accompany hepatic metastases (especially from renal cancer). More frequently, arterioportal shunting is the consequence of liver or tumor biopsy.

Inferior vena cava tumor thrombus occurs in HCC, malignant renal or adrenal tumors and primitive leiomyosarcoma of inferior vena cava or renal vein.[30] In contrast, portal and hepatic vein tumor thrombi have very high specificity for HCC. They can be easily differentiated from bland thrombus when they expand the caliber of the invaded vein or when they clearly show hypervascularity. Endovenous portal tumor invasion rarely occurs with hepatic metastases: only 1% of all patients presenting with metastases;[31,32] moreover, tumor casts due to metastases generally neither expand the vein caliber nor present as hypervascular.[31] Malignant endocrine tumors from the pancreas may lead to antegrade endoluminal invasion of superior mesenteric or splenic vein and portal trunk.[33,34] One must also take care to differentiate venous occlusion related to tumor invasion from portal flow reversal which is common in the cirrhotic liver.

Presence of a fibrous central scar in a liver tumor is considered highly specific for hyperplastic nodular hyperplasia; nevertheless, it may be present in HCC and fibrolamellar HCC.[35,36]

DETECTION RATE

It is a classical rule that hypervascular lesions of 0.5 cm in diameter can be detected by arteriography; by contrast, hypo- or isovascular tumors must be more than 2.0 cm in diameter to be detected.[37] It has been demonstrated that infusion techniques[5] and digital subtraction angiography[1] improve detection rate; but these two techniques carry a high false positive rate in cirrhotic patients since hypervascular HCC nodules cannot be differentiated from heterogeneous non specific contrast medium uptake associated with cirrhosis. The false positive rate for arteriography in detecting small HCC is around 22%.[38] False negatives are related to many intricate factors:

Table 12.1 – Angiographic detection rate of hepatocellular carcinoma to tumor size

	1 cm	2 cm	3 cm	5 cm
Takayasu *et al* [44]	45% ►	◄ 64% ►	◄ 93%	►
Choi *et al* [43]	◄ 74%	►		
	◄ 90%		►	
	◄ 96%			►
Takayasu *et al* [39]	55% ►	◄ 87%	►	
Kudo *et al* [2] **Conventional angiography**	25% ►	◄ 61% ►	◄ 80% ►	
DSA	33% ►	◄ 75% ►	◄ 100% ►	

i) the resolution of angiography may not be sufficient to demonstrate hypervascularity when nodules are too small or located in the left lobe and masked by bone vertebral structures,

ii) nodules may be isovascular as compared to the liver parenchyma,

iii) nodules may be poorly vascularized because of immature neovascularization.[24] This presentation often occurs in cases of well-differentiated HCC[25,39-41] and in tumors with diffuse fatty metamorphosis.[40-42]

Review of the angiographic literature reveals a wide variation in accuracy in detecting small HCC as a variety of techniques were used by the different authors. Accuracy of angiographic methods for detection of small HCC is 61 to 81%[2,39,43,44] (Table 12.1).

In conclusion, it is generally accepted that angiography is still a key investigation for diagnosis of small HCC and detection of small intrahepatic metastases, as well as frequently being the first step in effective intra-arterial tumor treatment.

REFERENCES

1. Bookstein J. Hepatocellular carcinoma: recent advances in diagnosis with iodized oil. *Radiology* 1985; **154**: 253-254

2. Kudo M, Tomita S, Tochio H, *et al*. Small hepatocellular carcinoma: diagnosis with US angiography with intra arterial CO_2 microbubbles. *Radiology* 1992; **182**: 155-160

3. Roche A, Schmit P, Medina F, Raynaud A, Lacombe P. The value of a portal study in determining the etiology of hepatic masses in adult. *Radiology* 1982; **143**: 387-393

4. Takayasu K, Itabashi M, Moriyama N. Hepatocellular carcinoma arising from the left diaphragm. *Clin Radiol* 1994; **49**: 579-581

5. Takashima T, Matsui O. Infusion hepatic angiography in the detection of small hepatocellular carcinoma. *Radiology* 1980; **136**: 321-325

6. Takashima S, Nakatsuka H, Nakamura K, *et al.* A new method of hepatic arteriography-balloon occluded hepatic arteriography. *Nippon Acta Radiol* 1984; **44**: 565-576

7. Okuda K, Musha H, Yoshida T, *et al.* Demonstration by celiac angiography of growing casts of hepatocellular carcinoma in the portal vein: the thread and streaks sign. *Radiology* 1975; **17**: 303-309

8. Kojiro M, Nakashima T. Pathology of hepatocellular carcinoma. In: Okuda K, Ishak J ed. *Neoplasms of the liver.* New-York: Springer-Verlag, 1987: 81-104

9. Freeny P, Baron R, Teefey S. Hepatocellular carcinoma: reduce frequency of typical findings with dynamic contrast enhanced CT in a non Asian population. *Radiology* 1992; **182**: 143-148

10. Tanaka K, Numata K, Okazaki H, *et al.* Diagnosis of portal vein thrombosis in patients with hepatocellular carcinoma: efficacy of color doppler sonography compared with angiography. *AJR* 1993; **160**: 1279-1283

11. Okuda K, Jinnouchi S, Nagasaki Y, *et al.* Angiographic demonstration of growth of hepatocellular carcinoma in the hepatic vein and inferior vena cava. *Radiology* 1977; **124**: 33-36

12. Jolly J, Delamarre J, Razafimahalo A, *et al.* Occult hepatocellular carcinoma in cirrhosis: value of US guided biopsy of portal vein system thrombus. *Abdom Imag* 1993; **18**: 344-346

13. Kanematsu M, Imaeda T, Minowa H, *et al.* Hepatocellular carcinoma with tumor thrombus in the inferior vena cava and right atrium. *Abdom Imag* 1994; **19**: 313-316

14. Okuda K, Musha H, Yamasaki T, *et al.* Angiographic demonstration of intra-hepatic arterioportal anastomoses in hepatocellular carcinoma. *Radiology* 1977; **122**: 53-58

15. Yamashita Y, Takahashi M, Baba Y, *et al.* Hepatocellular carcinoma with or without cirrhosis: comparison of CT and angiographic presentation in the US and Japan. *Abdom Imag* 1993; **18**: 168-175

16. Ros P, Murphy B, Buck J, *et al.* Encapsulated hepatocellular carcinoma: radiologic findings and pathologic correlation. *Gastrointest Radiol* 1990; **15**: 233-237

17. Nelson R, Chezmar J. Pathology and imaging of hepatocellular carcinoma neoplasms: are findings from Asian populations applicable to non-Asian groups? *AJR* 1993; **160**: 1188-1190

18. Otsuji M, Uchida H, Ohishi H. Dynamic computed tomography of the hepatocellular carcinoma with particular reference to capsule. *Jpn J Clin Radiol* 1983; **28**: 1465-1471

19. Okuda K, Obata H, Jinnouchi S, *et al.* Angiographic assessment of gross anatomy of hepatocellular carcinoma: comparison of celiac angiogram and liver pathology in 100 cases. *Radiology* 1977; **123**: 21-29

20. Okuda K, Peters R, Simson I. Gross anatomy features of hepatocellular carcinoma from three disparate geographic areas: proposal of a new classification. *Cancer* 1984; **54**: 2165-2173.

21. Karani J. Tumours: benign, primary malignant. In: Wilkins R, Nunnerley H ed. *Imaging of the liver, pancreas and spleen.* Blackwell, 1990: 172-186

22. Friedman A, Lichtenstein J, Goodman Z, Fishman E, Siegelman S, Dachman A. Fibrolamellar hepatocellular carcinoma. *Radiology* 1985; **157**: 583-587

23. Ohtomo K, Itai Y. Early diagnosis of hepatocellular carcinoma. In: Ferrucci J, Mathieu D ed. *Advances in hepatobiliary radiology.* St Louis: C.V. Mosby Company, 1990: 181-208

24. Kanai T, Hiroashi S, Upton M, *et al.* Pathology of small hepatocellular carcinoma: a proposal for a new gross classification. *Cancer* 1987; **60**: 810-819

25. Honda H, Ochiai K, Adachi E, *et al.* Hepatocellular carcinoma: correlations of CT, angiography and histopathologic findings. *Radiology* 1993; **189**:857-852

26. Vlahos L, Trakadas S, Gouliamos A, *et al.* Comparative study between US, CT, intraarterial digital substraction angiography and MRI in the differentiation of tumors of the liver. *Gastrointest Radiol* 1990; **15**:102-106

27. Choi B, Takayasu K, Han M. Small hepatocellular carcinoma and associated nodular lesions of the liver: pathology, pathogenesis and imaging findings. *AJR* 1993; **160**: 1177-1187

28. Matsui O, Kadoya M, Kameyama T, *et al.* Benign and malignant nodules in cirrhotic livers: distinction based on blood supply. *Radiology* 1991; **178**: 493-497

29. Adler J, Goodgold M, Mitty H, *et al.* Arteriovenous shunts involving the liver. *Radiology* 1978; **129**: 315-322

30. Subramanyam B, Balthazar E, Hilton S, *et al.* Hepatocellular carcinoma with venous invasion: sonographic angiographic correlation. *Radiology* 1984; **150**: 793-796

31. Heaston D, Chuang V, Wallace S, *et al.* Metastatic hepatic neoplasms: angiographic features of portal vein involvement. *AJR* 1981; **136**: 897-900

32. Araki T, Suda K, Sekikawa T, *et al.* Portal venous tumor thrombosis associated with gastric adenocarcinoma. *Radiology* 1990; **174**: 811-814

33. Bok E, Cho K, Williams D, *et al.* Venous involvement in islet cell tumors of the pancreas. *AJR* 1984; **142**: 319-322.

34. Roche A, Baert A, Thérasse E, Rigauts H, Marchal G. Endocrine tumors of the pancreas. In: Baert A ed. *Radiology of the pancreas.* Springer-Verlag, 1994: 197-234

35. Rummeny E, Weissleder R, Sironi S, *et al.* Central scar in primary liver tumors: MR features, specificity and pathologic correlations. *Radiology* 1989; **171**: 323-326

36. Mathieu D, Bruneton J, Drouillard J, *et al.* Hepatic adenomas and focal nodular hyperplasia: dynamic CT study. *Radiology* 1986; **160**: 53-58

37. Wallace S, Chuang V. Liver tumours: diagnosis and management. In: Herlinger M, Lunderquist A, Wallace S ed. *Clinical radiology of the liver.* New York: Marcel Decker Inc., 1983: 715-864

38. Sumida M, Ohto M, Ebara M, *et al.* Accuracy of angiography in the diagnosis of small hepatocellular carcinoma. *AJR* 1986; **147**: 531-536

39. Takayasu K, Moriyama N, Muramatsu Y, *et al.* The diagnosis of small hepatocellular carcinoma: efficacy of various imaging procedures in 100 patients. *AJR* 1990; **155**: 49-54

40. Yoshimatsu S, Inoue Y, Ibukuro K, *et al*. Hypovascular hepatocellular carcinoma undetected at angiography and CT with iodized oil. *Radiology* 1989; **171**: 343-347

41. Sonoda T, Shirabe K, Takenaka K, *et al*. Angiographically undetected small hepatocellular carcinoma: clinicopathological characteristics, follow-up and treatment. *Hepatology* 1989; **10**: 1003-1007

42. Yoshikawa J, Matsui O, Takashima T, *et al*. Fatty metamorphosis in hepatocellular carcinoma: radiologic features in 10 cases. *AJR* 1988; **151**: 717-720

43. Choi B, Park J, Kim B, *et al*. Small hepatocellular carcinoma: detection with sonography, computed tomography (CT), angiography and Lipiodol-CT. *Br J Radiol* 1989; **62**: 897-903

44. Takayasu K, Shima Y, Muramatsu Y, *et al*. Angiography of small hepatocellular carcinoma: analysis of 105 resected tumors. *AJR 1986*; **147**: 525-529

13

Computed tomography

O Matsui, M Kadoya, J Yosikawa and T Gabata

Computed tomography (CT) plays an important role in the screening, differential diagnosis, staging, and evaluation of the results of the treatment of hepatocellular carcinomas (HCC) because of its objectiveness in visualizing the relation between the lesions and the surrounding tissues, without being disturbed by intervening bones, air in the gut or lung, or dense fatty tissue. Recent advances of spiral CT greatly improved diagnostic accuracy and open a new era in the imaging diagnosis of HCCs. Now, a combination of CT and arteriography using spiral CT is the most sensitive and accurate diagnostic modality for HCCs.

In this chapter, we describe the ability and clinical usefulness of CT, especially spiral CT, in the diagnosis and treatment of HCCs.

TECHNIQUE

For the diagnosis of HCCs, both pre- and postcontrast CT are necessary, and, as far as possible, dynamic CT following intravenous bolus injection should be performed. The technique of contrast enhancement differs depending on the purpose of the study and the machines used.

Drip infusion

CT is performed immediately after the completion of drip infusion of 100-150 ml of 60% iodinated contrast medium. Contrast medium should be administered as quickly as possible to obtain good contrast between the tumor and surrounding liver parenchyma.

Incremental dynamic CT with intravenous bolus injection of contrast medium (dynamic CT)

This is the preferred CT technique for routine evaluation of HCCs. In this technique, 100-150 ml of 60% iodinated contrast medium is administered by a power injector before and during the incremental scanning of the liver. Contrast material is infused in either a monophasic or a biphasic mode. In the bipahsic mode, about half of the contrast medium is delivered at 2-4 ml/s, followed by the other half at 1 ml/s. In monophasic mode, contrast medium is infused at 2-3 ml/s. Dynamic CT during incremental movement of the table is carried out 30 to 40 seconds after the start of the injection of contrast medium and, by using conventional CT with 1 cm slice thicknesses and 2-second scan time, the entire liver can be scanned within 1.5-3 minutes. This techinique provides a sustained increase in hepatic parenchymal attenuation over 2 to 4 minutes of 45 Hounsfield units (HU).[1] For the assessment of the contrast enhancement characteristics of a single lesion, dynamic CT at the same level is performed, and is called a single level dynamic study. In dynamic CT with intravenous bolus contrast medium injection, the early scans (20-30 seconds following injection) show dense opacification of the abdominal aorta and its branches while later scans demonstrate the portal and venous systems clearly. However, considering the time required for injection and the long circulation pathway, terms such as "arterial-dominant" and "portal-dominant" phases have come into use.[2] Following the portal-dominant phase, contrast medium distributes over the whole body, and is also called the "equilibrium" phase. The injected contrast medium gradually disappears from the blood spaces and then distributes into interstitial tissues in the later equilibrium phase (delayed CT scan). The enhancement seen on delayed CT is called "delayed enhancement". With the conventional CT machine, it was impossible to obtain arterial-dominant phase images of the entire liver. However, after the introduction of spiral (or helical) CT, it has become easier to achieve them within breath holding, and has markedly improved the diagnostic ability of CT.[3] With spiral CT, a volume acquisition of the entire liver is accomplished within 20-30 seconds. Therefore, it is possible to obtain the relatively pure arterial- and portal-dominant phase images of the entire liver. With dynamic CT using spiral CT, typically 100-150 ml of contrast medium is injected at a rate of 2-3 ml/s. For the arterial-dominant phase of images, scanning can be initiated 30-40 seconds after the beginning of the contrast infusion. 7-10 mm/s table incrementation and 7-10 mm slice thickness are usually employed.[4,5] CT scanning immediately following the completion of dynamic study usually reflects the late portal-dominant (equilibrium) phase of images.

CT during or after intra-arterial contrast medium injection

The combined use of CT and arteriography is the most precise imaging method for the diagnosis of hepatic mass lesions. However, it is an invasive method and its indication should be considered the same as for hepatic angiography. There are three combinations of CT and arteriography: CT during the infusion of contrast medium into the hepatic artery (CT arteriography: CTA),[6] CT during arterial portography (CTAP)[7-9] and CT performed after intra-arterial injection of iodized poppyseed oil (Lipiodol: Guerbet Laboratories, France).[10]

In CTA, 10-15 ml of contrast medium is infused into the hepatic artery at a rate of 1-3 ml/s during the scanning of each slice of the liver. With the conventional CT machine, larger amounts of contrast medium and a slower rate are needed for acceptable CT arteriographic study of the entire liver. After the introduction of spiral CT, it has become possible to obtain high-quality CTA pictures of the entire liver during a single breath hold. In CTA using spiral CT, contrast medium is infused into the hepatic artery (from the proper or common hepatic artery is ideal, but if not possible, injection into the celiac artery is recommended) at a rate of 1-3 ml/s during the scanning of the entire liver with breath holding. The injection of contrast medium is initiated around 5 seconds before the start of scanning.

For CTAP using a conventional CT machine, 70-100 ml of contrast medium is injected via a catheter in the superior mesenteric artery at a rate of 0.5-1.5 ml/s during sequential scanning of the liver with incremental changes in the position of the table.[7-9,11,12] Usually 1 cm slice thicknesses, 1-2 second scanning time, and 1 cm table incrementation are employed and about 4-6 seconds scan-delay is needed between the scanning of each slice. Therefore, it takes 1-2.5 minutes to obtain CTAP images of the entire liver. The scanning is started around 20 seconds after the initiation of the infusion of contrast medium. Intra-arterial injection of a vasodilator such as prostaglandin E1 is carried out immediately before the contrast medium injection to overcome the laminal flow of the portal venous system. The infusion of the contrast medium is stopped around 20 seconds before the end of scanning.

In CTAP using a spiral CT system, almost the same scanning conditions as those of dynamic CT using a spiral CT machine are used.[13,14] Because the scanning time of the entire liver is 20-30 seconds, it is possible to reduce the amount of contrast medium injected or to increase the rate of infusion of contrast medium. Usually 50-100 ml of contrast medium is infused at a rate of 1-3 ml/s following the intra-arterial injection of vasodilator. Scanning is started 20-30 seconds after the begining of the injection of contrast medium. Other advantages of CTAP with a spiral CT machine are that there are no slice gaps and smooth 3D-reconstruction vascular images can be obtained.[14] Immediately following CTAP, we usually take another CT scan of the entire liver (delayed CT).

In Lipiodol CT, CT is performed 1-2 weeks following injection of 2-5 ml of Lipiodol into the proper hepatic artery. In our study, simple Lipiodol injection not followed by transcatheter arterial embolization (TAE) by gelatin sponge particles is not sufficiently diagnostic, because Lipiodol disappears from hepatic tumors relatively quickly.[15]

IMAGING MODALITIES FOR THE DIAGNOSIS OF HCC

Various imaging modalities are now available to diagnose HCC, such as US, CT, radionuclide scintigraphy, MRI, hepatic angiography, and a combination of CT or US and arteriography. Knowledge of the features of each method and selection of the suitable one in individual cases are necessary.

Usually, US is the first choice because it is noninvasive and widely availabile. CT is the second choice. Recent advances in spiral CT systems have enhanced the usefulness of CT examination. Dynamic CT using a spiral CT machine is very sensitive at detecting small classical HCCs (Fig. 13.1). MRI is not always necessary for the diagnosis of HCCs, although it has a unique ability in the differential diagnosis of hepatic mass lesions.[16-18] When some abnormality is found by noninvasive methods, hepatic angiography including a combination of CT and arteriography or US after the intra-arterial injection of carbon dioxide microbubbles (CO_2 US angiography)[19] is indicated to confirm the existence of HCC, to make a precise differential diagnosis, and to evaluate the extent of the disease (staging). CTA is useful for the visualization of the macroscopic pathology of the hepatic lesions and the evaluation of arterial vascularity of the small mass lesions. CTAP is the most sensitive technique in the detection of hypovascular hepatic tumors and intrahepatic portal venous obstruction and is effective in

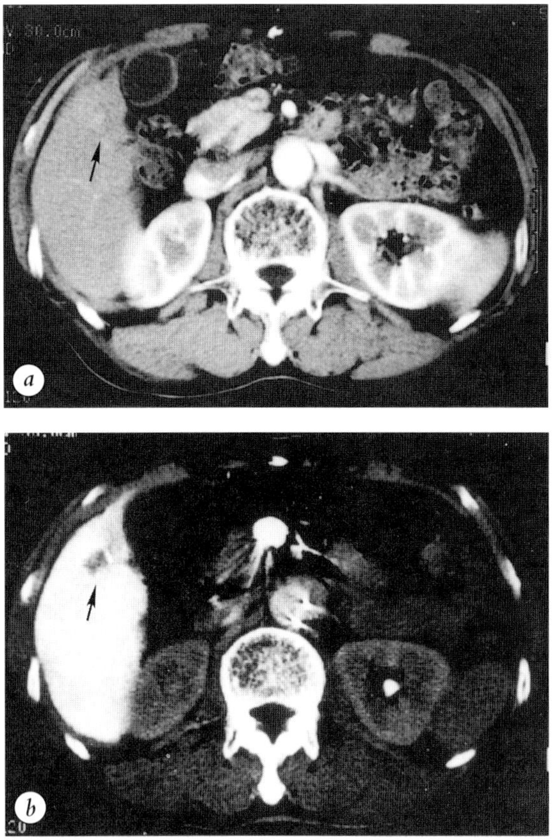

Figure 13.1 – Minute classical HCC detected firstly by dynamic CT using spiral CT system.

a) A minute staining is shown on arterial-dominant phase of dynamic CT (arrow). Both pre and postcontrast CT did not visualize it.

b) CT during arterial portography (CTAP) shows it as a definite hypodense area indicating intranodular portal perfusion defect (arrow).

determining segmental anatomy of the liver (Fig. 13.1).[20] CTAP using spiral CT may be the best modality for the preoperative evaluation of hepatic tumors including HCC.[11,14] However, the findings obtained by CTAP are usually nonspecific (Fig.13.1), and therefore CTAP findings should be carefully analyzed with reference to the finding of other imaging methods. Another problem of CTAP is the finding of various kinds of pseudolesions due to localized different portal flow caused by intrahepatic arterio-portal shunt, cystic venous drainage (S4, S5)[21], aberrant gastric venous drainage (S4, S1)[22] (Fig. 13.2), suspected venous drainage from the falciform ligament (S4), and so on. Lipiodol CT is the most sensitive in the detection of minute

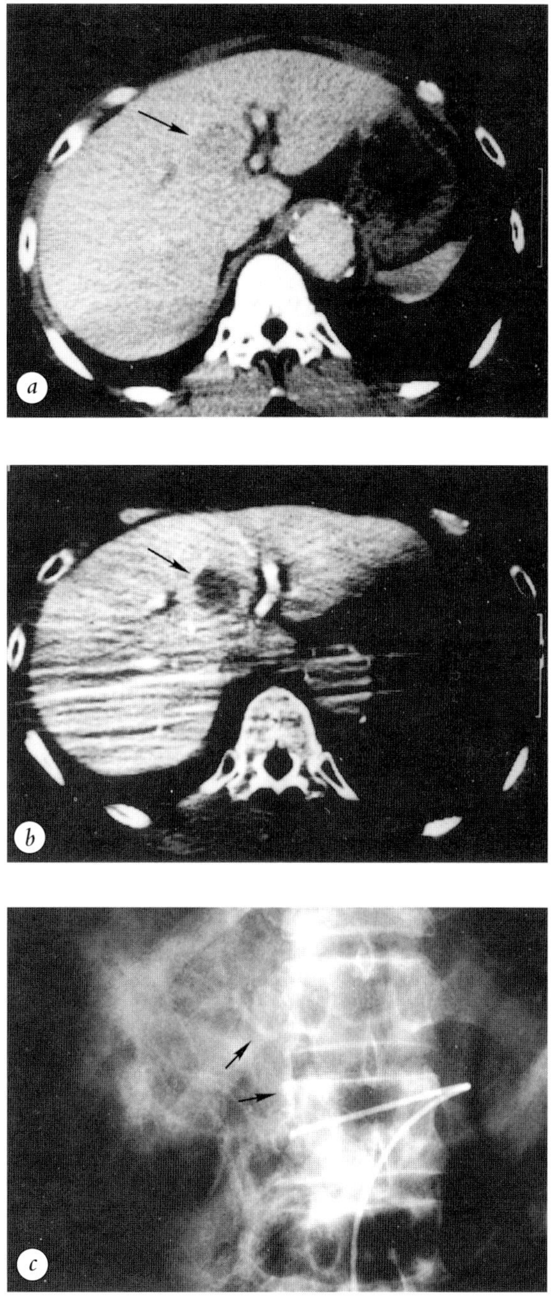

Figure 13.2 – Hyperplastic change seen in the area with aberrant right gastric venous drainage in cirrhotic liver.

a) Postcontrast CT shows slightly hypodense area in S4 (arrow).

b) CTAP shows it as a definite hypodense area (arrow).

c) Common hepatic arteriography shows the aberrant right gastric venous drainage into S4 (arrows).
(From *Radiology* 1995; **197**:345-349)

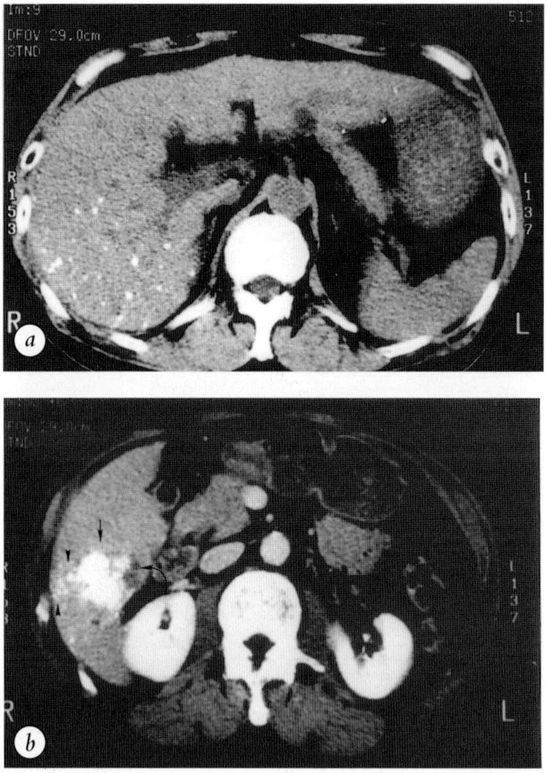

Figure 13.3 – Lipiodol CT obtained 2 months following transcatheter arterial embolization using Lipiodol and Gelfoam particles.

a) Precontrast CT shows multiple Lipiodol retentions in minutes intrahepatic metastases.

b) Postcontrast CT shows a small recurrent mass in the peripheral portion of the Lipiodol-filled main tumor (arrow). Minute daughter nodules are seen just adjacent to the main tumors (arrowheads). Viable portion is visualized as hypodense area (curved arrow).

hypervascular classical HCCs (Fig. 13.3). However, without combined TAE, its detection of hepatic tumors is not so reliable.[15] Lipiodol CT is mainly carried out for the evaluation of local recurrence of HCCs treated by TAE therapy (Fig. 13.3).

SCREENING OF HCC IN HIGH-RISK GROUPS

In major Japanese institutions, periodic screening examinations are performed in patients with liver cirrhosis or chronic hepatitis, especially when these are related to hepatitis B or C virus infection. α-Fetoprotein (AFP) measurement and US are carried out every 3 months. Usually, the detectability of well-differentiated HCCs by US is superior to that by CT.[23] However, dynamic CT, especially using spiral CT, is very sensitive in the detection of small hypervascular classical HCCs which should be treated as soon as possible (Fig. 13.1).[5] Therefore, we think that the periodic performance of dynamic CT using spiral CT will become very important.

HISTOLOGIC ASPECTS OF HCC IMPORTANT FOR CT DIAGNOSIS

Two types of human HCC are now recognized. One is *de novo* carcinogenesis. The other is stepwise development of HCC from adenomatous hyperplasia (AH), atypical AH, atypical AH with malignant foci, well-differentiated HCC to classical HCC (Edmondson's grade II or above) in a liver with cirrhosis or chronic hepatitis, especially in patients with hepatitis B or C virus infection.[24-26] The definition of these nodules associated with liver cirrhosis at our institution is as follows.[24] AH is considered to be a premalignant lesion and has been designated variably as dysplastic nodule, paraplastic nodule, macroregenerative nodule type II. AH is a grossly distinct and expansive nodular lesion larger than the surrounding regenerative nodules in the cirrhotic liver (>8 mm in the largest diameter) and consists of hepatocytes that are no different morphologically from the hepatocytes of the surrounding regenerative nodules and show no cellular or structural atypism. Atypical AH is defined as AH consisting of hepatocytes that have variable nuclear and structural atypia but are not overt carcinoma cells. However, some controversy still exists concerning the definite differentiation between early stage well-differentiated HCCs and atypical AHs with severe atypia (borderline lesion). Because the borderline lesions occasionally have microscopic HCC foci,[24,26] they are treated clinically as early stage cancer. Therefore, the precise differentiation between early stage well-differentiated HCC and borderline lesion is not always necessary.

Although the gross features of HCC vary depending on the size of the tumor and the presence or absence of liver cirrhosis, many advanced HCCs exhibit an expansile tumor growth with a combination of varying degrees of infiltrative tumor growth and intrahepatic metastasis.[27] Fibrous capsule and septa are gross pathological features in HCCs. These

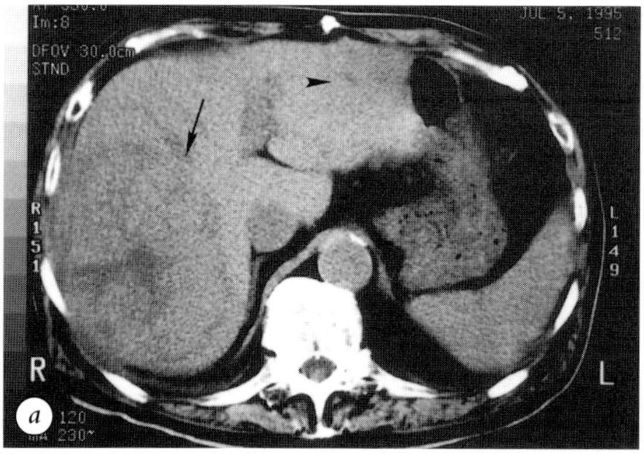

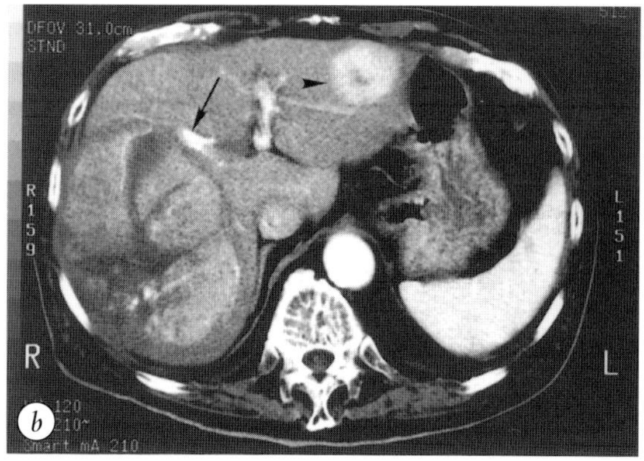

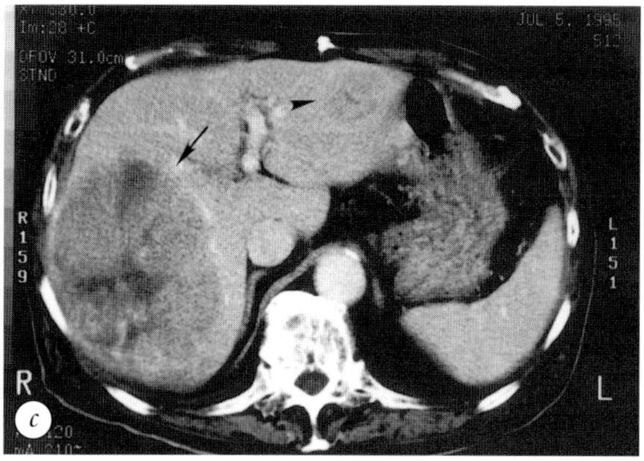

Figure 13.4 – Nodular type of advanced HCC.

a) Precontrast CT shows a giant hypodense nodule with surrounding more hypodense band (capsule) and internal mosaic architecture separated by hypodense septums (arrow). Another relatively small HCC is also demonstrated (arrowhead).

b) Arterial-dominant phase of dynamic CT shows dense staining in the tumors. Internal mosaic pattern is most clearly visualized in this phase (arrow and arrowhead).

c) Postcontrast CT shows enhanced capsule surrounding the tumors (arrow and arrowhead).

features are well-developed in classical HCCs larger than 2 cm, but are rarely seen in HCCs less than 1.5 cm. The advanced HCCs are classified into four major types: expansive type (single nodular and multinodular), infiltrative type, mixed expansive and infiltrative type, and diffuse type.[27] In advanced HCCs, extension of the tumor into the portal or hepatic veins is often seen (tumor thrombi). Small HCCs less than 3 cm in diameter usually show a nodular type configuration and are subdivided into four types: single nodular type, single nodular type with extranodular growth, contiguous multinodular type, and poorly demarcated nodular type.[28]

HCC shows various degrees of fatty metamorphosis histologically, especially small classical HCCs and well-differentiated HCCs. Fatty change is diffuse or focal, and the degree of fat deposition varies among components in a mosaic architecture.[27,29]

HCC cells often invade or flow into portal venules and grow within the lumen (tumor thrombus). In the advanced stage of HCC, tumor thrombi are occasionally demonstrated in major intrahepatic portal or hepatic veins and variously modify the macroscopic pathology and imaging findings.

CT FINDINGS FOR TYPICAL CLASSICAL HCC

Advanced HCC

The expansive type of HCC is sharply demarcated and usually single nodular or multinodular. Most HCCs of this type which are associated with liver cirrhosis have a fibrous capsule and internal mosaic architecture. These macroscopic features of the expansive type are very specific and their detection by imaging is almost certainly diagnostic of HCC. The fibrous capsule is seen as a thin circular hypodense band surrounding the tumor on precontrast CT and during the arterial-dominant phase of dynamic CT, and as a hyperdense band on postcontrast CT (Fig. 13.4). The internal mosaic architecture is characterized by components separated by thin bands (fibrous septum) with the same CT features as those of the fibrous capsule and with each component showing different densities on precontrast, dynamic

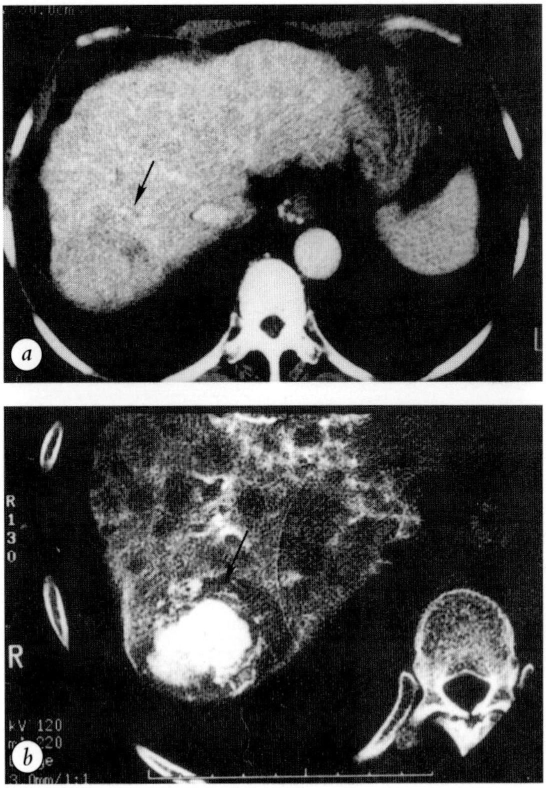

Figure 13.5 – CT arteriography (CTA) in a classical HCC.

a) Postcontrast CT shows a hypodense solid mass (arrow).

b) CTA shows macroscopic features (mosaic architecture) of the tumor clearly (arrow).

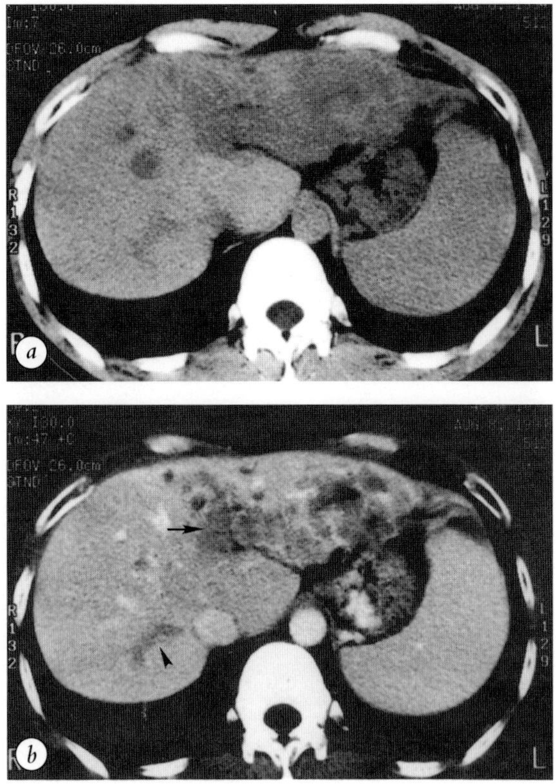

Figure 13.6 – Infiltrative type of advanced HCC

a) Precontrast CT shows diffuse hypodensity in S2 and S4 with unclear margin.

b) Postcontrast CT shows multiple scattered hypodense nodules with unclear margin in S2 and S4. Tumor thrombus in left portal vein (arrow) and right hepatic vein (arrowhead) are demonstrated as enhanced but hypodense mass lesion in each vessels.

and postcontrast CT (Fig. 13.4).[2,30] These macroscopic features are most precisely visualized by CTA (Fig. 13.5). Conversely, in the infiltrative type, the tumor-nontumor boundary is irregular and indistinct, neoplastic foci of varying sizes are fused to form larger foci distributed segmentally, and tumor thrombi in the portal veins are often associated (Fig. 13.6). This type of HCC occasionally demonstrates segmental uneven hypodense areas with unclear margins due to spreading tumors and/or Zhan's infarction caused by portal venous obstruction on precontrast CT (Fig. 13.6). The diffuse type shows numerous small nodules, 0.5-1.0 cm in diameter, scattered throughout the liver and which do not fuse with each other. Diffuse nodules are visualized as diffusely distributed small hypodense nodules on both pre- and postcontrast CT. This CT finding is very similar to that for regenerative nodules and diffuse metastases and it is not easy to differentiate these lesions without dynamic CT. In clinical practice, the frequency of this type is extremely rare. Small or minute daughter nodules adjacent to the main nodule are another macroscopic characteristic of HCC (Figs. 13.3, 7).

In addition to the morphological features described above, the hypervascular nature of HCCs is relatively specific. Typical classical HCCs are hyperdense in the arterial-dominant phase of dynamic CT and become hypodense in the portal-dominant or equilibrium phases (Figs. 13.4, 7).

Another histologic and imaging characteristic of advanced classical HCCs is their tendency to grow into neighboring intrahepatic portal veins and/or hepatic veins (tumor thrombus). Tumor thrombi in the major portal or hepatic veins are shown as a cast-like mass with soft tissue density within hypodense vessels on precontrast CT. On postcontrast CT, they appear as a hypodense mass in the well-enhanced vessel (Fig. 13.6). At the site of tumor thrombus, arterio-venous or arterio-portal (A-P) shunting are often seen, and it demonstrates marked hypervascularity and early visualization of portal or hepatic veins (Fig. 13.8). When a small solid mass is seen continuously from the HCC nodule along the portal tract or hepatic vein, the possibility of tumor thrombus should be considered (Fig. 13.6).

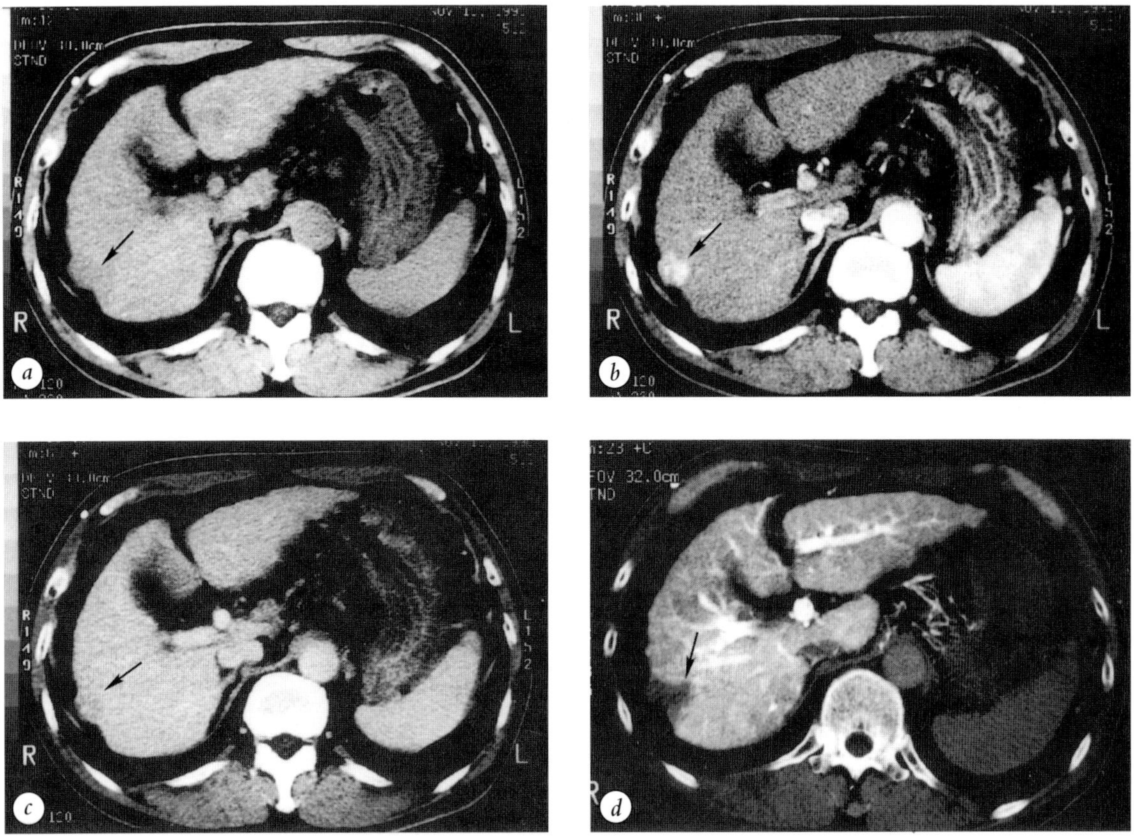

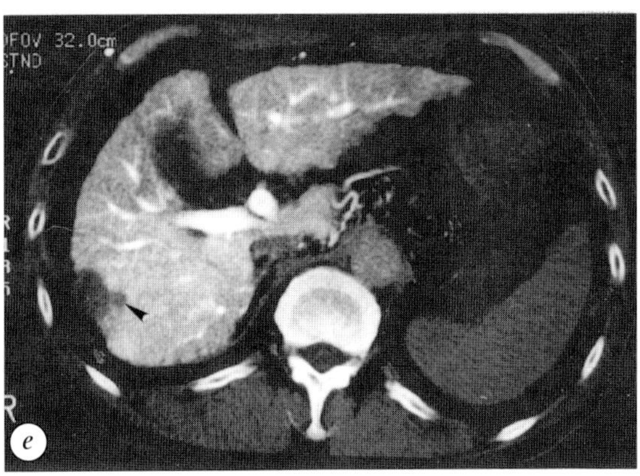

Figure 13.7 – Small advanced classical HCC.

a) Precontrast CT shows a hypodense nodule (arrow).

b) Arterial-dominant phase of dynamic CT shows definite staining with internal mosaic architectue in the tumor (arrow).

c) postcontrast CT shows it as a faintly hypodense nodule (arrow).

d, e) CTAP shows wedge-shaped perfusion defect which cover the upper portion of the tumor (arrow in *d*) and a minute daughter nodule just adjacent to the tumor (arrowhead in *e*).

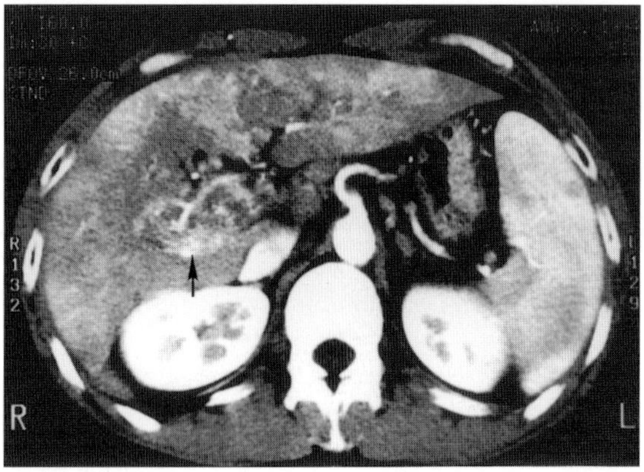

Figure 13.8 – Tumor thrombus in the portal vein shown by dynamic CT. Arterial-dominant phase of dynamic CT shows marked hypervascularity in the right portal vein (arrow). Peripheral segmental stainings due to portal venous obstruction are well-visualized.

The hepatic segment in which the feeding portal vein is obstructed demonstrates segmental staining[31,32] in the arterial-dominant phase of dynamic CT, probably due to arterial compensation for the decreased portal blood flow (Figs.13.8-10). When portal ischemia is severe and long-standing, the obstructed segment shows hypodensity relative to surrounding non-obstructed segments on precontrast CT (Fig. 13.6), and hyperdensity on postcontrast CT, probably due to fibrotic changes.

Intraperitoneal bleeding due to the rupture of the tumor is one of the most serious complications of advanced HCCs. Though rare it also occurs in small hypervascular HCCs. On CT, the ruptured HCC with internal hyperdensity due to fresh thrombus is usually seen at the peritoneal surface of the liver, mostly protruding from the surface (Fig. 13.11). Hyperdense ascites (hemoperitoneum) is commonly associated.

Small classical HCC

Almost all small classical HCCs have a nodular type of configuration. The macroscopic features of nodular small classical HCCs are the same as those described in the expansive type of HCC (Figs.13.4, 7, 9). According to our study,[17] around 90% of HCCs larger than 2 cm showed a fibrous capsule on macroscopic pathologic examination, 70% to 80% of which were demonstrated on imaging diagnosis. On the other hand, the capsule was seen in about 50% of the tumors less than 2 cm in diameter, was poorly developed in macroscopic examination, and was visualized on imaging examinations in less than 20% of cases (Fig. 13.1). The same study[17] focusing on the mosaic architecture gave similar results. When these macroscopic features are not seen, a small classical HCC is visualized as a non-specific hypervascular mass on CT.

Single nodular type with extranodular growth, contiguous multinodular type, and poorly demarcated nodular type of small HCC usually show a nodular configuration with an irregular or unclear margin.

Small classical HCCs occasionally show fat density in the tumor and it is almost certainly diagnostic for HCC or HCC-related lesion such as adenomatous

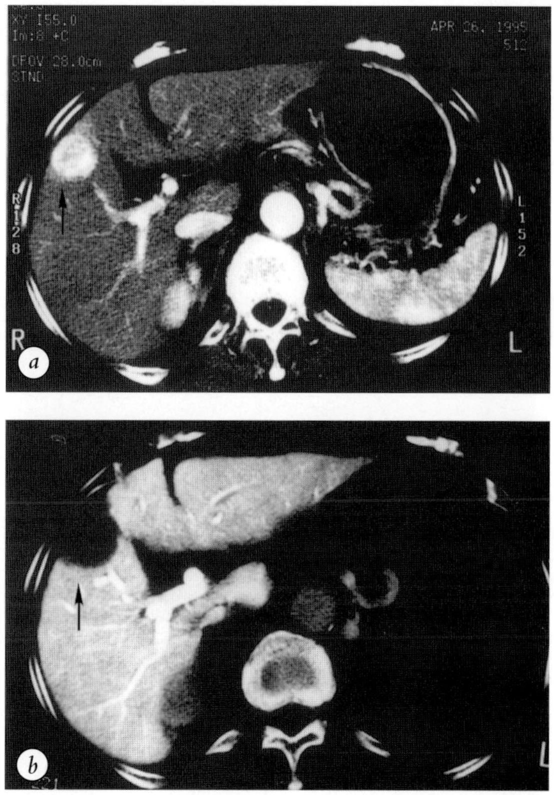

Figure 13.9 – Small classical HCC with surrounding segmental staining.

a) Arterial-dominant phase of dynamic CT shows well-opasified tumor with surrounding peripheral segmental staining (arrow).

b) CTAP shows fan-shaped portal perfusion defect peripheral to the tumor (arrow).

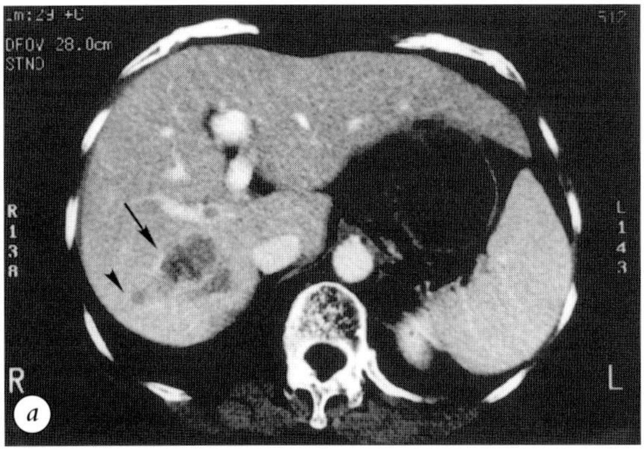

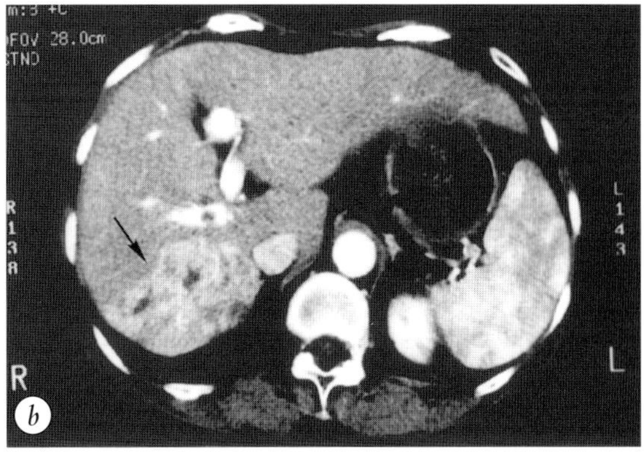

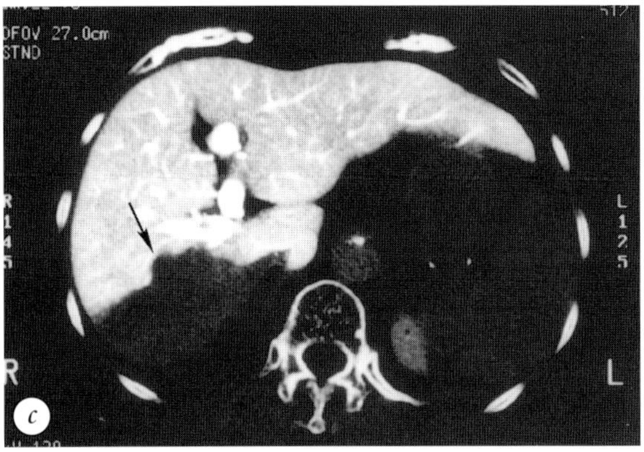

Figure 13.10 – Relatively small classical HCC with portal tumor thrombus.

a) Postcontrast CT shows a hypodense mass with internal mosaic architecture (arrow) and daughter nodule (arrowhead).

b) Arterial-dominant phase of dynamic CT shows definite staining in the entire S7 including the tumor (arrow).

c) CTAP shows wedge-shaped portal perfusion defect in the entire S7 including the tumor (arrow) due to tumor thrombus in the proximal portion of superior posterior intrahepatic portal vein.

hyperplasia in patients with high-risk for HCC (Fig. 13.12).[29]

DIFFERENTIAL DIAGNOSIS OF CLASSICAL HCC

CT findings indicating a fibrous capsule are also seen in hepatic adenomas, rarely in medullary metastatic or cholangiocellular carcinomas, and in non-epithelial hepatic tumors. Mosaic architecture separated by fibrous septa is pathognomonic for HCC, but care should be taken not to misdiagnose uneven CT densities in the tumors due to degeneration, necrosis or bleeding as a true mosaic pattern.

When the macroscopic features are lacking, classical HCCs must be differentiated from various other hypervascular hepatic mass lesions such as cavernous hemangioma, hypervascular metastasis, hepatic adenoma, focal nodular hyperplasia (FNH), and small A-P shunting. Among them, cavernous hemangioma is the most common. Cavernous hemangiomas are composed of vascular channels of various sizes separated by thin fibrous tissue. Therefore, they show almost the same density as that of the aorta with a clear margin on precontrast CT. On dynamic CT, cavernous hemangiomas show early peripheral enhancement and centripetal fill-in during the arterial-dominant phase and prolonged enhancement

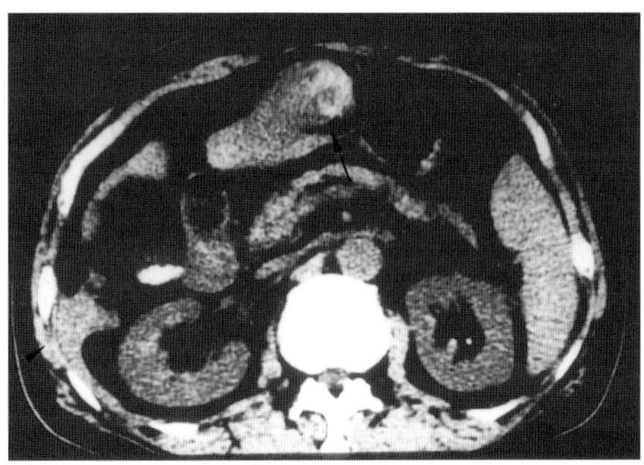

Figure 13.11. – Ruptured small HCC. Precontrast CT shows a hepodense mass with internal hyperdensity due to fresh blood clot protruded from the liver (arrow). Hemoperitoneum is shown as hyperdense intrperitoneal fluid (arrowhead).

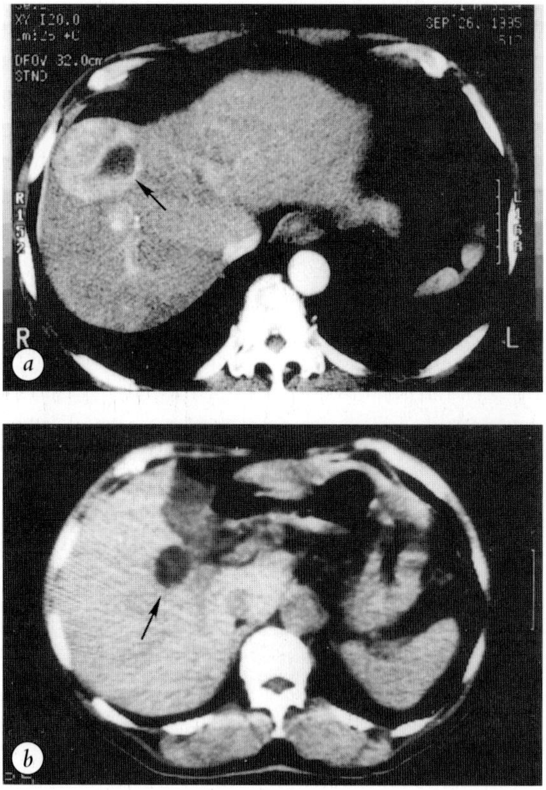

Figure 13.12 – Classical HCC with marked fatty metamorphosis. *a)* Arterial-dominant phase of dynamic CT shows a well-enhanced mass with internal definite hypodense portion (arrow). Fat deposition was confirmed by CT density and chemical shift imaging of MR imaging. *b)* Precontrast CT shows extremely hypodense mass with fat density (arrow).

in the delayed equilibrium phase.[2,33,34] On the other hand, classical HCC nodules are usually opacified throughout the entire tumor during the arterial-dominant phase and become hypodense in the equilibrium phase (Fig. 13.7). In cavernous hemangioma, the densities of the lesion are almost the same as those of the aorta throughout precontrast CT, the arterial-dominant phase of dynamic CT, and postcontrast CT. This fact is also very useful in CT diagnosis of cavernous hemangioma. Although this dynamic CT pattern is diagnostic, a conclusive diagnosis is not always possible for small lesions less than 1.5 cm in diameter and in which case MRI or arteriography should be performed.

Hypervascular metastatic liver cancers, usually from the medullary type of carcinomas, are occasionally difficult to differentiate from HCCs by imaging findings alone. Differentiation of hepatocellular adenoma from HCC by imaging diagnosis is impossible. However, when hepatic adenoma is seen in cirrhotic liver, it is impossible to differentiate from well-differentiated HCC even in the histology.

FNH typically contains a central stellate scar with radiating fibrous septa containing one or more large arteries and bile ducts, dividing the lesion into nodules. Visualization of this central vascular scar with radiating arteries (spoke-wheel pattern) is diagnostic. If the central scar is large enough to be visualized on CT, it appears hypodense on precontrast CT and the arterial-dominant phase of dynamic CT and hyperdense on postcontrast CT. However, when FNH is small, the differentiation from HCC by CT is not easy.

Small peripheral A-P shunting is occasionally seen in cirrhotic livers. On dynamic CT, it demonstrates small hyperdense nodules and its differentiation from small classical HCC is very important in clinical practice. It usually shows a wedge-shaped configuration and a portal venule can be seen in the center of the enhanced area. Without these features, the differentiation of small A-P shunting and small classical HCC may be impossible by CT or other imaging diagnosis. The area with A-P shunting is usually not demonstrated on pre- and postcontrast CT. However, when fatty liver is associated, this area may show focal sparing of fatty infiltration.

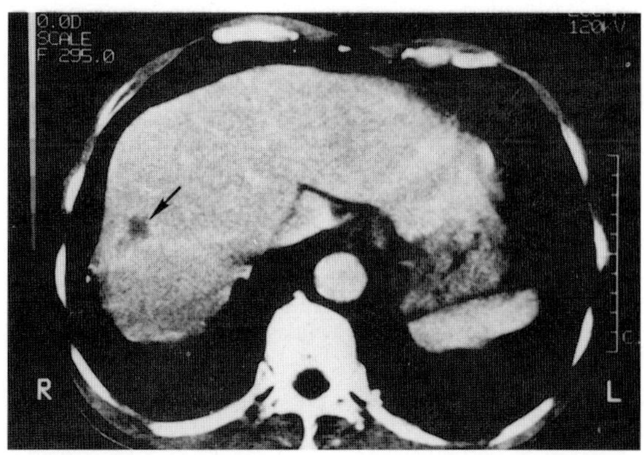

Figure 13.13 – Necrotic small classical HCC. Postcontrast CT shows a small unenhanced nodule with surrounding enhanced capsule (arrow).

CT FINDINGS AND DIFFERENTIAL DIAGNOSIS OF CLASSICAL HCC WITH ATYPICAL HISTOLOGIC FEATURES

The histopathology of HCCs varies depending on the combination of the following features: the structural pattern (trabecular, sclerosing, etc), and differences in the degree of cell differentiation, cytological variants (fatty change, clear cells, etc). The histologic characteristics modify the imaging findings differently and include HCCs with marked fatty metamorphosis, massive necrosis, abundant fibrous stroma (scirrhous type), sarcomatous change, and copper accumulation.

When fatty metamorphosis is severe, CT shows an attenuation value of less than -10 Hounsfield units (HU) in the tumor, making a specific diagnosis possible of the fat component.[29] When the degree of fat deposition differs among internal mosaic components, the mosaic architecture may be more clearly visualized and the diagnosis of HCC made (Fig. 13.12a). However, when it is diffuse in the tumor (Fig. 13.12b), such cases should be differentiated from lipomatous tumors such as lipoma, liposarcoma, angiomyolipoma, and myelolipoma and focal fatty change. The area of HCC with marked fat deposition is usually hypovascular (Fig 13.12a); therefore, it may be differentiated from extremely hypervascular angiomyelolipoma. However, the differentiation of HCC with marked fatty metamorphosis from other lipomatous tumors by CT is usually impossible. Focal fatty change is usually differentiated from true mass lesions by its segmental configuration.[35,36] However, when it is small, its differentiation from fatty HCC is difficult.

Spontaneous massive necrosis is not uncommonly seen in small HCCs with fibrous capsule, and is shown as a non-enhanced mass with enhanced capsule on postcontrast CT (Fig. 13.13). This CT finding is very similar to that of organized abcess or hematoma, other necrotic tumors, ciliated hepatic foregut cyst[37], and complicated cyst.

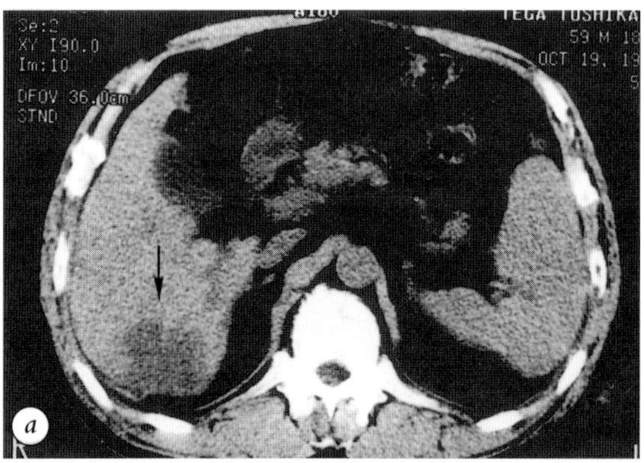

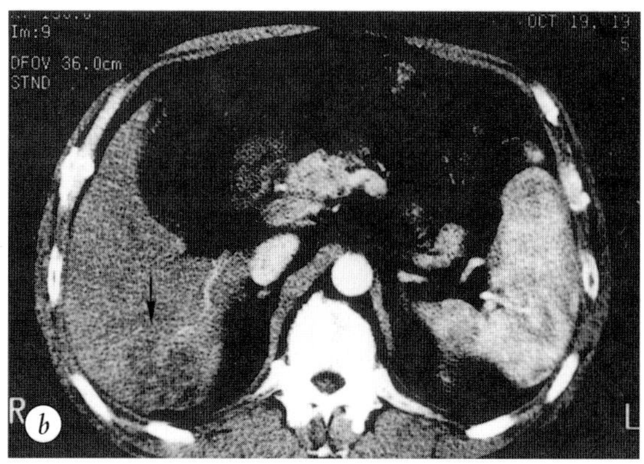

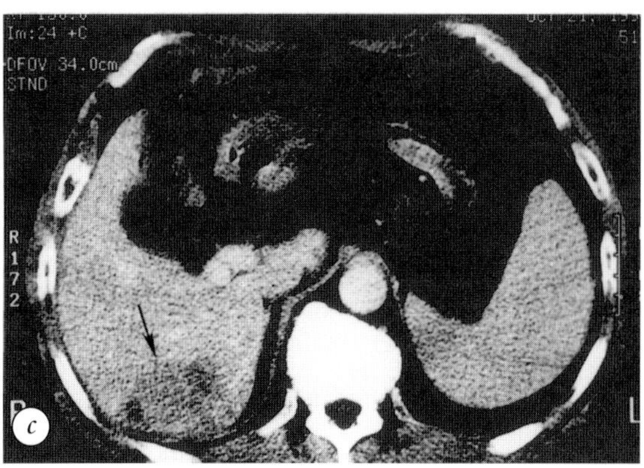

Figure 13.14 – Scirrhous type of classical HCC.

a) Percontrast CT shows a hypodense mass with irregular margin (arrow).

b) Arterial-dominant phase of dynamic CT shows no definite enhancement in the tumor (arrow).

c) Delayed CT shows delayed enhancement in the tumor (arrow).

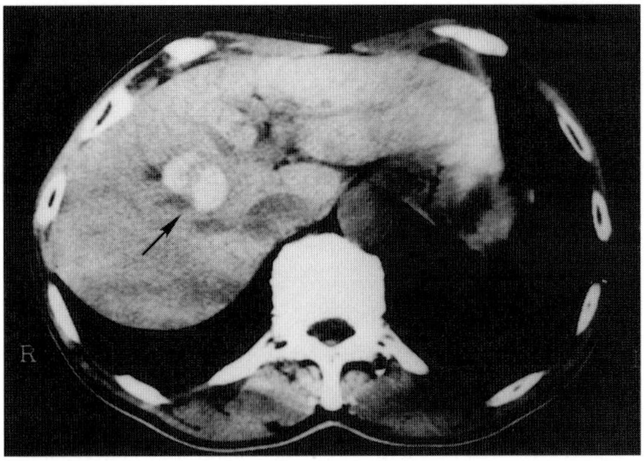

Figure 13.15 – Small classical HCC with marked copper accumulation. Precontrast CT shows a hyperdense mass relative to the surrounding liver parenchyma (arrow). (From *Radiology* 1991; **180**: 623-628).

Intratumoral hemorrhage is common histologically in classical HCCs. However, massive intratumoral or peritumoral hemorrhage in small HCCs is rare. When it occurs, it significantly modifies the imaging findings. Intratumoral or peritumoral hyperdensity due to fresh blood thrombus is seen on precontrast CT in the acute or subacute stage (Fig. 13.11). On postcontrast CT, the area with hemorrhage does not demonstrate enhancement.

HCCs with abundant fibrous stroma separating cords of tumor cells are called the scirrhous type according to the World Health Organization classification. This type of HCC demonstrates hypovascularity on the arterial-dominant phase of dynamic CT and delayed enhancement on delayed CT (Fig. 13.14). These CT findings are commonly seen among hepatic mass lesions with rich fibrous tissue such as confluent hepatic fibrosis in cirrhotic liver[38], granuloma, fibrous scar, cholangiocellular carcinoma, and metastases from scirrhous carcinomas.[39] Differential diagnosis among them is sometimes impossible by CT alone.

Copper accumulation is seen in 20-40% of HCCs. Copper is identified indirectly as copper-binding protein (CBP), stained black by orcein, and directly revealed by electron X-ray microanalyzer. Our investigation revealed that small HCCs with marked copper accumulation show hyperdensity (50 to 60 HU) on precontrast CT which is probably attributable to the abundant CBP in cancer cells (Fig. 13.15).[40]

HCCs with sarcomatous changes have been reported sporadically. Kojiro *et al* reported that about 4% of autopsy cases of HCCs show various degrees of sarcomatous change.[27] They are usually hypodense on precontrast and postcontrast CT, and hypo or avascular on the arterial-dominant phase of dynamic CT, and resemble cholangiocellular carcinoma, metastatic carcinoma, or scirrhous type of HCC except for on delayed enhancement.

Calcification in HCCs is rare (about 0.2% of our cases). Calcium deposits are usually seen in the necrotic area (dystrophic calcification). The pattern of calcification is non-specific, and when calcium deposits are seen in the cirrhotic liver, the possibility of HCC should always be kept in mind.

Intrahepatic portal vein obstruction due to tumor thrombus or compression by the tumor is common in advanced HCCs and not uncommon even in small HCCs. It modifies the imaging findings in several ways. As described above, the hepatic segment in which the feeding portal vein is obstructed shows denser staining than the non-obstructed segments (segmental staining) on dynamic CT, CTA and Lipiodol CT (Fig. 13.8-10). This segmental staining occasionally obscures the tumor staining in small HCCs, making the tumor appears larger than it

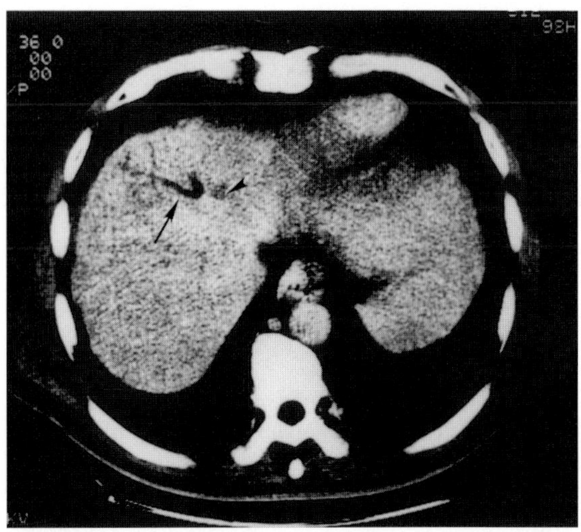

Figure 13.16 – Small HCC with bile duct growth. Post contrast CT shows dilated intrahepatic bile duct (arrow) and a small hypodense nodule (arrowhead).

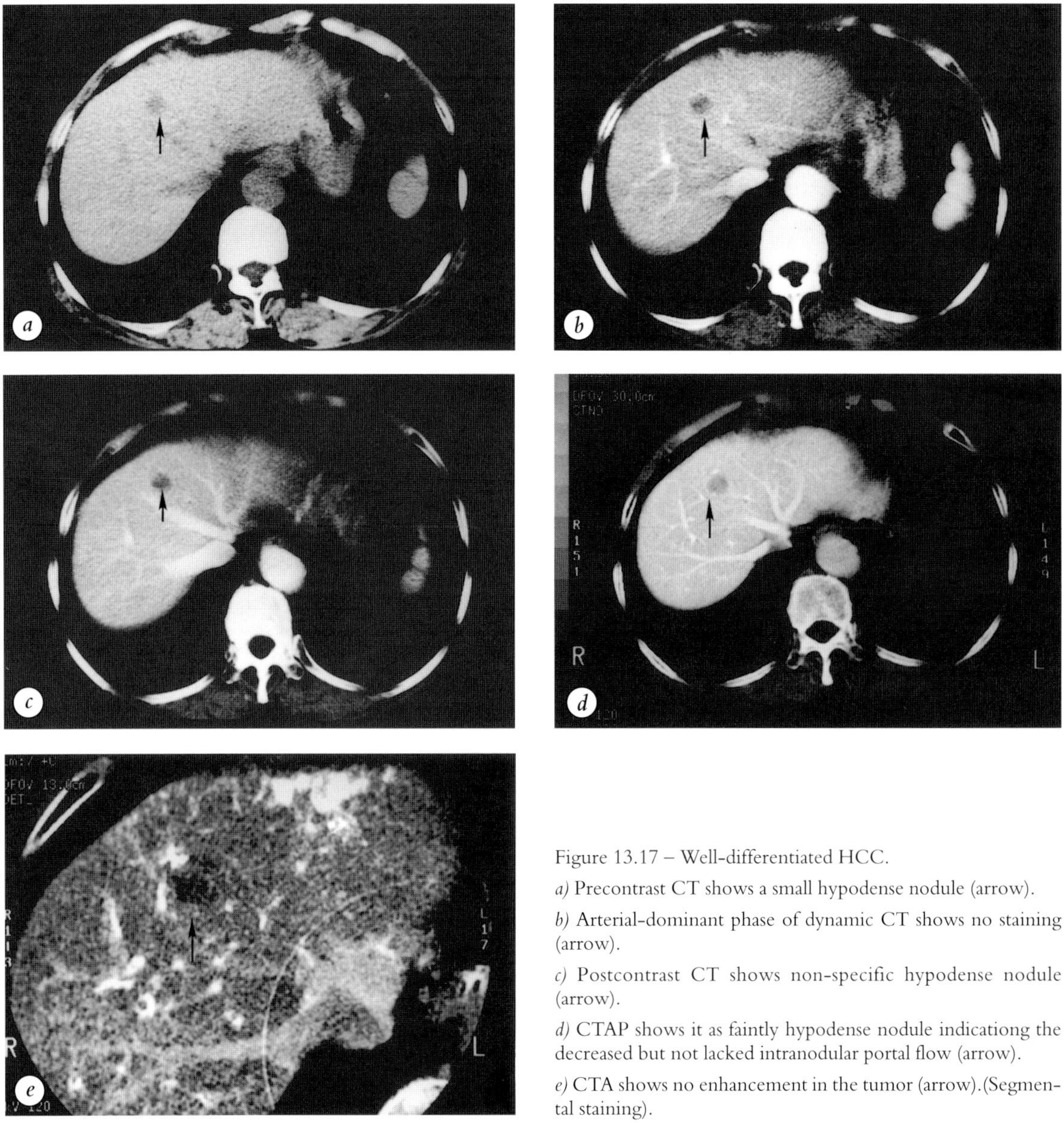

Figure 13.17 – Well-differentiated HCC.

a) Precontrast CT shows a small hypodense nodule (arrow).

b) Arterial-dominant phase of dynamic CT shows no staining (arrow).

c) Postcontrast CT shows non-specific hypodense nodule (arrow).

d) CTAP shows it as faintly hypodense nodule indicationg the decreased but not lacked intranodular portal flow (arrow).

e) CTA shows no enhancement in the tumor (arrow).(Segmental staining).

actually is or causing it to be missed altogether[31,32] (Fig. 13.10).

Tumor growth into the bile duct is found in 6% of autopsied HCCs[27] and can even be seen in small HCCs (Fig. 13.16). In such cases, differentiation from bile duct carcinoma is not easy by US or CT. A cast-like defect with smooth margin on direct cholangiography is an important imaging feature of HCC with tumor growth into the bile duct.

CT FINDINGS AND DIFFERENTIAL DIAGNOSIS OF WELL-DIFFERENTIATED HCC

Early stage well-differentiated HCCs are usually shown as nonspecific solid mass lesions on imaging tests[16,41,42] (Fig. 13.17). They show variable echogenicity on US and homogeneous hypodensity on precontarst CT. When fatty metamorphosis is moderate to marked throughout the tumor, they are visualized as definitely hyperechoic round nodules on US and extremely hypodense round nodules on CT. When fat deposition is uneven in the mass, the internal architecture becomes non- homogenous on imaging. On the arterial-dominant phase of dynamic CT, most of the well-differentiated HCCs do not demonstrate any staining or show only faint staining (Fig. 13.17). The capsule and internal mosaic architecture are rarely seen. Because of the imaging characteristics described above, it should be differentiated from many other hypovascular solid mass lesions. Among them, differentiation from other hepatocytic nodular lesions associated with liver cirrhosis, such as AH, is most important clinically. However, because precise differentiation is difficult, even with histology, we have been trying to estimate the grade of malignancy of hepatocytic nodular lesions, and found that the analysis of intranodular blood supply [41,43] and the signal intensity on MRI[16] are valuable for this purpose. Intranodular portal

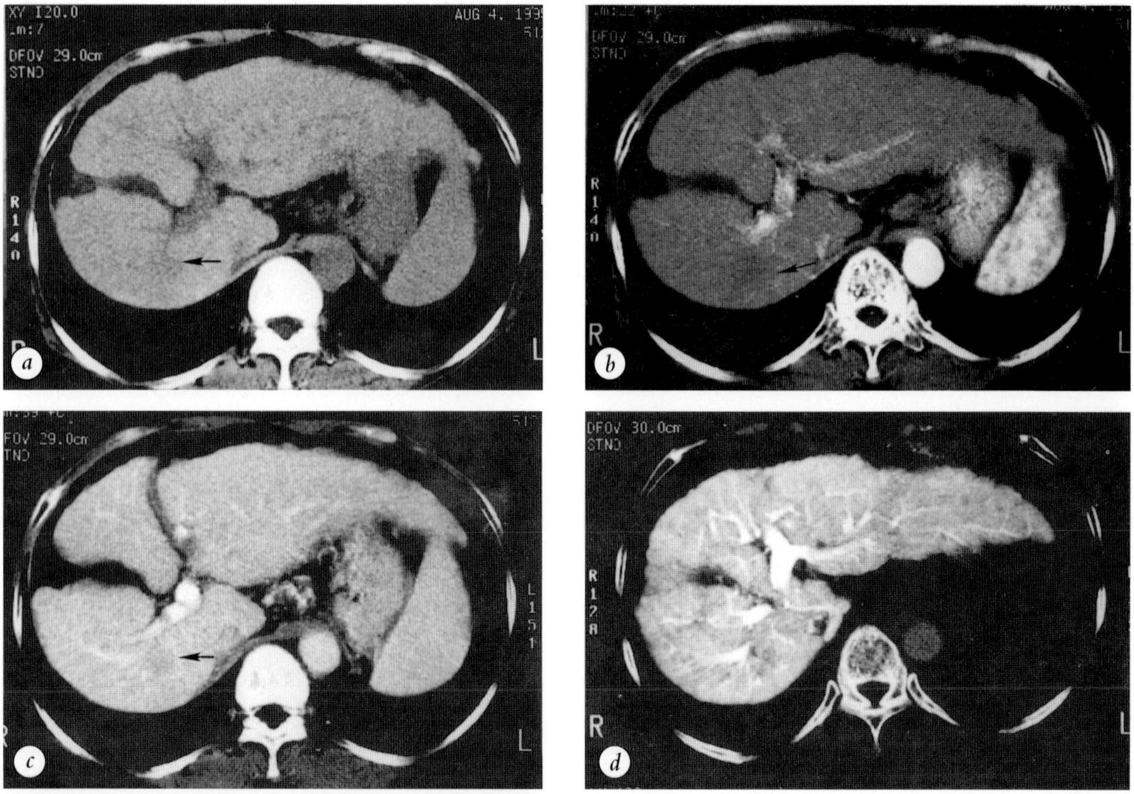

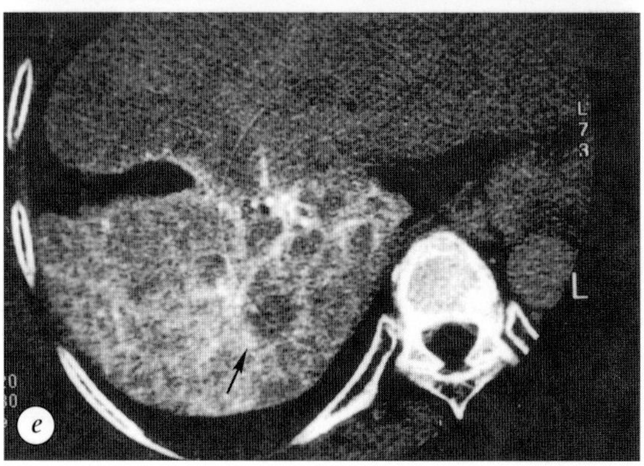

Figure 13.18 – Atypical adenomatous hyperplasia (AH).

a) Precontrast CT shows a faintly hypodense mass (arrow).

b) Arterial-dominant phase of dynamic CT shows no enhancement in the tumor (arrow).

c) Postcontrast CT shows it as a faint hypodense mass (arrow).

d) CTAP does not demonstrate it, because of abundant intranodular portal blood flow.

e) CTA shows no enhancement in the tumor (arrow).

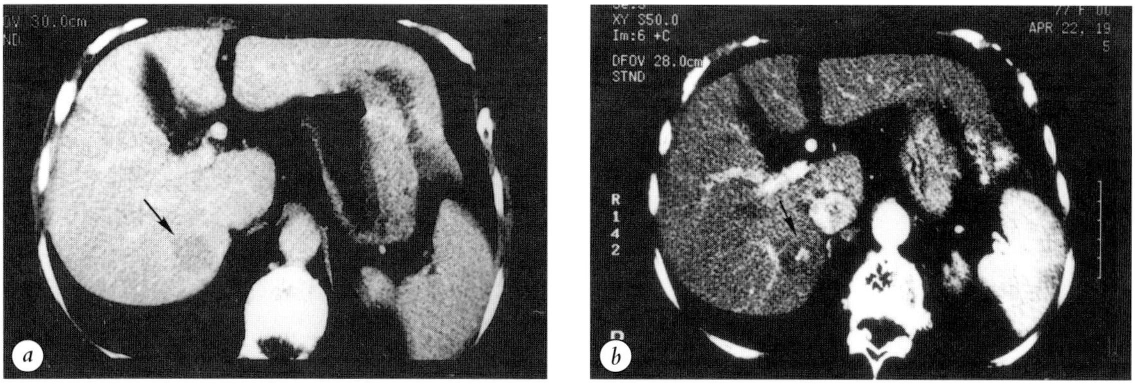

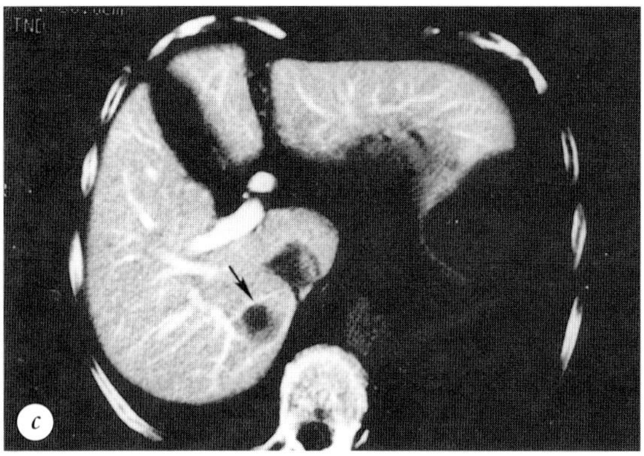

Figure 13.19 – AH with a malignant focus.

a) Postcontrast CT shows non-specific hypodense mass (arrow).

b) Arterial-dominant phase of dynamic CT shows a small well-enhanced portion in the non-enhanced mass (arrow).

c) CTAP shows a small portal perfusion defect in slightly hypodense mass (arrow).

supply can be evaluated only by CTAP. On CTAP, classical HCCs show definite hypodensity in the densely enhanced liver parenchyma (portal supply negative) (Figs. 13.1,7). By contrast, the majority of AHs are not visualized on CTAP (portal supply positive) (Fig. 13.18) and the majority of well-differentiated HCCs demonstrate faint hypodensity (portal supply decreased but not negative) (Fig. 13.17). On the other hand, an arterial supply (evaluated by dynamic CT, dynamic MRI, hepatic arteriography, or CO_2 US angiography) greater than that of the surrounding liver is verified in almost all classical HCCs (Figs. 13.1,7), in a quarter of well-differentiated HCCs, and in almost no AHs (Fig. 13.18). In AH with internal malignant foci, when one of the malignant foci is large enough to be detected by CT, a small portal perfusion defect may be demonstrated in a well-enhanced mass on CTAP and the area with portal perfusion defect may show enhancement on the arterial-dominant phase of dynamic CT and CTA (Fig. 13.19). This CT findings are also important in the diagnosis of early stage well-differentiated HCCs. However, care should be taken as almost the same pattern can be seen in well-differentiated HCC with internal classical HCC foci (early advanced HCC).[42]

The estimation of the grade of malignancy of the hepatocytic nodular lesions associated with liver cirrhosis by imaging diagnosis is very important clinically, because there are many hepatocytic nodules in cirrhotic livers which are not visualized by US, percutaneous biopsy for these small lesions is not always technically accurate, and histologic diagnosis of these nodules based on small specimens is not always reliable.

There are various kinds of focal liver parenchymal changes that mimick tumors (pseudotumor) in the liver, especially in cirrhotic livers. These include focal fatty change, focal sparing in fatty liver, and focal hyperplastic change. Their images are very similar to those of well-differentiated HCC and/or borderline lesions and, when they are seen in cirrhotic liver, the differentiation may be difficult. One of the important differential points is that these pseudotumors are commonly seen in the liver surrounding gallbladder fossa, the posterior aspect of segment IV, and adjacent to the falciform ligament. We revealed that these areas occasionally receive systemic venous drainage such as cystic venous drainage into liver parenchyma surrounding gallbladder fossa,[21] aberrant gastric venous drainage into the posterior aspect of segment IV[22], or from the veins from the abdominal wall to liver parenchyma adjacent to falciform ligament (unpublished data). Care should be taken to check if these areas show portal perfusion defect on CTAP, and possibly demonstrate early enhancement on dynamic CT due to relatively early venous return compared to the surrounding liver parenchyma.[44] We recently reported that hyperplastic change was occasionally seen in the focal area of liver parenchyma (posterior aspect of segment IV) which receives the aberrant gastric venous drainage in cirrhotic livers and differentiation between this hyperplastic change and well-differentiated HCC was difficult (Fig. 13.2).[44] To verify systemic venous drainage by arteriography, spiral CT with reconstruction technique, or CT during injection of contrast medium into gastric arteries or the cystic artery, is useful to avoid unnecessary biopsy or surgery during the imaging diagnosis of early stage HCCs.

CT STAGING OF HCC

Radiologic staging of HCC defines the extent and location of intrahepatic disease, involvement of surgically critical areas (portal hepatis, inferior vena cava, major bile ducts), and presence of extrahepatic disease.

For inoperable, far advanced HCCs, staging by US, CT and/or MRI is sufficient for patient management. However, for localized HCCs in which surgery or other local therapy such as percutaneous ethanol injection therapy (PEI) or subsegmental transcatheter arterial embolization[45] is being considered, more precise staging by arteriography, including a combination of CT and arteriography, especially CTAP, is recommended. The final preoperative staging should be performed by IOUS when surgery is carried out.

At first, the size and number of the tumors should be evaluated precisely. Intrahepatic metastases are usually hypervascular, and dynamic CT using the spiral system, dynamic multislice MRI, hepatic arteriography using digital subtraction angiography system, and Lipiodol CT are all extremely sensitive (Figs. 13.1, 3, 7). By these methods, minute nodules smaller than 5 mm can be visualized. CTAP is also very sensitive in detecting minute intrahepatic metastases because almost all of them lack a portal blood supply[8,9] (Fig. 13.7).

Vascular invasion including tumor thrombus in the portal vein should also be precisely evaluated because it is very important for surgery and prognosis. Invasion of the major veins is well diagnosed by US, CT, and MRI (Figs. 13.6, 8). However, for the detection of invasion of the peripheral portal veins, CTAP is necessary. CTAP visualizes the portal perfusion defect caused by portal thrombi as a wedge-shaped hypodense area including the tumor (Figs. 13.7, 10). When a portal perfusion defect is shown as a fan-shaped hypodense area on CTAP (Fig. 13.9), only compression of the portal venules is usually verified histologically. However, our previous study showed that the frequency of microscopic tumor thrombi is very high in fan-shaped portal perfusion defect.[20]

The segmental location of the lesion can be diagnosed in relation to the intrahepatic vessels by various imaging methods. However, when a small lesion is located at the boundary of the segments, it is not easy to determine segmental anatomy. Because CTAP can visualize intrahepatic portal and hepatic veins and the entire tumor most clearly, it may be the best imaging method for this purpose.[11,14,20]

Lymphatic metastases in HCC are seen in about 15% of autopsy cases, especially in the peripancreatic and hepatic hilar lymph nodes.[27] CT is useful for detecting these nodes.[46]

Extrahepatic hematogenous metastases were revealed in about 59% of autopsied HCCs. The lung was the most common site and the adrenal gland, gastrointestinal tract, bone, spleen, heart, and kidney were also involved (in order of decreasing frequency).[27] CT may be most valuable for the diagnosis of these extrahepatic metastases except for bone metastasis.

CT EVALUATION OF TREATMENT OF HCC

CT is the most widely used modality for the evaluation of the treatment of HCC.

After PEI, the area which shows no enhancement on dynamic CT and postcontrast CT is considered to reflect coagulation necrosis (Fig. 13.20). Therefore, if this non-enhanced area becomes larger than the size of the tumor before treatment, the therapeutic effect is evaluated as complete. However, in PEI, A-P shunting, portal vein thrombosis due to injected ethanol, and reactive changes are often seen in the surrounding liver and modify CT findings.[47] In the arterial-dominant phase of dynamic CT, various degrees of enhancement caused by these changes may be shown.

The coagulation necrosis brought about by TAE without Lipiodol is also well evaluated by dynamic CT or postcontrast CT. However, when Lipiodol is used as an embolic material, the precise evaluation of necrosis by CT is occasionally difficult, because of the partial volume effect or artifacts caused by dense Lipiodol accumulation. In our previous histologic study in surgically resected or autopsied HCCs following TAE therapy with Lipiodol or simple Lipiodol injection for diagnostic purpose, the mechanism of Lipiodol accumulation and retention in the tumor was considered to be as follows:

1. Lipiodol injected into the hepatic artery accumulates in the hepatic tumors in proportion to their vascularity.

2. Lipiodol is retained for more than 30 days in the necrotic areas of the tumor and liver parenchyma that arise from Lipiodol injection and TSE therapy.

3. Lipiodol mostly disappears within 20 days from non-necrotic areas of the tumor and liver parenchyma.[15]

Therefore, the area with Lipiodol retention on CT taken more than 30 days following TAE can be considered to be necrotic (Fig. 13 3). When Lipiodol retention is not seen regardless of the Lipiodol accumulation on CT obtained within a few days after TAE, viable residual tumor or recurrence should be considered (Fig. 13.3). Dynamic CT and postcontrast CT are also useful to confirm residual tumor or recurrence and should be performed (Fig. 13.3). If possible, dynamic MRI should be performed for the precise evaluation of the viable tumors after TAE with Lipiodol, because Lipiodol does not disturb the images and the contrast resolution of MRI is extremely high

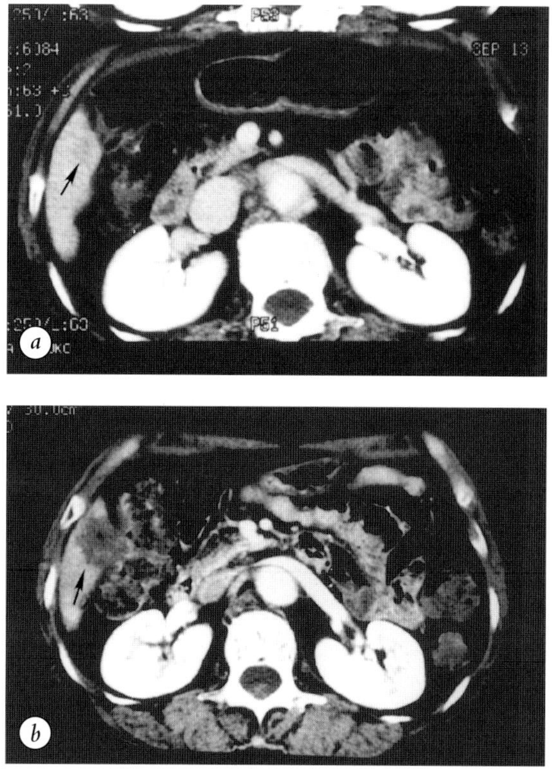

Figure 13.20 – Small HCC completely treated by PEI.

a) Postcontrast CT obtained before PEI shows enhanced small solid mass (arrow).

b) Postcontrast CT obtained following PEI shows definite enhanced area including the tumor and surrounding liver parenchyma (arrow).

REFERENCES

1. Foley WD, Berland LL, lawson TL, *et al*: Contrast enhancement technique for dynamic hepatic computed tomographic scanning. *Radiology* 1983; **147**:797-803

2. Itai Y. Imaging diagnosis with computed tomography. In: Okuda K, Ishak KG (eds) *Neoplasms of the Liver*. Springer-Verlag, Tokyo 1986, pp289-300.

3. Baron RL. Understanding and optimizing use of contrast material for CT of the liver. *AJR* 1994; **163**:323-331

4. Bluemke DA, Fishman EK: Spiral CT of the liver. *AJR* 1993; **160**:787-792

5. Ueda K, Kitagawa K, Kadoya M, *et al*: Detection of hypervascular hepatocellular carcinoma by using spiral volumetric CT: comparison of US and MR imaging. *Abdom Imaging* 1995; **20**:547-554

6. Prando A, Wallace S, Bernardino ME, Lindell MM: Computed tomographic arteriography of the liver. *Radiology* 1979; **130**:697-701

7. Matsui O, Kadoya M, Suzuki M, *et al*: Dynamic sequential computed tomography during arterial portography in the detection of hepatic neoplasms. *Radiology* 1983; **147**: 721-727

8. Matsui O, Takashima T, Kadoya M, *et al*: Dynamic computed tomography during arterial portography: the most sensitive examination for small hepatocellular carcinoma. *J Comput Assist Tomogr* 1985; **9**:19-24

9. Matsui O, Takashima T, Kadoya M, *et al*: Liver metastases from colorectal cancer: detection with CT during arterial portography. *Radiology* 1987; **165**:65-69

10. Ohishi H, Uchida H, Yoshimura H, *et al*: Hepatocellular carcinoma detected by iodized oil. Use of anticancer agents. *Radiology* 1985; **154**: 25-29

11. Nelson RC, Chezmar JL, Sugarbaker PH, *et al*: Preoperative localization of focal liver lesions to specific liver segments: utility of CT during arterial portography. *Radiology* 1990; **176**:89-94

12. Merine D, Takayasu K, Wako F: Detection of hepatocellular carcinoma: comparison of CT during arterial portography with CT after intraarterial injection of iodized oil. *Radiology* 1990; **175**:707-710

13. Bluemke DA, Soyer P, Chan B, *et al*: Spiral CT during arterial portography: techniques and applications. *Radiographics* 1995; **15**:633-637

14. Soyer P, Bluemke DA, Bliss DF, *et al*: Surgical segmental anatomy of the liver: demonstration with spiral CT during arterial portography and multiplanar reconstruction. *AJR* 1994; **163**:99-103

15. Matsui O, Takashima T, Kadoya M, *et al*: Mechanism of Lipiodol accumulation and retention in hepatic tumors: analysis in cases with simple lipiodol injection. *Nippon Acta Radiologica* 1987; **47**:1395-1404 [English abstract]

16. Matsui O, Kadoya M, Kameyama T, *et al*: Adenomatous hyperplastic nodules in the cirrhotic liver: differentiation from hepatocellular carcinomas with MR imaging. *Radiology* 1989; **173**:123-126

17. Kadoya M, Matsui O, Takashima T, Nonomura A: Hepatocellular carcinoma: Correlation of MR imaging and histopathologic findings. *Radiology* 1992; **183**: 819-825

18. Itai Y, Ohtomo K, Matsui O: Diagnosis of primary liver cancer using magnetic resonance imaging. In Tobe T, *et al* (eds): *Primary Liver Cancer in Japan*. Springer-Verlag, Tokyo 1992, p139-151

19. Kudo M, Tomita S, Tochio H, *et al*: Sonography with intraarterial infusion of carbon dioxide microbubbles (sonographic angiography): value in differential diagnosis of hepatic tumors. *AJR* 1992; **158**:65-74

20. Matsui O: Basic and clinical studies of dynamic sequential computed tomography during arterial portography in the diagnosis of hepatic cancers. *Nippon Acta radiologica* 1986; **46**: 335-359 [English abstract]

21. Matsui O, Takashima T, Kadoya M, *et al*: Staining in the liver surrounding gallbladder fossa on hepatic arteriography caused by increased cystic venous drainage. *Gastrointest Radiol* 1987; **12**:307-312

22. Matsui O, Takahashi S, Kadoya M, *et al*: Pseudolesion in segment IV of the liver at CT during arterial portography: correlation with aberrant gastric venous drainage. *Radiology* 1994; **193**:31-35

23. Honda H, Kaneko K, Maeda T, *et al*: Small hepatocellular carcinomas undetected on two-phased incremental computed tomography. Angiographic and clinicopathologic findings. *Invest Radiol* 1995; **30**:458-564

24. Nakanuma Y, Terada T, Ueda K, *et al*: Adenomatous hyperplasia of the liver as a precancerous lesion. *Liver* 1993; **13**: 1-9

25. Takayama T, Makuuchi M, Hirohashi S, *et al*: Malignant transformation of adenomatous hyperplasia to hepatocellular carcinoma. *Lancet* 1990; **336**: 1150-1153

26. Arakawa M, Kage M, Sugihara S *et al*: Emergence of malignant lesions within an adenomatous hyperplastic nodule in a cirrhotic liver. *Gastroenterology* 1986; **91**:198-208

27. Kojiro M, Nakashima T: Pathology of hepatocellular carcinoma. In Okuda K, Ishak KG(eds) *Neoplasm of the liver*. Springer-Verlag. Tokyo 1987, p81-104

28. Kanai T, Hirohashi S, Upton M, *et al*: Pathology of small hepatocellular carcinoma: a proposal for a new gross classification. *Cancer* 1987; **60**: 810-819

29. Yoshikawa J, Matsui O, Takashima T, *et al*: Fatty metamorphosis in hepatocellular carcinoma : radiologic features in 10 cases. *AJR* 1988; **151**: 717-720

30. Itai Y, Araki T, Furui S, *et al*: Differential diagnosis of hepatic masses on computed tomography: with particular reference to hepatocellular carcinoma. *J Comput Assist Tomogr* 1981; **5**:843-850

31. Matsui O, Takashima T, Kadoya M, *et al*: Segmental staining on hepatic arteriography as a sign of intrahepatic portal vein obstruction. *Radiology* 1984; **152**: 601-606

32. Itai Y, Moss AA, Goldberg HI: Transient attenuation difference of lobar or segmental distribution detected by dynamic computed tomography. *Radiology* 1982; **144**:31-35

33. Itai Y, Ohtomo K, Yamauchi T, *et al*: CT of hepatic masses: significance of prolonged enhancement and delayed enhancement. *AJR* 1986; **146**: 792-796

34. Itai Y, Furui S, Araki T, Yashiro N, Tasaka A: Computed tomography of cavernous hemangioma of the liver. *Radiology* 1980; **137**:149-155

35. Yoshikawa J, Matsui O, Takashima T, *et al*: Focal fatty change of the liver adjacent to the falciform ligament: CT and sonographic findings in five surgically confirmed cases. *AJR* 1987; **149**: 491-494,

36. Matsui O, Kadoya M, Takahashi S, *et al*: Focal sparing of segment IV in fatty livers shown by sonography and CT: correlation with aberrant gastric venous drainage. *AJR* 1995; **164**:1137-1140

37. Kadoya M, Matsui O, Yoshikawa J, *et al*: Ciliated hepatic foregut cyst: radiologic features. *Radiology* 1990; **175**: 475-477

38. Ohtomo K, Baron RJ, Dodd GD *et al*: Confluent hepatic fibrosis in advanced cirrhosis: Appearance at CT. *Radiology* 1993; **188**:31-35

39. Yoshikawa J, Matsui O, Kadoya M, *et al*: Delayed enhancement of fibrotic areas in hepatic masses: CT-pathologic correlation. *J Comput Assist Tomogr* 1992; **16**:206-211

40. Kitagawa K, Matsui O, Kadoya M, *et al*: Hepatocellular carcinomas with excessive copper accumulation: CT and MR findings. *Radiology* 1991; **180**: 623-628

41. Matsui O, Kadoya M, Kameyama T, *et al*: Benign and malignant nodules in the cirrhotic livers: Distinction based on blood supply. *Radiology* 1991; **178**: 493-497

42. Takayasu K, Muramatsu Y, Furukawa H, *et al*: Early hepatocellular carcinoma: appearance at CT during arterial portography and CT arteriography with pathologi correlation. *Radiology* 1995; **194**:101-105

43. Ueda K, Matsui O, Terada T, Nakanuma Y: Vascular supply in adenomatous hyperplasia of the liver and hepatocellular carcinoma: A morphometric study. *Human Pathology* 1992; **23**: 619-626

44. Matsui O, Kadoya M, Yoshikawa J, *et al*: Aberrant gastric venous drainage in cirrhotic livers: imaging findings in focal areas of liver parenchyma. *Radiology* 1995; **197**:345-349

45. Matsui O, Kadoya M, Yoshikawa J, *et al*: Small hepatocellular carcinoma: treatment with subsegmental transcatheter arterial embolization. *Radiology* 1993; **188**: 79-83

46. Araki T, Hihara T, Karikomi M, *et al*: Hepatocellular carcinoma: metastatic abdominal lymphnodes identified by computed tomography. *Gastrointest Radiol* 1988; **13**: 247-252,

47. Yoshikawa J, Matsui O, kadoya M, *et al*: Hepatocellular carcinoma: CT appearance of parenchymal changes after percutaneous ethanol injection therapy. *Radiology* 1995; **194**:107-111

14

Magnetic resonance imaging

A Del Maschio, E Angeli, A Vanzulli, F De Cobelli and S Sironi

Magnetic resonance imaging (MRI) of the liver has undergone rapid technical maturation and is already acknowledged as having an important role in clinical liver imaging.[1] Emerging applications include detection, characterization, staging, and follow-up of liver tumors.[1] Due to recent technical improvements such as the use of motion artifact suppression techniques, the development of MR contrast agents, and fast imaging techniques, MRI offers new capacities as a diagnostic imaging modality.[2,3]

The ability of MRI to detect and characterize abnormal tissues is based upon the ability of specific pulse sequence techniques to display differences in one or more MR tissue parameters.[4-7] Tissue parameters (relaxation times, hydrogen density, chemical shift, magnetic susceptibility, and motion) can influence image contrast to different degrees.[3,7-11] T1 and T2 relaxation time differences between liver and tumor are the most important parameters determining image contrast.[6,7] Hydrogen density usually has the least influence on image contrast as only fat and fluids differ significantly from other tissues. Chemical shift, defined as differences in resonance frequency of hydrogen atoms bound to different molecules, can be exploited as a source of image contrast by specialized imaging techniques.[11] Magnetic susceptibility of iron overloaded liver can contribute markedly to the MR image information. Motion in the form of blood flow is responsible for the superb delineation of blood vessels.[12] Capillary flow and diffusion contribute little to conventional MR image contrast unless magnetic contrast agents are administered.[12]

Tumor relaxation times show a wide range. However, some trends are evident and become manifest as differences in MR signal intensity. Biological variation of the same histologic tumor type can be attributed to individual variation in cellularity, necrosis, fibrosis, or fat content.[13,14] As a result, MR signal intensity varies among individual lesions in a single patient, and varies even more among different patients with the same tumor type. The standard deviation of relaxation times for any single histological type is often greater than the difference in the means between two different histologic types.[13,14]

Tumor detectability improves with increasing difference in tumor–liver relaxation times.[15,16] For example, tumors with long T1 and T2 relaxation times (metastases, hemangiomas) show higher tumor–liver contrast than tumors with T1 and T2 relaxation times similar to liver (hepatic adenoma, focal nodular hyperplasia, and hepatocellular carcinoma).[15,16]

The selection of a specific MR pulse sequence (spin echo, inversion recovery, gradient echo, etc) and its timing parameters (TR, TE, TI, flip angle) are the major determinants of image quality and tumor detectability. The diagnostic utility of any pulse sequence can be assessed by determining the signal-to-noise ratio (SNR) and the tumor–liver contrast-to-noise ratio (CNR).[5-7]

SNR is a quantitative parameter that generally correlates with image quality or anatomic resolution (not to be confused with spatial resolution or voxel dimensions).[4] The higher SNR, the better the anatomic resolution.[4] Anatomic resolution also can be assessed visually by inspection of an MR image. The less grainy the image and the sharper the vein–liver border, the better the anatomic resolution. The CNR is a quantitative parameter that generally correlates with lesion detectability.[4] Positive CNR values indicate hyperintensity and negative CNR hypointensity of the tumor relative to liver.[17] A priori, lesion detectability does not depend upon whether the lesion is bright or dark relative to adjacent normal tissue. Higher values (either negative or positive) indicate more conspicuous lesions. CNR values generally correlate with sensitivity in lesion detection and decreased threshold for detection of small tumors.[4]

Quantitative signal intensity measurements of liver, spleen, muscle, and other tissues can be obtained through "region of interest" software programs[16,17] These measurements are used to calculate SNR, CNR, or tissue-to-tissue signal intensity ratios for objective, analysis of nonanatomic image information.[15-17] In routine clinical imaging however, qualitative (visual) assessment of signal intensity is commonly performed by comparing signal intensity of hepatic tumors to reference tissues in the same slice.[15] For example, hepatocellular tumors tend to appear iso- or hyperintense relative to liver on T1 weighted sequences[13,18] Hemangiomas typically have the same signal intensity as CSF or gallbladder bile on heavily T2 weighted pulse sequences (TE > 150 ms), and metastases show a signal intensity similar to the spleen on all pulse sequences.[15,16]

Calculation of T1 and T2 relaxation times is an alternative quantitative method for characterizing tissue[16,17] Typically, signal intensity measurements from multiple pulse sequences are fitted to signal intensity equations of spin echo, inversion recovery, or gradient echo (GE) sequences. Due to the exponential nature of the intensity equations, the nonlinear curve fit improves using iterative algorithms and as many datapoints as possibile. Using a less than three-point fit, relaxation times derived from MR images show a wide variation. As for the ratios described above, calculated relaxation times have been applied primarily for scientific purposes.

In recent years, the use of paramagnetic contrast agents has improved the capability of MR imaging in the evaluation of primary liver tumor.[19-23] Gadopentetate dimeglumine is the primary intravenously administered paramagnetic contrast agent available for MR imaging. Gadopentetate dimeglumine acts as a vascular agent and causes T1 shortening, appearing hyperintense on T1 weighted images.[19,22] The contrast agent is quickly distributed to the extracellular compartment in both normal and abnormal liver tissues, a process that often requires the use of dynamic techniques such as T1 weighted gradient-echo imaging to detect the differential uptake between the lesion and the normal liver.[19-23] With the development of intravenously administered contrast agents specific for the liver reticuloendothelial system, such as superparamagnetic iron oxide and other agents that are excreted by hepatocytes into the biliary system,[24-26] MR imaging has the potential to replace functional radionuclide imaging of the liver as contrast material-enhanced MR images provide physiologic information as well as anatomic detail. Superparamagnetic iron oxide is a particulate agent that undergoes phagocytosis by the reticuloendothelial system and, therefore, is taken up by normal liver, fatty liver, and benign tumors containing Kupffer cells.[24-26] Use of superparamagnetic iron oxide results predominantly in T2 shortening, causing decreased signal intensity on images obtained with all pulse sequences, expecially T2 weighted sequences, which produce a marked decrease in the signal intensity of the normal liver.[24-26]

We believe that current development of liver-specific contrast agents will further enhance the utility of MR imaging for detection and characterization of focal liver lesions.

TECHNICAL ASPECTS

The study of liver pathology has been one of the main challenges for MRI because of the presence of image degradation due to motion artifacts, chemical-shift and flow artifacts, and sometimes poor intrinsic contrast between normal liver and lesions.

The introduction of artifact suppression techniques and the use of dynamic sequences during a bolus injection of paramagnetic contrast agent (Gadolinium DTPA) has largely overcome the problems described above and MR imaging of the upper abdomen has become one of the main diagnostic tools in everyday practice.

Newer contrast agents such as manganese-DPDP, Gadolinium-EOB or Gadolinium-BOPTA will further improve the capabilities of MR imaging in detecting focal liver lesions.

Spin echo technique

The spin echo technique is still the most frequently used sequence in the abdominal examination.

Using a short repetition time (TR, 200-500 ms) and a short echo time (TE, 15-20 ms) a good liver to lesion contrast is usually achieved in cases of secondary lesions,[4] but a suboptimal contrast can be obtained in some cases of primary liver tumors.[5-7]

It is important in **T1 weighted** spin echo imaging that T2 effects are minimized by minimizing the TE and that a TR that is shorter than the T1 of the tissues one wishes to contrast is chosen.

One effective method of artifact reduction in spin echo imaging is *signal averaging*; this method increases acquisition time and for this reason a maximum number of 2 to 4 acquisitions (NEX) is usually employed.[2]

Another effective method of respiratory movement artifact reduction in spin echo imaging is *respiratory ordered phase encoding*:[3] the data obtained from a respiratory monitoring device are used to reorder the sequence of phase encoding steps in the two dimensional Fourier transform imaging acquisition. By reordering the phase encoding steps according to the respiratory cycle, fewer ghosts are presented on the images. This method is particularly effective in T1 weighted spin echo sequences but less useful when T2 weighted images are acquired.

Spin echo **T2 weighted** imaging is acquired with long TR (longer then 2000 ms) and with intermediate (25-50 ms) and long (80-120 ms) echo time (TE). These sequences, especially when the magnet operates at high field strength, afford improved intraparenchymal contrast[5,6] and good sensitivity for lesion detection, but are frequently degraded by motion related artifacts and low signal-to-noise ratios.

One possible technique to reduce motion related artifact is *flow compensation*.[8,9,12] This technique shapes the readout gradient to compensate for velocity dependent phase shifts acquired by non-stationary nuclei during image acquisition.

Another way to compensate for image artifacts generated by pulsating blood is *spatial presaturation*: this technique employs 90° radiofrequence (RF) pulses outside the imaging volume to saturate the spins in blood vessels flowing into that volume.[27] In the abdomen, because the venous flow and the arterial flow occur in opposite directions, spatial presaturation is applied on both sides of the imaging volume to reduce unwanted signal arising in both the aorta and inferior vena cava.

When *flow compensation and spatial presaturation* are employed together, the vessels running perpendicular to the plane of acquisition are with low signal because of presaturation, whereas blood flowing within the plane of acquisition (i.e. portal vein) shows increased signal due to flow compensation.

Fast spin echo techniques

One relatively recent evolution of the spin echo technique is fast spin echo acquisition: in this technique a series of four, eight or more echoes are acquired after the initial excitation pulse. Several lines of the K space[5,8,28] are obtained during each TR while in conventional spin echo one single line is obtained.[29-31] This technique allows a marked reduction in acquisition time permitting the use of *respiratory triggering* and a higher number of NEX.

The image contrast is a combination of many different echo times and the overall contrast is established by the echo times of the central K space lines. The images obtained have some differences in comparison to conventional spin echo: the fat signal is more intense necessitating the use of *fat suppression techniques*[11,32] and the liver-to-lesion contrast can be lower in cases of primary liver tumors, but the time saving and the lower artifacts present on the image compensate for these drawbacks.

Gradient echo and fast gradient echo techniques

Gradient echo techniques represent another important component of the imaging approach to the upper abdomen. With these techniques the echo signal is obtained through the use of readout gradient reversal rather than using the 180° spin echo pulse.[33-35]

With this approach both TR and TE can be markedly shortened, allowing the acquisition of many slices in relatively short time. With high gradient amplitude (> 15 mT/m) and rapid switching time about 15 slices can be acquired in a single breath hold (20 s), permitting artifact free imaging of the liver and dynamic acquisitions during a bolus injection of contrast medium (e.g. Gadolinium-DTPA).

In gradient echo imaging the contrast is determined not only by TR and TE but also by the flip angle of the initial exciting pulse. For T1 weighted sequences, short TE (shorter than 10 ms) and large flip angles (more than 45°) are employed.[36]

The use of short repetition times result in residual transverse magnetization after each TR, with the buildup of a so called steady-state situation and reduction of the T1 effect of the acquisition. This residual transverse magnetization can be eliminated through the use of spoiler pulses (spoiled gradient echo techniques).[28]

The echo time determines also the appearance of signal suppression or of signal summation between the signal of water and the signal of fat in locations where the two substances are present in the same voxel:[10,37-39] at 1.5 T field strength the signal of water and the signal of fat are in opposite phase (signal suppression) at echo times of 2.1 ms, 6.3 ms and 10.5 ms, while the signals are in phase (signal summation) at echo times of 4.2 ms, 8.4 ms and 12.6 ms. The images obtained in opposite phase are recognizable due to the presence of a dark line at the interfaces between abdominal organs and intra-abdominal fat. This technique (chemical shift imaging) can be useful in characterizing areas of focal steatosis demonstrating a signal drop in areas of steatosis when opposite phase images are obtained.[38,39]

Gradient echo images are very flow sensitive because of flow related enhancement; so they can be used to evaluate hepatic vasculature patency.[34,35]

An evolution of gradient echo technique is the proprietary sequences called **Turbo-FLASH** (Siemens) in which the TR is reduced to less than 10 ms, lowering the number of phase encoding steps, and the TE is reduced acquiring only fractional echo sampling. Imaging times in the order of 300-1000 ms have been obtained with ultra rapid gradient echo techniques. With these very short imaging times the T1 contrast is partially lost and an inversion pulse is applied to give the sequence a strong T1 weighting.

Echo planar imaging (EPI) technique

Only recently gradient technology allowed the use of an ultrafast imaging technique called echo planar imaging.[40,41] With this technique most (multi-shot EPI) or all (single-shot EPI) of the information required to generate the image are collected following a single excitation. Images can be acquired in a period as short as 40 ms.

Depending on the TE employed, the degree of T2 weighting of the image can be varied. T1 weighting can be obtained through the use of a preparatory 180° inversion pulse at the beginning of the image acquisition.[42]

The use of single-shot EPI is strongly dependent on hardware performances because gradients with a slew rate of at least 150 T/m/s are to be employed. Moreover the accumulation of phase errors during the filling of the K space in a single acquisition can introduce important spatial distortions. Also the strong sensitivity to susceptibility artifacts limits the image quality in areas where tissue–air interfaces are present.[40,41]

The EPI acquisition can be split in different "shots",[41] so the drawbacks of the technique can be partially overcome, while mantaining a very good temporal resolution (about 20 s) and a strong T2 weighting. These sequences are still under investigation and their clinical utility has to be assessed.

Besides gradient technology, recent improvements have been made in the field of the receiver chain. The use of multiple receiver channels with multicoil systems (phased array coils) allow a great improvement in contrast-to-noise ratio, spatial and contrast resolution in upper abdomen studies.[43]

For liver imaging the *acquisition plane* is almost always axial; other planes (sagittal, coronal or oblique) are employed for particular clinical questions such as inferior vena cava or portal patency or for the detection of lesions in difficult areas such as the hepatic dome or the inferior margin of the liver.

The *slice thickness* is between 5 and 10 mm, ideally 7 mm, with an intersection gap of 0.5-2 mm.

The field of view (FOV) has to be tailored to the patient and to the sequence used: the smallest possible in standard sequences. When dynamic sequences are

Table 14.1 – Example of study protocol for MR imaging of liver

SEQ.	COIL	Plane	SEQ.	TR/TE	ETL	FOV	MTX	NEX	OPT.	TIME
Localizer	Ph. Array	Cor.	SE	200/15	NA	40 1 FOV	256*128	1	NO	20 sec
Axial FS	Ph. Array	Axial	FSE	5000-7000/120	16	35-40 1-3/4 FOV	256*224	2-3	RT, FS, FC, P, NFR	3-6 min
Dinamic x4 times	Ph. Array	Axial	2D Fast SPGR	100-175 /4,2	N/A	35-40 1-3/4 FOV	256*192	1	P	20-30 sec
Delayed	Ph. Array	Axial	2D Fast SPGR	100-175 /4,2	NA	35-40 1-3/4 FOV	256*192	1	P	20-30 sec

Note: RT = Respiratory triggering, FS = Fat suppression, FC = Flow compensation, P = Spatial presaturation, NPR = No false wrap employed the FOV has to be large enough to allow 3/4 sampling (rectangular matrix) without the "no phase wrap" option, so avoiding aliasing artifact.

MRI OF THE LIVER IN PATIENTS WITH SUSPECTED HCC

- Our imaging protocol (Table 14.1) starts with a coronal localizer acquired with standard spin echo in about 20 s. All the sequences are acquired with an abdominal multi-channel receiver coil (Torso phased array).
- The first diagnostic sequence is a respiratory triggered fast T2 sequence with fat suppression. We use a TR triggered to 1 or 2 respiratory cycles, depending on the respiratory frequency: the resulting TR must be in the range 5000-7000 ms. We use an effective TE of about 120 ms with an echo train of 16, a matrix size of 256 x 224, a field of view of 35 cm and 2 or 3 NEX. Fat saturation is always applied with frequency selective RF pulses to compensate for the different contrast intrinsic to fast spin echo sequences. The overall acquisition time varies between 3 and 6 min.
- After this sequence a spoiled gradient echo acquisition is prescribed (2D fast spoiled GRASS (SPGR)) with a TR of about 100-175 ms depending on the number of slices required. Minimum TE with the signal of water and the signal of fat in phase is applied (4.2 ms). A rectangular field of view (3/4) and 1 NEX, without foldover suppression is used. This sequence allows the acquisition of about 12-15 slices in the time of a breath hold (20 s).
- The same sequence, without repeating the prescanning procedures, is repeated 5 times during a bolus injection of a standard dose of Gadolinium DTPA.
- After about 5 minutes the same 2D fast SPGR sequence is acquired to rule out angiomatous lesions.

Our protocol is particularly useful in demonstrating small hypervascular lesions during the precocious (arterial) phases of Gadolinium injection, in order to detect satellite nodules or perilesional relapse in patients already treated for hepatocellular carcinoma.

IMAGING FINDINGS

Signal intensity

On MRI, the signal intensity pattern of nodular form of advanced HCC is somewhat nonspecific and variable. Advanced HCC generally demonstrates moderate reduction of signal intensity on T1 weighted images (Fig. 14.1a), and signal increase on T2 weighted images[1,13-15,18] (Fig. 14.1b). These features are similar to metastases and other types of benign and malignant tumors, and relate to long T1 and T2 relaxation times, due to increased water content in the tumor.[15, 17]

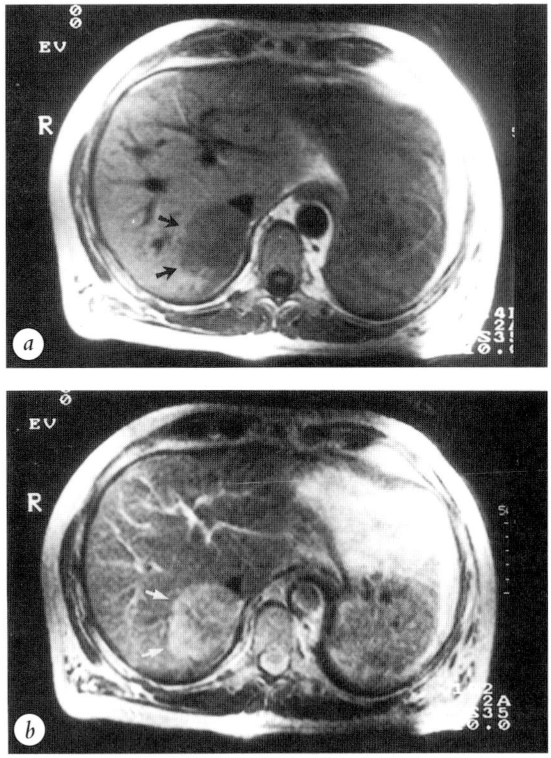

Figure 14.1 –

a) Axial SE T1 weighted image.

b) Axial SE T2 weighted image.

In *a)* HCC lesion (arrows) typically shows low signal intensity relative to liver. In *b)* the same lesion (arrows) has high signal intensity. This represents the most common signal intensity pattern of HCC on conventional SE sequences.

T1 weighted images

Marked hypointensity on T1 weighted images may be found in highly fibrotic lesions.[14] Well-differentiated and early HCCs are often isointense (Fig. 14.2) on T1 weighted images and may show an hyperintense (Fig.14.3) pattern in about 30-50% of patients.[1,14,44-47] High signal intensity on T1 weight-

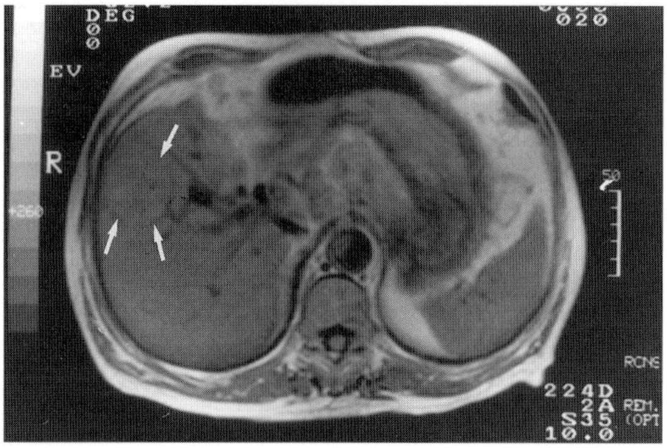

Figure 14.2 –

Axial SE T1 weighted image demontrates a primary liver tumor (HCC) which shows signal intensity similar to that of the surrounding liver parenchima. At the periphery of the tumor is evident a thin layer of low signal intensity, corresponding to the capsule (arrows).

ed images may be determined by tumor fatty changes,[1,13,14] high glycogen content,[48] intratumoral copper,[49,50] or hemorrhagic necrosis. Hemorrhagic necrosis is generally observable in large, undifferentiated HCCs (Fig. 14.4a,b). Fat and glycogen are more common in small, well-differentiated HCCs, probably reflecting a defective release of these components by partially functioning hepatocytes (Fig. 14.5a-c). These features are not completely characteristic of small HCC, and can be found in the early stage of hepatic carcinogenesis like regenerating nodules or adenomatous hyperplasia, as well as in benign hepatic lesions like adenomas, focal nodular hyperplasia (FNH), and lipomas. The increased signal intensity from fat deposits in the tumor cells is more evident at higher field strengths than at low field strengths;[13] chemical shift imaging (phase contrast technique with gradient echo imaging)[13] may be useful to differentiate fatty from hemorrhagic degeneration.

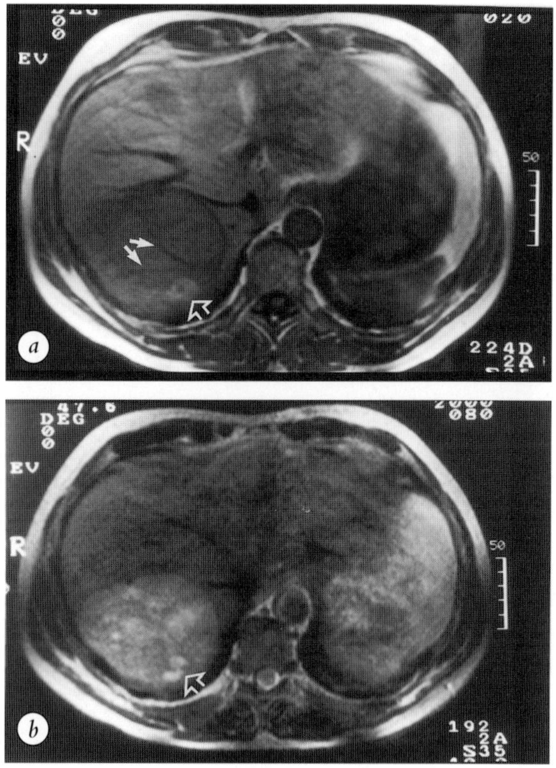

Figure 14.4 –

a) Axial SE T1 weighted image.

b) Axial SE T2 weighted image.

In *a)* and *b)* a large tumor is detectable as hypointense and hyperintense mass on SE T1 and T2 weighted images, respectively. On both images a intratumoral area of high signal intensity is visible, corresponding to hemorrhagic focus (open arrow). Furthermore on T1 weighted images intratumoral septae can be detected as thin bands of low signal intensity (small arrows).

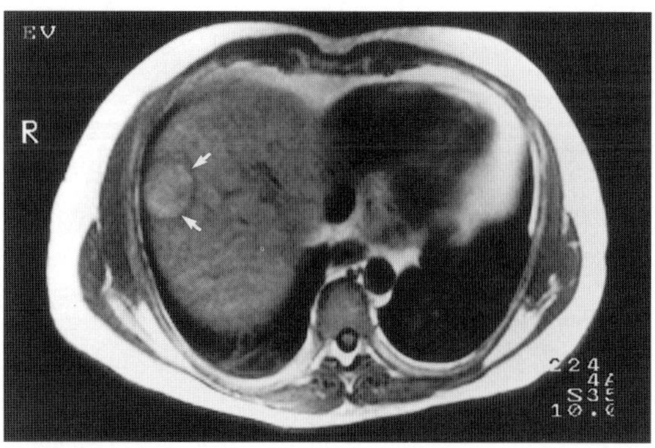

Figure 14.3 –

Axial SE T1 weighted image shows HCC lesion of high signal intensity relative to liver; the peripheral capsule is also present (arrows).

Because of the abnormal low signal of iron overloaded liver, variable grade of lesion hyperintensity relative to surrounding parenchyma is a common finding of HCC superimposed on hemochromatosis, on all sequences[51] (Fig. 14.6a,b).

T2 weighted images

Most HCCs (about 90%) appear hyperintense on T2 weighted images[13,14] (Figs. 14.1b, 4b, 6b); only about 10% may have an isointense pattern, generally when well differentiated (Edmonson grade 1 HCC)[13,52] (Fig. 14.7a,b). In fact, histologic studies seem to indicate that the signal intensity on T2 weighted images correlates with the grade of malignancy in nodular lesions of cirrhotic liver.[13,52] When comparing signal intensities of different histologic patterns of HCC, no significant difference can be observed between the trabecular and pseudoglandular forms of tumors; nevertheless, marked hyperintensity due to increased tumor extracellular water can be found in some HCCs with pseudoglandular pattern[13,53] (Fig.14.8). Furthermore, localized

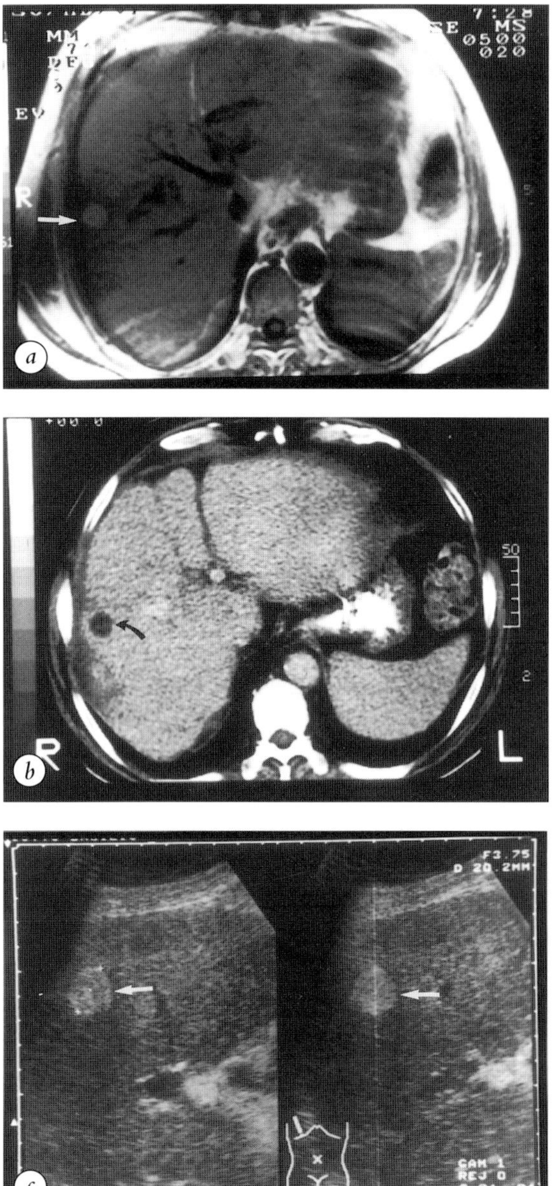

Figure 14.5 –

a) Axial SE T1 weighted image.

b) Contrast-enhanced CT scan.

c) Ultrasound scans.

In *a)* a small rounded HCC lesion shows high signal intensity compared to liver due to fat degeneration of tumor tissue (arrow). In *b)* corresponding CT image reveales an area of low attenuation which is typical of fat tissue (arrow). In *c)* the lesion is of high echogenicity relative to liver (arrows).

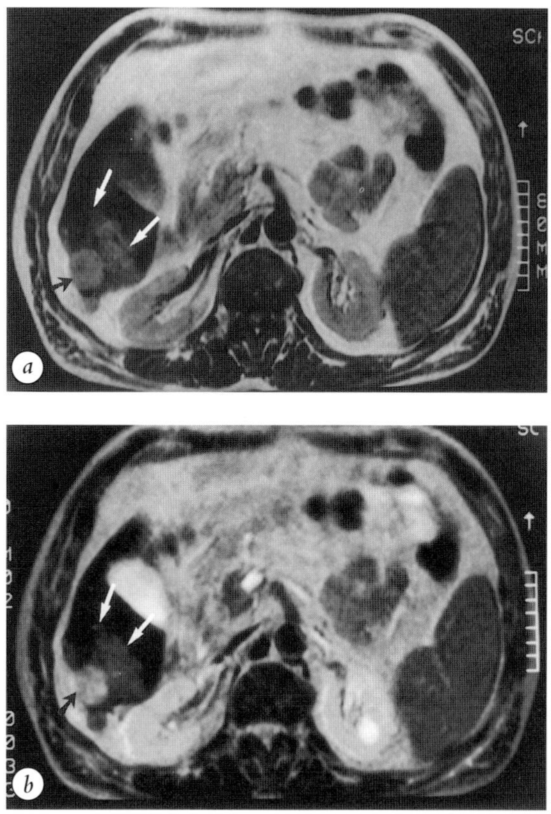

Figure 14.6 –

a) Axial SE T1 weighted image.

b) Axial SE T2 weighted image.

In *a)* and *b)* the HCC lesion appears as a mass of high signal intensity (black arrow). The adjacent liver parenchima has abnormal low signal intensity due to hemocromatosis. A perilesional area of relative high signal intensity can be seen on both images; such finding corresponds to edema (white arrows).

hyperintense foci on T2 weighted images can be found in large tumors with peliotic changes of intratumoral sinusoids.[13,53] Conversely, few (about 2-3%) HCCs with spontaneous coagulation necrosis may be observed as hypointense lesions on T2 weighted images.[13]

Morphologic features

HCC can be frequently recognized and differentiated from other hepatic lesions by means of typical morphologic features, which often correspond to specific histologic structures. The most important features of HCC are internal heterogeneity, intratumoral septa and/or scar, capsule, daughter nodules and vascular invasion.

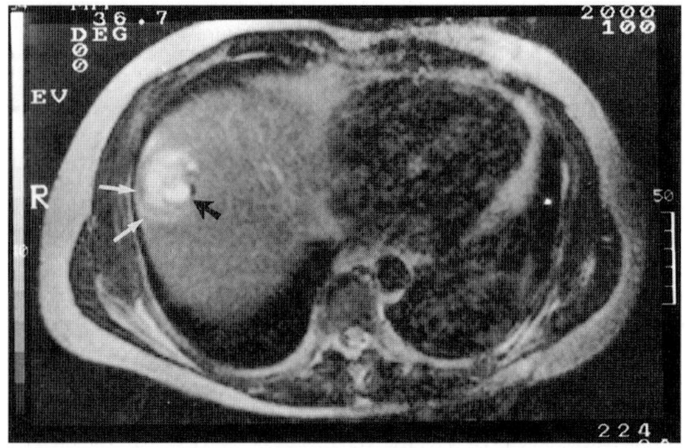

Figure 14.8 – Axial SE T2 weighted image. A HCC lesion of marked high signal intensity (black arrow) due to increased tumoral water content corresponds to pseudo-glandular pattern. At the periphery of the lesion a double-layered rim (an hypointense inner layer surrounded by an hyperintense outer layer) is evident (white arrows).

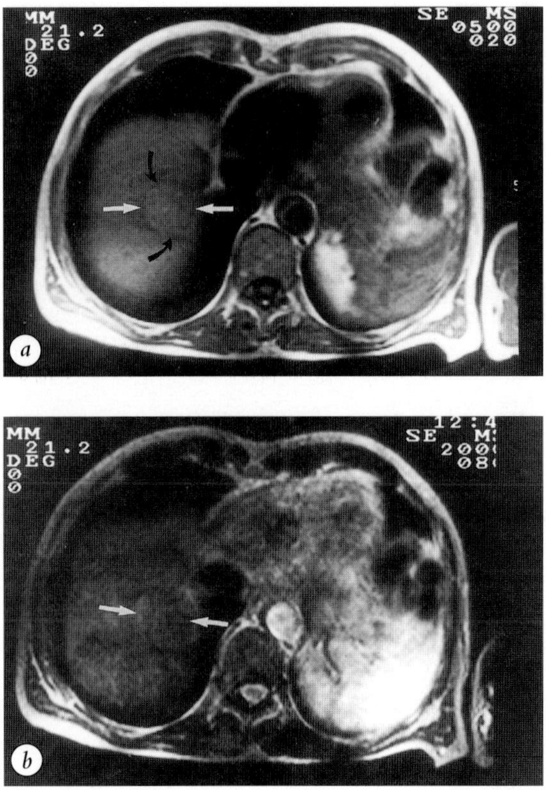

Figure 14.7 –

a) Axial SE T1 weighted image.

b) Axial SE T2 weighted image.

On both images the HCC lesion appears as isointense mass relative to liver (white arrows). On T1 weighted image the capsular structure is also appreciable (black arrows).

Internal heterogeneity

The great majority (92%) of hepatic lesions with non-homogeneous signal intensity are malignant.[15] Internal heterogeneity is a common feature at gross examination (from 50% to 80% in tumors larger than 3 cm).[13,15] Especially on T2 weighted images, a "mosaic" or a "nodule-within-nodule" pattern of signal intensity can be observed, due to the presence of multiple iso-hyperintense tumoral foci, sometimes at different carcinogenetic stages, spared into areas of low-signal, noncancerous regenerative liver tissue, siderotic nodules or coagulative necrosis[51,54-56] (Fig. 14.9a-c).

Septa/scar

A mosaic pattern can be observed in the presence of intratumoral septa, depicted as thin linear-like structures, hypointense on all sequences[18] (Figs. 14.4a,b, 10). Presence of intratumoral septa may account for a bad response to PEI, due to uneven intratumoral ethanol diffusion. In some hepatic tumors a central scar can be identified. Fibrous scars are more commonly seen in fibrolamellar HCCs, as central stellate or cleft-like structures, hypointense on all sequences. On occasion, an inflammatory scar can be detected in HCC, appearing hypointense on T1 weighted images and hyperintense on T2 weighted images, because of increased free water, with long T1 and T2 relaxation times.[57] These scar features are

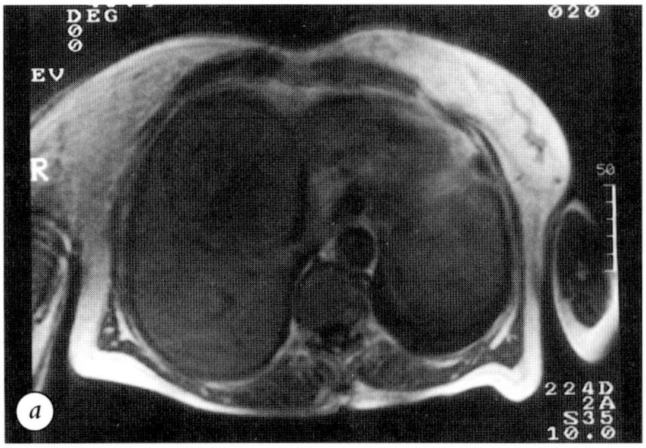

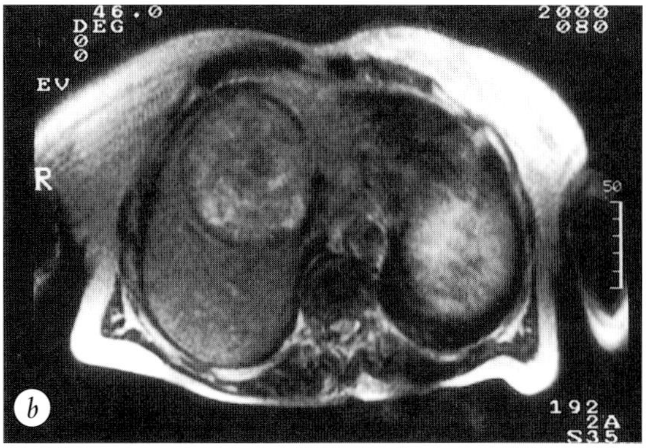

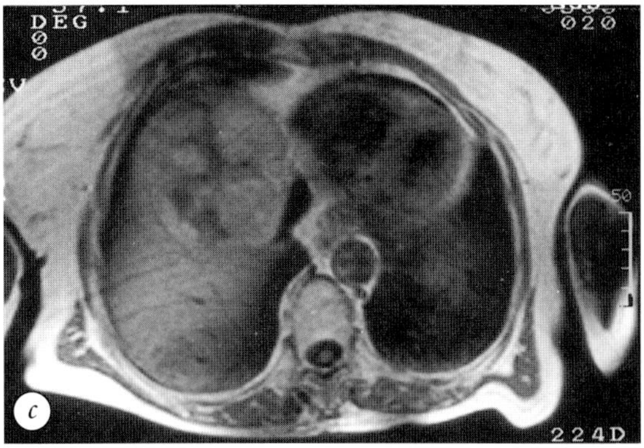

Figure 14.9 –

a) Axial SE T1 weighted image.

b) Axial SE T2 weighted image.

c) Axial Gadolinium-enhanced SE T1 weighted image.

In all MR images an inhomogeneous signal intensity pattern corresponds to internal heterogeneity of the HCC. This finding is commonly found especially at pathologic examination of large lesion.

indistinguishable from those of vascular scars, frequently detected in FNH, and a reliable differentiation of malignant from benign tumors cannot be exclusively based upon this sign[57] (Fig. 14.11a, b).

Capsule

Capsular formation is an important characteristic feature of the nodular form of HCC (Figs. 14.2, 3, 4a,b, 7b, 9a-c, 11a). Capsule is identified at pathologic examination in about 80 % of HCCs; higher frequencies of detection are reported for lesions larger than 2 cm (about 90-95%) than in small HCCs (54% for lesions smaller than 2.0 cm).[13] Capsule is a common feature of slow-growing, well-differentiated HCC,[18] and is associated with a better prognosis. Capsule thickness increases as the tumor grows, but is generally between 0.5 and 5 mm. It is a specific feature of hepatocellular neoplasms: therefore it can also be seen in benign hepatic tumors, like adenomas. Tumor capsules of benign and malignant lesions are indistinguishable on histology and MR imaging, both being produced by the compression of normal hepatic parenchyma by tumor growth.[13,54]

MR imaging is more sensitive than any other imaging technique in detecting HCC capsule.[14] The MR detection rate of tumor capsule seems to be higher in Asian populations (66%),[13](42%)[14,18] than in American populations (24%).[1] Capsule is more easily depicted on T1 weighted images as a low-intensity

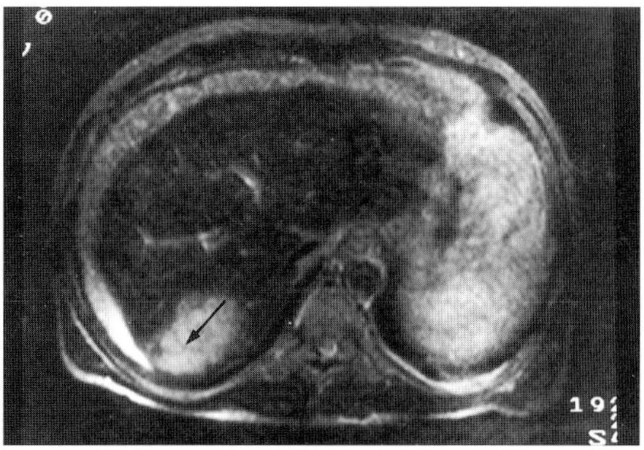

Figure 14.10 –

Axial SE T2 weighted image. The HCC lesion appears as hyperintense mass relative to liver; intratumoral septae can be detected as thin bands of low signal intensity (arrow).

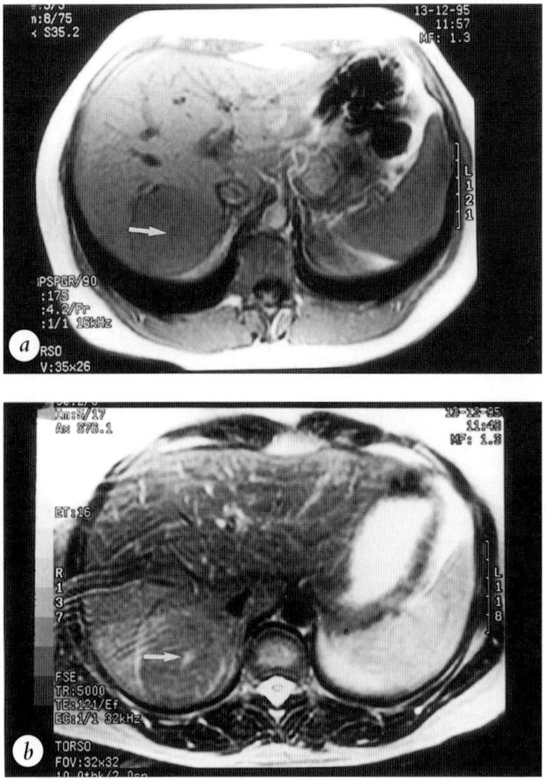

Figure 14.11 –

a) Axial SE T1 weighted image.

b) Axial SE T2 weighted image.

In a) a large HCC lesion shows low signal intensity; centrally a small area of lower signal intensity corresponds to central scar tissue (arrow). In b) the HCC lesion is isointense to liver and the central scar (arrow) is of high signal intensity due to inflammatory tissue.

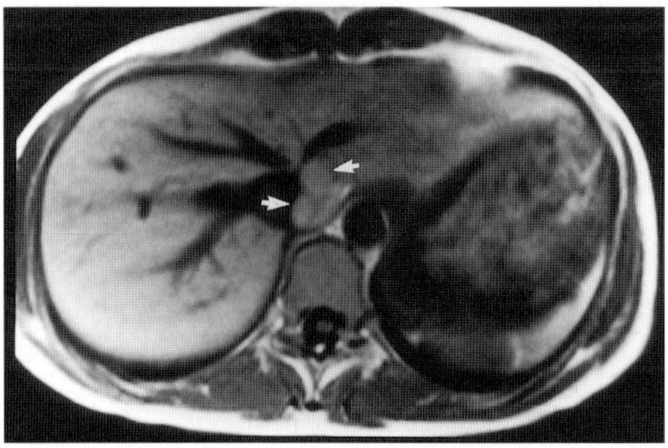

Figure 14.12 – Axial SE T1 weighted image demonstrates an adenoma with peripheral capsule (arrows).

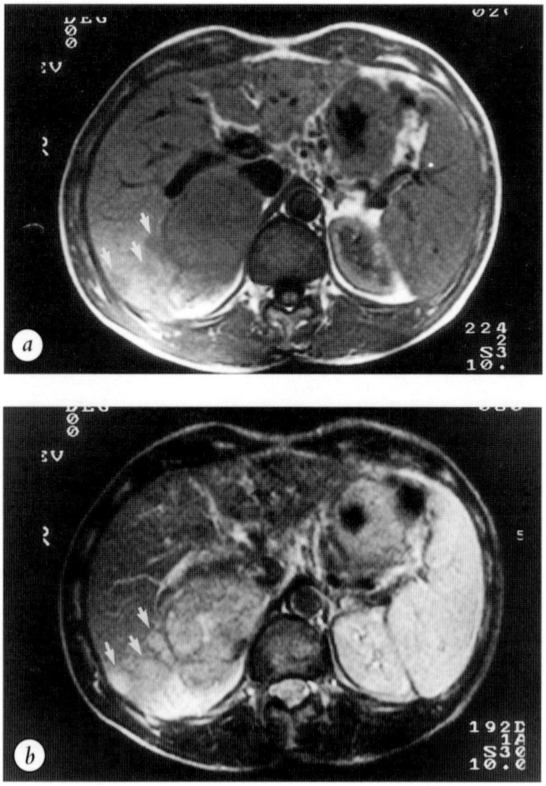

Figure 14.13 –

a) Axial SE T1 weighted image.

b) Axial SE T2 weighted image.

Large HCC lesion is easily detectable on both images. The presence of small daugther nodules (arrows) is also evident: these appear as low signal intensity and high signal intensity lesions close to the main tumor on T1 and T2 weighted images, respectively.

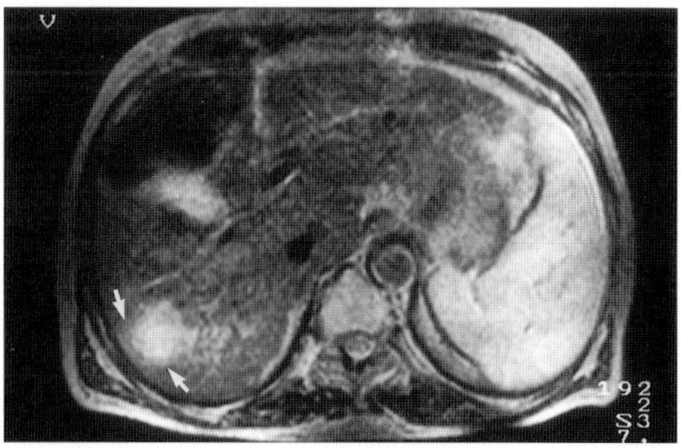

Figure 14.14 – Axial SE T2 weighted image shows high signal intensity HCC-tumor with peripheral edema (arrows).

band; in about 50% of detected cases, a capsule may be demonstrated also on T2 weighted images as a single hypointense (Fig. 14.4b) ring or as a double layered structure (an hypointense inner layer surrounded by an hyperintense outer layer)[13, 18] (Fig. 14.8). Histologic studies reveal that the inner low-intensity band corresponds to fibrotic tissue and the outer high intensity band represents a water rich layer with compressed small vessels or newly formed biliary ducts.[14,18] Although suggestive of HCC, detection of a tumor capsule is not completely specific, because it may be observed in cases of hepatic adenoma[1] (Fig. 14.12). Furthermore, a low-signal rim reflecting the hepatic parenchyma compressed by the tumor has been observed on SE T1 weighted images in 4% of patients with metastatic colorectal adenocarcinoma.[14,58]

The delineation of a tumor capsule is important not only for differential diagnosis with all the other hepatic malignancies, but also from a therapeutic point of view. TAE and PEI have been reported to be more effective in encapsulated than in noncapsulated forms of HCC.

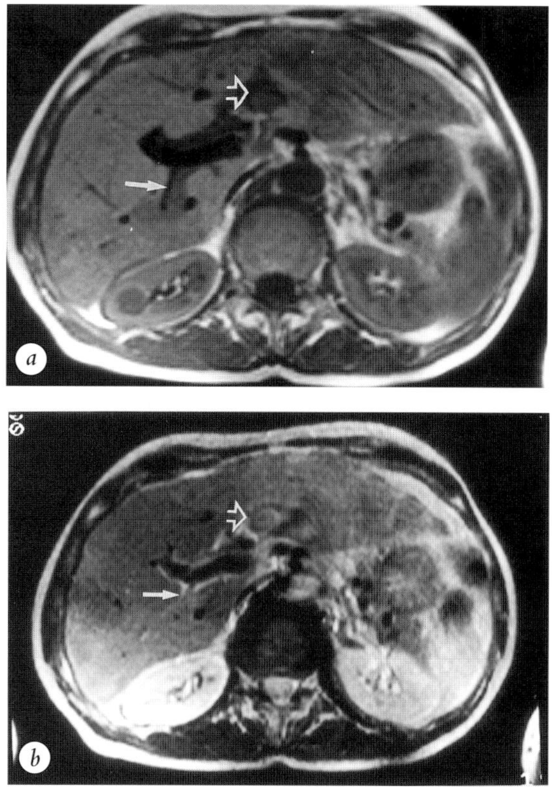

Figure 14.15 –
a) Axial SE T1 weighted image.
b) Axial SE T2 weighted image.
MR images show neoplastic thrombosis of the main left branch of portal vein (open arrow). The same finding is also present in the posterior segment of the right branch of portal vein (arrow). In both cases a soft tissue mass is visible inside the venous structure.

Daughter nodules

Daughter nodules adjacent to the primary tumor can be found in patients with advanced HCC; they typically show signal intensities similar to the primary tumor[18] (Fig. 14.13a,b).

Edema

Edema is a diagnostic feature generally associated with malignant hepatic lesions and may be observed in up to 29% of HCCs[1] (Figs. 14.6a,b, 14). Edema can be seen on T2 weighted images as an hyperintense band surrounding the nodule, or as an area extending from an apex at the tumor to a broad base at the liver capsule, reflecting the anatomic distribution of venous or lymphatic blockage.[59]

Vascular invasion

Vascular invasion is a common feature of diffuse or infiltrating forms of HCC (Fig. 14.15a,b). A focal loss of the void signal characteristic of normal flow in portal or hepatic veins suggests the diagnosis on conventional spin echo images;[55] MR image interpretation may be equivocal in the presence of slow venous flow due to tumoral compression. A segmental edema evident as an hyperintense signal on T2 weighted images may be occasionally observed[1] (Figs. 14.15b, 16a,b). Flow sensitive gradient echo sequences may also be used to confirm the venous thrombosis.[12]

Diffuse HCC

The diffuse form of HCC may be difficult to differentiate from marked tissue changes due to cirrhosis, both on US and CT studies. In doubtful cases, MR imaging may demonstrate wide signal anomalies of the liver, often with segmental or lobar distribution, more evident as large hyperintense areas on T2 weighted images[1] (Fig. 14.16a,b).

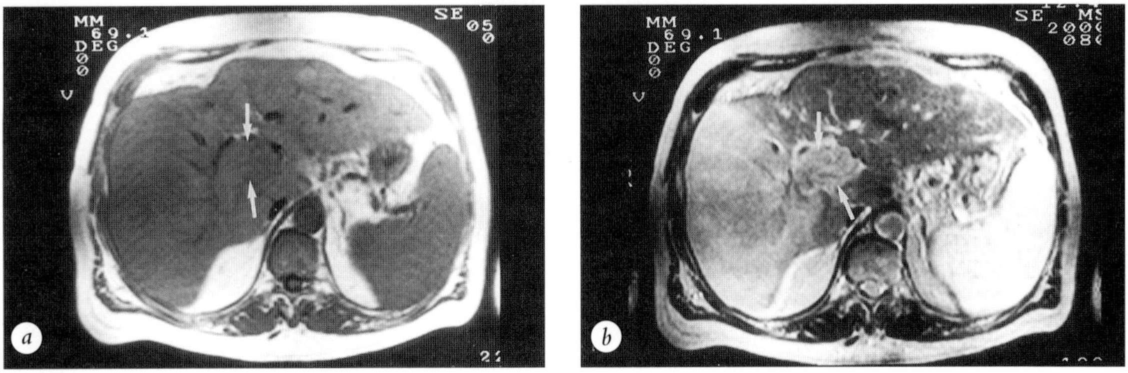

Figure 14.16 –

a) Axial SE T1 weighted image.

b) Axial SE T2 weighted image.

On both images diffuse infiltrative HCC lesion with neoplastic thrombosis of portal vein is detectable (arrows).

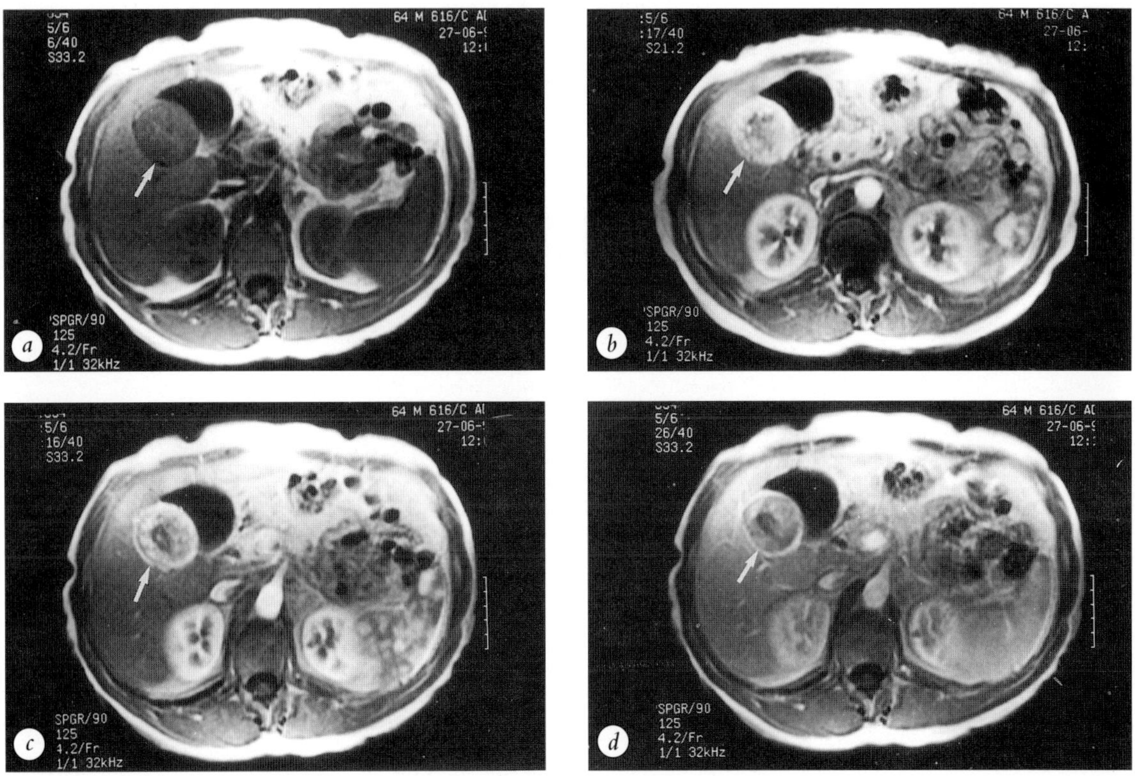

Figure 14.17 –

a) Axial Fast Multiplanar Spoiled GRASS (FMSPGR) image before Gadolinium injection.

b-d) Gadolinium-enhanced dynamic MR study performed at 30, 60 and 120 seconds after start of contrast material injection.

In *a)* the lesion (arrow) has low signal intensity to liver. On dynamic imaging the lesion shows different degrees of enhancement. The early peak (30") of enhancement is typical of HCC lesions.

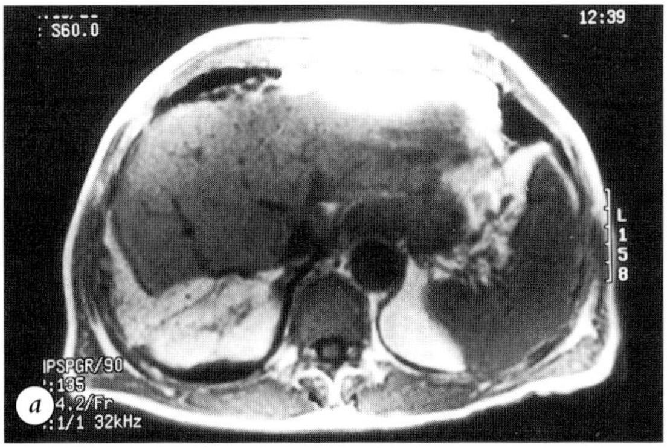

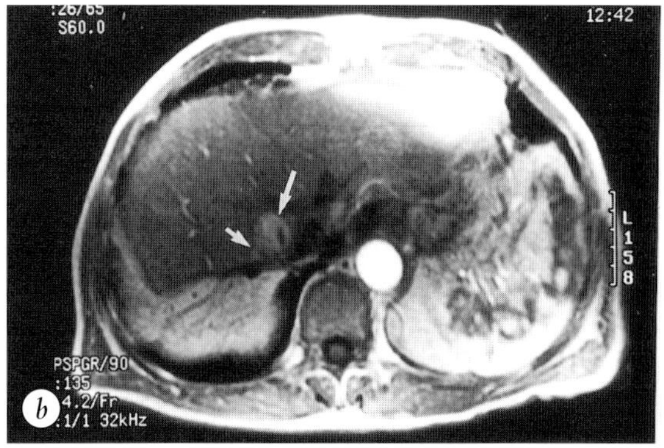

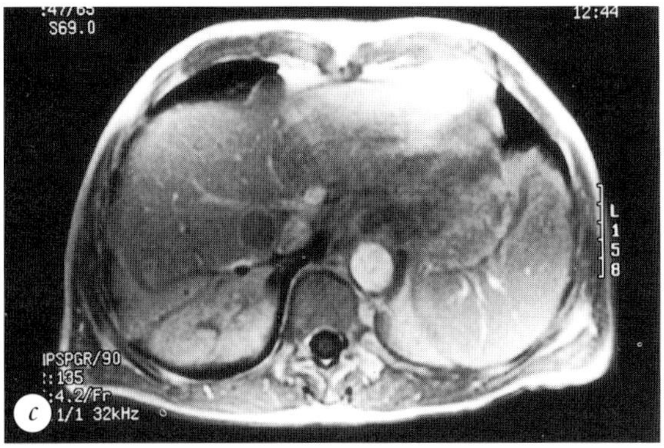

Figure 14.18 –

a) Axial Fast Multiplanar Spoiled GRASS (FMSPGR) image before Gadolinium injection.

b,c) Gadolinium-enhanced dynamic MR study performed at 30 and 90 seconds after start of contrast material injection.

The main lesion (large arrow) and a small daughter nodule (small arrow) are confidently detectable only on dynamic images.

Vascularity

HCCs are generally hypervascular tumors, predominantly supplied by the hepatic arterial system; as a result of heterogeneous internal architecture, necrotic hypovascular areas may be observed especially in large tumors.[1,23,46,47,62,63]

Dynamic MRI scanning, provided by fast imaging techniques following a bolus of Gd DTPA, has recently permitted the evaluation of the contrast enhancement pattern of HCC.[60-63] The degree of enhancement on dynamic gadolinium-enhanced images corresponds to the degree of vascularity of the lesion.[23,46,47,62,63] Depending on different sequences and contrast material doses, from 57%[46] to 86%[19] to 100%[20,21] of HCCs show variable grades of hyperintensity in relation to the normal liver parenchyma in the first minute after injection of Gd DTPA; the peak of tumoral enhancement is reached about 45 seconds after the injection, with a maximum lesion-to-liver contrast at 10-15 seconds (Figs. 14.17a-c, 18a,b). A nodule-within-nodule appearance can be observed in 27% of small (<3 cm) HCCs in the early arterial phase of the enhancement (1minute);[19] heterogeneous enhancement can be seen in 66-86% of HCCs.[19,46]

After the first minute, tumor enhancement decreases gradually and lesions tend to approach isointensity in relation to surrounding parenchyma.[19-23]

On delayed images (2-5 minutes), late capsular enhancement may be observed in 43%-55% of HCC[19,23,47] (Figs. 14.17d, 18c); this phenomenon is attributed to the large extracellular spaces of the capsular region, which include vascular lakes within the compressed liver parenchyma.[23]

DIFFERENTIAL DIAGNOSIS

Development of HCC, in countries with high prevalence of hepatic virus infections, is usually associated with chronic liver disease, such as chronic active hepatitis or cirrhosis. It is therefore necessary to differentiate between the nodular lesions commonly detectable in these conditions. The carcinogenesis in the cirrhotic liver has been recently described as a multistep process from frankly benign regenerative nodules to overt malignant HCC. The spectrum of

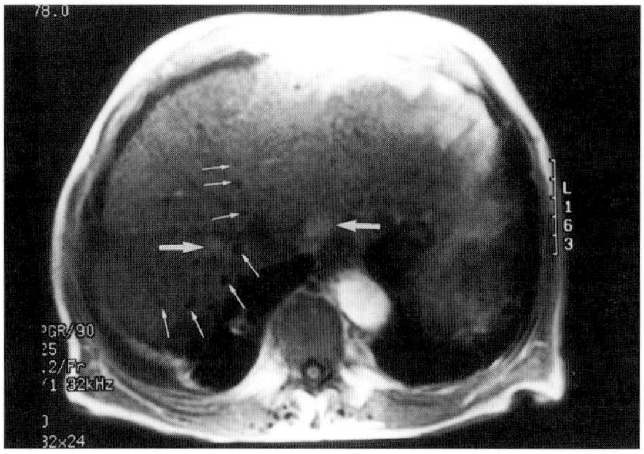

Figure 14.19 – Gadolinium-enhanced dynamic MR study performed at 30 seconds after injection of gadolinium shows two hypervascular lesions (large arrows) of high signal intensity and several hypointense regenerative nodules (small arrows).

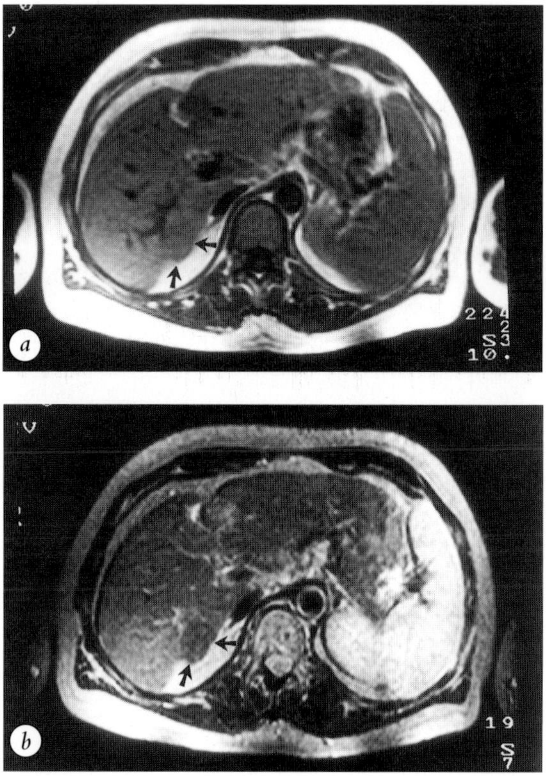

Figure 14.20 –

a) Axial SE T1 weighted image.

b) Axial SE T2 weighted image.

The lesion which appears isointense in *a)* and hypointense in *b)* corresponds to adenomatous hyperplasia (arrows).

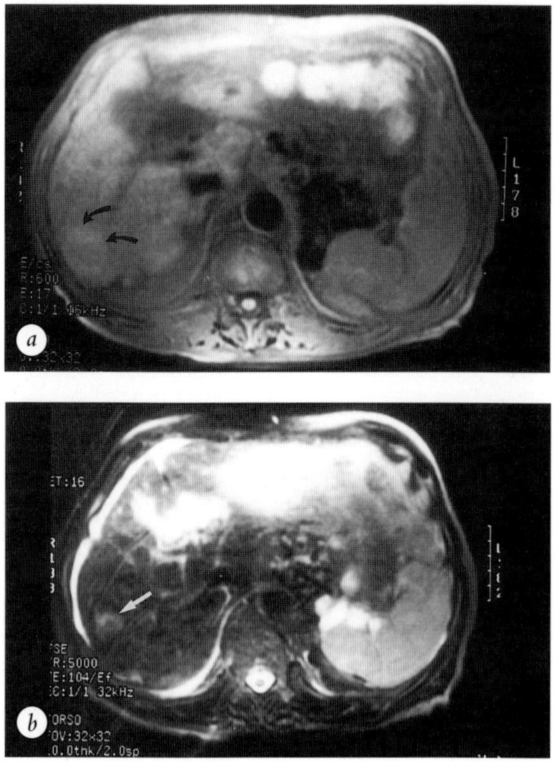

Figure 14.21 –

a) Axial fat-suppressed SE T1 weighted image.

b) Axial SE T2 weighted image.

In *a)* a lesion of low signal intensity surrounded by hyperintense pattern (arrows) is an early advanced HCC. In *b)* the same lesion is slighlty hyperintense.

focal nodular lesions includes, in order of increasing malignancy, large regenerative nodule, adenomatous hyperplasia, atypical adenomatous hyperplasia, early HCC and early advanced HCC.

Moreover, in the United States and many western countries, HCC may arise from a relatively normal liver, and differential diagnosis should include all other benign or malignant nodular lesions commonly affecting the liver, such as cyst, hemangioma, FNH, adenoma, cholangiocarcinoma and metastases.

Regenerative nodules

Regenerative nodules are a common feature of liver cirrhosis at gross pathologic examination. On MR images they may appear as small hypointense nodular lesions on both T1 and T2 weighted images.[64-66] They can be easily differentiated from HCCs, which

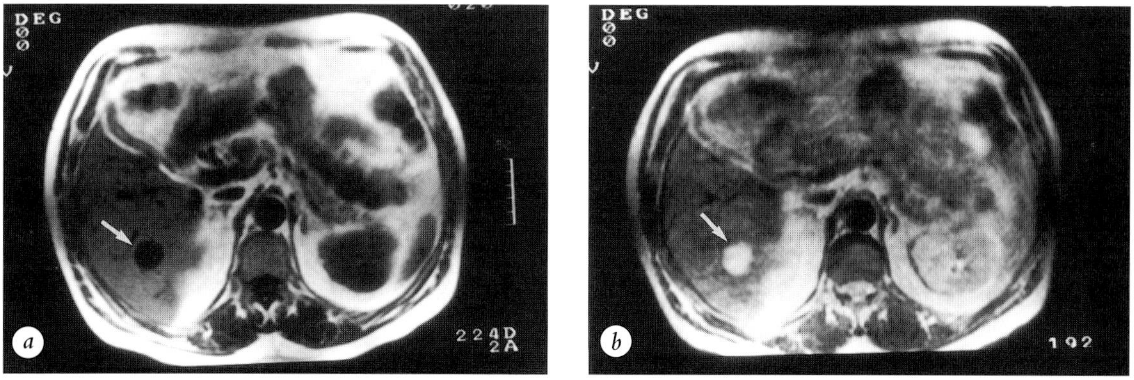

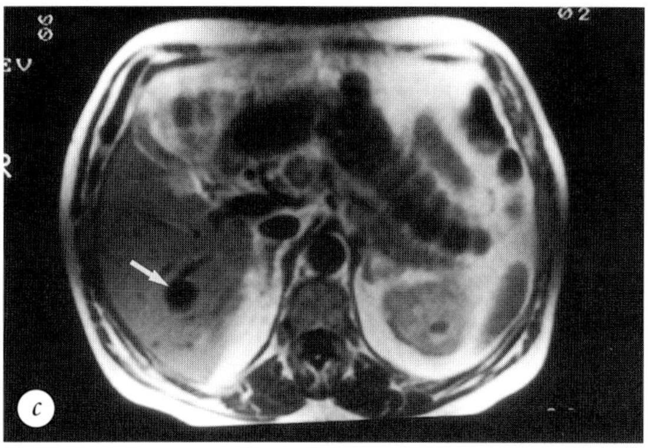

Figure 14.22 –

a) Axial SE T1 weighted image.

b) Axial SE T2 weighted image.

c) Axial Gadolinium-enhanced SE T1 weighted image.

On T1 weighted images before and after gadolinium injection the lesion (arrow) shows homogeneous low signal intensity and high signal intensity on T2 weighted images; this pattern is typical of cystic lesion.

appear with high signal intensity on T2 weighted images. In another study[67] regenerating nodules were better detectable on gradient echo (GRE) images, using short TE. Many regenerating nodules are observed as hypovascular-hypointense nodules in the early phase of gadolinium-enhanced images (Fig. 14.19). Pathologic studies have shown hemosiderin deposits in many of these nodules, partially accounting for the low signal because of magnetic susceptibility effects.[65] Internal heterogeneity is a morphologic feature useful for distinguishing HCC from large regenerative nodules.[51]

Adenomatous hyperplasia

Adenomatous hyperplasia is a large regenerative nodule with dysplastic histology.[68] Due to histologic similarity, the signal characteristics resemble those of well-differentiated HCC, being iso-hyperintense on T1 weighted images and isointense or slightly hypointense on T2 weighted images[51] (Fig. 14.20a,b). Unlike malignant lesions, adenomatous hyperplasia has smooth margins and lacks a capsule. Enhancing features are generally similar to surrounding liver, due to a prevalent portal vein vascular supply.[51,68]

Early HCC

Early HCC is defined as a nodule of adenomatous hyperplasia containing several areas of well-differentiated HCCs; these areas are not large enough to be recognized macroscopically. Early HCC shows a hyper- or isointense pattern on T1 weighted images and an isointense pattern on T2 weighted images.[44,52] Consequently, in 50 % of cases, early HCC cannot be detected due to isointensity on both T1 and T2 weighted images. Nevertheless, early HCC may be distinguished from overt HCC which demonstrates an hyperintense pattern on T2 weighted images, and has no pseudocapsule.[44,52]

Early advanced HCC (HCC with early components)

Early advanced HCC has been recently considered a transitional tumor between early HCC and advanced HCC, and is generally associated with them in

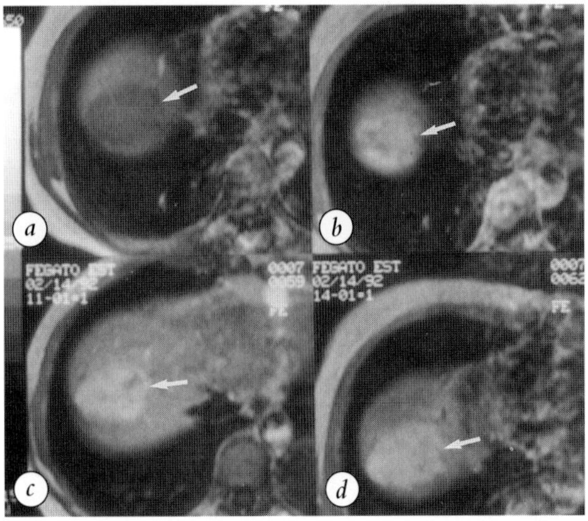

Figure 14.23 – Dynamic MR study performed before and at 30 and 120 seconds and 8 minutes after start of contrast material injection. On GRE T1 image before gadolinium injection *a)* the hemangioma is of low signal intensity to liver; *b,c)* dynamic MR scanning after administration of Gd-DTPA shows early peripheral enhancement, with *d)* centripetal progression and late complete filling.

patients with chronic liver disease. It consists of advanced HCC, large enough to be detected at gross examination, within early HCC;[6] on dynamic MR study early advanced HCC usually shows hypervascularity.[70] Early advanced HCC may have a dominant early component with small overt HCC nodules, showing a nodule-within-nodule appearance at gross examination and on MR images (central hypointensity surrounded by hyperintensity on T1 weighted images; central hyperintensity on T2 weighted images) (Fig. 14.21a,b). In more advanced cases a larger overt HCC nodule with scanty early components at the periphery is evident: on MRI only overt HCC nodules can be recognized as an hyperintense area on T2 weighted images.[51]

Cyst

The diagnosis of simple cysts is generally easy and highly specific by means of sonography. Due to the long T1 and T2 relaxation times of water, a cyst is typically hypointense on T1 weighted images and strongly hyperintense on T2 weighted images (Fig. 14.22a,b). These features can be similar to those of hepatic hemangioma. These two benign lesions can be easily differentiated on gadolinium-enhanced images, that demonstrate lack of enhancement of cyst[63] (Fig. 14.22c).

Cavernous hemangioma

Cavernous hemangioma appears as a low-intensity lesion on T1 weighted images, and has homogeneous high signal intensity on T2 weighted images[16,17] (Fig. 14.23a,b); this feature depends on long T1 and T2 relaxation times due to rich fluid content. Because of extremely long T2 relaxation times (150±45 ms at 0.6 T), a cut-off value of 88 ms has been proposed for differentiating between cavernous hemangioma and HCC at 1.5 T MR examination.[16,17] Other morphologic criteria can be useful: cavernous hemangiomas have sharp, lobular margins and lack hypointense capsule or peripheral edema. Dynamic MR scanning after administration of Gd DTPA shows early peripheral enhancement, with centripetal progression and late (5-30 minutes) complete filling[19-22,63] (Fig. 14.23). Persistent hyperintensity on T1 weighted delayed scanning is a specific feature and differentiates hemangioma from all the other hepatic nodular lesions.[19-22]

FNH

This benign tumor shows typical low lesion-to-liver contrast on plain T1 weighted and T2 weighted images, appearing isointense (46%) or slightly hypointense (54%) relative to the liver parenchyma on T1 images (this feature is more evident on GRE images) and isointense (43%) or slightly hyperintense (57%) on T2 weighted images[47] (Fig. 14.24a,b). Capsule is not evident, while a central vascular scar can be seen in 43% of FNH on T1 weighted images (hypointense) and 32% on T2 weighted images (hyperintense) (Fig. 14.24a,b). As for HCC, on dynamic MRI a strong peak of enhancement can be seen about 45 seconds after bolus injection of Gd

DTPA, with a maximum lesion-to-liver contrast at 15 seconds; studies with ultrafast dynamic MRI after bolus injection of Gd DTPA[21] report that enhancement tends to be slightly stronger and earlier than that of HCC (Fig. 14.24c). Unlike HCC, enhancement is homogeneous in 96% of FNHs. Central scarring can be seen as central nonenhancing areas in 75% of FNHs in the early enhancing phase, but with a late enhancement in the late phase (1-8 min)[47] (Fig. 14.24d).

Adenoma

Differential diagnosis between hepatic adenoma and well-differentiated HCC may be very difficult because of similar morphologic features (Fig. 14.12) (iso-hyperintensity on T1 weighted images, variable presentation on T2 weighted images, internal heterogeneity due to necrosis and/or hemorrhage, possibly hypointense capsule or central scarring, early enhancement at dynamic MR study).[71] Clinical data (young age, female sex, absence of liver dysfunction, oral contraceptive use) may help the diagnosis.

Cholangiocarcinoma

The MRI features of cholangiocarcinoma are similar to those of other tumors, being hypointense on T1 weighted images and hyperintense on T2 weighted images.[72] Peripheral cholangiocarcinoma generally presents as a large mass, but, differently from HCC, hyperintensity on T1 weighted images and capsular formation are very uncommon features (Fig. 14.25a).

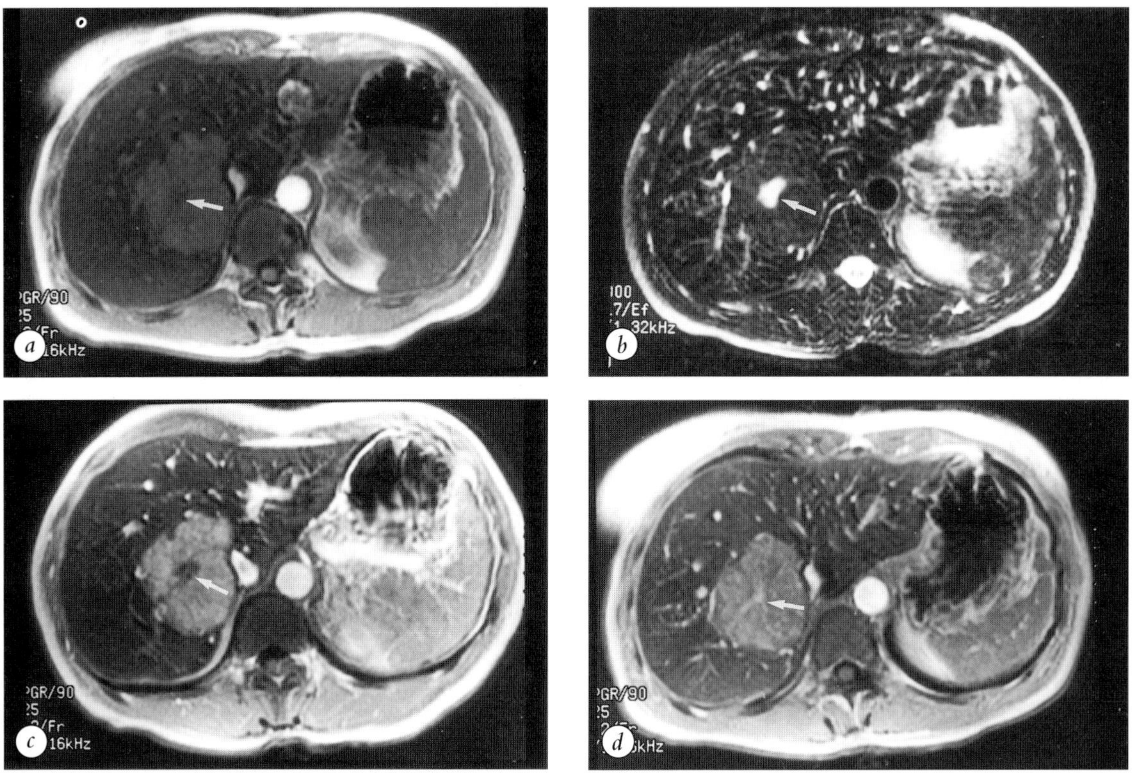

Figure 14.24 –

a) Axial Fast Multiplanar Spoiled GRASS (FMSPGR) image before Gadolinium injection.

b) Axial FSE T2 weighted image.

c,d) Gadolinium-enhanced dynamic MR study performed at 30 and 120 seconds after start of contrast material injection.

In *a)* a large FNH shows high signal intensity relative to the adjacent liver parenchima with low signal intensity due to hemocromatosis; centrally a small area of low signal intensity corresponds to scar (arrow). Caval and aorta hyperintensity is due to the inflow phenomena. In *b)* the HCC lesion is isointense to liver and the central scar is of high signal intensity (vascular scar) (arrow). On dynamic early phase, the lesion shows marked enhancement. The central scar (arrow), unenhanced in the early phase, demonstrates high signal intensity on the delayed phase.

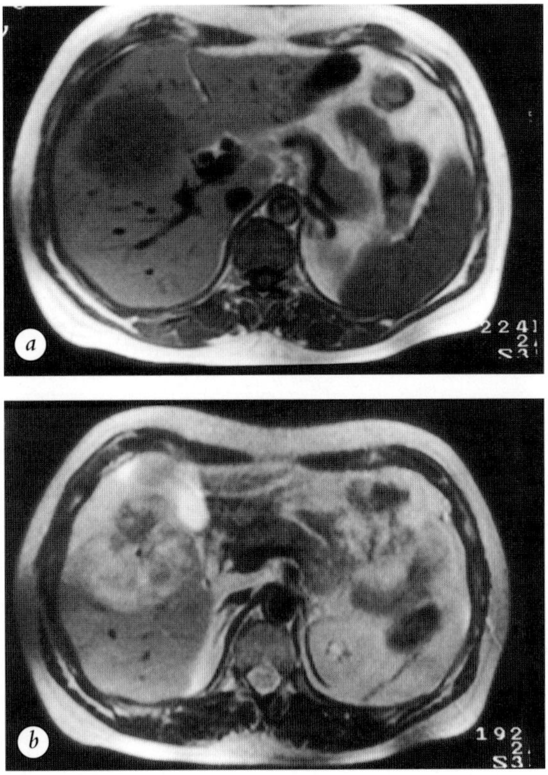

Figure 14.25 –

a) Axial SE T1 weighted image.

b) Axial gadolinium-enhanced SE T1 weighted image.

The cholangiocarcinoma shows aspecific hypointense pattern in *a)* In *b)* the lesion shows moderate enhancement with incomplete central filling. The capsule is no evident on both images.

After administration of Gd DTPA, a moderate peripheral enhancement may be observed, with late centripetal progression, but without a complete filling of necrotic central areas[73] (Fig. 14.25b). Central (hilar) cholangiocarcinoma is commonly associated with biliary dilation and infiltration of portal vessels, leading to segmental or lobar atrophy.

Metastases

Metastases may present with a wide spectrum of different signal intensities and morphologic features, sometimes mimicking those of HCC.[58] Regarding signal intensity, non-homogeneous T1 hypointensity and T2 hyperintensity are the most common features[17] (Fig. 14.26a,b); hyperintensity on T1 weighted images has been described in cases of metastatic melanoma, because of the paramagnetic effect of melanin; central liquefactive necrosis is relatively common, leading to a target configuration on T2 weighted images[58]). In some lesions, generally from colorectal carcinoma, central areas of decreased signal intensity may be observed on T2 weighted images, due to coagulative necrosis and fibrosis.[58] Capsule and/or scars are rarely encountered; peritumoral edema (hyperintense on T2 images) may occur due to vascular or biliary obstruction[1,59] (Fig. 14.26b). Most metastases are hypovascular, and thus may be easily distinguished from HCCs in the early arterial phase of contrast enhancement on dynamic MRI scanning; moderate peripheral contrast enhancement may be observed in the venous phase, sometimes with a tendency to slow central filling on delayed images.[19,21] Hypervascular metastases (from endocrine tumors like carcinoids, islet cell tumors and

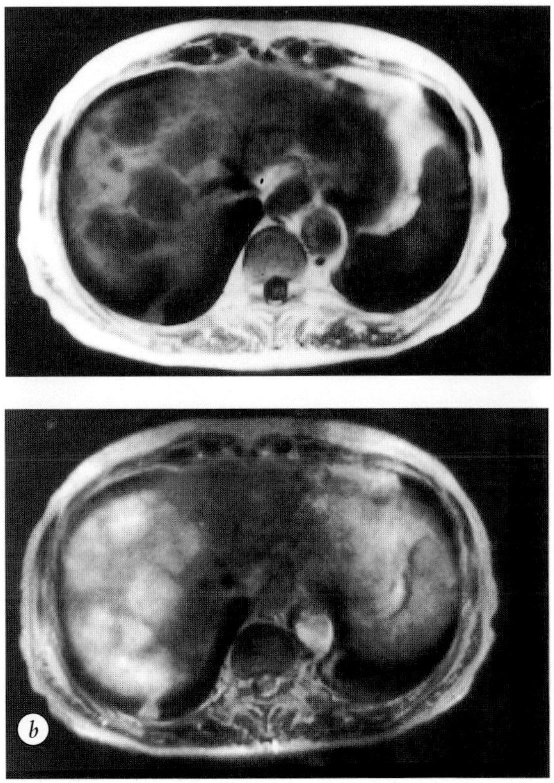

Figure 14.26 –

a) Axial SE T1 weighted image.

b) Axial SE T2 weighted image.

Multiple metastases from colorectal adenocarcinoma demonstrate low signal intensity in *a)* and high signal intensity in *b)*. In *b)* peripheral edema is evident.

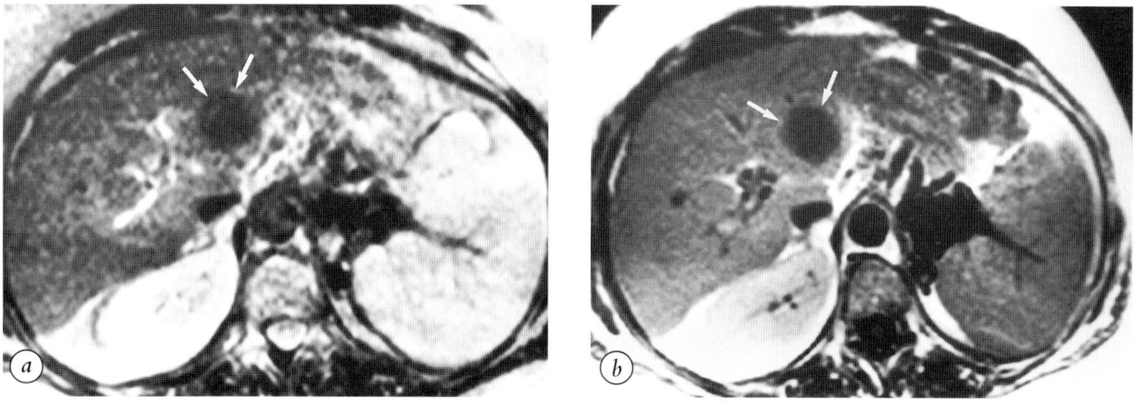

Figure 14.27 –
a) Axial SE T2 weighted image.
b) Axial gadolinium-enhanced SE T1 weighted image.
HCC completely necrotic after PEI therapy (arrow). In *a)* the lesion is displayed as focal hypointensity and in *b)* the lesion shows lack of enhancement.

pheochromocytomas) may have early arterial enhancement, thus being difficult to distinguish from HCC.[47]

In summary, the combined use of T1 and T2 weighted pulse sequences, followed by a dynamic MRI study, may allow the accurate detection of HCC. A differential diagnosis from most of the other benign and malignant hepatic lesions is provided by the ability of MR imaging to identify specific morphologic features such as fatty degeneration, capsule, peritumoral edema and vascular invasion.

FOLLOW-UP OF TREATED HCC

Even though surgical resection is considered the preferred therapeutic treatment for HCC, in recent years new therapeutic procedures have been introduced such as percutaneous ethanol injection (PEI) under US guidance and transarterial embolization (TAE) with ultrafluid liposoluble contrast medium (Lipiodol), chemotherapeutic agent and gelatin sponge.[74-89]

Recently, several reports[90-100] indicated that MR imaging may have a role in the follow-up evaluation of HCC lesions treated with PEI or with TAE therapy. In fact MR imaging seems to be able to assess the presence or absence of residual tumor tissue after treatment or conversely to indicate complete tumor regression.[90-100]

On follow-up of PEI treatment using unenhanced T2 weighted images, the finding of uniform hypointensity of the treated lesion corresponds to complete tumor necrosis[91] (Fig. 14.27). On the same images, the finding of persistent hyperintensity of the lesion corresponds to the presence of residual viable tumor.[91] The reason for hypointensity on T2 weighted images in necrotic tumors after ethanol injection has been previously investigated.[91] This finding seems to be related to a decrease of free water in coagulative necrotic tissue relative to liver parenchyma.

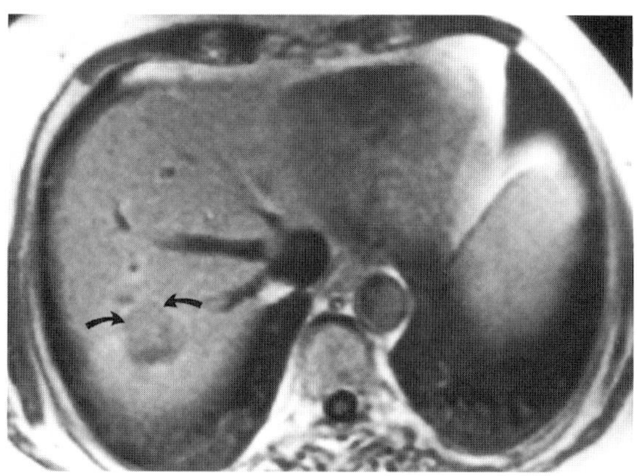

Figure 14.28 – Axial gadolinium-enhanced SE T1 weighted image. HCC in which complete necrosis was not obtained with PEI, confirmed at surgical specimen. The lesion is displayed as a mass with enhancement due to the residual viable tumor (arrow).

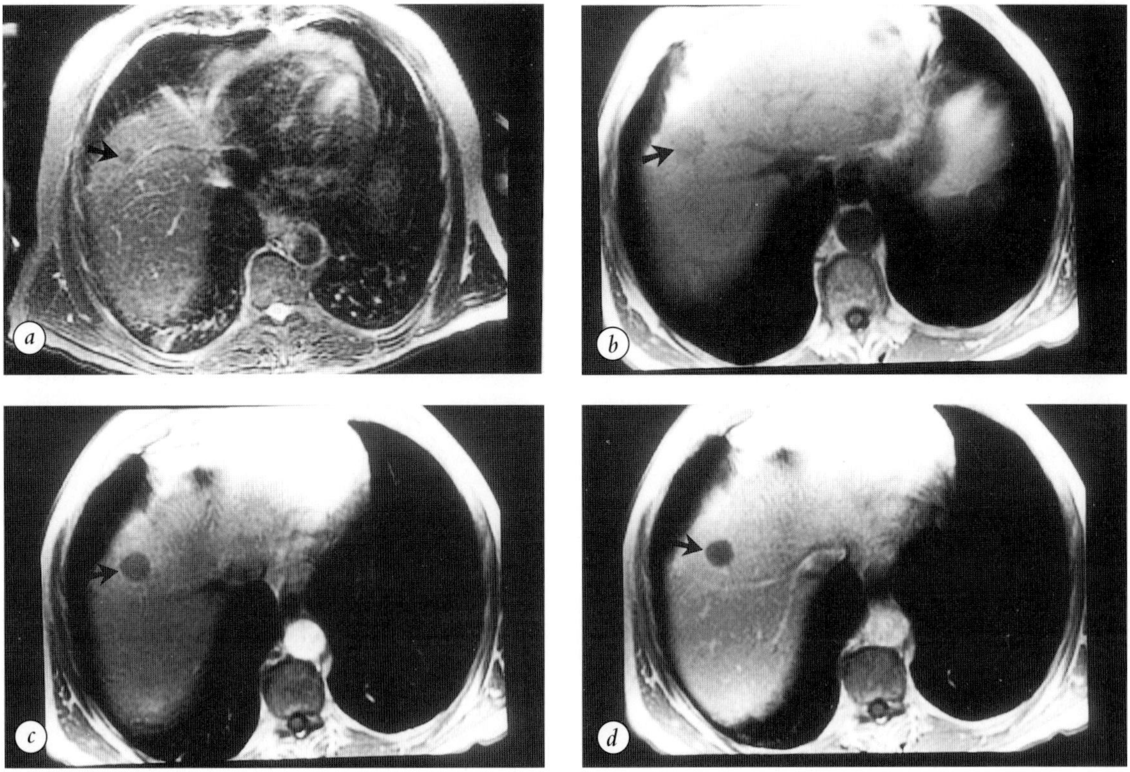

Figure 14.29 –

a) Axial SE T2 weighted image.

b) Axial Fast Multiplanar Spoiled GRASS (FMSPGR) image before Gadolinium injection.

c,d) Gadolinium-enhanced dynamic MR study performed at 30 and 90 seconds after start of contrast material injection.

HCC completely necrotic after TAE therapy (arrow). In *a)* at 12-month follow-up, the lesion appears as focal hypointensity. In *b)* the lesion is slighlty hypointense relative to liver. In the contrast-enhanced dynamic images the tumor shows lack of enhancement.

The presence of an inflammatory reaction at the periphery of the necrotic area may also mimic residual tumor, as it shows high signal intensity on T2 weighted images.[91]

For a more accurate evaluation of the outcome of therapy, contrast-enhanced MR studies are extremely useful[92,96-99] (Fig. 14.28). When viable neoplastic tissue is still present after treatment, gadolinium-enhanced T1 weighted SE images as well as dynamic contrast-enhanced MRI studies show the presence of nodular or crescentic enhancing areas[92,96-99] (Fig. 14.28). Concerning follow-up of TAE treatment, on T2 weighted unenhanced images at short term follow-up an increase in lesion signal intensity is usually observed;[90,99] it has been suggested that this finding can be due to the presence of an intralesional hemorrhagic component related to the embolization procedure.[90,97,99] At later follow-up, lesions which were treated successfully revealed the appearance of progressive and persistent hypointensity[99] (Fig. 14.29). The change, between short and medium-long term follow-up on T2 weighted images, from hyperintensity to a progressive hypointensity seems to be related to the evolution of the initial hemorrhagic necrotic process towards a later phase of coagulative necrosis.[99] On post treatment contrast enhanced dynamic images, the lack of enhancement corresponds to complete necrosis (Fig. 14.29), while the persistence of areas of enhancement usually corresponds to residual viable neoplastic tissue[92,93,96-99] (Fig. 14.30). In the evaluation of HCC lesions treated with PEI or with TAE, a thin enhancing halo can be observed on contrast enhanced T1 weighted images: such a

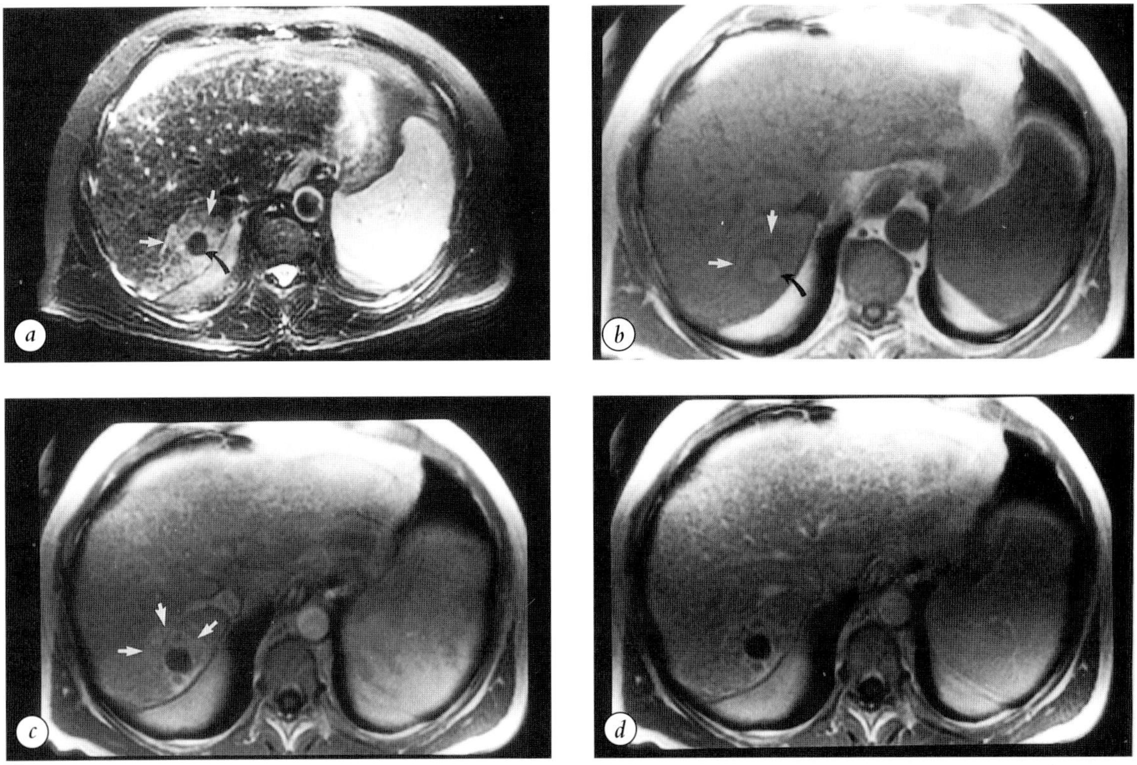

Figure 14.30 –

a) Axial SE T2 weighted image.

b) Axial Fast Multiplanar Spoiled GRASS (FMSPGR) image before Gadolinium injection.

c,d) Gadolinium-enhanced dynamic MR study performed at 30 and 90 seconds after start of contrast material injection.

HCC in which complete necrotic degeneration was not obtained with TAE. In *a)* the lesion is displayed as a mass of central low signal intensity (black arrow) with hyperintense peripheral portions (white arrows). In *b)* the mass is slighlty hyperintense (black arrow) relative to liver with perilesional hypointensity (white arrow). In *c)* the lesion still shows enhancement at the periphery (arrows). In *d)* the enhanced area is no more evident.

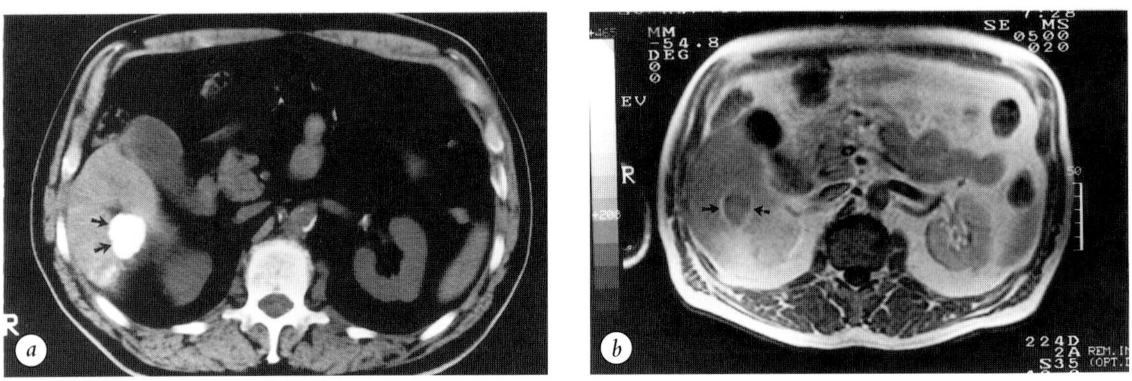

Figure 14.31 –

a) CT-Lipiodol image.

b) Axial gadolinium-enhanced SE T1 weighted image.

HCC completely degenerated after TAE treatment. On Lipiodol-CT, the lesion shows homogeneous Lipiodol accumulation (arrows). In a) the tumor shows lack of enhancement with a thin regular enhancing halo at the periphery, due to the inflammatory reaction (arrows).

finding usually indicates the presence of an inflammatory reaction along the periphery of the necrotic area[92,99] (Fig. 14.31).

The signal intensity features of the treated lesions observed on enhanced T1 weighted MRI images closely parallel the attenuation features decribed with contrast-enhanced CT scans.[91] This similarity between enhanced CT and enhanced MRI imaging patterns may result because gadolinium has pharmacokinetic and biodistribution properties similar to those of iodinated contrast agents.[91]

In assessing the outcome of PEI treatment, several studies indicated that MR imaging and CT may have similar accuracy.[91,99,100] For evaluating the therapeutic effect of TAE, however, MRI imaging shows a definite advantage, in that the independence of MRI signal intensity from the retention of iodized oil in the tumor allows a more confidential assessment of the response to treatment, particularly in lesions which show incomplete retention of iodized oil on CT.[99, 100]

In conclusion, we believe that MRI imaging could be considered a very accurate examination to select those patients suspected of partial ineffectivenes of PEI or TAE therapy who are suitable for further diagnostic and therapeutic procedures.

REFERENCES

1. Rummeny E, Weissleder R, Stark DD, *et al.* Primary liver tumors: diagnosis by MR imaging. *AJR* 1989; **152**:63-72
2. Hahn PF, Ferrucci JT. Motion artifact reduction with fast spin echo imaging. *Radiology* 1987; **168**: 183-191
3. Bailes DR, Gilderdale DJ, Bydder GM, *et al.* Technical note. Respiratory ordered phase enconding (ROPE): a method for reducing respiratory motion artifacts in MR imaging. *J Comput Assist Tomogr* 1985; **9**:835-838
4. Edelstein WA, Bottomely PA, Hart HR, Smith LS. Signal, noise, and contrast in nuclear magnetic resonance (NMR) imaging. *J Comput Assist Tomogr* 1983; **7**:391-401
5. Henkelman RM, Hardy P, Poon PY, Bronskell MJ. Optimal pulse sequence for imaging hepatic metastases. *Radiology* 1986; **161**:727-731
6. Foley WD, Kneeland JB, Cates JD, *et al.* Contrast optimization for the detection of focal hepatic lesions by MRI at 1.5 T. *AJR* 1987; **149**:1155-1160
7. Spritzer CE, Baker ME, Blinder RA, Herfkens RJ. Comparison of short repetition time (TE) and long TR/TE spin echo pulse sequences for detecting hepatic metastases at 1.5T. *Abstr Radiol* 1987; **165**(p): 202
8. Haacke EM, Lenz GW. Improving MR image quality in the presence of motion by using rephasing gradients. *AJR* 1987; **148**:1251-1258
9. Pattany PM, Phillips JJ, Chiu CL, et al. Motion artifact suppression technique (MAST) for MR imaging. *J Comput Assist Tomogr* 1987; **11**:369-377
10. Rosen BR, Carta EA, Pykett IL. Proton chemical shift imaging: an evaluation of its clinical potential using an in vivo fatty liver model. *Radiology* 1985; **154**:469-472
11. Chan TW, Listerud J, Kressel HY. Combined chemical shift selective and echo offset imaging for fat suppression: theory and initial clinical experience. *Radiology* 1991; **181**: 41-45
12. Higgins CB. The vascular System. In: Higgins CB, Hricak, Helms CA, eds. *Magnetic Resonance Imaging of the Body.* 2nd ed. New York, NY: Raven, 1992; 629-678
13. Kadoya M, Matsui O, Takashima T, Nonomura A. Hepatocellular carcinoma: Correlation of MR imaging and histopathologic findings. *Radiology* 1992; **183**:819-825
14. Ebara M, Ohto M, Watanabe Y, *et al.* Diagnosis of small hepatocellular carcinoma: Correlation of MR imaging and tumor histologic studies. *Radiology* 1986; **159**:371-377
15. Brown J, Lee JM, Lee JK, *et al.* Focal hepatic lesions: Differentiation with MR imaging at 0.5 T. *Radiology* 1991; **179**:675-679
16. Ohmoto K, Itai Y, Yoshida H, *et al.* MR differentiation of hepatocellular carcinoma from cavernous hemangioma: Complementary roles of FLASH and T2 values. *AJR* 1989; **152**:505-507
17. Lombardo DM, Baker ME, Spritzer CS, Blinder R, Meyers W, Herfkens RJ. Hepatic hemangioma vs metastases: MR differentiation at 1.5T. *AJR* 1990; **155**: 55-59
18. Itoh K, Nishimura K, Togashi K, *et al.* Hepatocellular Carcinoma: MR Imaging. *Radiology* 1987; **164**:21-25
19. Yoshida H, Itai Y, Ohmoto K, *et al.* Small hepatocellular carcinoma and cavernous hemangioma: Differentiation with dynamic FLASH MR imaging with Gd-DTPA. *Radiology* 1989; **171**:339-342
20. Olivetti L, Grazioli L, Maroldi R, Matricardi L, Milanesio L. Dynamic contrast-enhanced MR imaging of focal liver lesions. *Radiol Med* 1992; **83**: 353-360
21. Villa A, Moro G, Genovese E, *et al.* Dynamic study of nodular hepatic lesions with ultrafast sequences and fast intravenous bolus injection of Gd-DTPA. *Radiol Med* 1993; **85**:352-363
22. Mirowitz S, Lee JK, Gutierrez E, *et al.* Dynamic Gadolinium-enhanced rapid acquisition spin-echo MR imaging of the liver. *Radiology* 1991; **179**: 371-376
23. Ohtomo K, Itai Y, Yoshikawa K, *et al.* Hepatic tumors: dynamic MR imaging. *Radiology* 1987; **163**:27-31
24. Marchal G, Van Hecke P, Demaerel P, *et al.* Detection of liver metastases with superparamagnetic iron oxide in 15 patients: results of MR imaging at 1.5T. *AJR* 1989; **152**:771-775
25. Saini S, Stark DD, Hahn PF, *et al.* Ferrite particles: a superparamagnetic MR contrast agent for enhanced detection of liver carcinoma. *Radiology* 1987; **162**:217-222
26. Hahn PF, Stark DD, Weissleder R, *et al.* Clinical application of superparamagnetic iron oxide to MR imaging of tissue perfusion in vascular liver tumors. *Radiology* 1990; **174**: 361-366

27. Felmlee JP, Ehman RL. Spatial presaturation: a method for suppressing flow artifacts and improving depiction of vascular anatomy in MR imaging. *Radiology* 1987; **164**:559-564

28. Crawley AP, Wood ML, Henkleman RM. Elimination of transverse coherences in FLASH MRI. *J Magn Reson Imag* 1988; **8**:248-260

·29. Henning J, Navreth A, Friedburg H. RARE imaging: a fast imaging method for clinical MR. *J Magn Reson Imag* 1986; **3**:823-833

30. Henning J, Friedburg H. Clinical applications and methodological developments of the RARE technique. *Magn Reson Imag* 1988; **6**:391-395

31. Melki PS, Mulkerr RV, Panych LP, Jolesz FA. Comparing the FAISE method with conventional dual echo sequences. *J Magn Reson Imag* 1991; **1**:319-326

32. Schwartz L, Seltzer S, Tempany C, *et al.* Prospective comparison of T2-weighted fast spin echo, with and without fat suppression, and conventional spin-echo pulse sequences in the upper abdomen. *Radiology* 1993; **189**:411-416

33. Edelman RR, Hahn PF, Buxton R, *et al.* Rapid MR imaging with suspended respiration: clinical application in the liver. *Radiology* 1986; **161**: 125-131

34. Haase A, Frahm J, Matthaci D, *et al.* FLASH imaging: rapid NMR imaging using low flip angle pulses. *J Magn Reson Imaging* 1986; **67**: 258-266

35. Mills TC, Orthendahl DA, Hylton NM, *et al.* Partial flip angle MR imaging. *Radiology* 1987: **162**: 531-539

36. Wehrli FW. Fast scan magnetic resonance. *Magn Reson Q* 1990; **6**(3):165-230

37. Dixon WT. Simple proton spectroscopic imaging. *Radiology* 1984; **153**:189-194

38. Lee JKT, Dixon WT, Ling D, *et al.* Fatty infiltration of the liver: demonstration by proton spectroscopic imaging. Preliminary observations. *Radiology* 1984; **156**:429-433

39. Heiken JP, Lee JKT, Dixon WT. Fatty infiltration of the liver evaluation by proton spectroscopic imaging. *Radiology* 1985; **157**: 707-710

40. Pykett IL, Rzedzian RR. Instant images of the body by magnetic resonance. *Magn Reson Med* 1987; **5**:563-571

41. Stehling MJ, Howseman AM, Ordidge RJ, *et al.* Whole body echo planar imaging at 0.5 T. *Radiology* 1989; **170**:257-263

42. Weisskopf RM. Improved hard pulse sequences for frequency selective presaturation in magnetic resonance. *J Magn Reson Imag* 1990; **86**:170-175

43. Campeau NG, Johnson CD, Felmlee JP, *et al.* MR imaging of the abdomen with a phased-array multicoil: prospective clinical evaluation. *Radiology* 1995;**195**:769-776

44. Muramatsu Y, Nawano S, Takayasu K, *et al.* Early hepatocellular carcinoma: MR imaging. *Radiology* 1991; **181**:209-213

45. Rosenthal RE, Davis PL. MR imaging of hepatocellular carcinoma at 1.5 T. *J Magn Reson Imag* 1991; **1**:212-216

46. Mahfouz AE, Hamm B, Wolf KJ. Dynamic gadopentate dimeglumine-enhanced MR imaging of hepatocellular carcinoma. *Eur Radiol* 1993; **3**: 453-458

47. Mahfouz AE, Hamm B, Taupitz M, Wolf KJ. Hypervascular liver lesions: differentiation of focal nodular hyperplasia from malignant tumors with dynamic gadolinium-enhanced MR imaging. *Radiology* 1993; **186**:133-138

48. Bartolozzi C, Lencioni R, Caramella D, Paolicchi A, Russo R, Romani R. Correlations between magnetic resonance imaging and histopathologic findings in hepatocellular carcinoma. *Radiol Med* 1994; **87**: 90-95

49. Ebara M, Watanabe S, Kita K, *et al*: MR Imaging of small hepatocellular carcinoma: Effect of intratumoral copper content on signal intensity. *Radiology* 1991; **180**: 617-621

50. Kitagawa K, Matsui O, Kadoya M, *et al.* Hepatocellular carcinomas with excessive copper accumulation: CT and MR findings. *Radiology* 1991; **180**:623-628

51. Mitchell DG, Rubin R, Siegelman E, *et al.* Hepatocellular carcinoma within siderotic regenerative nodules: the "nodule-within-nodule" sign on MR images. *Radiology* 1991; **178**:101-103

52. Inoue E, Kuroda C, Fujita M, *et al.* MR features of various grades of small hepatocellular carcinoma. *J Comput Assist Tomogr* 1993; **17**(1) :75-79

53. Ohtomo K, Itai Y, Matuoka Y, *et al.* Hepatocellular carcinoma: MR appearence mimicking cavernous hemangioma. *J Comput Assist Tomogr* 1990; **14**: 650-652

54. Choi BI, Lee GK, Kim St, *et al.* Mosaic pattern of encapsulated hepatocellular carcinoma: correlation of magnetic resonance imaging and pathology. *Gastrointest Radiol* 1990; **15**: 238-240

55. Itai Y, Ohtomo K, Furui S, *et al.* MR imaging of hepatocellular carcinoma. *J Comput Assist Tomogr* 1986; **10**:963-968.

56. Terada T, Kadoya M, Nakanuma Y, et al. Iron-accumulating adenomatous hyperplastic nodule with malignant foci in the cirrhotic liver. *Cancer* 1990; **65**:1994-2000

57. Rummeny E, Weissleder R, Sironi S, *et al.* Central scars in primary liver tumors: MR featutes, specificity, and pathologic correlation. *Radiology* 1989; **171**:323-326

58. Outwater E, Tomaszewski JE, Daly JM, *et al.* Hepatic colorectal metastases: correlation of MR imaging and pathologic appearance. *Radiology* 1991; **180**: 327-332

59. Itai Y, Ohtomo K, Kokubo T, *et al.* Segmental intensity differences in the liver on MR images: a sign of intrahepatic portal flow stoppage. *Radiology* 1988; **167**:17-19

60. Kim T, Murakami T, Oi H, *et al.* Detection of hypervascular hepatocellular carcinoma by dynamic spiral CT. *J Comput Assist Tomogr* 1995; **19**(6) :948-954

61. Ito K, Choji T, Nakada T, Nakanishi T, Kurokawa F, Okita K. Multislice dynamic MRI of hepatic tumors. *J Comput Assist Tomogr* 1993; **17**(3): 390-396

62. Imaeda T, Mochizuki R, Kanematsu M, *et al.* Hemodynamics of small hepatocellular carcinoma (5 cm or less in diameter): cases with discrepant findings between dynamic MR images and hepatic arteriograms. *Abdom Imag* 1995; **20**:534-540

63. Semelka RC, Shoenut JP, Kroeker MA, *et al.* Focal liver disease: comparison of dynamic contrast-enhanced CT and T2-weighted fat-suppressed, FLASH, and dynamic gadolinium-enhanced MR imaging at 1.5T. *Radiology* 1992; **184**: 687-694

64. Itai Y, Ohnishi S, Ohtomo K, *et al.* Regenerating nodules of liver cirrhosis: MR imaging. *Radiology* 1987; **165**:419-423

65. Ohtomo K, Itai Y, Ohtomo Y, *et al.* Regenerating nodules of liver cirrhosis: MR imaging with pathologic correlation. *AJR* 1990; **154**:505-507

66. Ferrucci JL. Liver tumor imaging: current concepts. *AJR* 1990;**155**: 473-484

67. Murakami T, Kuroda C, Marukawa T, *et al.* Regenerating nodules in hepatic cirrhosis: MR findings with pathologic correlation. *AJR* 1990; **155**: 1227-1232

68. Matsui O, Kadoya M, Takashima T, *et al.* Adenomatous hyperplastic nodules in cirrhotic livers: differentiation from hepatocellular carcinoma with MR imaging. *Radiology* 1989; **173**:123-126

69. Winter III TC, Takayasu K, Muramatsu Y, *et al.* Early advanced hepatocellular carcinoma: evaluation of CT and MR appearance with pathologic correlation. *Radiology* 1994; **192**: 379-387

70. Matsui O, Kadoya M, Takashima T, *et al.* Benign and malignant nodules in cirrhotic livers: distinction based on blood supply. *Radiology* 1991; **178**: 493-497

71. Gabata T, Matsui O, Kadoya M, *et al.* MR imaging of hepatic adenoma. *AJR* 1990; **155**: 1009-1011

72. Dooms G, Kerlan R, Hricak H, *et al.* Cholangiocarcinoma: Imaging by MR. *Radiology* 1986; **159**: 89-84

73. Fan Z, Yamashita Y, Harada M, *et al.* Intrahepatic cholangiocarcinoma: Spin-echo and contrast-enhanced dynamic MR imaging. *AJR* 1993; **161**:313-317

74. Kanematsu T, Matsumata T, Shirabe K, *et al.* A comparative study of hepatic resection and transcatheter arterial embolization for the treatment of primary hepatocellular carcinoma. *Cancer* 1993; **71**:2181-2186

75. Farmer D, Rosove M, Shaked A, Busuttil R. Current treatment modalities for hepatocellular carcinoma. *Ann Surg* 1994; **219**: 236-247.

76. Livraghi T, Bolondi L, Lazzaroni S, *et al.* Percutaneous ethanol injection in the treatment of hepatocellular carcinoma in cirrhosis: a study on 207 patients. *Cancer* 1992; **69**: 925-929.

77. Livraghi T, Vettori C. Percutaneous ethanol injection therapy of hepatoma. *Cardiovasc Intervent Radiol* 1990; **13**: 146-152.

78. Shiina S, Tagawa K, Unuma T, *et al.* Percutaneous ethanol injection therapy for the treatment of hepatocellular carcinoma: analysis of 77 patients. *AJR* 1990; **155**: 1221-1226.

79. Shiina S, Tagawa K, Unuma T, *et al.* Percutaneous ethanol injection therapy for hepatocellular carcinoma: a histopathologic study. *Cancer* 1991; **681**: 524-1530.

80. Takayasu K, Shina Y, Maramatsu T, *et al.* Hepatocellular carcinoma: treatment with intra-arterial iodized-oil with and without chemo therapeutic agents. *Radiology* 1987; **162**: 345-351.

81. Yamada R, Sato M, Kawabata M, *et al.* Hepatic artery embolization in 120 patients with unresectable hepatoma. *Radiology* 1984; **148**:397-401.

82. Nakao N, Kamino K, Miura K, Takayasu Y, Ohnishi M, Miura T. Transcatheter arterial embolization in hepatocellular carcinoma: a long-term follow-up. *Radiat Med* 1992; **10**:13-18.

83. Uchida H, Ohishi H, Matsuo N, *et al.* Transcatheter hepatic segmental arterial embolization using Lipiodol mixed with an anticancer drug and Gelfoam particles for hepatocellular carcinoma. *Cardiovasc Intervent Radiol* 1990; **13**:140-145.

84. Matsui O, Kadoya M, Yoshikawa J, *et al.* Small hepatocellular carcinoma: treatment with subsegmental transcatheter arterial embolization. *Radiology* 1993; **188:** 79-83.

85. Choi B, Kim H, Han J, *et al.* Therapeutic effect of transcatheter oily chemoembolization therapy for encapsulated nodular hepatocellular carcinoma: CT and pathologic findings. *Radiology* 1992; **182**:709-713.

86. Sakurai M, Okamura J, Kuroda J, *et al.* Transcatheter chemoembolization effective for treating hepatocellular carcinoma: a histopathologic study. *Cancer* 1984; **54**:387-392.

87. Tanaka K, Nakamura S, Numata K, *et al.* Hepatocellular carcinoma: Treatment with percutaneous ethanol injection and transcatheter arterial embolization. *Radiology*1992; **185**:457-460.

88. Tanaka K, Okazaki H, Nakamura S, *et al.* Hepatocellular carcinoma: Treatments with a combination therapy of transcatheter arterial embolization and percutaneous ethanol injection. *Radiology* 1991; **179**:713-717.

89. Lencioni R, Bartolozzi C, Caramella D. Treatment of small hepatocellular carcinoma with percutaneous ethanol injection: analysis of prognostic factors in 105 Western patients. *Cancer* 1995; **76**: 1737-1746.

90. Yoshioka H, Nakagawa K, Shindou H, *et al.* MR imaging of the liver before and after transcatheter hepatic chemoembolization for hepatocellular carcinoma. *Acta Radiologica* 1990; **31**:63-67

91. Sironi S, Livraghi T, Angeli E, *et al.* Small hepatocellular carcinoma: MR follow-up of treatment with PEI. *Radiology* 1993; **187**:119-123

92. Sironi S, De Cobelli F, Livraghi T, *et al.* Small hepatocellular carcinoma treated with percutaneous ethanol injection: unenhanced and Gadolinium-enhanced MR imaging findings. *Radiology* 1994; **192**:407-412

93. Bartolozzi C, Lencioni R, Caramella D, Falaschi F, Cioni R, Di Conscio G. Hepatocellular carcinoma: CT and MR features after transcatheter arterial embolization and percutaneous ethanol injection. *Radiology* 1994; **191**:123-128

94. Yoshikawa K, Yashiro N, Kokubo T, *et al.* MR imaging of hepatoma treated by embolization. *J. Comput Assist Tomogr* 1986; **10**:973

95. Marakami T, Nakamura H, Tsuda K, *et al.* Treatment of hepatocellular carcinoma by Chemoembolization: Evaluation with 3DFT MR imaging. *AJR* 1993; **160**:295-299

96. Bartolozzi C, Lencioni R, Caramella D, Mazzeo S, Ciancia EM. Treatment of hepatocellular carcinoma with percutaneous ethanol injection: evaluation with contrast-enhanced MR imaging. *AJR* 1994;**162**:827-831

97. Marukawa T, Harada K, Kuruda C *et al.* MRI of the resected hepatocellular carcinoma specimens following trans-catheter arterial embolization. Comparison with pathologic findings. The 5th Asian Oceanian Congress of Radiology (ab) 1987, 147

98. Yamashita Y, Yoshimatsu S, Sumi M, Harada M, Takahashi M. Dynamic MR imaging of hepatoma treated by transcatheter arterial embolization therapy. *Acta Radiol* 1993; **34**:303-308

99. Castrucci M, De Cobelli F, Sironi S, Salvioni M, Del Maschio A. MR Imaging in the follow-up of hepatocellular carcinoma (HCC) treated with transarterial chemoembolization (TACE). *Abdom Imaging* 1996; in press

100. Marakami T, Nakamura H, Hori S, *et al.* Detection of viable tumor cells in hepatocellular carcinoma following transcatheter arterial chemoembolization with iodized oil. *Acta Radiol* 1993; **34**:399-403

15

Scintigraphy

M Kudo

The use of scintigraphy has decreased for the purpose of diagnosing hepatocellular carcinoma (HCC) since its resolution capacity is inferior to those of other imaging modalities, such as ultrasound (US), computed tomography (CT), or magnetic resonance imaging (MRI). However, scintigraphy has the unique characteristic of being a functional diagnostic tool rather than a morphologic diagnostic tool. Therefore, the clarification of the features of each scintigraphic procedure and its proper application to the differential diagnosis of hepatic tumors make possible the differentiation of the tumor based on the functional approach. In this chapter, the concept of the newly developed functional approach of hepatic scintigraphy, the present status of scintigraphic diagnosis, and future prospects in the diagnosis of HCC are described.

TECHNIQUE

Liver Imaging (Table 15.1)

Colloid liver scan

With recent advances in several imaging modalities, the role of colloid liver scan in the detection of HCC has drastically changed. The size of the HCC nodule that can be detected by planar colloid scan is 2-3 cm when it is located at the liver surface and 3-4 cm when in a deep location. This relatively poor resolution capability is the main reason that colloid liver scan is no longer routinely used for the detection of HCC. However, with the introduction of single-photon emission computed tomography (SPECT), the resolution capability has been markedly improved (Fig. 15.1). HCC nodules as small as 1.5 cm in

Table 15.1— Scintigraphy of liver tumors

Technique	Radioisotope	Accumulation site (mechanism)
Liver imaging		
Colloid liver scan	Tc-99m-phylate	Kupffer cell (RES*)
	Tc-99m-Sn colloid	Kupffer cell (RES*)
Hepatobiliary scan	Tc-99m-PMT	Hepatocyte, biliary duct
	Tc-99m-HIDA	Hepatodyte, biliary duct
Hepatocyte receptor scan	Tc-99m-NGA	Hepatocyte ASGP** receptor
	Tc-99m-GSA	Hepatocyte ASGP** receptor
Tumor imaging		
RBC scan	Tc-99m-RBC	
	Tc-99m-HSA	
blood-flow scan (dynamic scan)		Blood flow
blood-pool scan (delayed scan)		Blood volume (pooling)
Hepatic tumor-specific scan		
Gallium scan	^{67}Ga-citrate	HCC,metastasis, inflammation
Delayed hepatobiliary scan	Tc-99m-PMT	HCC
Bone-seeking scan	Tc-99m-MDP	Calcified metastatic cancer
PET scan	^{18}FDG	HCC, metastasis

*= Reticuloendothelium system **=Asialoglycoprotein receptor

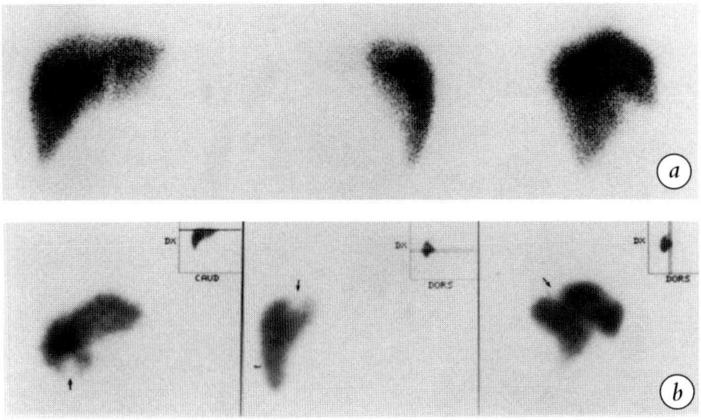

Figure 15.1 – Hepatocellular carcinoma.

a) Planar image of colloid liver scan. No focal defect is demonstrated.

b) In the same patient, single-photon emission CT (SPECT) colloid liver scan reveals an apparent focal defect at the anterosuperior segment of the right lobe, compatible with the findings in hepatocellular carcinoma.

diameter can be detected by colloid SPECT scan.[1] Even though its sensitivity in detecting small lesions less than 2 cm in diameter is inferior to that of US, CT, or MRI, the colloid SPECT scan may complement US for small nodules located in the subdiaphragmatic regions, where the US beam does not penetrate. The reported detection rate of small HCC less than 5 cm in diameter using the combination of colloid SPECT and US is as high as 94% (47/50), higher than that using US alone (80%).[1]

Hepatobiliary scan

It is well known that hepatobiliary agents including Tc-99m-Sn-pyridoxil-5-methyltryptophan (PMT) are sometimes taken up by HCC (Fig. 15.2) and its distant metastases as visualized with the delayed scan obtained at intervals ranging from 1 to 8 hours after injection.[2-8] The mechanism postulated to account for these findings is that HCC that concentrate hepatobiliary agents are well-differentiated, so it is possible that they produce bile, but they cannot excrete it because they lack functioning biliary ducts.[7] The positive rate of this technique in HCC is approximately 60%.[7] These HCC lesions are, therefore, initially less intensely radioactive relative to the normal parenchyma, but gradually become relatively more intensely radioactive as the normal liver excretes the agent.

The nodules which present hot spots on the delayed hepatobiliary scan include focal nodular hyperplasia (FNH) or hepatocellular adenoma (HA) in addition to HCC. However, both FNH and HA occur in the non-cirrhotic liver as contrasted with HCC, which is usually associated with liver cirrhosis. Therefore, the specificity of delayed hepatobiliary scan for the diagnosis of HCC is nearly 100% when considered together with the clinical information as to whether or not associated liver cirrhosis is present.

The distant metastases of HCC, such as lung or bone metastases, present intense accumulation of this imaging agent. Therefore, this technique is clinically useful in the determination of whether or not an extrahepatic tumor is a metastasis of HCC.

Hepatocyte receptor scan

Asialoglycoprotein (ASGP) receptor is a hepatocyte surface receptor, specific to serum ASGP.[9] An analog ligand of ASGP can be obtained by attaching the galactosyl unit to human serum albumin. The resulting compound is galactosyl neoglycoalbumin (NGA), which when radiolabeled becomes a member of a new class of diagnostic agents called receptor-binding radiopharmaceuticals.

Tc-99m-labeled NGA was first developed in the United States, and it subsequently became available in Europe as well. In Japan, Tc-99m labeled GSA has been commercially available for routine clinical use since 1992. Hepatic receptor scintigraphy is, therefore, performed with intravenous injection of Tc-99m GSA or Tc-99m NGA.[10,11]

The ASGP receptor is present in the normally functioning hepatocyte,[9] whereas it does not exist in cancer cells.[12] Therefore, focal defect is demonstrated by ASGP receptor scintigraphy in HCC.[13] On the other hand, macroregenerating nodule and adenomatous hyperplastic (AH) nodule contain intranodular

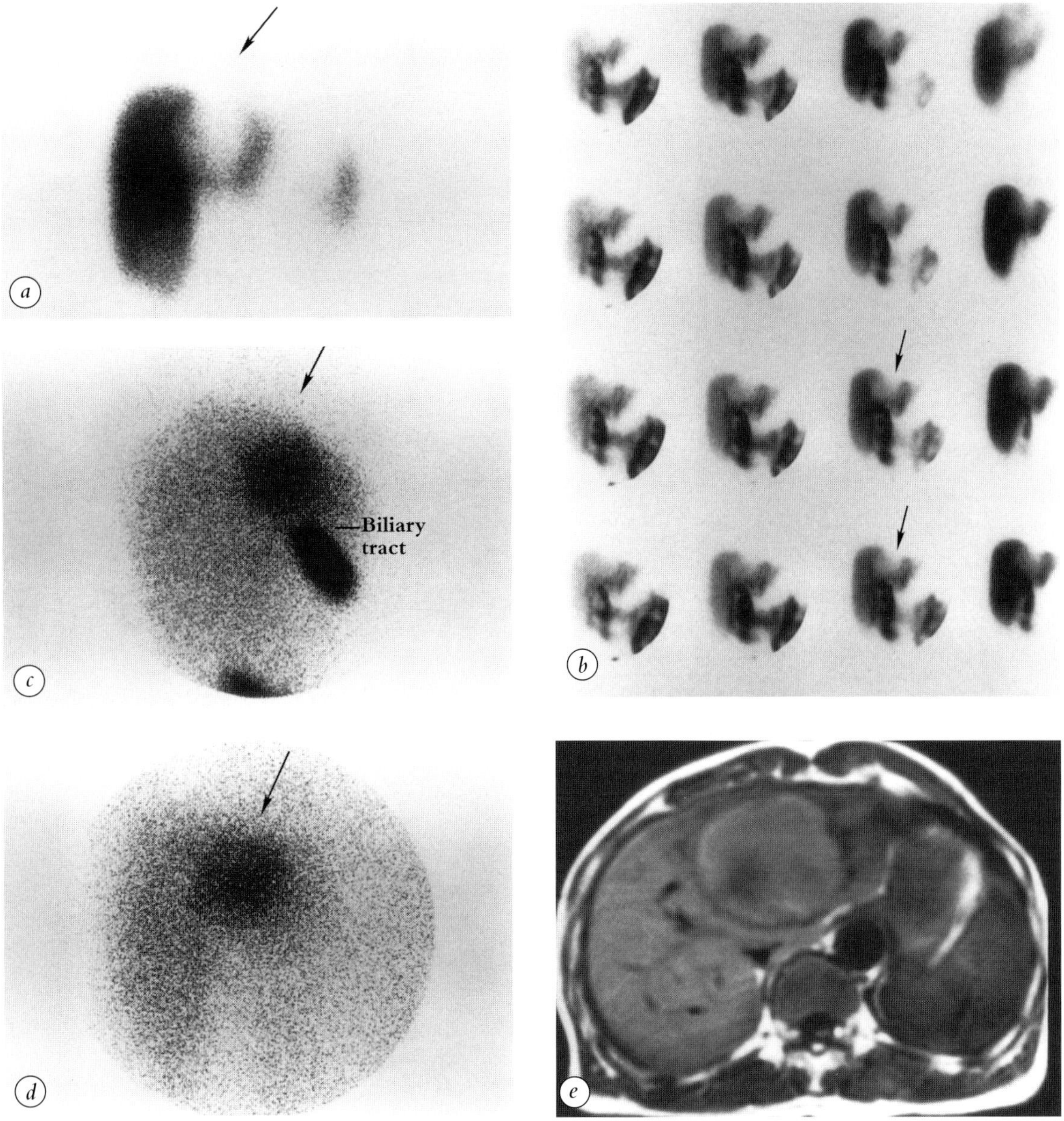

Figure 15.2 – Hepatocellular carcinoma on hepatobiliary and Ga scan.

a) A focal defect is seen on colloid liver scan at the left lobe of the liver.

b) Hepatobiliary scan (Tc-99m-Sn-pyridoxil-5-methyltryptophan) dynamic image shows a focal defect at the left lobe of the liver.

c) On the hepatobiliary scan at the delayed phase (6 hours post injection), however, intense accumulation can be seen at the left lobe, indicative of the diagnosis of hepatocellular carcinoma (HCC).

d) Intense accumulation is also observed by the Ga-67 citrate scanning.

e) MRI also shows appearance compatible with HCC.

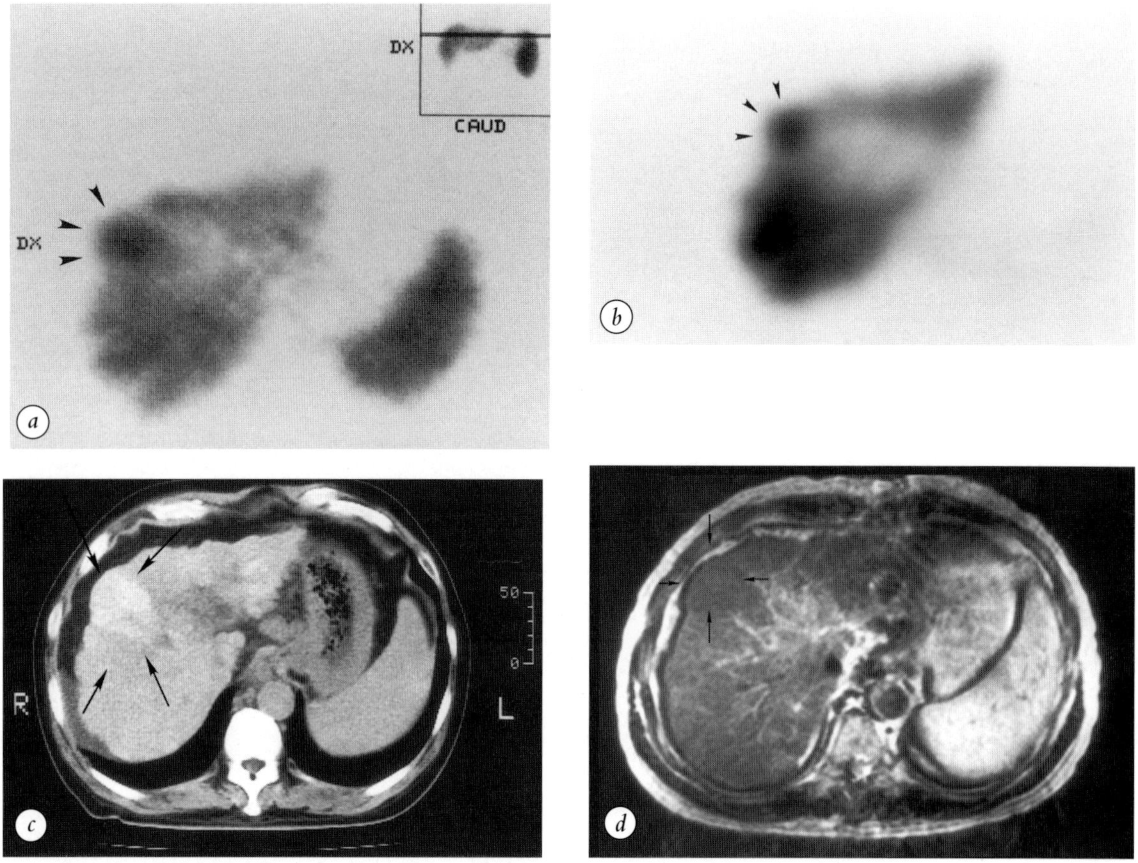

Figure 15.3 – Adenomatous hyperplasia on receptor SPECT.

a) On the colloid liver SPECT scan, intense accumulation is demonstrated at segment 8 in a patient with liver cirrhosis (arrows).

b) Marked accumulation is also demonstrated using the receptor SPECT scan at the same region, suggesting the diagnosis of adenomatous hyperplasia (arrows).

c) Plain CT scan discloses a high-density nodule at the same region (arrows).

d) T2-weighted MR image depicts a hypo-intense nodule at segment 8, compatible with the diagnosis of adenomatous hyperplasia (arrows).

normally functioning hepatocytes. Thus, Tc-NGA or Tc-GSA uptake within the hepatic nodule is a specific finding of a benign nodule, especially AH (Fig. 15.3), which is a preneoplastic nodule. This technique therefore plays a very important role in the differential diagnosis between HCC and premalignant lesions in the cirrhotic liver.

Tumor imaging

Delayed red blood cell scan

Previous studies have demonstrated that Tc-99m-labeled red blood cell (RBC) scanning is an accurate method for differentiating hepatic hemangioma from HCC and other hepatic malignancies, with the sensitivity of this technique being significantly improved with the addition of SPECT.[14-18] SPECT imaging allows improved contrast enhancement, as well as improved size/shape definition afforded by tomographic deletion of superimposed structures, permitting the lesion activity on delayed images to be separated from that of overlying liver tissues.[14,15]

Due to this added capability labeled RBC SPECT imaging can be used routinely to detect hemangiomas greater than 2.0 cm in size, and to identify hemangiomas as small as 1.0 cm when located at the hepatic periphery. It is important that SPECT interpretation involves direct association with the corresponding tomographic image (CT or US), especially when evaluating centrally located hemangiomas that may be situated near major intrahepatic vessels. The specificity and positive predictive value of labeled RBC SPECT scanning approaches 100%.[16]

Gallium-67 scan

Approximately 90% of HCC tumors show uptake of gallium-67 equal to or higher than that of surrounding liver tissues (Fig. 15.2) according to the literature.[19] However, small HCC tumors less than 2 cm in diameter, which are easily detectable by modern imaging modalities such as US, CT or MRI, rarely show a positive result on gallium-67 scan. In addition, gallium-67 accumulates not only in malignant tumors but also in other pathological conditions, such as regenerative nodules, FNH, adenomas, metastases, lymphomas, and abscesses,[20] possibly due to binding of a Ga-67-transferrin complex to transferrin receptors. Therefore, the Ga-67 scan is rarely used to diagnose HCC in the clinical setting. The Ga-67 scan might be useful in the evaluation of the therapeutic response of HCC.

Positron emission tomography

Positron emission tomography (PET) using fluorine-18-fluorodeoxyglucose (FDG) is useful in monitoring the treatment response after interventional therapy for HCC (Fig. 15.4).[21-23] Torizuka *et al.*[23] found that FDG-PET was useful in the characterization of the tumor, assessment of the therapeutic effect, confirmation of *in vitro* enzymatic activity of glucose metabolism, and histological grading of HCC. Although PET is not a routinely available technique at present, it is a promising method for assessing the treatment effect and quite accurately monitoring the recurrence after a therapeutic procedure for HCC.

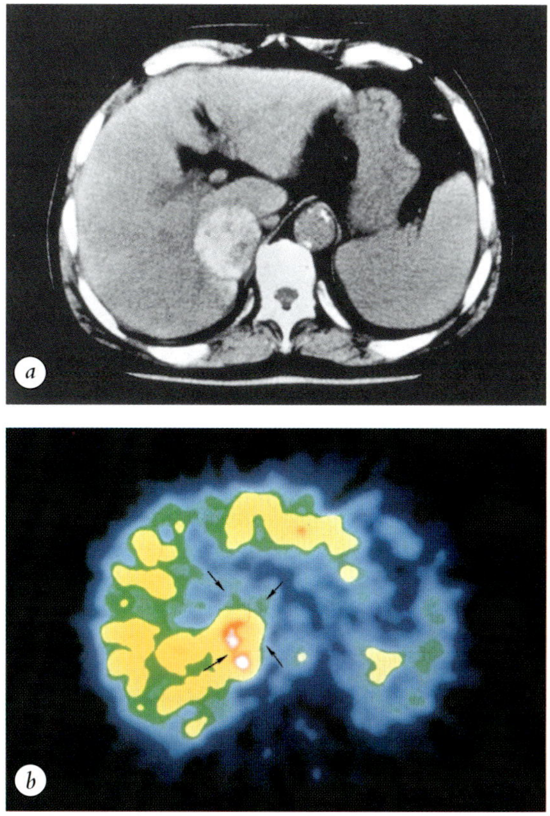

Figure 15.4 – Hepatocellular carcinoma on FDG-PET.

a) HCC after transcatheter arterial embolization with Lipiodol and anticancer drugs. The high-density tumor as depicted by Lipiodol retention is evident at segment 1. Good therapeutic response can be expected based on this finding.

b) However, intense accumulation is demonstrated by the FDG-PET study (arrows), suggesting that this HCC nodule is still viable. Tumor viability was subsequently confirmed with further evaluation. FDG-PET is useful in the evaluation of therapeutic response after interventional therapy for HCC. [Courtesy of Drs. T Torizuka and N Tamaki, Kyoto University, Japan].

DIFFERENTIAL DIAGNOSIS, FOCAL NODULAR HYPERPLASIA

Focal nodular hyperplasia (FNH) is a non-tumorous hyperplastic nodule, occurring in the non-cirrhotic liver, which is typically seen in women aged 20-50. Since FNH is a hypervascular nodule, it is sometimes very difficult to differentiate it from HCC even by dynamic CT or angiography. Colloid liver scan is believed to be useful in the diagnosis of FNH.[24-26] Of FNH lesions, one third each present preferential accumulation of colloidal isotope, iso-uptake (Fig. 15.5), and focal defect on colloid liver scan. For the accurate detection of colloid uptake within the nodule, it is very important to interpret the colloid SPECT image by reference to the associated tomographic images, such as those acquired by US, CT or MRI. When colloidal uptake is present within a tumor found in non-cirrhotic liver, the possibility of FNH is quite high.

FNH also shows intense accumulation on hepatobiliary scan (Fig.15.5), which is useful in the

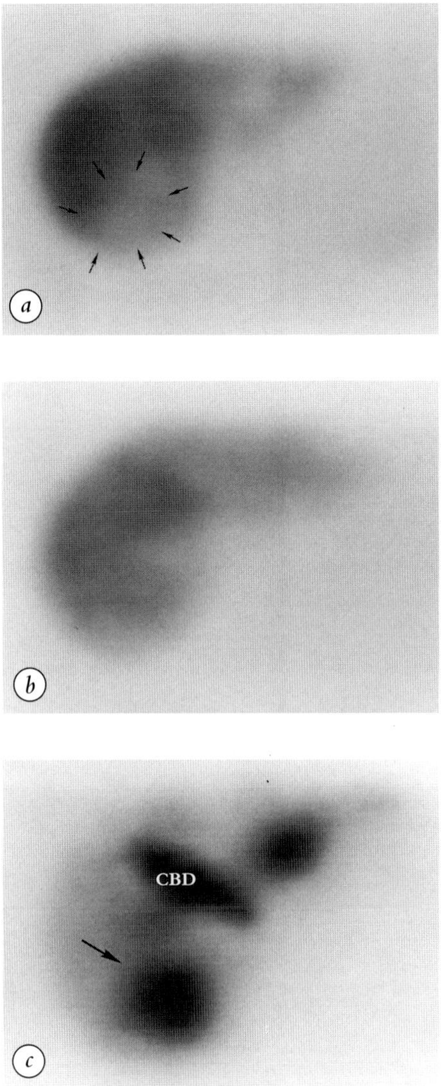

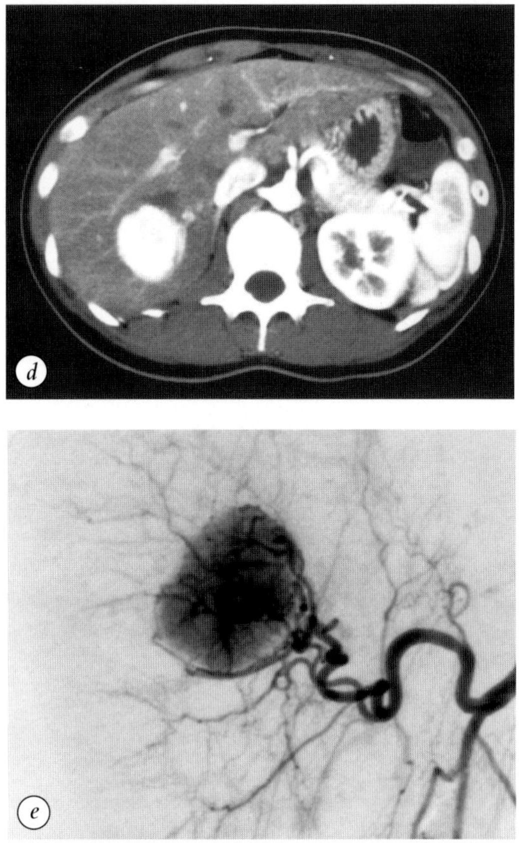

Figure 15.5 – Focal nodular hyperplasia (FNH) on hepatobiliary SPECT.

a) A focal defect is demonstrated by the colloid liver scan (arrows).

b) Iso-uptake can be seen using receptor SPECT scanning.

c) Marked accumulation of the hepatobiliary agent can be seen on the delayed SPECT scan (arrow).

d) Hypervascularity is evident upon the dynamic CT study.

e) Angiography reveals spoke-wheel sign, the most specific finding for FNH.

diagnosis and differentiation. However, it cannot be differentiated from hepatic adenoma, which also presents intense accumulation on hepatobiliary scan.

Hepatocellular adenoma

Hepatocellular adenoma (HA) is a benign hepatic neoplasm originated from hepatocytes, with a predilection to occur in women aged 30-40 years old. It is sometimes very difficult to differentiate it from HCC since its angiographic finding of hypervascularity is similar to that of HCC. Previous reports as to the characteristic findings in HA on colloid liver scan indicated decreased uptake or focal defect because of the absence of Kupffer cells within the nodule.[26,27] However, more recent reports revealed that HA frequently contains Kupffer cells within the tumor, and therefore, intense accumulation can be demonstrated in some cases.[28-30] Accordingly, HA should be included in the differential diagnosis when intense accumulation is observed within a nodule in a non-cirrhotic liver.

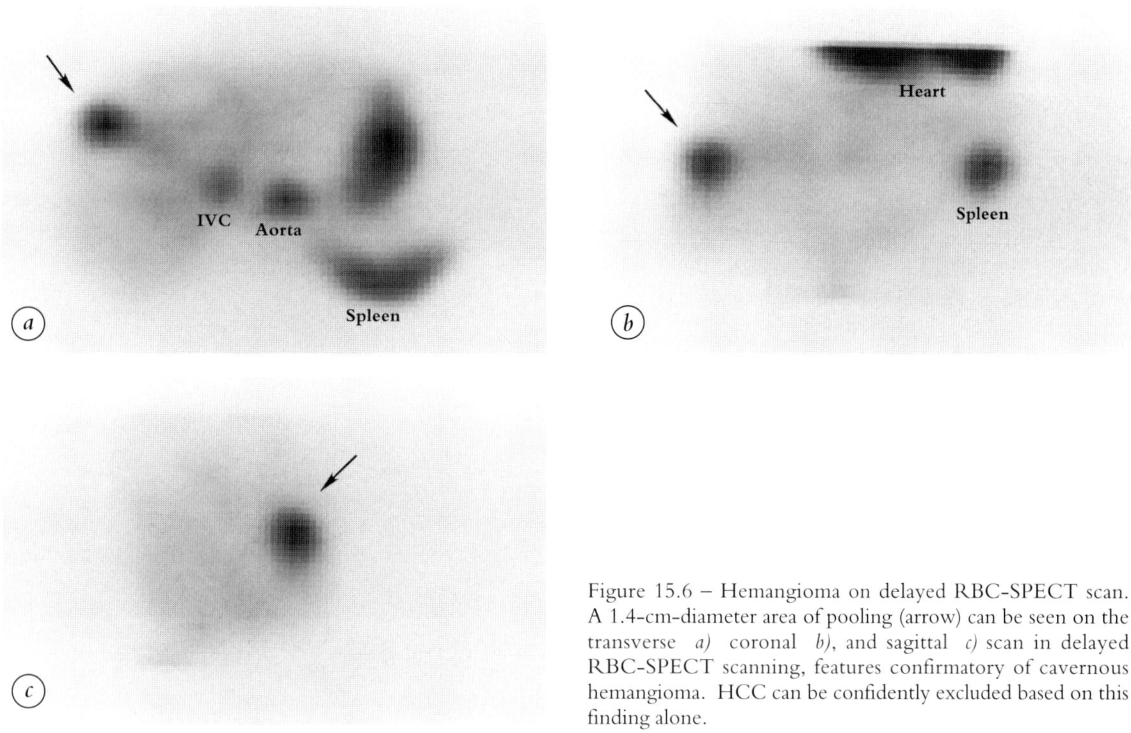

Figure 15.6 – Hemangioma on delayed RBC-SPECT scan. A 1.4-cm-diameter area of pooling (arrow) can be seen on the transverse *a)* coronal *b)*, and sagittal *c)* scan in delayed RBC-SPECT scanning, features confirmatory of cavernous hemangioma. HCC can be confidently excluded based on this finding alone.

Marked retention of a hepatobiliary agent is also a characteristic finding for HA.

Adenomatous hyperplasia

Adenomatous hyperplasia (AH) is a precancerous hyperplastic lesion, associated with liver cirrhosis.[31] Histologically, it is very difficult to differentiate it from well-differentiated HCC since similar pathologic findings such as hypercellularity or increased nuclear cytoplasm ratio are observed in both AH and well-differentiated HCC.[32] In order to differentiate the two, one must confirm normal functioning of the hepatocytes with normal receptor function within the tumor. AH can be demonstrated by intense accumulation in receptor scintigraphy.

Intense accumulation is also demonstrated by colloid liver scan since AH contains Kupffer cells as well.

Hemangioma

Well-differentiated HCC with fatty change often shows an hyperechoic pattern on ultrasonography, similar to that of hemangioma. Differentiation by ultrasonography alone is practically impossible, especially when associated liver cirrhosis is present. In such cases, delayed RBC-SPECT imaging provides very important information in the confirmation of hemangioma. If a positive result is obtained, well-differentiated HCC can be definitely ruled out using this technique alone (Fig. 15.6).

While the overall accuracy of MRI is slightly greater than that of delayed RBC-SPECT scan for the diagnosis of hemangiomas,[18,33] the differences appear most pronounced in certain specific lesions based on size and location. Labeled RBC-SPECT scan has limited sensitivity in routinely detecting hemangiomas less than 2.0 cm, as well as those 2.5 cm or less adjacent to major intrahepatic vessels or the heart. MRI satisfactorily characterizes small hemangiomas 1.0 to 2.0 cm in size. The limitations of MRI include the considerable cost and the incapacity to differentiate hemangiomas from hypervascular metastases. Therefore, RBC-SPECT scan seems to be the method of choice for diagnosing a hemangioma larger than 2.0 cm, and MRI may serve as a complementary tool to SPECT for the diagnosis of a small hemangioma less than 2.0 cm or a lesion located adjacent to the heart and/or major intrahepatic vessels.[32]

CONCLUSION

Scintigraphy, which was previously performed for screening HCC, is no longer performed routinely in the clinical setting because of the rapid progress in US, CT, and MRI technology. However, since scintigraphy provides unique information as to the function of the tumor, it sometimes plays an important role in the confirmatory and/or differential diagnosis of hepatic tumors by demonstrating the functional characteristics of the distinctive components constituting the specific type of tumor, such as HCC, FNH, adenoma, hemangioma, or adenomatous hyperplasia.

It is very important to keep in mind that functional diagnosis using scintigraphy is sometimes more useful than morphological diagnostic procedures, such as US, CT, and MRI. However, in order to perform scintigraphic studies most effectively in the diagnosis of hepatic tumors, one should be aware of the characteristic function or features of each tumor. An understanding of the type of radioisotope needed to demonstrate such characteristics is also crucial. Finally, SPECT imaging is mandatory in order to corroborate the other tomographic images.

In conclusion, it is emphasized that the role of scintigraphy has been drastically changed during the last decade, from that of a screening test to a diagnostic one, or from a morphological diagnostic tool to a functional and confirmatory tool in the diagnosis of hepatic tumors.

REFERENCES

1. Kudo M, Hirasa M, Takakuwa H, *et al.* Small hepatocellular carcinomas in chronic liver disease: detection with SPECT. *Radiology* 1986; **159**: 697-703
2. Utz JA, Lull RJ, Anderson JH, *et al.* Hepatoma visualization with 99mTc-pyridoxylidene glutamate. *J Nucl Med* 1980; **21**: 747-749
3. Lee VW, O'Brien MJ, Devereux DF, *et al.* Hepatocellular carcinoma: uptake of 99mTc-IDA in primary tumor and metastasis. *AJR* 1984; **143**: 57-61
4. Vincent LM, Renner JB: Uptake of hepatobiliary agents by hepatocellular carcinoma. *AJR* 1984; **143**: 1119-1120
5. Hasegawa Y, Nakano S, Ibuka K, *et al.* The importance of delayed imaging in the study of hepatoma with a new hepatobiliary agent. *J Nucl Med* 1984; **25**: 1122-1126
6. Hasegawa Y, Nakano S, Ibuka K, *et al.* Concentration of Tc-99m-Sn-pyridoxil-5-methyltryptophan, a biliary agent, in distant metastases of hepatomas. *Eur J Nucl Med* 1985; **10**: 255-258
7. Calvet X, Pons F, Bruix J, *et al.* Technetium-99m DISIDA hepatobiliary agent in diagnosis of hepatocellular carcinoma: relationship between detectability and tumor differentiation. *J Nucl Med* 1988; **29**: 1916-1920
8. Hasegawa, Nakano S, Ibuka K, *et al.* Specific diagnosis of hepatocellular carcinoma by delayed hepatobiliary imaging. *Cancer* 1986; **57**: 230-236
9. Ashwell G, Steer CJ. Hepatic recognition and catabolism of serum glycoproteins. *JAMA* 1981; **246**: 2358-2364
10. Kudo M, Washino K, Yamamichi Y, Ikekubo K. Synthesis and radiolabeling of galactosyl human serum albumin. *Method Enzymol* 1994; **247**: 383-394
11. Kudo M, Vera DR, Stadalnik RC Hepatic receptor imaging using radiolabeled asialoglycoprotein analogs. In: *Neoglycoconjugates: Preparation and Applications,* Edited by Yuan C Lee, Academic Press, New York, 1994, pp373-402
12. Stockert RJ, Becker FF. Diminished hepatic binding protein for desialylated glycoproteins during chemical hepatocarcinogenesis. *Cancer Res* 1980; **40**: 3632-3634
13. Kurtaran A, Li SR, Raderer M, *et al.* Technetium-99m-galactosyl-neoglycoalbumin combined with iodine-123-tyr-(A14)-insulin visualizes human hepatocellular carcinomas. *J Nucl Med* 1995; **36**: 1875-1881
14. Brodsky RI, Friedman AC, Maurer AH, Radecki PP, Caroline DF. Hepatic cavernous hemangioma: diagnosis with 99mTc-labeled red cells and single-photon emission CT. *AJR* 1987; **148**: 125-129
15. Tumeh SS, Benson C, Nagel JS, English RJ, Holman BL. Cavernous hemangioma of the liver: detection with single-photon emission computed tomography. *Radiology* 1987; **164**: 353-356
16. Kudo M, Ikekubo K, Yamamoto K, *et al*: Distinction between hemangioma of the liver and hepatocellular carcinoma: value of labeled RBC SPECT scanning. *AJR* 1989; **152**: 977-983
17. Moinuddin M, Allison JR, Montgomery JH, Rockett JF, McMurray JM. Scintigraphic diagnosis of hepatic hemangioma: its role in the management of hepatic mass lesions. *AJR* 1985;**145**: 223-228
18. Birnbaum BA, Weinreb JC, Megibow AJ, *et al.* Definitive diagnosis of hepatic hemangiomas: MR imaging versus Tc-99m-labeled red blood cell SPECT. *Radiology* 1990; **176**: 95-101
19. Silberstein EB, McAfee JG. *Differential Diagnosis in Nuclear Medicine,* McGraw-Hill Book Company, New York, 1984.
20. Cornelius EA, Afferburg CE. Problems in the imaging diagnosis of hepatoma. *Clin Nucl Med* 1984; **9**: 30-38
21. Torizuka T, Tamaki N, Inokuma T, *et al.* Value of fluorine-18-FDG-PET to monitor hepatocellular carcinoma after interventional therapy. *J Nucl Med* 1994; **35**: 1965-1969
22. Okazumi S, Isono K, Enomoto K, *et al.* Evaluation of liver tumors using fluorine-18-fluorodeoxy-glucose PET. characterization of tumor and assessment of effect of treatment. *J Nucl Med* 1992; **33**: 333-339.
23. Torizuka T, Tamaki N, Inokuma T, *et al.* In vivo assessment of glucose metabolism in hepatocellular carcinoma with FDG-PET. *J Nucl Med* 1995; **36**: 1811-1817

24. Welch TJ, Sheedy PHII, Johnson CM, *et al*: Focal nodular hyperplasia and hepatic adenoma: Comparison of angiography, CT, US and scintigraphy. *Radiology* 1985; **156**: 593-595

25. Sandler MA, Petrocelli RP, Marks DS, Lopez R: Ultrasonic features and radionuclide correlation in liver cell adenoma and focal nodular hyperplasia, *Radiology* 1980; **135**: 393-397

26. Sorensen TI, Baden H: Benign hepatocellular tumors. *Scand J Gastroenterol* 1975; **10**: 113-119

27. Casarella WJ, Knowles DM, Wolf M, *et al:* Focal nodular hyperplasia and liver cell adenoma: radiologic and pathologic differentiation. *AJR* 1978; **131**: 393-402

28. Lubbers PR, Ros PR, Goodman ZD, Ishak KG: Accumulation of Technetium-99m sulfur colloid by hepatocellular adenoma: scintigraphic pathologic correlation. *AJR* 1987; **148**: 1105-1108

29. Goodman ZD, Ulrika VW, Lubbers PR, *et al*: Kupffer cells in hepatocellular adenomas. *Am J Surg Pathol* 1987; **11**: 191-196

30. Sackett JF, Mosental WT, House RK, *et al*: Scintillation scanning of liver cell adenoma. *AJR* 1971; **113**: 56-60

31. Edmondson HA: Benign epithelial tumors and tumors-like lesions of the liver. In: *Hepatocellular carcinoma*, Edited by Okuda K and Peters RL, John Wiley and Sons, New York, 1976, p309-p330

32. Sakamoto M, Hirohashi S, Shimosato Y. Early stages of multistep hepatocarcinogenesis: adenomatous hyperplasia and early hepatocellular carcinoma. *Hum Pathol* 1991; **22**: 172-178

33. Birnbaum BA, Weinreb JC. Hepatic hemangioma: a comparison of 99mTc-labeled red blood cell SPECT and MRI for definitive diagnosis. In: *Liver Imaging*, Edited by Ferrucci JT and Stark DD, Andover Medical Publishers, Boston, 1990, p201-p208

16

Comparison of different imaging techniques

BI Choi

A variety of imaging modalities, including US, CT, MR, nuclear medicine, and angiography are currently used in evaluating patients with known or suspected HCC. Further technological advancement will undoubtedly have a major impact on liver tumor imaging. Increased speed of data acquisition and consequently shorter scan times in CT (spiral imaging) and MR (echo planar) should show further improvement in spatial resolution by further limiting motion artifacts. Development of new contrast materials for liver tumor imaging in US and MR may improve tumor detection by increasing the contrast between the tumor and the surrounding liver parenchyma.[1] Evaluation of the liver may be performed by multiple modalities. It is important to obtain the diagnostic study appropriate for the patient's clinical situation. Also, it is important that the most efficacious techniques are used to perform any imaging study in order that the greatest information is obtained by that particular diagnostic modality.

Many studies have addressed how best to define a suspected liver cancer by the various imaging methods. Review of previous reports reveals a wide variation in accuracy for US, CT and angiography in liver imaging, as a variety of techniques, scanners and protocols were used for each technique. The advantages and disadvantages of each modality are determined by a combination of factors including resolution, safety, reproducibility, cost and availability. The interrelationship between these imaging modalities must be understood in order to use each modality effectively and efficiently.

The purpose of this chapter is to present the detectability and important imaging characteristics of HCCs and precancerous lesions associated with liver cirrhosis with the variety of diagnostic imaging techniques currently available. The advantages, pitfalls, and the role of these imaging techniques will also be discussed.

DETECTION OF HCC

The pathogenesis of HCC occurs by at least two separate and distinct pathways. In the United States and other Western countries, HCC may arise *de novo* from a relatively normal liver without a background of macroregenerative nodules.[2-9] However, in the Far East, HCC almost always develops by means of a multistep process in patients with chronic liver disease.[4,6,8,10-12]

With advances in surgical techniques in patients with chronic liver disease, particularly cirrhosis, resected liver specimens sometimes show small nodular lesions without features of definite cancer in addition to the main HCC. These small nodular lesions were classified as adenomatous hyperplasia or other synonyms.[13-15]

Some of these lesions show severe atypia, and currently they are considered to be precancerous lesions and early stages of cancers.[16] The lesions vary histologically, from frankly benign, large regenerating nodules to equivocally malignant nodules to nodules containing obvious malignant foci. In hepatocarcinogenesis of the cirrhotic liver, a regenerating nodule might be the first step in the development of HCC, going through phases of adenomatous hyperplasia, early HCC, early advanced HCC, and finally advanced HCC in a multistep fashion.[8,12]

Advanced (overt) HCC

Early detection of HCC is important, since the most effective treatment for HCC is surgical resection or local ablation therapy when the tumor is small. Fortunately, recent advances in liver imaging techniques have facilitated the detection of small HCCs.[17-21] As the capability of detecting small HCCs has increased, the definition of small tumors has changed, from a solitary tumor less than 4.5 cm to a tumor less than 2 cm in diameter.[22-24] Until now, the definition of a small HCC was based not on pathophysiologic criteria, but on the ability to detect the tumor.

With the widespread use of imaging techniques, the number of asymptomatic cases diagnosed has increased considerably.[17-20,25-28] Another factor contributing to early detection and diagnosis is the HCC screening program, which includes monitoring of serum levels of α-fetoprotein and follow-up imaging, mainly US, in patients with chronic liver disease.[25-29]

The numerous imaging techniques available for detecting small HCCs and regional differences have resulted in various diagnostic standards and comparative studies.[17,20,30-35] The relative efficacies of various techniques for detecting HCCs less than

3 cm in diameter have been evaluated. Review of previous reports reveals a wide variation in accuracy for US, CT and angiography, as a variety of techniques, scanners, and protocols were used for each technique. The sensitivity for detecting HCCs less than 3 cm in diameter is 55-98% with US,[20,30,32,33,36,37] 46-84% with CT,[20,30,32,33,36-38] 61-81% with angiography,[20,30,37,38] 82% with CT arteriography,[33] 86-91% with CT arterial portography,[33,36] 71-96% with iodized oil CT,[30-33,36] 86% with sonographic angiography,[31] and 94-96% with intraoperative US (Fig. 16.1).[32,33,38] In most comparative analyses, the sensitivities of intraoperative US, CT arterial portography, and iodized oil CT (Fig. 16.2) are significantly higher than those of US, CT or angiography (Table 16.1).[30, 32,36]

Spiral (helical or volumetric) CT is the latest advance in rapid scanning techniques. Spiral CT is a new technology that couples continuous tube rotation

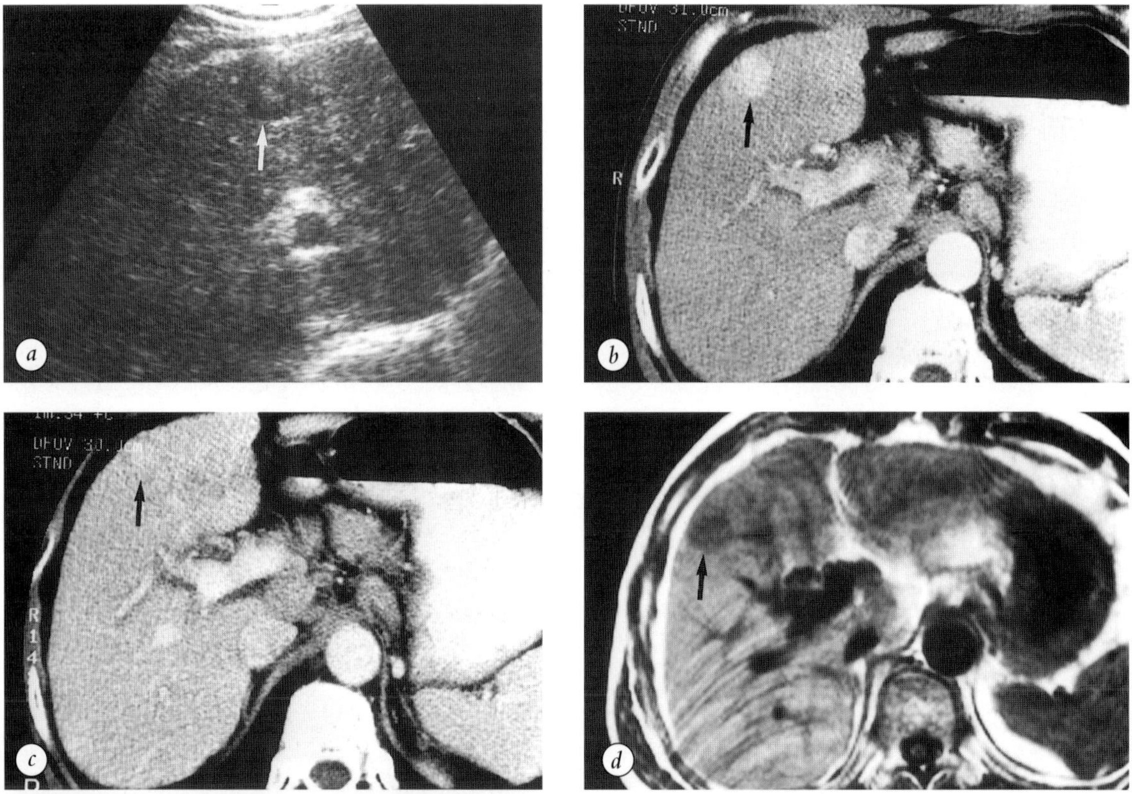

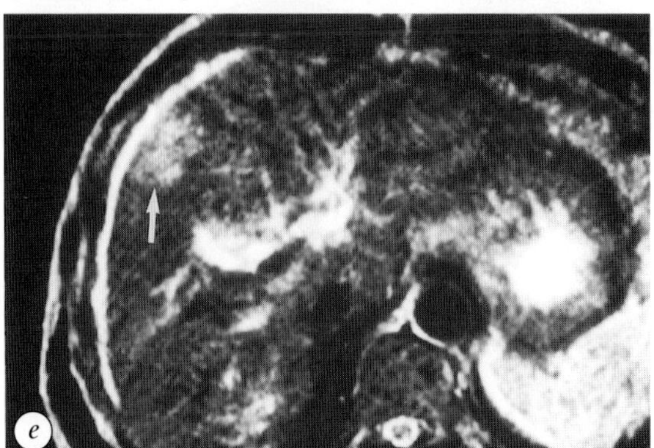

Figure 16.1 – A small advanced HCC identified with various imaging techniques in a 49-year-old man.

a) Sonogram of the liver shows round hypoechoic mass (arrow) in segment 8 of the liver.

b) CT scan in the arterial dominant phase of dynamic CT shows highly enhancing mass (arrow) in segment 8 of the liver.

c) CT scan in the portal dominant phase shows suspicious low-attenuating mass (arrow) in the same area.

d) T1-weighted MR image (600/17) demonstrates hypointense mass (arrow) in the same area.

e) T2-weighted MR image (2500/80) demonstrates hyperintense mass (arrow) in the same area.

Table 16.1 – Detection rates (%) of various imaging techniques for small advanced hepatocellular carcinomas less than 3 cm

Author	Year	SPECT	Sonography	CT	Angiography	CTA	CTAP	L-CT	IOUS	MR
Kudo *et al*[20]	1986	57	70	47	80					
Hayashi *et al*[38]	1987			67	61				94	
Matsui *et al*[36]	1988		55	46	63		86	71		
Choi *et al*[30]	1989		66	74	81			96		
Takayasu *et al*[33]	1990		84	84	81	82	91	93	96	
Ohto *et al*[37]	1992		98	75	81					79

CTA = CT arteriography   CTAP = CT arterial portography   L-CT = Lipiodol CT   IOUS = Intraoperative sonography

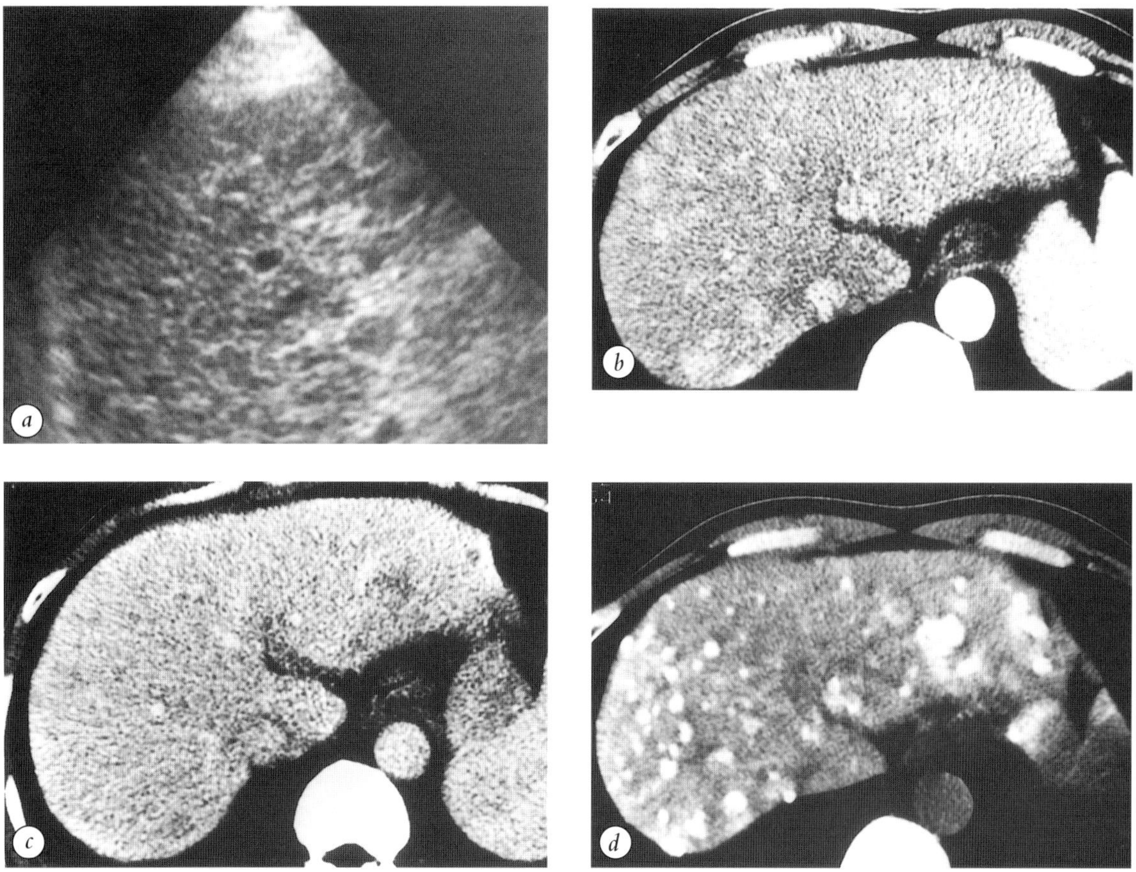

Figure 16.2 – Multinodular advanced HCC demonstrated differently with different CT techniques in a 58-year-old man.

a) Sonogram of the liver shows diffuse coarse liver with multiple, suspicious, tiny, hypoechoic nodules scattered in the entire liver.

b) CT scan in the arterial dominant phase with spiral CT shows multiple high-attenuation nodules in the entire liver.

c) CT scan in the portal dominant phase shows several suspicious low-attenuation nodules in both hepatic lobes. The arterial phase is better than the portal venous phase in detecting hepatic nodules.

d) CT scan with iodized oil shows numerous small hepatic nodules with retention of Lipiodol in the entire liver. Lipiodol CT is the most sensitive technique for detecting intrahepatic metastatic nodules of HCC in this case.

with continuous table feed, thus enabling volumetric acquisitions to be obtained during a single breath-holding period.[39-42]

The continuous data acquisition with spiral CT gives three advantages in hepatic imaging compared with standard incremental CT: (a) the potential for improved lesion detection due to both elimination of respiratory misregistration and retrospective image reconstruction at arbitrary positions along the z axis,[43] (b) improved lesion densitometry due to imaging the liver while intravenous contrast material is at its peak level,[25] and (c) production of high-quality multiplanar images.[41] Spiral CT with smaller interscan spacing increases confidence in detection and overall detection rate of focal liver lesions.[44] Therefore, spiral CT has the potential for improved detection of HCC (Fig. 16.1b,c). Several reports have described the advantages of spiral CT in detecting HCCs,[43,45] however, further controlled studies are needed.

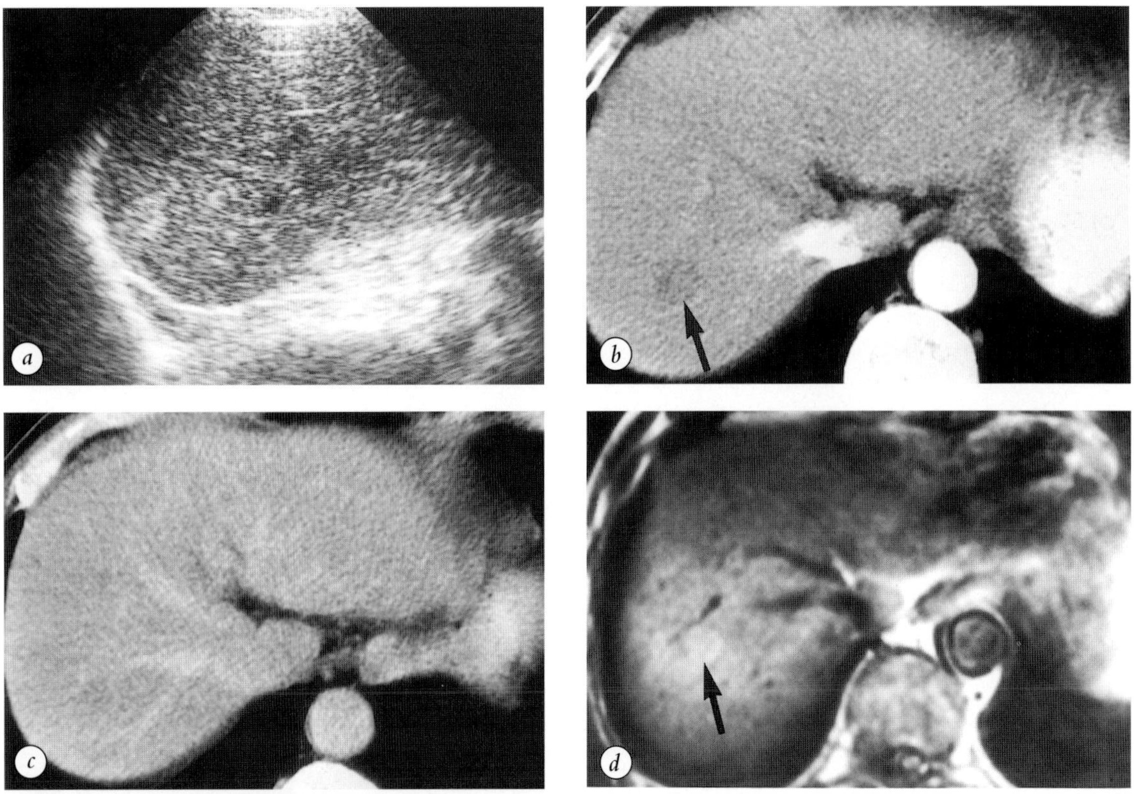

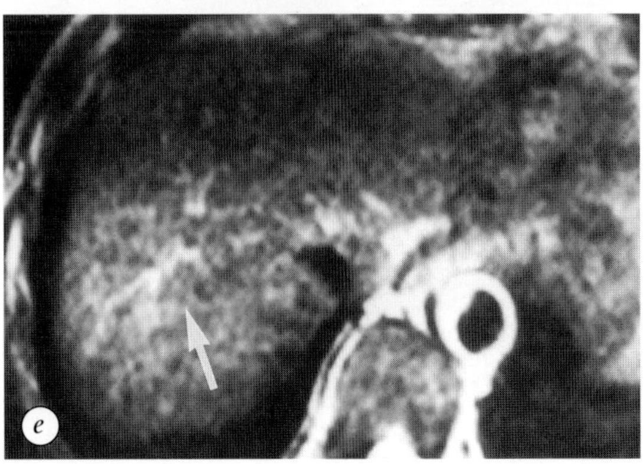

Figure 16.3 – A denomatous hyperplasia in a 62-year-old man.

a) Sonogram of the liver shows an ovoid hyperechoic mass in right upper liver.

b) CT scan in the arterial dominant phase of spiral CT shows suspicious low-attenuation mass (arrow) in segment 7 of the liver.

c) CT scan in the portal dominant phase of spiral CT shows no demonstrable mass.

d) T1-weighted MR image (600/30) demonstrates a slightly hyperintense nodule (arrow) in segment 7 of the liver.

e) T2-weighted MR image (2000/60) demonstrates a suspicious hypointense nodule (arrow) in segment 7 of the liver.

Recently, several investigators[46-48] have compared MR imaging with CT in the evaluation of focal hepatic lesions of all varieties. Although controversy exists about which imaging technique is more accurate and which should be the method of choice, current studies suggest that MR imaging and contrast-enhanced CT are comparable in the detection of hepatic tumors.[48-50] One comparative study of CT and MR imaging in a large population of patients with HCCs smaller than 3 cm shows that MR imaging (79%) is similar to CT (75%) in detecting small HCCs (Fig. 16.1).[37]

Associated nodular lesions

Adenomatous hyperplasia

Screening procedures, including periodic US and CT evaluations and measurement of serum levels of α-fetoprotein in patients with chronic liver disease, enable the detection of small HCCs. Noncancerous nodular lesions also such as adenomatous hyperplasia are being detected more often.[8,16,51-53] Most areas of adenomatous hyperplasia without malignant foci are small, less than 1.2 cm in diameter.[8,51] On sonograms, particularly intraoperative sonograms, they are frequently found as a lesion associated with advanced HCC and usually appear as an hypoechoic mass. Typical adenomatous hyperplasias usually are not detected with angiography and do not enhance on CT scans, even on CT arteriograms. Because these lesions are difficult to detect, the efficacy of imaging techniques for evaluation of these lesions has not been established. According to recent data,[54] the overall sensitivity for detecting adenomatous hyperplasia was 23% with US,. 4% with CT, 0% with angiography, 25% with CT arteriography, 40% with CT arterial portography, and 54% with intraoperative US (Fig. 16.3).

Early HCC (adenomatous hyperplasia with malignant foci)

Adenomatous hyperplasia can be accompanied by cancerous foci, and this type of lesion has been defined as adenomatous hyperplasia with malignant foci, which is thought to be an early form of HCC. The definition of adenomatous hyperplasia with malignant foci remains controversial,[8,12,16,55,56] and the definite histologic boundary with nodular lesions associated with liver cirrhosis is not yet clear.[8,12,16]

Early HCCs are also small, with mean diameters less than 1.7 cm.[8,12,53,57,58] Therefore, detection is difficult, and the efficacy of imaging techniques for evaluation of these lesions has not been well established. Recent studies[54,57,58] indicate an overall sensitivity of 64% for US, 56-58% for CT, 31% for angiography, 50-70% for CT arteriography, 66-71% for CT arterial portography, and 88% for intraoperative US (Fig. 16.4 a-c).

Early advanced HCC

Early advanced HCC is advanced HCC within early HCC. Pathologically, it consists of a definite cancerous nodule of advanced HCC (Edmondson grade II or higher) that is large enough to be detected at gross examination, surrounded by a rim of early HCC (Edmondson grade I).[12,59] On cut surface examination, the early component of early advanced HCC is relatively flat and red-yellow to yellow in color. The advanced component is usually but not always distinct as a discrete nodular lesion that often bulges out from the surface of the surrounding liver at gross examination.[12]

A recent study[12] indicated an overall sensitivity of 81% for CT, 83% for MR, 100% for CT arteriography, 86% for CT arterial portography, and 63% for iodized oil CT (Fig. 16.5). Standard CT and MR imaging had essentially equivalent sensitivities for the detection of early advanced HCC. However, lesion conspicuity was generally better with CT. T1-weighted MR images seem to be superior to T2-weighted images in the detection of early advanced HCC, which is probably secondary to advantages in detecting the early component of early advanced HCC. The sensitivity of T1-weighted imaging was slightly greater than that of T2-weighted imaging (72% vs 61%).[12] The 100% sensitivities reported for CT arteriography are likely to be artificially elevated as a result of both the relatively small number of patients in these categories and an element of selection bias since standard CT and MR imaging were the initial diagnostic tests of choice and other imaging modalities were usually performed only after these two modalities showed a suspicious lesion.[12]

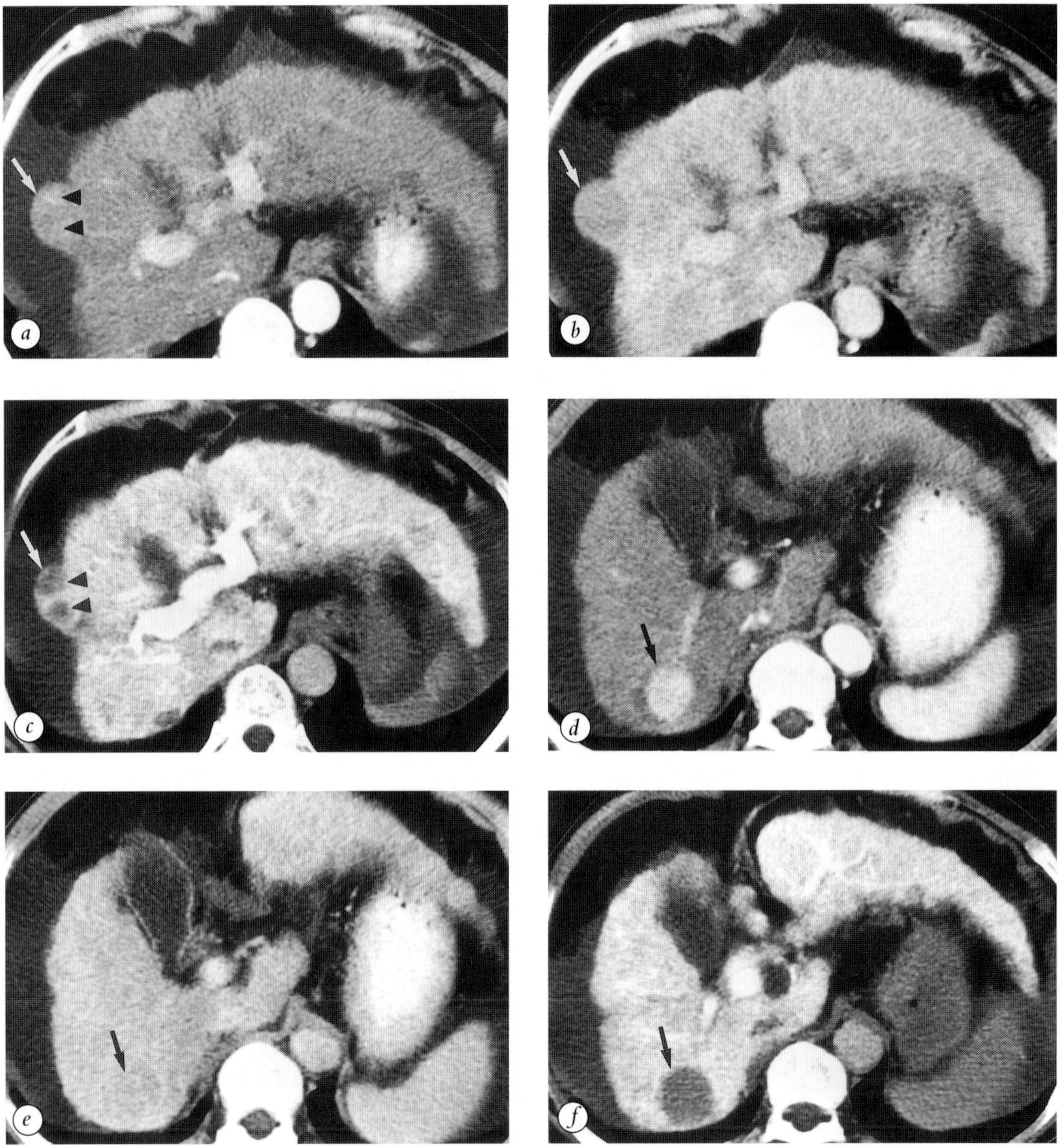

Figure 16.4 – An early HCC associated with an advanced small HCC in a 54-year-old woman.

a) CT scan in the arterial dominant phase with spiral CT shows exophytic mass (arrow) with two high-attenuating nodules (arrowheads) in segment 5 of the liver. Liver is contracted and nodular. Ascites is also seen.

b) CT scan in the late phase shows exophytic mass with slight low-attenuation.

c) CT arterial portogram shows two filling defects (arrowheads) in exophytic mass (arrow), indicating partial defect of portal blood supply in the tumor. Therefore, the tumor is considered to be an adenomatous hyperplasia with malignant foci, so called early HCC.

d) An advanced small HCC associated with the early HCC in figure 4a-c. CT scan in the arterial phase with spiral CT shows highly enhancing mass (arrow) in segment 6 of the liver, indicating blood supply from the hepatic artery.

e) CT scan in the late phase shows iso-attenuating mass (arrow) in segment 6 of the liver.

f) CT arterial portogram shows round filling defect (arrow) in the same area, indicating no portal blood supply. Therefore, the tumor is advanced HCC even though the tumor is small.

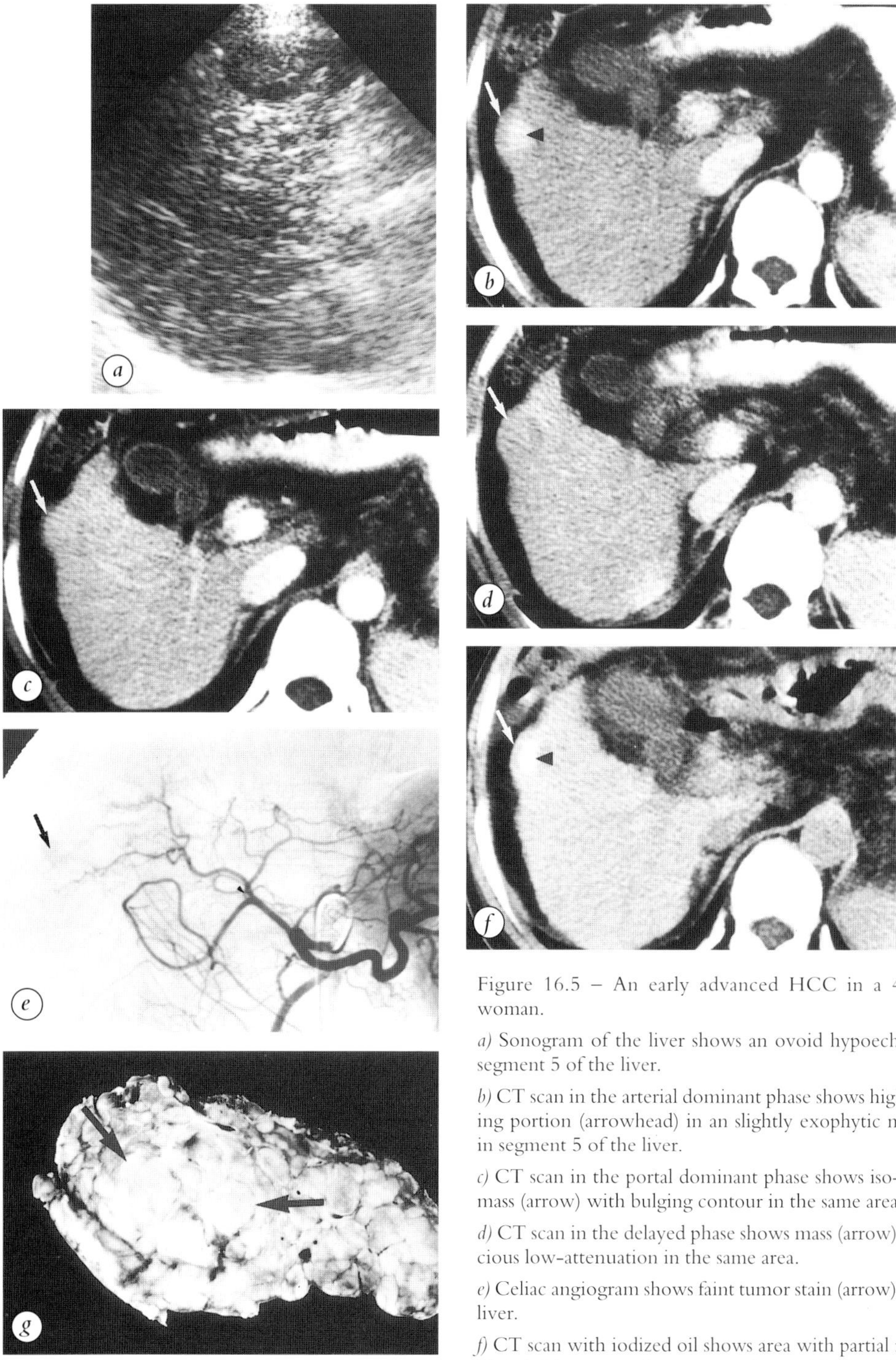

Figure 16.5 – An early advanced HCC in a 46-year-old woman.

a) Sonogram of the liver shows an ovoid hypoechoic mass in segment 5 of the liver.

b) CT scan in the arterial dominant phase shows highly enhancing portion (arrowhead) in an slightly exophytic mass (arrow) in segment 5 of the liver.

c) CT scan in the portal dominant phase shows iso-attenuating mass (arrow) with bulging contour in the same area.

d) CT scan in the delayed phase shows mass (arrow) with suspicious low-attenuation in the same area.

e) Celiac angiogram shows faint tumor stain (arrow) in the right liver.

f) CT scan with iodized oil shows area with partial retention of Lipiodol (arrowhead), corresponding to highly enhancing portion in Fig. 5a, in slightly exophytic mass (arrow).

g) Cut surface of the resected specimen shows a yellow mass (arrows) without a fibrous capsule measuring 2 cm in diameter. At histopathologic examination, well-differentiated HCC was seen with central focal area of advanced HCC.

DIAGNOSIS OF HCC

Cancer is thought to develop through a multistep process that includes initiation, promotion, and progression.[12,60] This sequence includes activation of multiple oncogenes and suppression of multiple tumor suppressor genes.[12] It has recently been revealed that, particularly in the presence of chronic liver disease, human HCC shows an obvious multistep progression through clonal expansion and subclonal progression. Sakamoto *et al*[60] believe that HCC provides a good model for studying the multiple progressive steps in human tumorigenesis.

The spectrum of focal nodular lesions in patients with chronic liver disease ranges from regenerating to advanced HCC. Several reports[8,12,51-55,57,58,61,62] describe the imaging appearance of these nodular lesions associated with liver cirrhosis, including regenerating nodules, adenomatous hyperplasia, early HCC and early advanced HCC, reflecting progress in the qualitative diagnosis of small HCCs and associated small nodular liver lesions.

The distinction between malignant and benign nodules is important clinically because surgical resection is the most effective treatment of small malignant nodules whereas surgery is not necessary for benign nodules.[8,12]

Advanced (overt) HCC

On sonograms, the pattern of echogenicity of HCCs is diverse. However, most small HCCs are hypoechoic (Fig. 16.1a), in contrast to advanced HCCs, which are mostly hyperechoic.[27,29,63,64] Pathologically, resected specimens of hypoechoic HCCs have solid tumor tissue without necrosis. Nonliquefactive necrosis, hemorrhage, fatty change, interstitial fibrosis, and sinusoidal dilatation were thought to produce hyperechogenicity.[8,26] A thin, peripheral, hypoechoic halo, which corresponds to a fibrous capsule in resected specimens, is one of the characteristic findings of small HCCs.[65] Other characteristic sonographic findings of small HCCs are lateral shadowing, probably related to the fibrous capsule of the tumor,[29] posterior acoustic enhancement, and mosaic pattern.[8,66] Doppler US can provide information on blood flow that is useful in differential diagnosis of HCC and other liver tumors.[67,68]

Dynamic contrast-enhanced sonographic angiography with intraarterial infusion of CO_2 microbubbles, a contrast material for sonographic examinations, is a newly developed imaging tool that is a combination of US and angiography.[31,69] Sonographic angiography shows a hyperechoic pattern in typical HCC, as compared with a marginal spotty hyperechoic pattern for hemangioma and an internal spotty hyperechoic pattern for fibrous granuloma.[69] With this imaging technique, although most uniform or mosaic hypervascular nodules are HCC, the same vascular pattern is occasionally observed in metastases or lymphomas, as reported previously.[31] Therefore, it would be inappropriate to diagnose HCC on the basis of imaging findings alone when this imaging technique is used. However, the technique is useful for the accurate depiction of vascularity within a tumor and provides information that is valuable in planning treatment.[31] When surgical resection is not indicated, transcatheter arterial embolization therapy or intraarterial infusion of chemotherapeutic agents mixed with iodized oil is effective for treatment of hypervascular HCC, whereas such therapy would not be effective for treatment of isovascular or hypovascular HCC. Percutaneous injection of ethanol is indicated for such nodules.[8]

Intraoperative US not only can show small HCCs but also characteristic features, and is thought to be the final step of preoperative staging of HCC.[32]

On conventional CT scans, most small HCCs appear as relatively well defined, low-attenuation masses, and when the HCC is encapsulated, the capsule shows ring-like contrast enhancement. However, the conventional CT appearance of HCCs is often similar to that of other hepatic tumors and is nonspecific.[70,71]

Dynamic CT has made possible analysis of the dynamic distribution of contrast material in the normal liver and in hepatic masses.[72,73]

The majority of HCCs are hypervascular, and tumors enhance rapidly but then quickly become less dense than the surrounding liver (Fig. 16.1b,c).[73] These findings correlate well with the angiographic features of hypervascular hepatic tumors other than cavernous hemangiomas (Fig. 16.2).[73] In encapsulated small HCCs, prolonged enhancement of the capsule occurs. Attenuation is higher than that of the liver in the delayed phase.[72] HCCs larger than 3 cm in diameter tend to have a mosaic pattern (Fig. 16.6), whereas smaller HCCs do not.[66] Fatty metamorphosis or steatosis, which is seen on a CT scan as a focal zone of tissue within a tumor that has the same CT appearance or negative Hounsfield numbers as fat, has been described as a specific feature of HCC.[74,75] Recently, Freeny *et al*[9] reported a low frequency of typical findings with CT in a non-Asian population. However, another recent study[76] reported the similar frequencies of the typical findings of HCCs in non-Asian population to those reported with Asian patients. Reported morphologic differences between non-Asian and Asian patients with HCC may be due to differences in underlying liver disease, tumor size, and histologic grade.[76]

CT arteriography and CT arterial portography consist of obtaining rapid CT scans during a bolus injection of contrast material administered through a transfemoral catheter with its tip located in the hepatic artery (arteriography) or the superior mesenteric artery (arterial portography). The value of CT arteriography or CT arterial portography in the detection of HCC lies in the differences in perfusion between normal liver (blood supply from the hepatic artery only).[77] Most HCCs are seen as enhancing masses on CT arteriograms and as filling defects on CT scans obtained during arterial portography, because most of these tumors have no portal supply (Fig. 16.4d-f).[52]

Infusion of iodized poppy seed oil (Lipiodol) at angiography was introduced for the treatment of HCC, as Lipiodol accumulates in a tumor and can be combined with lipophilic anticancerous agents. CT with iodized oil is useful for differentiating small HCCs from regenerating nodules (Fig. 16.2d). Another benefit is that CT with iodized oil can be used to evaluate the therapeutic effect of transcatheter oily chemoembolization therapy of HCCs, particularly in cases of encapsulated small nodular HCCs.[78]

The morphologic characteristics and the signal intensity of tumors on MR images can be used to establish criteria for the diagnosis of small HCCs (Fig. 16.1d,e). MR images show a capsule in 24-56% of small HCCs,[21,74,78] and relatively T1-weighted and T2-weighted spin-echo (SE) images show heterogeneous internal architecture in most HCCs. The capsule of an HCC tumor has a low intensity relative

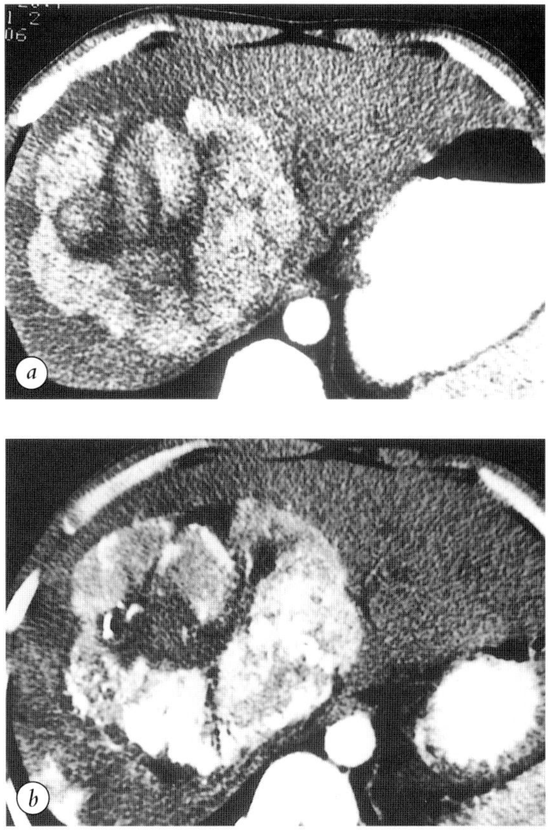

Figure 16.6 – An advanced HCC with mosaic pattern in a 51-year-old man.

a) CT scan in the arterial dominant phase shows a well-defined, lobulated mass with several compartments having different attenuation.

b) CT scan with iodized oil shows dense retention of Lipiodol in compartments with high attenuation in *a)*. Area with low-attenuation within the mass does not show retention of Lipiodol, indicating necrotic or fibrotic portion.

to the liver on both T1- and T2-weighted images because fibrous tissue does not have enough mobile protons. MR imaging is superior to CT for showing capsules. T1-weighted images were superior to CT scans or T2-weighted images for showing the capsule.[74,79,80] Fatty degeneration of HCC is a common pathologic feature,[16,74,81,82] and this change could be detected on the basis of isointensity or high intensity on T1-weighted SE images or on the basis of decrease in the tumor/liver ratio of intensity on phase-contrast images.[82,83] Accumulation of copper as one of the causes of the high-intensity pattern on T1-weighted images of small HCCs is still controversial.[84,85] The mosaic pattern reflects a configuration of multiple compartments of the same or different attenuations or intensities within the tumor. T2-weighted images were superior to CT scans or T1-weighted images in showing the mosaic pattern of HCC.[80]

Weinmann *et al*[86] reported that the pharmacokinetic behavior of IV-delivered gadopentetate dimeglumine was similar to that of well-known iodinated contrast agents. Ohtomo *et al*[87] stated that the features of HCCs on dynamic MR images corresponded well to the features on single-level dynamic CT scans. Dynamic MR imaging is a useful method for assessment of the hemodynamics of small HCCs and may replace dynamic CT if fast imaging methods with multisection modes and better contrast agents are developed because of the inherently greater contrast resolution of MR.

Adenomatous hyperplasia

On sonograms, adenomatous hyperplasias have a hypoechoic and hyperechoic pattern, and the findings are similar to those of regenerating nodules or small HCCs (Figs. 16.3a, 7a).[88] The lesions are not usually detected with conventional CT or CT arterial portography, because typical adenomatous hyperplasia, which has almost the same histologic features as regenerating nodules and which contains multiple portal tracts, shows almost the same volume of portal flow as does the surrounding cirrhotic liver (Fig. 16.7b,c).[52] The usefulness of MR imaging was described by Matsui *et al*.[51] Adenomatous hyperplasias without atypia were hypointense on T2-weighted images and hyperintense on T1-weighted images, for unknown reasons (Figs. 16.3d,e, 7e,f). This combination of intensities on T1- and T2-weighted images is a finding specific to adenomatous hyperplasia. The pathologic factors that constitute signal intensities in adenomatous hyperplasias should be studied further.

Early HCC

Early HCC is defined as a nodular lesion that shows no substantial alteration of hepatic architecture and frequently contains a portal structure. The tumor usually occurs in patients with chronic liver disease, especially cirrhosis. The color of the cut surface of early HCC is mostly reddish yellow to yellow. Microscopically, cancer cells are very well differentiated, corresponding to grade I according to Edmondson's classification of HCC.[89] Early HCC has an increased cell density with little atypia and frequent fatty changes.[56,57]

The term early is used to indicate that the lesion corresponds to the early stage of hepatocarcinogenesis and does not imply a good clinical prognosis after treatment. Early HCC is presumed to be an intermediate step between adenomatous hyperplasia and early advanced HCC in the multistep progression of hepatocarcinogenesis.[16,58]

The precise diagnosis of early HCC is not always easy. Sonograms usually show a hypoechoic mass without evidence of a capsule or mosaic pattern, closely resembling adenomatous hyperplasia.[88,90]

In a recent study,[57] the most common CT pattern of early HCC was isoattenuation on unenhanced, early enhanced, and late enhanced CT scans (iso-iso-iso). These lesions were not detectable on CT scans because neither a low-attenuation ring on unenhanced CT scans nor a high-attenuation ring around the lesion on late enhanced CT scans was seen.

Early HCC is usually hypovascular. Matsui *et al*[52] found that intranodular portal blood flow tends to decrease as the grade of malignancy increases. Unlike adenomatous hyperplasia, almost all HCCs of Edmondson grade 2 or greater had a definite decrease in the intranodular portal supply on CT scans obtained during arterial portography. In intermediate lesions, such as early HCC, and well-differentiated (grade 1) HCC, the intranodular portal blood supply tended to decrease progressively as the grade of malignancy increased, whereas the intranodular hepatic arterial supply increased (Figs. 16.4,7). Unlike early HCCs, adenomatous hyperplasias are not visualized on a CT scan obtained during arterial portography because of portal blood flow in the lesions.[52] The relationship between the portal and arterial blood supplies in the hepatocytic lesions found in the cirrhotic liver was considered to be reciprocal at imaging.[52] Therefore, the combination of CT arteriography and CT arterial portography is more accurate than either alone in determining the nature of the nodular lesions associated with liver cirrhosis.[52,58]

On MR images, early HCC mainly has a hyper- or isointense pattern on T1-weighted images and a hypo- or isointense pattern on T2-weighted images (Fig 16.7j,k).[12,53] Sometimes, early HCC has a unique MR appearance, consisting of a mostly low-intensity nodule with a small focus of intermediate or high intensity on T2-weighted images.[12,51,55] The relationship between progression of malignant disease and signal-intensity pattern for early stages of HCC has not been fully studied.

Early advanced HCC

Pathologically, early advanced HCC consists of a definite cancerous nodule of HCC that is large enough to be detected at gross examination surrounded by early HCC.[12,59,60] Rim *et al*[59] concluded that early advanced HCC has been shown conclusively to be a transitional tumor between early HCC and advanced HCC. Other terms used for early advanced HCC include HCC with early components,[53] overt HCC with early components,[8] advanced HCC in early HCC,[60] nodule-in-nodule lesion,[59] and adenomatous hyperplasia with malignant foci with macroscopic tumor nodules.[53] The mean diameter of early advanced HCCs (2.0 cm) was substantially larger than that of early HCCs (1.4 cm).[59] As might be expected in this multistep model of hepatocarcinogenesis, the proportion of early advanced HCCs to early HCCs increased with tumor diameter.[91]

A recent study[12] described two types of imaging characteristics of early advanced HCC. A nodule-in-nodule appearance was identified in approximately one-third to one-half of cases (Fig. 16.5). Signal behavior of early and advanced components of early advanced HCC followed the expected behaviors of isolated early HCC and isolated advanced HCC, respectively.[12] The inner nodule represents the advanced component and the peripheral margin (general component) the early component. The early component of early advanced HCC tended to be hypoattenuating or hypointense at early enhanced CT (Fig. 16.5b), CT arteriography, and T2-weighted MR imaging, and hyperintense at T1-weighted MR imaging. Conversely, the advanced component tended to be hyperattenuating or hyperintense at early enhanced CT (Fig. 16.5b), CT arteriography, and T2-weighted MR imaging, and hypointense at T1-weighted MR imaging.[12]

If a nodule-in-nodule appearance was not seen on images, it was not possible to determine with certainty whether the general component of the lesion that was visualized at imaging represented the early component, the advanced component, or the entire lesion of early advanced HCC. For example, the visualized homogeneous lesion could correspond to the early component of the early advanced HCC that is directly adjacent to an undetected, isointense nodule of advanced HCC or vice versa.[12]

ROLE OF IMAGING TECHNIQUES IN TREATMENT PLANNING

Early detection of HCC is important because early treatment, either surgical resection or local ablation, of these tumors is the most effective. Therefore, screening and regular follow-up with imaging techniques have been introduced in patients at high risk for HCC.[7]

The role of US and CT in the screening of HCCs are complementary. US has become a major screening technique in Asian populations because high sensitivity of real-time US for detection of these tumors has been established.[25-29] Furthermore, the simplicity and flexibility of real-time US have made it a major tool for guiding diagnostic aspiration and therapeutic procedures for HCC. CT is also an accurate, relatively noninvasive technique used to evaluate HCC, and it is a complementary screening technique when clinical questions cannot be answered with US. With CT, not only can the extent of the HCC be defined more accurately, but the extrahepatic spread of disease can be better defined.[8,91]

If nodules are considered inoperable because screening procedures indicate multiplicity, vascular invasion, or extrahepatic metastasis, sonographically guided percutaneous biopsy is performed to allow a final diagnosis based on histologic findings in addition to the imaging findings. If nodules are potentially operable, MR imaging is used to characterize them further. Color flow Doppler imaging also is useful in the characterization of liver tumors. However, color Doppler imaging is not yet satisfactory for routine examination of the liver, where the blood flow is slow especially in deeply seated tumor.[8]

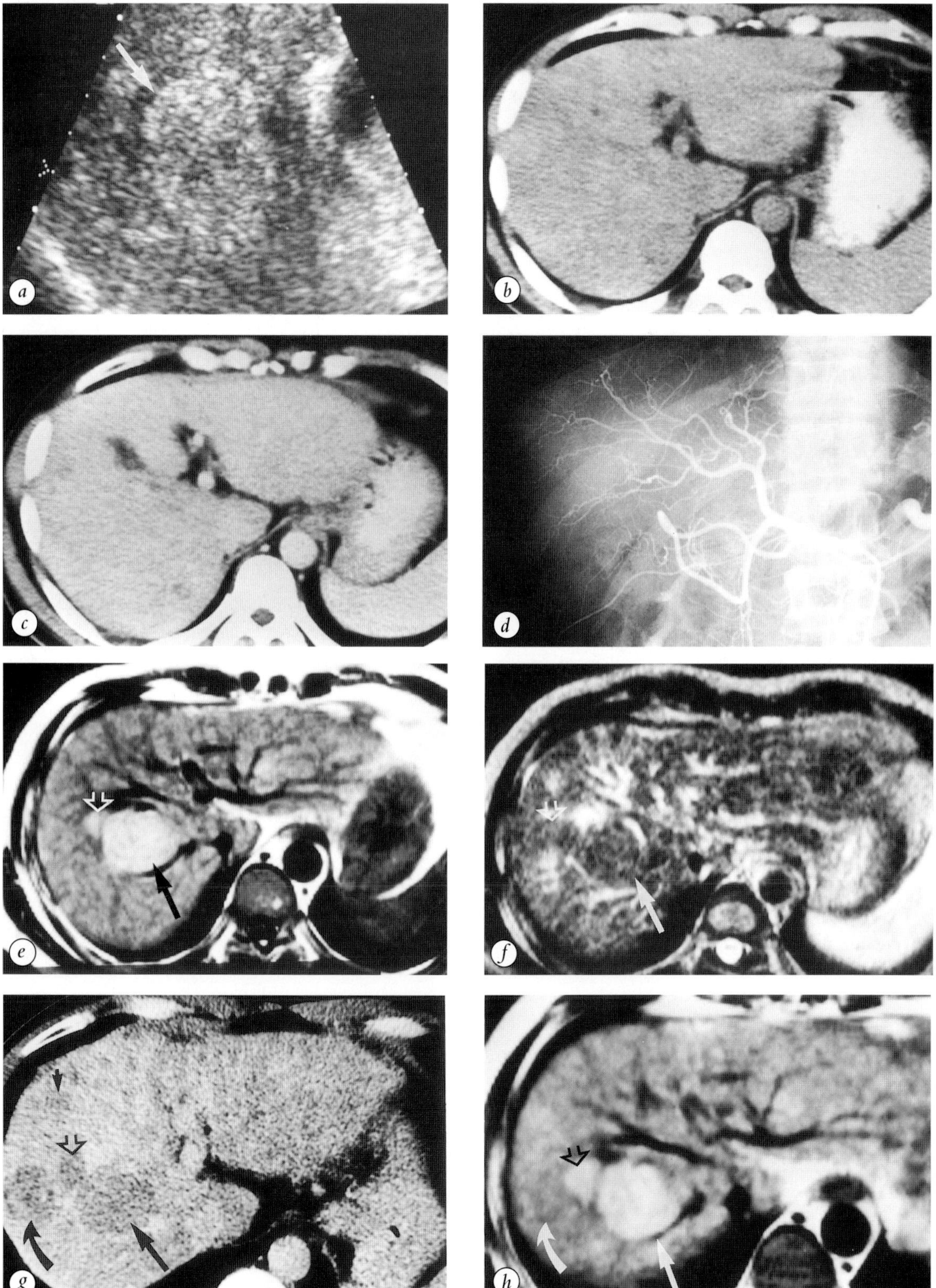
a
b
c
d
e
f
g
h

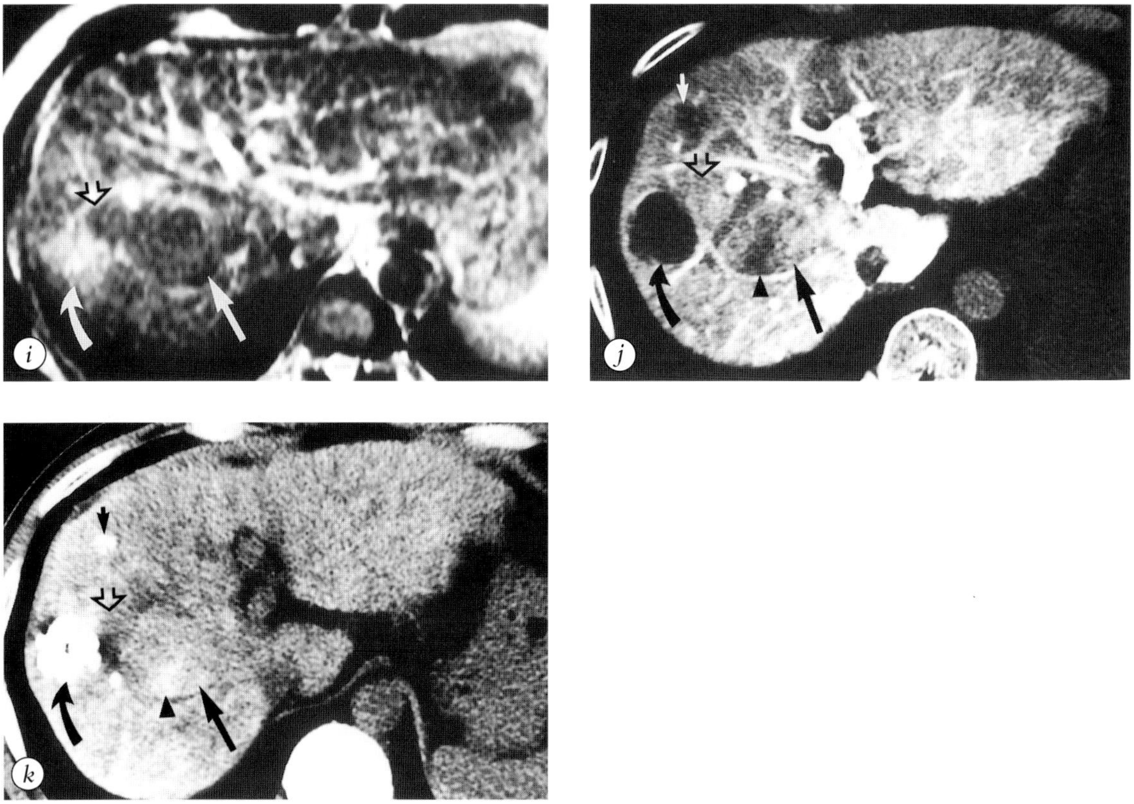

Figure 16.7 – Typical example of hepatocarcinogenesis from an adenomatous hyperplasia *(a-f)* to an early HCC and advanced HCC *(g-k)* during 12-month-follow-up period in a 45-year-old man.

a) Initial sonogram of the liver shows slightly hyperechoic mass without definite capsule (arrow) in the right liver.

b) Initial unenhanced CT scan shows no definite mass in the liver.

c) Initial contrast-enhanced CT scan also shows no definite mass in the liver.

d) Initial hepatic angiogram shows no evidence of thumor in the liver.

e) Initial T1-weighted MR image (550/15) shows two masses with high intensity (arrow & open arrow), in the right liver.

f) Initial T2-weighted MR image (2300/120) shows two masses with low intensity (arrow & open arrow) in the same area, consistent with adenomatous hyperplasia.

g) Conventional contrast-enhanced CT scan 12 month after the initial studies shows three masses (arrow, arrowhead, & curved arrow), and one suspicious mass (short arrow) in the right liver.

h) T1-weighted MR image (550/15) shows two masses with high intensity (arrow & open arrow), and one mass with suspicious low intensity (curved arrow).

i) T2-weighted MR image (2000/80) shows two masses with low intensity (arrow & open arrow), and one mass with high intensity (curved arrow). Therefore, the mass indicated by curved arrow is considered to be an advanced HCC.

j) CT arterial portogram shows complete defect of portal flow in the mass indicated by curved arrow, partial defect (arrowhead) in the mass indicated by arrow, and no defect in the mass indicated by open arrow. Therefore, the mass indicated by curved arrow is consistent with advanced HCC ; the mass indicated by arrow, early HCC ; and the mass indicated by open arrow, adenomatous hyperplasia. Another defect area (short arrow) of portal flow is also seen, indicating advanced HCC.

k) CT scan after infusion of iodized oil shows dense complete retention of Lipiodol in two masses (short arrow & curved arrow), indicating advanced HCC ; parteal retention (arrowhead) of Lipiodol in one mass (arrow), indicating early HCC ; and no retention of Lipodol in one mass (open arrow), indicating adenomatous hyperplasia. These findings on Lipiodol CT scan correspond well to those on CT arterial portogram *(j)*

If the nodules are small and appear benign (such as regenerating nodules or adenomatous hyperplasia) on MR images, currently, interval serial scanning is the only practical method of follow-up. In such cases, final diagnosis based on histologic findings alone after percutaneous biopsy is difficult because entire pathologic specimens are needed for the histologic diagnosis.

If imaging findings suggest nodules are malignant, staging of the nodules by using CT arterial portography, CT with iodized oil, or sonographic angiography is necessary. At present, CT arterial portography appears to be one of the most accurate approaches for detecting an intrahepatic tumor and defining its extent.[8,92] CT with iodized oil is one of the most sensitive methods for detecting small hypervascular HCCs. Sonographic angiography is considered extremely sensitive for identifying the vascular pattern of the tumor even if the tumor is small. The selection of techniques for staging might be different because the decision as to which imaging techniques are state-of the-art and the levels of familiarity with various techniques vary among institutions.[8]

If imaging findings indicate that surgery is inadvisable, percutaneous biopsy is performed for further treatment planning. If the nodules are potentially resectable, intraoperative US is necessary for confirmation and for determination of the best operative method because small nodules may not be seen or palpated from the surface of the liver. Intraoperative US, which was first used by Makuuchi *et al*[93] in the diagnosis of HCCs, rarely produces blind areas, because scanning during surgery is not disturbed by the ribs, lung, or bowel, and the distortion and weakening of the ultrasound beam caused by the abdominal wall can be avoided.

CONCLUSIONS

Recent advances in various imaging techniques have facilitated the detection of small HCCs, with a marked improvement in the prognosis of these lesions. The tumors are usually detected by means of periodic US or CT in patients with chronic liver disease. Accurate tumor staging can be done preoperatively by using CT arterial portography, CT with iodized oil, or dynamic contrast-enhanced sonographic angiography. In addition, satisfactory hepatic resection can be done by using intraoperative US to detect tumors and visualize spatial relationships between tumors and adjacent hepatic vessels, thus improving the surgical results.[8]

These improvements have led to an increase in the detection of other hepatic nodular lesions such as regenerating nodules, adenomatous hyperplasia, atypical adenomatous hyperplasia, early HCCs, and early advanced HCCs in the cirrhotic liver. Because of the recent rapid evolution of knowledge regarding these small nodular lesions of the liver, the terminology used has been somewhat variable and confusing.[12] Although the definitions of adenomatous hyperplasia, early HCCs, and early advanced HCCs are still controversial, the concept of these borderline lesions is expected to prevail gradually.

Some of those lesions are malignant nodules; therefore, the distinction between benign and malignant nodules is important clinically. Recently, CT arterial portography, CT arteriography, and MR imaging have played important roles in differentiating these hepatic nodular lesions. However, most adenomatous hyperplasias and early HCCs are quite small and cannot be easily detected preoperatively, and they are, therefore, difficult to follow up. Data on their clinical course are lacking, and their biological behavior has not been analyzed in detail. Whether such lesions are premalignant or already malignant can be determined when more knowledge of their biologic behavior has been accumulated. Further study of these nodular lesions with imaging techniques is essential.[8]

In addition, at this time, the clinical significance of the imaging diagnosis of these nodular lesions is uncertain. More research must be performed to ascertain whether any significant correlation exists between the different steps of HCC and the clinical outcome.[8,12]

REFERENCES

1. Kane RA. Liver imaging update. *Semin Ultrasound CT MR*.1992;**13**:311-312
2. Kondo Y. Differential diagnosis of early hepatocellular carcinoma. In: Okuda K, Tobe T, Kitagawa T, eds. *Early detectionn and treatment of liver cancer. Gann Monograph on Cancer Research*, vol. 38. London, England: Taylor & Francis, 1991;39-50
3. Kojiro M, Sugihara S, Nakashima O. Pathomorphologic characteristics of early hepatocellular carcinoma. In: Okuda K, Tobe T, Kitagawa T, eds. *Early detection and treatment of liver cancer. Gann Monograph on Cancer Research*, vol. 38. London, England: Taylor & Francis, 1991;29-37
4. Ferrell L, Wright T, Lake J, Roberts J, Ascher N. Incidence and diagnostic features of macroregenerative nodules vs. small hepatocellular carcinoma in cirrhotic livers. *Hepatology* 1992;**16**:1372-1381
5. Kenmochi K, Sugihara S, Kojiro M. Relationship of histologic grade of hepatocellular carcinoma (HCC) to tumor size, and demonstration of tumor cells of multiple different grades in single small HCC. *Liver* 1987;**7**:18-26
6. Sakamoto M, Hirohashi S, Shimosato Y. Early stages of multistep hepatocarcinogenesis: adenomatous hyperplasia and early hepatocellular carcinoma. *Hum Pathol* 1991;**22**:172-178
7. Arakawa M, Sugihara S, Kenmochi K, *et al* Small mass lesions in cirrhosis: transition from benign adenomatous hyperplasia to hepatocellular carcinoma? *J Gastroenterol Hepatol* 1986;**1**:3-14
8. Choi BI, Takayasu K, Han MC. Small hepatocellular carcinomas and associated nodular lesions of the liver: pathology, pathogenesis, and imaging findings. *AJR* 1993;**160**:1177-1187
9. Freeny PC, Baron RL, Teefey SA. Hepatocellular carcinoma: reduced frequency of typical findings with dynamic contrast-enhanced CT in a non-Asian population. *Radiology* 1992;**182**:143-148
10. Tsuda H, Hirohashi S, Shimosato Y, Terada M, Hasegawa H. Clonal origin of atypical adenomatous hyperplasia of the liver and clonal identity with hepatocellular carcinoma. *Gastroenterology* 1988;**95**:1664-1666
11. Takayama T, Makuuchi M, Hirohashi S, *et al* Malignant transformation of adenomatous hyperplasia to hepatocellular carcinoma. *Lancet* 1990;**336**:1150-1153
12. Winter TC III, Takayasu K, Muramatsu Y, *et al* Early advanced carcinoma: evaluation of CT and MR appearance with pathologic correlation. *Radiology* 1994;**192**:379-387
13. Peters RL. Pathology of hepatocellular carcinoma. In: Okuda K, Peters RL, eds. *Hepatocellular carcinoma*. New York: Wiley, 1976;107-168
14. Ohta G, Nakanuma Y. Comparative study of three nodular lesions in cirrhosis: adenomatoid hyperplasia, adenomatoid hyperplasia with intermediate lesion and small hepatocellular carcinoma. In: Okuda K, Ishak KG, eds. *Neoplasms of the liver*. Tokyo: Springer, 1987;177-188
15. Furuya K, Nakamura M, Yamamoto Y, Togei K, Otsuka H. Macroregenerative nodule of the liver: a clinicopathologic study of 345 autopsy cases of chronic liver disease. *Cancer* 1988; **61**:99-105
16. Sakamoto M, Hirohashi S, Shimosato Y. Early stages of multistep hepatocarcinogenesis: adenomatous hyperplasia and early hepatocellular carcinoma. *Hum Pathol* 1991; **22**:172-178
17. Takashima T, Matsui O, Suzuki M, Ida M. Diagnosis and screening of small hepatocellular carcinoma: comparison of radionuclide imaging, ultrasound, computed tomography, hepatic angiography, and alpha-feto-protein assay. *Radiology* 1985; **145**:635-638
18. Maringhini A, Cottone M, Sciarrino E, *et al* Ultrasonographic and radionuclide detection of hepatocellular carcinoma in cirrhotics with low alpha-fetoprotein levels. *Cancer* 1984; **54**: 2924-2926
19. Takayasu K, Shima Y, Muramatsu Y, *et al* Angiography of small hepatocellular carcinomas: analysis of 105 resected tumors. *AJR* 1986;**147**:525-529
20. Kudo M, Hirasa M, Takakuwa H, *et al* Small hepatocellular carcinomas in chronic liver disease: detection with SPECT. *Radiology* 1986;**159**:697-703
21. Choi BI, Han MC, Kim CW. Small hepatocellular carcinoma versus small cavernous hemangioma: differentiation with MR imaging at 2.0 T. *Radiology* 1990;**176**:103-106
22. Okuda K, Nakashima T, Obata H, Kubo Y. Clinicopathological studies of minute hepatocellular carcinoma: analysis of 20 cases, including 4 with hepatic resection. *Gastroenterology* 1977;**73**:109-115
23. Chen DS, Sheu JC, Sung JL, *et al* Small hepatocellular carcinoma: a clinicopathological study in thirteen patients. *Gastroenterology* 1982;**83**:1109-1119
24. Liver Cancer Study Group of Japan. The size of tumor occupying ratio and distant metastases. In: The general rules for the clinical and pathological study of primary liver cancer. Tokyo: Kanehara, 1987:18
25. Sheu JC, Sung JL, Chen DS, *et al* Early detection of hepatocellular carcinoma by real-time ultrasonography: a prospective study. *Cancer* 1985;**56**:660-666
26. Tanaka S, Kitamura T, Nakanishi K, *et al* Effectiveness of periodic checkup by ultrasonography for the early diagnosis of hepatocellular carcinoma. *Cancer* 1990;**66**:2210-2214
27. Sheu JC, Sung JL, Chen DS, *et al* Ultrasonography of small hepatic tumors using high-resolution linear-array real-time instruments. *Radiology* 1984;**150**:797-802
28. Tanaka S, Kitamura T, Nakanishi K, *et al* Recent advances in ultrasonographic diagnosis of hepatocellular carcinoma. *Cancer* 1989;**63**:1313-1317
29. Choi BI, Kim CW, Han MC, *et al* Sonographic characteristics of small hepatocellular carcinoma. *Gastrointest Radiol* 1989;**14**:255-261
30. Choi BI, Park JH, Kim BH, *et al* Small hepatocellular carcinoma: detection with sonography, computed tomography (CT), angiography and Lipiodol-CT. *Br J Radiol* 1989;**62**:897-901
31. Kudo M, Tomita S, Tochio H, *et al* Small hepatocellular carcinoma: diagnosis with US angiography with intraarterial CO_2 microbubbles. *Radiology* 1992;**182**:155-160
32. Choi BI, Han JK, Song IS, *et al* Intraoperative sonography of hepatocellular carcinoma: detection of lesions and validity in surgical resection. *Gastrointest Radiol* 1991;**16**:329-333
33. Takayasu K, Moriyama N, Muramatsu Y, *et al* The diagnosis of small hepatocellular carcinomas: efficacy of various imaging procedures in 100 patients. *AJR* 1990;**155**:49-54
34. Merine D, Takayasu K, Wakao F. Detection of hepatocellular carcinoma: comparison of CT during arterial portography with CT after intraarterial injection of iodized oil. *Radiology* 1990;**175**:707-710
35. Miller WJ, Federle MP, Campbell WL. Diagnosis and staging of hepatocellular carcinoma: comparison of CT and sonography in 36 liver transplantation patients. *AJR* 1991;**157**:303-306

36. Matsui O, Kameyama T, Yoshikawa J, *et al* Angiographic diagnosis of hepatocellular carcinoma including CT arteriography and CT arterial portography [in Japanese]. *J Med Imaging* 1988;**8**:1289-1300

37. Ohto M, Kondo F, Ebara M. Pathology, diagnosis, and treatment for small liver cancer. In: Tobe T, Kameda H, Okudaira M, *et al* eds. *Primary liver cancer in Japan*. Tokyo: Spinger-Verlag, 1992;129-138

38. Hayashi N, Yamamoto K, Tamaki N, *et al* Metastatic nodules of hepatocellular carcinoma: detection with angiography, CT and US. *Radiology* 1987;**165**:61-63

39. Rubin GD, Dake MD, Napel SA, McDonnell CH, Jeffrey RB Jr. Three dimensional spiral CT angiography of the abdomen: initial clinical experience. *Radiology* 1993;**186**:147-152

40. Zeman RK, Fox SH, Silverman PM, *et al* Helical (Spiral) CT of the abdomen. *AJR* 1993;**160**:719-725

41. Heiken JP, Brink JA, Vannier MW. Spiral (helical) CT. *Radiology* 1993;**189**:647-656

42. Bluemke D, Fishman EK. Spiral CT of the liver. *AJR* 1993;**160**:787-792

43. Choi BI, Shin YM, Han JK, Chung JW, Park JH, Han MC. Focal hepatic nodules after transcatheter oily chemoembolization: detection with spiral CT versus conventional CT. *Abdom Imaging* 1996;**21:**33-36

44. Urban BA, Fishman EK, Kuhlman JE, *et al* Detection of focal hepatic lesions with spiral CT: comparison of 4- and 8-mm interval spacing. *AJR* 1993;**160**:783-785

45. Choi BI, Cho JM, Han JK, Choi DS, Han MC. Sprial CT for the detection of hepatocellular carcinoma: relative value of arterial and late phase scanning. *Abdom Imaging* 1996 (in press)

46. Heiken JP, Weyman PF, Lee JKT, *et al* Detection of focal hepatic masses: prospective evaluation with CT, delayed CT, CT during arterial portography, and MR imaging. *Radiology* 1989;**171**:47-51

47. Nelson RC, Chezmar JL, Sugarbaker PH, Bernardino ME. Hepatic tumor: comparison of CT during arterial portography, delayed CT and MR imaging for preoperative evaluation. *Radiology* 1989;**172**:27-34

48. Nelson RC, Chezmar JL, Steinberg HV, *et al* Focal hepatic lesions: detection by dynamic and delayed computed tomography versus short TE/TR spin echo and fast field echo magnetic resonance imaging. *Gastrointest Radiol* 1988;**13**:115-122

49. Barakos JA, Goldberg HI, Brown JJ, Gilbert TJ. Comparison of computed tomography and magnetic resonance imaging in the evaluation of focal hepatic lesions. *Gastrointest Radiol* 1990;**15**:93-101

50. Vlachos L, Trakadas S, Gouliamos A, *et al* Comparative study between ultrasound, computed tomography, intra-arterial digital subtraction angiography, and magnetic resonance imaging in the differentiation of tumors of the liver. *Gastrointest Radiol* 1990;**15**:102-106

51. Matsui D, Kadoya M, Kameyama T, *et al* Adenomatous hyperplastic nodules in the cirrhotic liver: differentiation from hepatocellular carcinoma with MR imaging. *Radiology* 1989; **173**:123-126

52. Matsui O, Kadoya M, Kameyama T, *et al* Benign and malignant nodules in cirrhotic livers: distinction based on blood supply. *Radiology* 1991;**178**:493-497

53. Muramatsu Y, Nawano S, Takayasu K, *et al* Early hepatocellular carcinoma: MR imaging. *Radiology* 1991;**181**:209-213

54. Takayasu K, Makuuchi M, Hirohashi S, *et al* Imaging of adenomatous hyperplastic lesions containing and not containing hepatocellular carcinoma in the liver [in Japanese]. *Nippon Shokakibyo Gakkai Zasshi* 1989;**86**:2404-2412

55. Mitchell DG, Rubin R, Siegelman ES, Burk DL Jr, Rifkin MD. Hepatocellular carcinoma within siderotic regenerative nodules: appearance as a nodule within a nodule on MR imaging. *Radiology* 1991;**178**:101-103

56. Kanai T, Hirohashi S, Upton MP, *et al* Pathology of hepatocellular carcinoma: a proposal for a new gross classification. *Cancer* 1987;**60**:810-819

57. Takayasu K, Furukawa, Wakao F, *et al* CT diagnosis of early hepatocellular carcinoma: sensitivity, findings, and CT-pathologic correlation. *AJR* 1995;**164**:885-890

58. Takayasu K, Muramatsu Y, Furukawa H, *et al* Early hepatocellular carcinoma: appearance at CT during arterial portography and CT arteriography with pathologic correlation. *Radiology* 1995;**194**:101-105

59. Rim K, Sakamoto M, Watanabe H, *et al* Pathology and DNA cytophotometry of small hepatocellular carcinoma with a nodule-in-nodule appearance: evidence for stepwise progression of hepatocellular carcinoma. *Jpn J Clin Oncol* 1992;**23**:26-33

60. Sakamoto M, Ino Y, Fujii T, Hirohashi S. Phenotype change in tumor vessels associated with the progression of hepatocellular carcinoma. *Jpn J Clin Oncol* 1993;**23**:98-104

61. Itai Y, Ohnishi S, Ohtomo K, *et al* Regenerating nodules of liver cirrhosis: MR imaging. *Radiology* 1987;**165**:419-423

62. Ohtomo K, Itai Y, Ohtomo Y, *et al* Regenerating nodules of liver cirrhosis: MR imaging with pathologic correlation. *AJR* 1990;**154**:505-507

63. Sheu JC, Chen DS, Sung JL, *et al* Hepatocellular carcinoma: US evolution in the early state. *Radiology* 1985;**154**:463-467

64. Cottone M, Marcino MP, Maringhini A, *et al* Ultrasound in the diagnosis of hepatocellular carcinoma associated with cirrhosis. *Radiology* 1983;**147**:517-519

65. Okuda K, Musha H, Nakajima Y, *et al* Clinicopathologic features of encapsulated hepatocellular carcinoma: a study of 26 cases. *Cancer* 1977;**40**:1240-1245

66. Yoshida T, Matsue H, Okazaki N, *et al* Ultrasonographic differentiation of hepatocellular carcinoma from metastatic liver tumor. *J Clin Ultrasound* 1987;**15**:431-437

67. Taylor KJW, Ramos I, Carter D, Morse SS, Snower D, Fortune K. Correlation of Doppler US tumor signals with neovascular morphologic features. *Radiology* 1988;**166**:57-62

68. Tanaka S, Kitamura T, Fujita M, Nakanishi K, Okuda S. Color Doppler flow imaging of liver tumors. *AJR* 1990;**154** :509-514

69. Matsuda Y, Yabuuchi I. Hepatic tumors: US contrast enhancement with CO_2 microbubbles. *Radiology* 1986;**161**:701-705

70. Itai Y, Nishikawa J, Tasaka A. Computed tomography in the evaluation of hepatocellular carcinoma. *Radiology* 1979; **131**:165-170

71. Moss AA, Schrumpf J, Schnyder P, Korobkin M, Shimshak RR. Computed tomography of focal hepatic lesions: a blind clinical evaluation of the effect of contrast enhancement. *Radiology* 1979;**131**:427-430

72. Itai Y, Ohtomo K, Kokubo T, *et al* CT of hepatic masses: significance of prolonged and delayed enhancement. *AJR* 1986;**146**:729-733

73. Araki T, Itai Y, Furui S, Tasaka A. Dynamic CT densitometry of hepatic tumors. AJR 1980;**135**:1037-1043

74. Ebara M, Ohto M, Watanabe Y, *et al* Diagnosis of small hepatocellular carcinoma: correlation of MR imaging and histologic studies. *Radiology* 1986;**159**:371-377

75. Yoshikawa J, Matsui O, Takashima T, *et al* Fatty metamorphosis in hepatocellular carcinoma: radiologic features in 10 cases. *AJR* 1988;**151**:717-720

76. Stevens WR, Johnson CD, Stephens DH, Batts KP. CT findings in hepatocellular carcinoma: correlation of tumor characteristics with causative factors, tumor size, and histologic tumor grade. *Radiology* 1994;**191**:531-537

77. Freeny PC, Marks WM. Computed tomographic arteriography of the liver. *Radiology* 1983;**148**:193-197

78. Choi BI, Kim HC, Han JK, *et al* Therapeutic effect of transcatheter oily chemoembolization therapy for encapsulated nodular hepatocellular carcinoma: CT and pathologic findings. *Radiology* 1992;**182**:709-713

79. Itoh K, Nishimura K, Togashi K, *et al* Hepatocellular carcinoma: MR imaging. *Radiology* 1987;**164**:21-25

80. Choi BI, Lee GK, Kim ST, Han MC. Mosaic pattern of encapsulated hepatocellular carcinoma: correlation of magnetic resonance imaging and pathology. *Gastrointest Radiol* 1990; **15**:238-240

81. Brown JJ, Lee JM, Lee JKT, Lom KJV, Malchow SC. Focal hepatic lesions: differentiation with MR imaging at 0.5 T. *Radiology* 1991;**179**:675-679

82. Martin J, Sentis M, Zidan A, *et al*. Fatty metamorphosis of hepatocellular carcinoma: detection with chemical shift gradient-echo MR imaging. *Radiology* 1995;**195**:125-130

83. Rosenthal RE, Davis PL. MR imaging of hepatocellular carcinoma at 1.5 tesla. *Gastrointest Radiol* 1992;**17**:49-52

84. Ebara M, Watanabe S, Kita K, *et al* MR imaging of small hepatocellular carcinoma: effect of intratumoral copper content on signal intensity. *Radiology* 1991;**180**:617-621

85. Kitagawa K, Matsui O, Kadoya M, *et al* Hepatocellular carcinomas with excessive copper accumulation: CT and MR findings. *Radiology* 1991;**180**:623-628

86. Weinmann HJ, Brasch RC, Press WR, *et al* Characteristics of gadolinium-DTPA complex: a potential NMR contrast agent. *AJR* 1984;**142**:619-624

87. Ohtomo K, Itai Y, Yoshikawa K, *et al* Hepatic tumors: dynamic MR imaging. *Radiology* 1987;**163**:27-31

88. Tanaka S, Kitamura T, Fujita M, Kasugai H, Inoue A, Ishiguro S. Small hepatocellular carcinoma: differentiation from adenomatous hyperplastic nodule with color Doppler flow imaging. *Radiology* 1992;**182**:161-165

89. Edmondson HA, Steiner PE. Primary carcinoma of liver: study of 100 cases among 48,900 necropsies. *Cancer* 1954;**7**:462-503

90. Watanabe H, Hirohashi S, Sakamoto M, *et al* New macroscopic subtype of small hepatocellular carcinoma-common type in early type-and histological consideration of the multistep progression of HCC [in Japanese]. Kanzo 1990;**31**:1267-1273

91. Laberge JM, Laing FC, Federle MP, Jeffrey RB Jr, Lim RC. Hepatocellular carcinoma: assessment of resectability by computed tomography and ultrasound. *Radiology* 1984;**152**:485-490

92. Ferrucci JT. Liver tumor imaging: current concepts. *Radiol Clin North Am* 1994;**32**:39-54

93. Makuuchi M, Hasegawa H, Yamazaki S. Intraoperative ultrasonic examination for liver surgery and new concepts in partial hepatectomy [in Japanese]. *Gekachiryo* 1981;**44**:579-586

17

Laparoscopy

L Buscarini and E Buscarini

Laparoscopy allows examination of a large part of the liver: however, the posterior segments are not visible. A lesion deeply located in the right lobe (obviously invisible) can be detected by palpation with a sonde. However, in the past, the application of laparoscopy to the diagnosis of hepatocellular carcinoma (HCC) has not been large because of the lack of any laboratory or imaging element to detect the tumor. The technique, being an invasive one, is not acceptable as a screening method. Large series of laparoscopies have included a small number of HCCs (120 cases out of 6000 laparoscopies).[1] The use of modern imaging techniques has reduced the need for laparoscopic examination, particularly for the detection of liver tumors, even though in Italy[2] the percentage of laparoscopies performed to diagnose primary malignant tumor of the liver was the same in the period 1973-74 (3%) and 1980-1981 (3.9%), that is before and after the introduction of US. The ability to obtain a tissue sample or a cell sample by US guided biopsy, after an initial period where laparoscopy was employed to validate the procedure, has further lowered the number of laparoscopies for HCC diagnosis.[3]

Laparoscopy can supplement US examination but its detection rate for HCC is less than that of US[4] (Table 17.1). In a series of 174 patients with HCC, the sensitivity of laparoscopy was found to be 69.5% (46 examinations) while sensitivity of US carried out in all patients was 98%.[5] However, the combination of US, US guided biopsy and laparoscopy represents the most efficient diagnostic tool for nodular pathology of the liver: in 20 patients with HCC 13 were diagnosed by laparoscopy; 17 by fine needle biospsy (FNB); and all 20 by the combination of both techniques.[6]

Table 17.1 – Detection rate of laparoscopy and US in 54 patients with HCC.[3]

Laparoscopy	Ultrasonography	
	single tumor	multiple tumors
No tumor	5	5
Single tumor	15	8
Multiple tumors	7	14

Table 17.2 – Distribution of 42 laparoscopies according to the indication.[10]

Indications	Number of laparoscopies
First diagnosis	8
Correction of false negatives of US-guided FNB	6
Check of true positives of US guided FNB *	13
Presurgical staging	15

* This indication pertained to the first period after introduction of US guided FNB.

INDICATIONS

The indications for laparoscopy can be summarized as follows:

1. diagnosis: if the mass lesion is superficially located and the result of imaging techniques is not definitive; or if there is a lack of correlation between the imaging and/or biopsy findings and the clinical condition. Sometimes, for particular histological features, the material obtained by a fine needle can be inadequate. In these cases, if the lesion is superficial, the use of a large needle is more advisable under laparoscopic control. As laparoscopic biopsy samples under direct vision, postbioptic bleeding can be monitored and stopped by inserting a fibrin cartridge in the bioptic hole or by using electrocautery.

2. in cases in a therapeutic program, laparoscopic examination is advisable to detect the presence of cirrhosis; to detect other nodules at the liver surface which are missed by other imaging techniques; to identify extrahepatic spread namely peritoneal and diaphragmatic metastases which are easily identified by laparoscopic examination, unlike with US or CT.[7,8] As such laparoscopy can be very useful as a preliminary step to liver transplantation. A staging laparotomy is not advisable, because the surgical mortality of OLT is higher in patients who have undergone such an operation.[9]

In a consecutive series of 157 patients with HCC diagnosed from 1982 to 1988 (by using either imaging techniques or US-guided FNB), laparoscopy was performed in 42 cases.[10] The indications are summarized in Table 17.2.

In the above applications, laparoscopy can be of a great importance, avoiding unnecessary delay in diagnosis and eliminating dangerous laparotomy. [11]

TECHNIQUE

Diagnostic laparoscopy is usually performed under local anesthesia. The introduction of the laparoscope requires a previous abdominal insufflation with carbon dioxide in order to create a real space for the examination. A direct view through the laparoscope is possible but a videocamera adapted to the eye-piece of the laparoscope projects the images of the explored field on the monitor. This practice solves sterility problems, enabling the co-worker to participate in the manoeuver and facilitating teaching.

For a methodic examination of the superior surface of the liver, the laparoscopic bed is basculated on the right to better explore the left portion of the left lobe and in turn, on the left, to examine the lateral part of the right lobe. In the Vanti-Trendelenburg position the liver dome can be well explored. The inferior surface of the liver has to be raised by a sonde (introduced through the channel of the operative laparoscope or through a second entrance), tract by tract in order to perform a complete examination of this part of the liver. The sonde moreover allows the presence of a hard zone under the surface to be detected and this can correspond to a mass lesion. The examination should be recorded, so it is possible to review the images whenever needed. For more detailed documentation still photographs can be taken.

Liver biopsy is carried out through the channel of the operative laparoscope; the needle is directed on the prefixed point and then the biopsy is taken. For laparoscopic biopsy, large needles are generally used, either tru-cut or Menghini needles. However, the use of cytologic sampling, under laparoscopic control, has been shown to be effective for the diagnosis of HCC.[12,13]

The advantages of laparoscopic biopsy are: the needle obviously avoids any superficial vessel (which in cirrhotic livers can be represented by large superficial varices); the sampling is adequate and the biopsy can be easily repeated if no heavy bleeding follows the first sampling. If bleeding persists, it is possible to stop the bleeding by a simple compression using the sonde, or by inserting a fibrin cartridge or by using electrocautery. The fibrin cartridge can be observed by US at the end of laparoscopy: it appears as a thick hyperechoic line and its detection can mark the site biopsied.

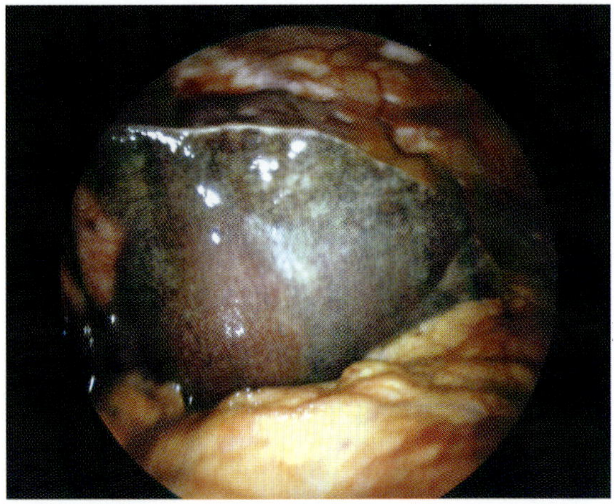

Figure 17. 1 - HCC in non cirrhotic liver. The tumor bulges into the inferior surface of the liver; the color is due to bile retention. Parietal peritoneum shows minute gray nodules of metastatic origin.

LAPAROSCOPIC FINDINGS

HCC without cirrhosis: in western and far eastern countries, HCC can infrequently arise in non cirrhotic livers. The tumor, if superficially located, can appear as a nodule of a different color or as a plaque. In some cases, it is possible to find multiple nodules bulging from the surface of the liver. When the tumor is deeply located, the presence of HCC can be suspected by observing a simple modification of the surface convexity (Fig 17.1). The tumor can diffusely infiltrate the liver. Generally HCC in normal liver is recognized when the disease is advanced (apart from accidental discovery); in these situations, imaging techniques easily identify the tumor. The use of laparoscopy is advised to correct a false negative US-guided biopsy or for pre-treatment staging. The presence of metastases on parietal peritoneum is easily detected as minute gray or whitish nodules (Fig 17.1).

In HCC in cirrhotics liver volume is generally enlarged. Laparoscopy can show the presence of cirrhosis, by simple inspection of the surface, identifying micronodular, macronodular or mixed nodularity forms. Moreover laparoscopy can assess the presence

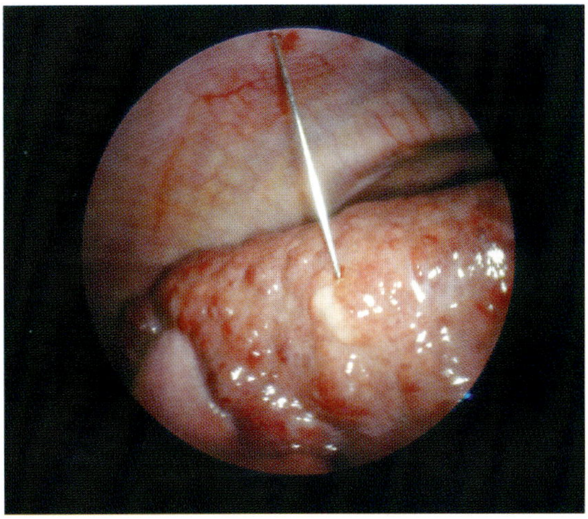

Figure 17.2 - Micronodular cirrhosis. A very minute yellow nodule is visible on the right lobe near the needle tip. Biopsy showed HCC (occasional diagnosis).

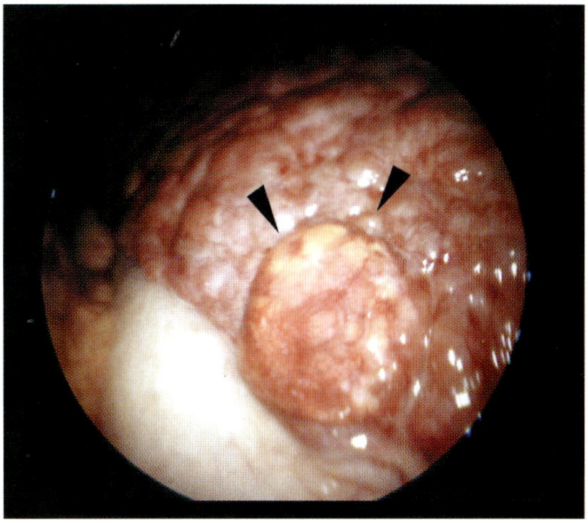

Figure 17.3 - A nodule of 3 cm bulges on the surface in a cirrhotic liver (right lobe); the surface of the nodule is quite similar to that of surrounding liver

of portal hypertension, identifying the presence of varices on the liver surface; recognizing a patent umbilical vein; evaluating the vascular system of parietal peritoneum, stomach, colon, omentum, gallbladder. The occurrence of hemorrhagic ascites in cirrhotic patient strongly suggests the presence of HCC.

HCC can be detected in very early phase as a minute yellow nodule, maintaining the same volume as the surrounding nodules (Fig. 17.2). In these cases only laparoscopic examination can allow identification, and offer the possibility of sampling. These lesions show histologic evidence of fatty change, in some cases presenting histologic features of borderline lesions. In a series of 22 patients (10 with HCC and 12 with borderline lesions) with the laparoscopic finding of a minute yellow nodule, the tumor was detected by US in only 5 cases.[14] This aspect however, is not specific because small foci of fatty infiltration, granulomas, hamartomas and metastases can have an identical appearance.

Usually the tumor presents as a small (2-3 cm in diameter), medium sized or large nodule bulging from the surface (Fig. 17.3), which can maintain the same aspect as the surrounding liver (in this case a certain macroscopic diagnosis is impossible) or it can appear with different aspects and colors with green areas due to accumulation of bile pigments, and red

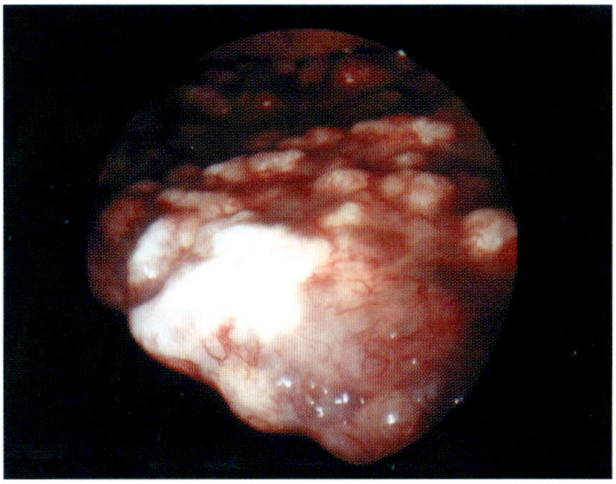

Figure 17.4 - The surface of the liver presents many gray-yellow nodules 1 cm in diameter; near the margin a gray tumoral plaque is evident.

nodules due to the presence of hemorrhagic foci. The tumor can present an abnormal vascularity over all of its surface or can be bordered by a ring of irregular caliber and tortuous vessels or appear as a reddish-yellowish hemispherical nodule with mildly increased vascularity.[15] The tumor can present gray areas as expressions of necrosis, but as the growth of HCC is generally slow, a mass with a central crater is really uncommon, being more characteristic of liver metastases. In some cases the tumor is multinodular, the nodules being identical (Fig. 17.4).

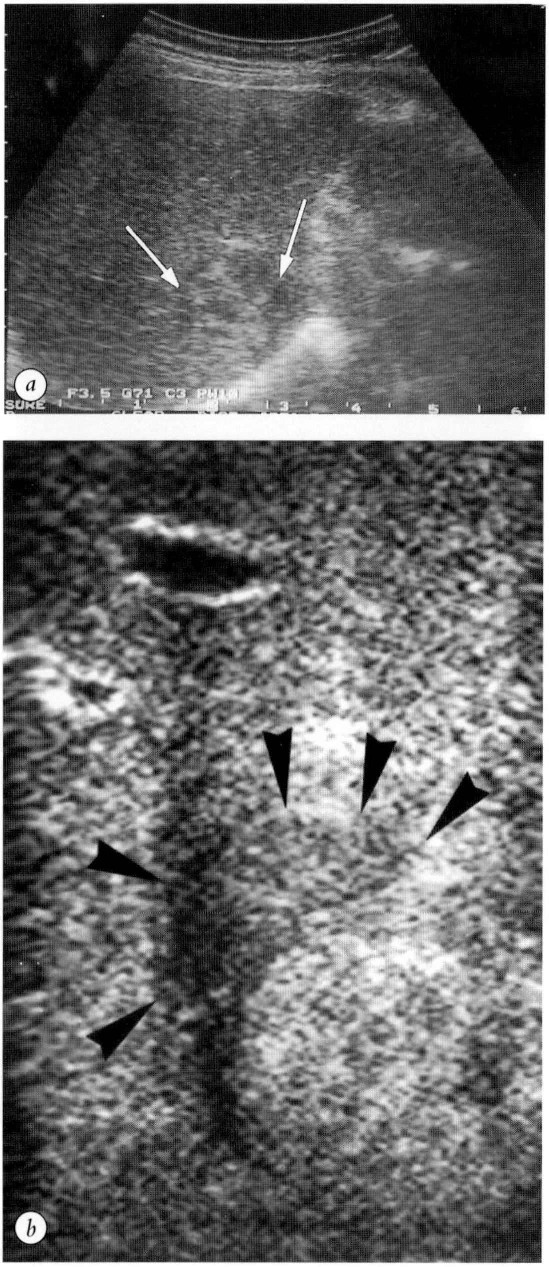

Figure 17.5 –

a) US shows a 3 cms nodule with mixed echopattern and poorly demarcated boundary (arrows).

b) Laparoscopic-US demonstrates a capsular disruption with an hypoechoic nodule (arrowheads) growing from the hyperechoic main nodule.

Dysplastic nodules (according to a new classification[16]) can have the same aspect as HCC and the exclusion of malignancy requires biopsy. However even the histologic diagnosis is very difficult either because the bioptic sampling involves only a small part of the tumor or due to the difficulty of histologic examination.[17]

Complications

Laparoscopic complications can arise from performing the pneumoperitoneum, the entrance of the trocar and finally for biopsy. The complication rate is very low. Tumoral seeding at the incision site of the trocar has been described after laparoscopy in a patient with HCC.[18]

LAPAROSCOPIC SONOGRAPHY

The use of US laparoscopy for staging of HCC has been proposed.[19,20] These preliminary experiences were gained using sector scanning prototypes. Now some sonographic 5-7.5 MHz frequency probes (linear, convex or sector) are commercially available. The tip of the probe is flexible, allowing better exploration.

The technique requires the introduction of the laparoscope above the umbilicus or 2-3 cm to the left and, under laparoscopic control, the introduction of a second trocar (5-6 cm to the right of the umbilicus up to the right anterior axillary line) for insertion of the sonographic probe. To complete a detailed exploration of the liver, the entrance site of the laparoscope and sonographic probe must be interchanged.

Liver exploration is performed by obtaining a strict contact between the sonographic probe and liver surface; the contact is facilitated by probe flexibility. The exploration, as described for the laparoscopic exam, is performed tract by tract by longitudinal and oblique scans. The exploration of the posterior segments can be performed by locating the probe in the subdiaphragmatic zone and moving it from the right to the left up to the falciform ligament. A crucial phase of the exploration is the identification of the portal pedicle and its branches, hepatic veins and biliary tree. The hepatic hilum exploration is performed by placing the probe laterally to the falciform ligament with longitudinal scan and moving the probe the full range of its movement (about 180°). In this way it is possible to identify hepatic veins, portal pedicle and common bile duct. Laparoscopic exploration in some instances can be completed by placing the probe in the inferior liver surface. Any movement of the probe must be performed gently and under continuous and steady laparoscopic control.

The main indication for US laparoscopy in HCC is pretherapeutic staging which is particularly important when the therapeutic program has a curative intent, independent of the type of treatment.[21] In the evaluation of patients with primary liver cancer laparoscopic sonography shows vascular involvement or intrahepatic metastases or diaphragmatic metastases, indicating if the tumor is not resectable.[22] In any case, any laparoscopic exam performed in an oncologic context should be completed by laparoscopic US. In this way an invasive technique (laparoscopy) will be utilized to its fullest potential.

The detection rate of laparoscopic sonography is very high, similar to intraoperative sonography, but up to now there have been no comparative studies between laparoscopic sonography,[23]and conventional US. Some important features such as disruption of the hypoechoic halo and presence of microsatellites, are very easily identified (Fig. 17.5). The possibility of combining use of the probe with echo-color Doppler will improve the study of venous involvement.

Characteristics of HCC are the same as those found with conventional US examination: small tumors appear generally hypoechoic and large tumors tend to appear as an hyperechoic mass or show a mixed echopattern. Some of the small HCCs show an increased echointensity without histologic signs of fatty change.[24] Laparoscopic ultrasonography moreover can correct some false positive diagnoses made by US.[19] Finally laparoscopic ultrasonography guided procedures allow biopsy to achieve pathologic diagnosis[19,25]and ethanol injection to treat, in selected cases, nonresectable lesions.[26]

REFERENCES

1. Dagnini G. *La laparoscopia*.1978 Padova: Piccin.
2. Gandolfi L, Rossi A, Leo P, Solmi L, Muratori R. Indications for laparoscopy before and after the introduction of ultrasonography. *Gastrointest Endosc* 1985; **31**: 1-3
3. Buscarini L, Sbolli G, Civardi G *et al.* Does ultrasonically guided biopsy modify indications to laparoscopy in hepatology? *Acta Endoscop* 1987; **17**: 85-88
4. Gandolfi L, Muratori R, Solmi L, Rossi A, Leo P. Laparoscopy compared with ultrasonography in the diagnosis of hepatocellular carcinoma. *Gastrointest Endosc* 1989; **35**: 508:511
5. Buscarini L, Fornari F, Canaletti R *et al.* Diagnostic aspects and follow-up of 174 cases of hepatocellular carcinoma. Second report. *Oncology* 1991; **48**: 26-30
6. Fornari F, Rapaccini GL, Cavanna L *et al.* Diagnosis of hepatic lesions: ultrasonically guided fine needle biopsy or laparoscopy? *Gastrointest Endosc* 1988; **34**: 231-234
7. Easter DW, Cuschieri A, Nathanson LK, Lavelle-Jones M. The utility of diagnostic laparoscopy for abdominal disorders. Audit of 120 patients. *Arch Surg* 1992; **127**: 379-383
8. Lightdale CJ. Laparoscopy for cancer staging. *Endoscopy* 1992; **24**: 682-686
9. McPeake JR, O'Grady JG, Zaman S *et al.* Liver transplantation for primary hepatocellular carcinoma: tumour size and number determine outcome. *J Hepatol* 1993; **18**: 226-234.
10. Buscarini L, Sbolli G, Civardi G, Cavanna L, Di Stasi M, Fornari F. Actual role of laparoscopy for diagnosis of hepatocellular carcinoma. *Acta Endoscop* 1989; **19**: 261-268.
11. Buscarini L, Di Stasi M, Buscarini E *et al.* Clinical presentation, diagnostic work-up and therapeutic choices in two consecutive series of patients with hepatocellular carcinoma. *Oncology* 1996;**53**:204-209
12. Jeffers L, Spiegiman G, Reddy R *et al.* Laparoscopically directed fine needle aspiration for the diagnosis of hepatocellular carcinoma: a safe and accurate technique. *Gastrointest Endosc* 1988; **34**: 235-237
13. Cussò X, Marti-Vicente A, Monés-Xiol J, Vilardell F. Laparoscopic cytology - an evaluation. *Endoscopy* 1988; **20**: 102-103
14. Kameda Y, Shinji Y. Early detection of hepatocellular carcinoma by laparoscopy: yellow nodules as diagnostic indicators. *Gastrointest Endosc* 1992; **38**: 554-559
15. Chen DS, Sheu JC, Sung JL *et al.* Small hepatocellular carcinoma - A clinicopathological study in thirteen patients. *Gastroenterology* 1982; **83**: 1109-1119
16. Summary of recommendations developed by an international working party, supported by the World Congress of Gastroenterology, Los Angeles 1994. Terminology of chronic hepatitis, hepatic allograft rejection, and nodular lesions of the liver. *Am J Gastroenterol* 1994; **89:**5177-5181
17. Buscarini L, Fornari F, Cavanna L. Diagnostic problem of hyperplastic regenerative nodule in cirrhotic liver. *Acta Endoscop* 1987; **17**: 233-239
18. Ishida H, Dohzono T, Furukawa Y, Kobayashi M, Tsuneoka K. Laparoscopy and biopsy in the diagnosis of malignant intra-abdominal tumors. *Endoscopy* 1984; **16**: 140-142
19. Okita K, Kodama T, Oda M, Takemoto T. Laparoscopic ultrasonography. Diagnosis of liver and pancreatic cancer. *Scand J Gastroenterol* 1994; **19** (suppl 94): 91-100
20. Fornari F, Civardi G, Cavanna L *et al.* Laparoscopic ultrasonography in the study of liver diseases. *Surg Endosc* 1989; **3**: 33-37
21. McIntyre RC, Stiegman GV, Pearlman NW. Update on laparoscopic ultrasonography. *Endosc Surg* 1994; **2**: 149-152

22. Cuesta MA, Meijer S, Borgstein PJ, Sibinga Mulder L, Sikkenk AC. Laparoscopic ultrasonography for hepatobiliary and pancreatic malignancy. *Br J Surg* 1993; **80**: 1571-1574

23. Baron RL. Detection of liver neoplasms: techniques and outcomes. *Abdom Imaging* 1994; **19**: 320-324

24. Fukuda M, Hirata K, Mima S. Preliminary evaluation of sonolaparoscopy in the diagnosis of liver diseases. *Endoscopy* 1992; **24**: 701-708.

25. Bonhof JA, Linhart P, Bettendorf U, Holper H. Liver biopsy by laparoscopic sonography. A case report demonstrating a new technique. *Endoscopy* 1984; **16**: 237-239

26. Cavina E, Goletti O, Buccianti P. Echolaparoscopy: an indispensable procedure for laparoscopic surgery. *Endosc Surg* 1994; **2**: 143-148.

18

Computer assisted image management

C Bartolozzi, D Caramella and R Lencioni

Screening programs for early detection of HCC in patients with chronic liver disease have been established in several institutions.[1,2] These programs involve the acquisition, storage and management of large number of image and amounts of text data, that require the use of information management systems.[3-5]

Radiologic information systems, that are available in almost every hospital, are inadequate for assisting in this task since only demographic data and examination reports can be managed. The lack of integration with digital image archives and clinical data such as those concerning hepatic function serum indices and tumor markers reduces the usefulness of this type of system. Such limitations appear even greater when a diagnosis of HCC is suspected and consequently additional data concerning imaging studies and pathological results of biopsy specimens must be entered into the system.

When a nonsurgical treatment strategy is selected, the input of information is particularly relevant and complex, as data from several sources must be obtained and carefully integrated in order to support the decision-making process. At the end of treatment imaging studies are performed to indefinitely monitor patients for early detection of tumor recurrences. In fact, close follow-up can never be suspended in patients with HCC as the risk of developing new lesions actually increases with time.[6-8] This peculiarity further stresses the information management system in that it requires large storage capacity and long-term consistency. In order to efficiently manage the information that is produced over this very long time-frame, centers that are following a large number of patients frequently rely on computer-assisted systems for comprehensive management of the relevant data.[9,10]

Such systems are required to provide an homogeneous environment for integrating clinical and radiological data, no matter if they are produced and stored in different locations, and to make them available at the right time to the physician that has to make the clinical decision. In particular, data concerning all previous diagnostic and therapeutic steps must be accessible to ensure correct management of the patient.

PATIENT MANAGEMENT AT THE UNIVERSITY OF PISA

At our institution, a full-scale screening program for early detection of HCC was started in January 1991. To be enrolled in this program, patients are required to have histologic confirmation of chronic liver disease. Patients with liver cirrhosis undergo US examinations and AFP level measurements at 4-6 month intervals, whereas those with chronic hepatitis are examined every 12 months.

When a nodular lesion is depicted at US, US-guided FNB is performed to enable histologic diagnosis.[11] Patients with histologically proven HCC undergo full clinical assessment and are further studied with color Doppler US, CT, and MR[12,13] to accurately define the extent of the tumor and establish eligibility for surgical or nonsurgical therapies, such as TAE, PEI and combined TAE and PEI, following standardized criteria adopted at our institution.[14-16]

The outcome of treatment is checked by AFP level measurement, color Doppler US, and CT or MR.[17-23] In the case of persistent tumor after treatment, additional therapeutic sessions are performed and the response to therapy is again verified with repeated AFP level measurement, color Doppler US, and CT or MR. The follow-up schedule includes US, color Doppler US, and AFP level measurement at 3-4 month intervals, and CT or MR at 6-8 month intervals. Clinical assessment is routinely performed every 3-4 months, if clinical status does not require more frequent evaluations or hospitalization.

The general scheme for patient recruitment entails three different criteria:

a) patients in whom screening, diagnosis, staging, therapy, and follow-up are all performed at the University of Pisa;

b) patients in whom screening and diagnosis are performed in affiliated hospitals, while staging, therapy, and follow-up are carried out at the University of Pisa;

c) patients in whom screening and diagnosis are performed in affiliated hospitals, while staging, therapy, and follow-up are shared between the affiliated hospitals and the University of Pisa.

Overall, in the last 5 years nearly 1,000 new cases of HCC were diagnosed at our institution or affiliated hospitals and more than 600 patients were enrolled for interventional treatment protocols.

INFORMATION FLOW

To illustrate the information generation and flow concerning the diagnostic and therapeutic management of HCC patients, let us consider the example of a patient in whom a 5 cm nodule is detected during a screening US examination.

Six to 10 US images (corresponding to 1.5-2.5 MByte) are usually sufficient to demonstrate the anatomic location of the lesion, the relationship between the lesion and the main vascular structures of the liver, and the characteristics of the lesion at grayscale and color Doppler US. The documentation of the FNB procedure may require two additional US images (corresponding to 0.5 MByte).

If HCC is pathologically confirmed, unenhanced and double-phase contrast-enhanced spiral CT or unenhanced and contrast-enhanced dynamic MR are done to further define the characteristics of the lesion, i.e. presence of tumor capsule, vascular invasion, or intrahepatic metastatic nodules. For that purpose, after selection of the most relevant images, the data that have to be stored may be limited to 6-12 MByte (12-18 CT images or 16-24 MR images).

In the case of an uninodular encapsulated tumor 5 cm in diameter, performing a single TAE session followed by PEI may be an appropriate treatment schedule.[15,24,25] The TAE session includes a preliminary angiographic study of the liver (6 angiographic images, corresponding to 1.5 MByte), catheterization of the segmental or subsegmental arteries feeding the tumor bearing area (4 angiographic images, corresponding to 1 MByte), injection of the anticancer-in-oil emulsion and embolic material, and a post-procedure angiographic control (4 angiographic images, corresponding to 1 MByte). Evaluation of the response to TAE includes repeated spiral CT or MR images with use of unenhanced and contrast-enhanced studies (again, no less than 6-10 MByte of image data must be selected for permanent storage). Completion of treatment with PEI is usually obtained in 6-8 sessions that require the acquisition of 36-48 gray scale and color Doppler US images (9-12 MByte). Final assessment of the outcome of combined TAE and PEI necessitates repeated unenhanced and contrast-enhanced spiral CT or unenhanced and contrast-enhanced dynamic MR (6-10 additional MByte of image data).

Summing up, in this example, in which complete response to therapy was assumed (no need for additional diagnostic or therapeutic procedures), the overall amount of image data may range between 32.5 and 50.5 MByte. Of course, 18-30 additional MByte/year are required for subsequent follow-up examinations (US and color Doppler US at 3-month intervals, and CT or MR at 6-month intervals). Therefore, without considering the input of text data (e.g. clinical and laboratory data, pathological and radiological reports, etc.), that do not require significant disk space, in this example up to about 50 MByte of image data may be necessary for documenting the diagnosis and treatment of a single lesion in a single patient.

SYSTEM REQUIREMENTS

A full scale hospital-wide picture archiving and communication system is certainly able to meet the requirements of the information generation and distribution process that has been described. However, such systems are relatively limited in number and their high cost prevents their widespread use outside selected university settings.[26, 27]

Therefore, for many institutions it may be more attractive to implement a small scale system specifically built for managing the data that are produced in the peculiar clinical scenario of the diagnosis and treatment of patients with HCC. If this solution is chosen, and a dedicated system for HCC is implemented, another strategic decision has to be made concerning the type of data transmission. Offline media, such as digital optical cards or magneto-optical disks may be used as a personal image and data repository that is kept under the direct responsibility of the patient.[28, 29]

As an alternative, networked systems may be installed at a higher cost, but also with better security and ready availability of data. Moreover, networked systems allow the exchange of information among physicians without requiring the actual presence of the patient. The extension of the network must vary to fit the needs of a single hospital (local area network), a more complex and distributed hospital institution (metropolitan area network), or a main central hospital having several affiliated hospitals that cooperatively manage patients with HCC (wide area network).[30-32]

In all cases images and data have to be entered into the system: for demographic and clinical data, integration with the radiology and hospital information systems must be foreseen. For image acquisition, secondary capture should be considered only when a direct digital acquisition according to the DICOM standard cannot be implemented.[33, 34]

The type of information exchange supported by the system must be appropriate to the needs of different physicians who are involved at different times and who undertake different roles in the clinical management of HCC patients and may be one of two types. On one hand, the system may provide an asynchronous information exchange, based on the mailbox metaphor: the data are sent now to be retrieved later by the receiver at his or her convenience.[35] On the other hand, interactive information exchange requires the simultaneous presence of all the interlocutors, with a more natural dialog but with the organizational disadvantage of requiring coordination of different physicians' time-schedules.

DATA MANAGEMENT AT THE UNIVERSITY OF PISA

The Department of Radiology of the University of Pisa is divided in two main radiological units: the first located in Santa Chiara Hospital, and the second in Cisanello Hospital, which are about 6 km apart. The two radiological units have different functional specializations: in Santa Chiara Hospital conventional radiographic examinations, angiographic procedures (including TAE), US and color Doppler US examinations, and US-guided interventional procedures (FNB, PEI) are performed. In Cisanello Hospital, spiral CT and MR examinations are performed. In each of the two units an Ethernet local area network for the acquisition and local management of diagnostic images has been installed. The two local area networks are connected by a metropolitan area network that was implemented in the framework of a national project.

The integrated system that we are using for intrainstitutional information exchange is based on a standard UNIX platform and on a software application enabling the import of images acquired with CT, MR, US, color Doppler US, and angiography, and to encapsulate them in multimedia messages for asynchronous as well as interactive communication (Figs 18.1, 2). The system allows a communication similar to a multimedia mail service: it is possible to send text, images, digitized voice and video recording of operations. The radiologist receiving the message can visualize the text and image information as well as replay the recorded operations and hear the attached vocal comment.

Recently, we investigated the cost-effectiveness of the intrainstitutional information exchange used by diagnostic and interventional radiologists involved in the management of HCC and operating in the two sites of our Department.[36] To assess the cost-effectiveness of intrainstitutional teleradiology, a comparison was made between the costs of one-year utilization of the system and the savings with respect to a conventional environment (costs of film production, film handling and transportation, and personnel costs).

The cost of the workstations was calculated as follows: acquisition cost, divided by the utilization rate and by the yearly depreciation rate. Since the two workstations were not only used for intrainstitutional teleradiology, but also for remote expert consultation and for Internet access, 33% utilization rate was assumed. Moreover, considering the rapid obsolescence of electronic equipment, a 25% yearly depreciation rate was assumed. Using this method, yearly hardware cost for the intrainstitutional teleradiology application were one twelfth of the initial cost of the two workstations, that is 2,600 ECU ($3,460).

In the one-year period that we considered for this study, the system was used 156 times, with an overall amount of transmitted data of 250 MByte, corresponding to a mean amount of transmitted information per session of 1.7 MByte (this relatively low amount of digital data is due to the fact that both lossless and clinical compression were always used). In

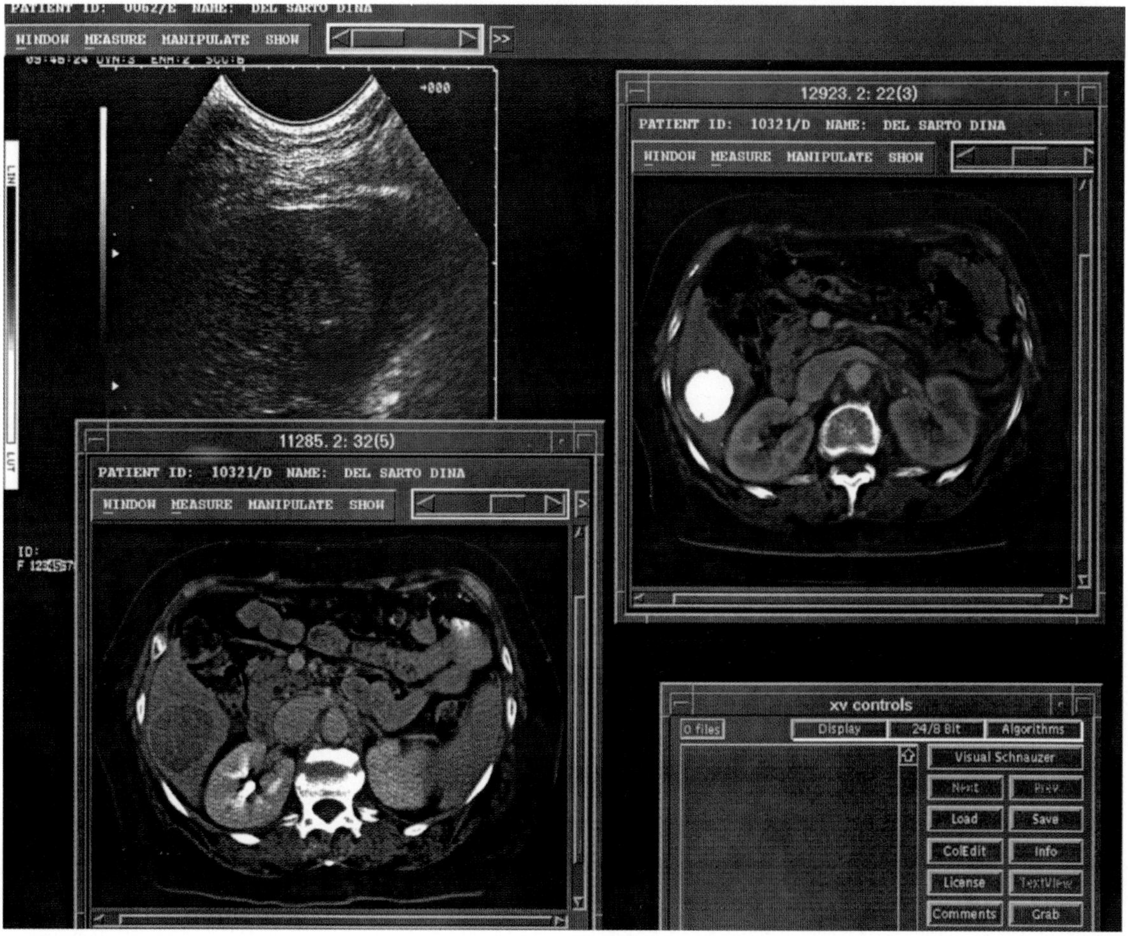

Figure 18.1 – Computer-assisted image management system. Display of a multimedia message showing the US-guided FNB image (top left), the pretreatment CT (bottom left) and the post-treatment CT after Lipiodol-TAE (right). The window on the bottom right of the screen contains commands for image visualization and processing.

our case, the network was available at no cost, because the link was provided within the framework of a national project. However, assuming a cost of 2.5 ECU ($3.3)/MByte, the transmission cost can be estimated in 625 ECU ($825).

Personnel cost is mainly related to the time spent by radiology residents in the training phase, and in the actual operating phase. Overall, the extra time spent by residents for intrainstitutional teleradiology was calculated as being about 1 man hour per session. The corresponding economic value of such activities in the one-year period considered was 1,200 ECU ($1600).

The use of the intrainstitutional teleradiology system avoided printing extra copies, with a consequent estimated saving of about 3 films per session with an overall saving of about 2,200 ECU ($2,920). Savings in terms of film handling and transportation were estimated to be 2 ECU ($2.6)/film with an overall additional saving of 900 ECU ($1,200).

The increased efficiency of image and data communication allowed experienced senior staff to reduce the time needed for consultation of previous images and for reporting. We estimated that time-saving for experienced senior staff was about 20 minutes for

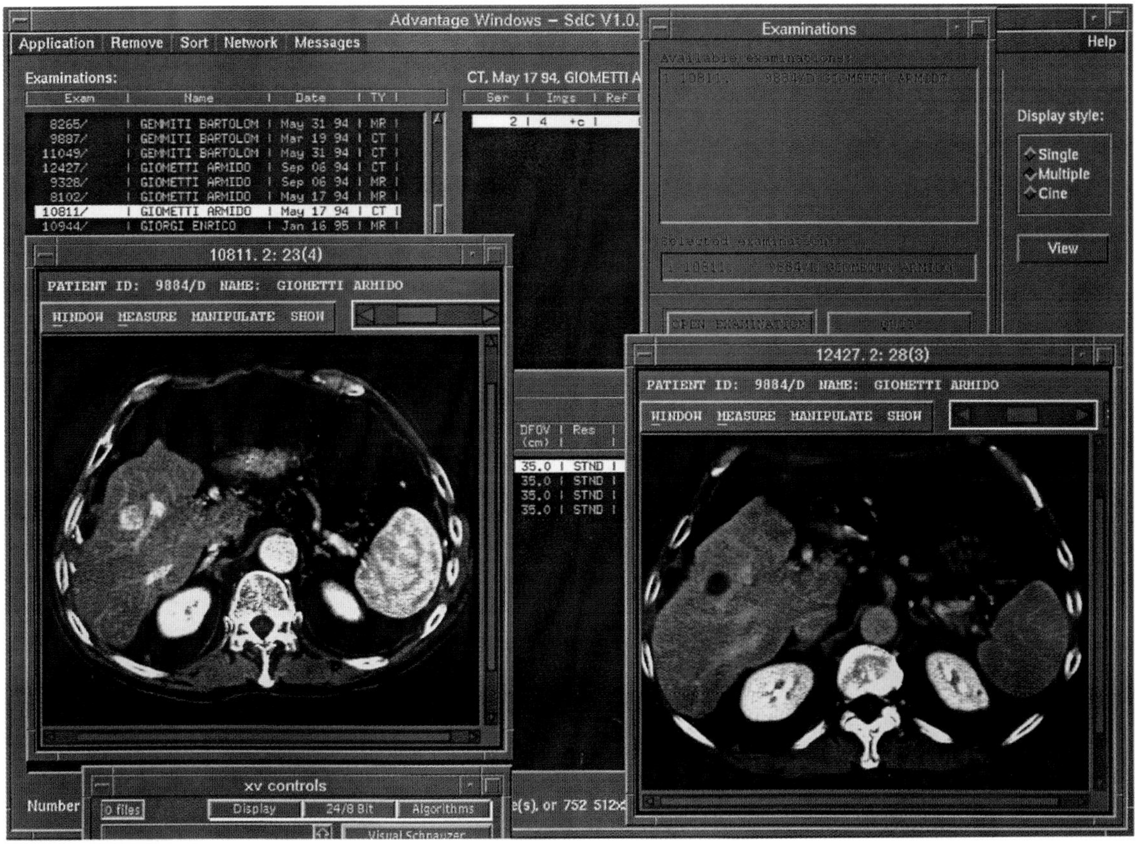

Figure 18.2 – Computer-assisted image management system. Display of a multimedia message including pretreatment CT (left) showing a small HCC, and CT after ablation of the tumor by PEI (right). The window on the top left of the screen contains the database of HCC patients.

each of the teleradiology sessions, corresponding to an economic saving of 1,250 ECU ($1660).

Although in our study overall costs (4,425 ECU) ($5,885) slightly exceeded estimated benefits (4,350 ECU) ($5,780), there are still many indications that cost savings within the health-care sector can be achieved by using telematics. However, all cost-effectiveness assessments should be performed over the long term, so as not to view initial technological cost as totally additional with respect to the conventional management of medicine. Moreover, benefits have to be evaluated from the veiwpoint of all medical institutes and disciplines. In fact, not only the monetary benefits for the department of radiology should be taken into consideration, but also some additional benefit that although not immediately apparent - the so called "hidden benefits" - may have an impact on the patient and on the hospital as a whole.

Organizational benefits include the possibility of sharing a common archive, with a distributed access and update of the clinical and radiologic data. Moreover, the accurate selection of the relevant images reduces the need for retrieving large number of images. There are also important benefits with regard to patient management. In fact the patient is not required to take care of any logistical problem concerning the keeping of medical records and radiologic images. At the same time, the patient's perception is of a highly organized group, that works as a single unit, although operating at two distant sites.

In our opinion, both these elements could explain the very low drop-out rate (less than 3%) in the series of patients included in our HCC program. This is one of the most relevant "hidden" benefits of our computer-assisted image management.

From our experience we concluded that although systems for data and image management cannot be justified solely on the basis of economic benefits, they may nevertheless allow increased intrainstitutional efficiency, requiring only limited additional resources. In particular we believe that such an approach could be usefully inplemented when architectural and logistical problems are present (e.g. a distributed hospital), when homogeneous series of patients require repeated diagnostic and interventional procedures, and when close follow-up of patients is necessary.

Planned evolution of the system

Our system performed well in the initial testing period. There are, however, several features that are being carefully considered to enhance its overall functionality. In particular, full integration with the radiologic information system will be implemented in order to allow the seamless import of data concerning patient demographics and radiologic reports.

A connection with selected clinical wards in the two hospitals is planned to enhance collaboration, but was impaired until now by the lack of a hospital-wide network. This problem should be solved in the near future by the installation of a fiberoptic network in both hospitals, that will still be connected through the metropolitan area network.

Affiliated hospitals have been occasionally reached by using the Internet for sending a small number of images and clinical information. However, a drawback of this transmission modality stemmed from our decision not to include demographic data on the patients in order to protect the confidentiality of the information. It may be expected that in the future better network security will allow the transmission of confidential information over the Internet. As an alternative the use of ISDN lines may be considered for establishing a more stable link between our center and the affiliated hospitals.

An interesting application of our system has been its use for teleconsultation with other centers active in this field. In recent years we have had teleconsultation sessions with the Department of Radiology of the University of Florence and the Department of Radiology of the University of Utrecht. In the future, new connections will be established since we expect this activity may be useful for a more confident diagnosis as well as for the selection of the most appropriate therapeutic strategy in difficult clinical cases. Moreover, the educational value has to be considered of sharing different experiences and approaches for better and more comprehensive patient care.

REFERENCES

1. Colombo M, De Franchis R, Del Ninno E, *et al* Hepatocellular carcinoma in Italian patients with cirrhosis. *N Engl J Med* 1991; **325**: 675-680.
2. Cottone M, Turri M, Caltagirone M, *et al* Screening for hepatocellular carcinoma in patients with Child's A cirrhosis: an 8-year prospective study by ultrasound and alphafetoprotein. *J Hepatol* 1994; **21**: 1029-1034.
3. Caramella D, Lencioni R, Mazzeo S, Bartolozzi C. Transmission of radiological images using broadband communications. *Eur Radiol* 1994; **4**: 377-381.
4. Scherrer JR. Communications: future needs and present solutions. *Int J Biomed Comput* 1995; **39**: 47-52.
5. Breant CM, Taira RK, Huang HK. Interfacing aspects between the picture archiving communications systems, radiology information systems, and hospital information systems. *J Digit Imaging* 1993; **6**: 88-94.
6. Belghiti J, Panis Y, Farges O, Benhamou JP, Fekete F. Intrahepatic recurrence after resection of hepatocellular carcinoma complicating cirrhosis *Ann Surg* 1992; **214**: 114-117.
7. Livraghi T, Giorgio A, Marin G, *et al*. Hepatocellular carcinoma and cirrhosis in 746 patients: long-term results of percutaneous ethanol injection. *Radiology* 1995; **197**: 101-108.
8. Bartolozzi C, Lencioni R. Ethanol injection for the treatment of hepatic tumours. *Eur Radiol* 1996; **6** (in press).
9. Kondoh H, Ikezoe J, Inamura K, Kuroda C, Kozuka T. Developing a new picture archiving and communication system for the new Osaka University Hospital. *J Digit Imaging* 1994; **7**:172-176.
10. Osteaux M, Van den Broek R, Temmerman Y, Wein B. Medical requirements for clinical integration. In: Osteaux M (ed). *A second generation PACS concept*. Berlin: Springer Verlag 1992: 23-43
11. Lencioni R, Caramella D, Bartolozzi C. Percutaneous biopsy of liver tumors with color Doppler US guidance. *Abdom Imag* 1995; **20**: 206-208.
12. Bartolozzi C, Lencioni R, Caramella D, Palla A, Bassi AM, Di Candio G. Small hepatocellular carcinoma: detection with US, CT, MR imaging, DSA, and Lipiodol-CT. *Acta Radiol* 1996; **37**: 69-74.
13. Lencioni R, Mascalchi M, Caramella D, Bartolozzi C. Small hepatocellular carcinoma: differentiation from adenomatous

hyperplasia with color Doppler US and dynamic Gd-DTPA-enhanced MR imaging. *Abdom Imag* 1996; **21**: 41-48.

14. Lencioni R, Vignali C, Caramella D, Cioni R, Mazzeo S, Bartolozzi C. Transcatheter arterial embolization followed by percutaneous ethanol injection in the treatment of hepatocellular carcinoma. *Cardiovasc Intervent Radiol* 1994; **17**: 70-75.
15. Bartolozzi C, Lencioni R, Caramella D, *et al* Treatment of large hepatocellular carcinoma: transcatheter arterial chemoembolization combined with percutaneous ethanol injection versus repeated transcatheter arterial chemoembolization. *Radiology* 1995; **197**: 812-818.
16. Lencioni R, Bartolozzi C, Caramella D, *et al* Treatment of small hepatocellular carcinoma with percutaneous ethanol injection. Analysis of prognostic factors in 105 Western patients. *Cancer* 1995; **76**: 1737-1746.
17. Lencioni R, Caramella D, Sanguinetti F, Battolla L, Falaschi F, Bartolozzi C. Portal vein thrombosis after percutaneous ethanol injection for hepatocellular carcinoma: value of color Doppler sonography in distinguishing chemical and tumor thrombi. *AJR* 1995; **164**: 1125-1130.
18. Lencioni R, Caramella D, Bartolozzi C. Hepatocellular carcinoma: use of color Doppler US to evaluate response to treatment with percutaneous ethanol injection. *Radiology* 1995; **194**: 113-118.
19. Lencioni R, Caramella D, Bartolozzi C. Response of hepatocellular carcinoma to percutaneous ethanol injection: CT and MR evaluation. *J Comput Assist Tomogr* 1993; **17**: 723-729.
20. Bartolozzi C, Lencioni R, Caramella D, Falaschi F, Cioni R, Di Coscio G. Hepatocellular carcinoma: CT and MR features after transcatheter arterial embolization and percutaneous ethanol injection. *Radiology* 1994; **191**: 123-128.
21. Lencioni R, Caramella D, Vignali C, Russo R, Paolicchi A, Bartolozzi C. Lipiodol-TC in the detection of tumor persistence in hepatocellular carcinoma treated with percutaneous ethanol injection therapy. *Acta Radiol* 1994; **35**: 323-328.
22. Bartolozzi C, Lencioni R, Caramella D, Mazzeo S, Ciancia EM. Treatment of hepatocellular carcinoma with percutaneous ethanol injection: evaluation with contrast-enhanced MR imaging. *AJR* 1994; **162**: 827-831.
23. Lencioni R, Mascalchi M, Paolicchi A, Zampa V. Breath-hold spin-echo MR imaging for evaluation of dynamic enhancement of native and treated hepatocellular carcinoma after intravenous Gd-DTPA administration. *MAGMA* 1995; **3**: 151-156.
24. Tanaka K, Nakamura S, Numata K, *et al*. Hepatocellular carcinoma: treatment with percutaneous ethanol injection and transcatheter arterial embolization. *Radiology* 1992; **185**: 457-460.
25. Koda M, Okamoto K, Miyoshi Y, *et al* Combination therapy with transcatheter arterial embolization and percutaneous ethanol injection for advanced hepatocellular carcinoma. *Hepatogastroenterology* 1994; **41**: 25-29.
26. Wiltgen M, Gell G, Graif E, *et al*. An integrated picture archiving and communications system-radiology information system in a radiological department. *J Digit Imaging* 1993; **6**: 16-24.
27. Schilling RB. Inforad: computers for clinical practice and education in Radiology. Teleradiology, information transfer, and PACS: implications for diagnostic imaging in the 1990s. *RadioGraphics* 1993; **13**: 683-686.
28. Langer M, Buitrago-Tellez CH, Schulze C, Gufler H, Mundinger A, Kommos F. Digital optical card. A promising technology for documentation and communication of images. *Acta Radiol* 1995; **36**: 674-678.
29. Ando Y, Hashimoto S. A standard data format for medical information in the IS & C system. *Comput Methods Programs Biomed* 1994; **43**: 27-36.
30. Stewart BK. Local area network topologies, media and routing. *RadioGraphics* 1992; **12**: 549-566.
31. Dwyer SJ III, Stewart BK, Sayre JW *et al*. Wide area network strategies for teleradiology systems. *RadioGraphics* 1992; **12**: 567-576.
32. Huang HK, Arenson RL, Dillon WP, Lou SL, Bazzill T, Wong AWK. Asynchronous transfer mode technology for radiologic image communication. *AJR* 1995; **164**: 1533-1536.
33. Bidgood WD Jr, Horii SC. PACS mini refresher course: introduction to the ACR-NEMA DICOM standard. *RadioGraphics* 1992; **12**: 345-353.
34. Mattheus R. European standardization efforts: an important framework for medical imaging. *Eur J Radiol* 1993; **17**: 28-37.
35. Bellon E, van Cleynenbreugel J, Suetens P, *et al* Multimedia E-mail systems for computer assisted radiological communication. *Med Info* 1994; **19**: 139-148.
36. Bartolozzi C, Caramella D, Lencioni R, *et al*. Cost-effectiveness of intrainstitutional information exchange in the diagnostic and therapeutical management of patients with hepatocellular carcinoma. *Acad Radiol* 1996; **3**: 577-579

19

Biopsy
Section 1: Technique

T Livraghi

A fine needle is one with an external diameter of <1 mm, that is a gauge >19.[1] Fine needle biopsy (FNB) is the procedure of choice for establishing and confirming the diagnosis of HCC. In fact, the diagnostic accuracy of FNB has proved in comparative prospective studies to be equal or superior to that of 14-16 gauge needles.[2-5] Furthermore, FNB can be handled in the outpatient clinic and is therefore less costly, is better tolerated by the patient, has a lower complications rate[6] and, since it allows more than one pass, permits the sampling of several areas of a lesion, an important point when more than one degree of differentiation may be present.

PREPARATION OF PATIENT

As this is an invasive procedure the patient's informed consent must be obtained. When possible, FNB should be done as soon as the lesion is detected, first because the patient will be less alarmed when the biopsy is seen as a follow-on from US, whereas if he is recalled he will certainly be more anxious, and second for the practical reason that this obviates another appointment and a second US or CT scan.

Mode of hospitalization

Unless the patient is already on the ward, our practice is to conduct FNB in the outpatient clinic (the rule at our center), keeping the patient under observation in the adjacent waiting room for two hours afterwards. This we consider sufficient for any bleeding, revealed by discomfort or pain in the right hypochondrium and/or restlessness, to become apparent. Before he goes home the patient always has a second US scan to detect any evidence of fluid. He must be accompanied by a responsible person, who is given the ward telephone number.

Premedication

Premedication is unnecessary unless the patient is unusually anxious, in which case he receives mild sedatives and anticholinergics (in adults Valium 10 mg + atropine 0.5 mg IM; in the elderly atropine 0.5 mg IM). The patient should anyway be reassured that he will feel only a little discomfort.

Coagulation tests

It has not been demonstrated that routine laboratory tests for coagulation changes (PT, PTT, PC) limit the risk of bleeding any more than a history of a tendency to bleed.[7,8] Indeed, it was emphasized in one study that liver FNB in patients whose coagulation tests were unfavourable involved no additional risks.[9] However, one could not act on such evidence if only for medicolegal reasons, since bleeding is known to be by far the most frequent complication of biopsy and the most frequent cause of death. An explanation of this discordance might be that, while coagulation abnormalities, almost the rule in liver disease, do not constitute a real risk over large numbers, they may be a real risk in an individual should the needle pierce a large blood vessel running along the capsule or along the surface of superficial HCC.

The minimum values required at our center are 40,000/mm^3 PC, 40% PT and within normal range for PTT.

With regard to aspirin and antiaggregants generally and to heparin calcium at low doses, although nothing has been published on the subject, we postpone FNB for a few days as a precaution.

PROCEDURE

Choice of needles and preparation of material

An aspiration needle yields material for smear cytology (SC) and a cutting needle material for microhistology (MH). The procedure for performing biopsy depends on the type of needle and so too does the mode of preparation of the resulting material.

Aspiration needles have a tip shaped like a flute mouthpiece, angled at 25°-30°, designed to slip clean through the tissues with the least possible damage. The steps in the procedure are: 1) insertion of needle into the target, 2) withdrawal of the stylet, 3) connection to a syringe, 4) aspiration, best if facilitated by a pistol-shaped grip, 5) simultaneous up-and-down movement with an excursion of about 1 cm in order to free the cells from the stroma, 6) release of the syringe plunger, 7) withdrawal.

There are several models of cutting needle, mostly of the Menghini type or modified Tru-cut needles, automatic or non automatic. The sample obtained with a cutting needle obviously gives a more faithful picture of the tissue and so makes the pathologist's task easier. The cost is some ten times that of an aspi-

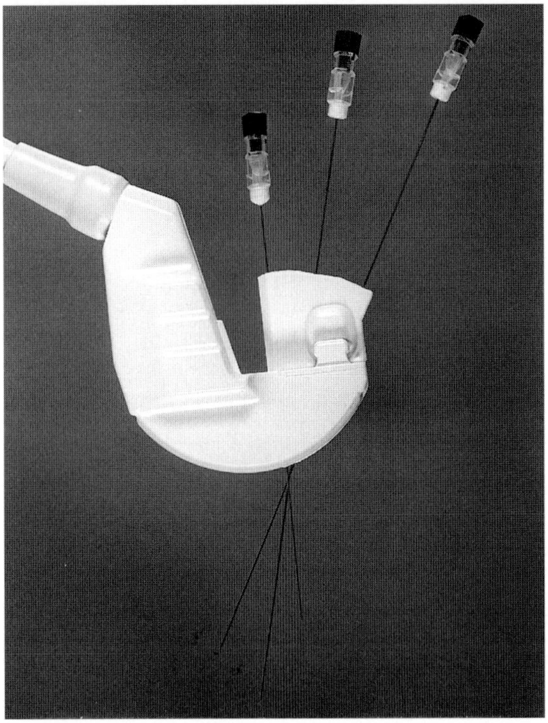

Figure 19.1 – 3.5 MHz convex biopsy probe with eccentric channel for perpendicular trajectories.

ration needle. By aiming the needle carefully before hitting the target one can sample tissue both from inside and outside the lesion in a single pass and so compare the two, which is of great importance in well-differentiated lesions.

The choice of needle type depends chiefly on the pathologist's expertise and experience, bearing in mind the superior yield of cutting needles in small lesions, which are usually well differentiated.[10] If the material supplied by an aspiration needle is plentiful, it can be prepared for inclusion cytology, that is as for ordinary histology.[11]

Guidance systems

US definitely has the edge over CT in guiding FNB, being quicker, simpler and less costly. Furthermore, US allows real-time monitoring of the needle's position and so with small lesions one is sure of hitting the target accurately. A second US scan after FNB to exclude bleeding takes only a few minutes and in any case is performed for HCC detection. At our center only one patient out of 535 underwent FNB under CT guidance, though at centers with little experience of interventional US the preference is for CT guidance.

US guidance

FNB can be performed by the so-called free-hand technique[12,13] or by using probes or biopsy devices.

FREE-HAND TECHNIQUE

Any type of probe may be used with this technique. The probe should be covered with plasticized fabric or with a sterile rubber sheath, the needle inserted alongside at the appropriate angle and monitored as far as the target. The drawbacks of this technique are the difficulty of reaching the target in some cases, e.g. when the approach has to be very oblique, and the training needed for gauging the angle at which the needle has to be inserted.

USING PROBES OR BIOPSY DEVICES

To solve the problem of centering free-hand easy guidance systems have been devised that enable even a beginner to be very precise. He needs only make the target coincide, with an electronic marker (line or channel) on the US monitor, which corresponds to the trajectory of the needle. Purpose-made probes, linear or convex, for tracking oblique or perpendicular trajectories are available (Fig. 19.1), as are guidance devices that can be fitted onto normal convex or sector probes for oblique trajectories (Fig. 19.2). Using the perpendicular approach, one can reach targets accessible only with difficulty, if at all, by an oblique approach, as for example when the only path of entry is a narrow intercostal "window". Another disadvantage of the oblique approach is the risk of the needle deviating from the planned trajectory, especially in the case of a hard cirrhotic liver or when the angle is very obtuse. However, there is a great difference in price between a guidance device and a biopsy probe.

EXECUTION

The depth of the target can easily be calculated with electronic calipers. The shortest distance is usually the best path for the needle. Only in a few circumstances is a different path chosen, nearly always to avoid areas or structures at risk. If the lesion is not homogeneous, each of the tissue components should be sampled. Biopsy of the outermost portion has the dual

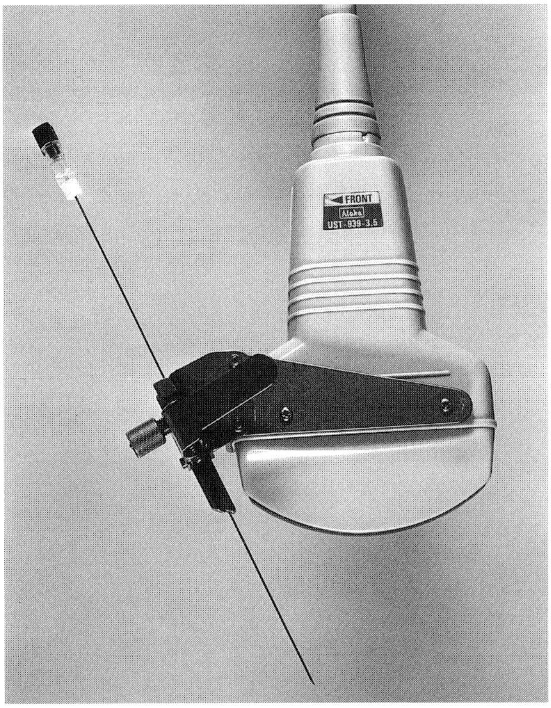

Figure 19.2 – Convex biopsy probe with lateral device.

advantage of avoiding the necrosis usually present in the innermost portion and of sampling the border between healthy and diseased tissue. Any US-detectable lesion may be sampled by FNB, the only exception being a lesion dorsal to the gallbladder, in which case a fatty meal may be given before the procedure in an attempt to reduce its bulk. The patient fasts for several hours beforehand. The designated area is disinfected with iodized alcohol, which is also used as contact medium. We do not give local anesthetics or make an incision in the skin. After placing the patient in the left lateral decubitus we use an intercostal approach, when possible, as this calls for little cooperation on the part of the patient. The subcostal approach is preferred for superficial lesions of the right lobe and the epigastric approach for those of the left lobe. We prefer to perform FNB under apnea, asking the patient to hold his breath at the respiratory phase during which the lesion was imaged best at the centering stage. Should more time be needed, fine needles are anyway flexible enough to allow the procedure to be done at any point in the respiratory cycle (Fig. 19.3). Two passes are usually made, if possible in different areas of the lesion.

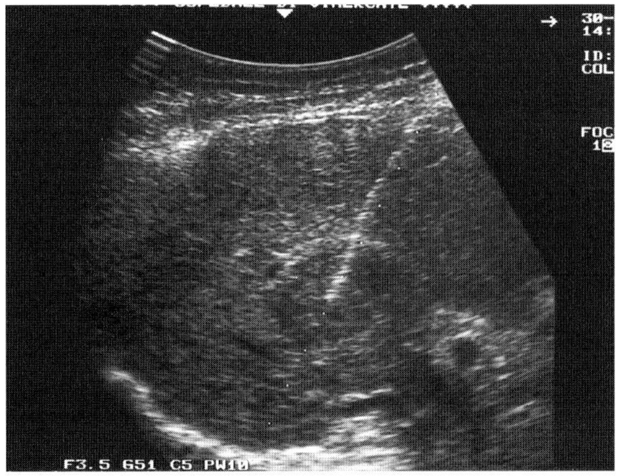

Figure 19.3 – 22G aspiration needle positioned inside an HCC by intercostal approach. The flexibility of the needle during the respiratory excursion is clear.

CT guidance

While US guidance can be handled by a single operator, CT calls for good organization and cooperation between technical and medical staff. A radiopaque landmark that does not produce artifacts, such as a thin copper grid, is applied to the skin to cover the entire scanning field. Preliminary scans are taken in the same position and at the same point in the respiratory cycle so that the best position for FNB may be chosen. It is important to remember that when a lesion is close to the diaphragm, the choise of respiratory phase is crucial. Unless critical structures lie in the way, it is best to choose the shortest vertical line from percutaneous landmark to lesion (Fig. 19.4). Antiseptic preparation of the skin is followed by administration of local anesthetics. A needle cannula is inserted into the superficial tissues and several scans are taken to check that the position is correct. The FNB needle fitted with a stop adjusted to the depth of the lesion is then threaded into the cannula and centering is again checked. For cranied lesions the triangulation procedure must be used to avoid the pleura.[14,15] A right-angled triangle is plotted on the monitor, its vertices representing the lesion. The entry angle is calculated with a goniometer.

RESULTS

The diagnostic accuracy of HCC by FNB is very high, ranging from 84% to 100%.[16-20] These data

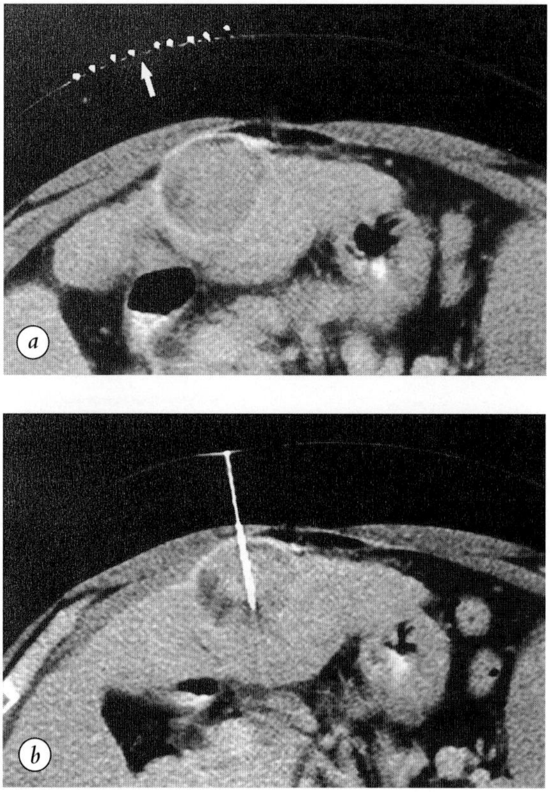

Figure 19.4 –

a) The arrow marks the thin grid lying on the surface of the abdomen, facilitating the centre of the lesion.

b) The scan confirms correct centering

have been obtained by SC, MH and the two combined. There is, however, no consensus as to which of these techniques is preferable, or when, and so every center does as it thinks best. SC alone has the advantage of low cost but the disadvantage of difficulty in the diagnosis of well-differentiated HCC; thus in doubtful or negative cases the patient has to be recalled for MH. MH has higher diagnostic accuracy than SC but its cost is higher too and its retrieval rate is sometimes lower in cases of partially necrotic HCC. The two combined (and hence two needles) ensure higher diagnostic reliability but carry higher costs and much unnecessary duplication.

In a comparative study of 112 consecutive patients we retrieved too little material in 7% with SC and in 13% with MH, false negatives in 8% with SC and in 2% with MH, generic malignancy in 10% of cases with SC and in 1% with MH, correct typing in 74% with SC and in 82% with MH. The two combined yielded a retrieval rate of 98.2% and correct typing in 93.7% of cases with only 3 false negatives.[18]

FNB can also be used to demonstrate the neoplastic origin of portal thrombi, with a high degree of reliability.[21,22] We use this FNB when HCC is diffuse, badly/or not detectable by imaging.

COMPLICATIONS

FNB is a low-risk procedure. In a multicenter study of 2,021 FNB of liver for metastases and HCC mortality was zero and the complication rate 0.5% with only two cases of bleeding that required transfusion.[23] In other, more general, studies of abdominal FNB mortality ranged form 0.10% to 0.03%.[24-27] In all, taking these series together plus some case reports, 21 deaths have been reported after FNB of focal liver lesions including 7 in HCC from bleeding. The data place HCC among the relatively high-risk diseases. Concomitant risk factors include a tendency to bleed secondary to cirrhosis, an abundant tumor blood supply and a superficial site. It is therefore essential to exclude severe blood coagulation abnormalities, to avoid direct puncture of the lesion, seeking, where possible, a trajectory that leaves healthy parenchyma between and to avoid too many passes. Some case reports mention the possibility of seeding.[28–31] In our series of 535 patients who underwent FNB, there were no fatalities; in 210 patients who had PEI with a total of 2,568 injections,[32] only one case required transfusion, and 3 cases seeded on the peritoneal wall, all in poorly differentiated HCC.

CONCLUSION

In capable hands FNB under US guidance is a simple, rapid, low-cost, low-risk procedure that can be carried out in the outpatient clinic. However, in the past decade new imaging possibilities have raised questions about the importance and role of FNB in the diagnosis of HCC. Indeed, at some centers with vast experience of HCC in cirrhosis the diagnosis is established by imaging alone, that is, when US, CT and/or MRI or angiography agree, with recourse to FNB only in doubtful cases or to secure additional information, such as the degree of differentiation or index of cell proliferation, possibly useful in evaluating the prognosis. One reason for this noninvasive stance is the desire to minimize the chances of seeding, especially in candidates for OLT, in whom the subsequent immunodepression might carry the risk of relapse. It is anyway common practice to avoid biopsy in patients with chronic liver disease presenting a lesion with the morphology characteristic of HCC and a high level of AFP (>200 ng/ml) or of DCP, or if serial US screening reveals a previously undetected lesion suggestive of HCC. It is therefore difficult to lay down a rule as to when FNB is indicated. Common sense suggests that at centers of great expertise the responsibility for making the choice should be left to them and that elsewhere FNB should performed always, except in the two instances mentioned above.

REFERENCES

1. Livraghi T, Damascelli B, Lombardi C, Spagnoli I. Risk in fine needle abdominal biopsy. *J Clin Ultrasound* 1983; **11**: 77-81
2. Jacobsen GK, Gammelgaard J, Fuglo M. Coarse needle biopsy versus fine needle aspiration biopsy in the diagnosis of focal lesions of the liver: ultrasonically guided needle biopsy in suspected hepatic malignancy. *Acta Cytol* 1983; **27**: 152-156
3. Bell DA, Carr CP, Szyfelbein WB. Fine needle aspiration cytology of focal liver lesion: results obtained with examination of both cytologic and histologic preparations. *Acta Cytol* 1986; **30**: 397-402
4. Glenthoj A, Sehested M, Torp-Pedersen S. Diagnostic reliability of histological and cytological fine needle biopsies from focal liver lesions. *Histopathology* 1989; **15**: 375-383
5. Jonasson JG, Wang HE, Porter DH, Tyagi G, Ducatman BS.Image-directed percutaneous biopsy. A comparison of cytologic and histologic findings. *Cancer* 1992; **70**: 2187-2191
6. Piccinino F, Sagnelli E, Pasquale G, Giusti G. Complications following percutaneous liver biopsy. A multicenter retrospective study on 68.276 biopsies. *J Hepatol* 1986; **2**: 165-173
7. Gazelle SG, Haaga JR, Rowland DY. Effect of needle gauge, level of anticoagulation, and target organ on bleeding associated with aspiration biopsy. *Radiology* 1992; **183**: 509-513
8. Silverman SG, Mueller PR, Pfister RC. Hemostatic evaluation before abdominal interventions: an overview and proposal. *AJR* 1990; **154**:233-238
9. Caturelli E, Squillante MM, Andriulli A *et al.* Fine-needle liver biopsy in patients with severely impaired coagulation. *Liver* 1993; **13**: 270-273
10. Kondo F, Ebara M, Sugiura N *et al.* Histological features and clinical course of large regenerative nodules: evaluation of their precancerous potentiality. *Hepatology* 1990; **12**: 592-598
11. Livraghi T, Pilotti S, Ravetto C, Sangalli G, Solbiati L. Inclusion-cytology versus smear-cytology in fine needle abdominal biopsy. *Eur J Radiol* 1985; **5**: 111-114
12. Bret PM, Fond A, Bretagnolle M, Labadie M, Bret P, Buffard P. Une technique simple de guidage des ponctions percutanée par l'echographie en temps réel. *J Radiol* 1982; **63**: 363-365
13. Livraghi T. A simple no-cost technique for real-time biopsy. *J Clin Ultrasound* 1984; **12**: 60-62
14. Gerzof SG. Triagulation: indirect CT guidance for abscess drainage. *AJR* 1981; **137**: 1080-1081
15. Van Sonnerberg E, Witterberg J, Ferrucci JT Jr *et al.* Triangulation method for percutaneous needle guidance: the angled approach to upper abdominal masses. *AJR* 1981; **137**: 757-761
16. Bret PM, Labadie M, Bretagnolle M *et al.* Hepatocellular carcinoma: diagnosis by percutaneous fine needle biopsy. *Gastrointest Radiol* 1988; **13**: 253-255
17. Roget L, Richard PH, Selles M *et al.* Valeur de la cytoponction échoguidée dans le diagnostic du carcinome hépatocellulaire. *J Radiol* 1989; **70**: 75-78
18. Sangalli G, Livraghi T, Giordano F. Fine needle biopsy of hepatocellular carcinoma: improvement in diagnosis by microhistology. *Gastroenterology* 1989; **96**: 524-526
19. Cohen MB, Haber MM, Holly EA, Ahn DK, Bottles K, Stoloff AC. Cytologic criteria to distinguish hepatocellular carcinoma from nonneoplastic liver. *Am J Clin Pathol* 1991; **95**: 125-130
20. Sbolli G, Fornari F, Civardi G *et al.* Role of ultrasound guided fine needle aspiration biopsy in the diagnosis of hepatocellular carcinoma. *Gut* 1990; **31**: 1303-1305
21. Livraghi T, Corti D, Sangalli G. Fine needle biopsy of a patent umbilical vein thrombus demonstrates hepatocellular carcinoma. *Diag Imag* 1983; **52**: 332-334
22. Dodd GD, Carr BI. Percutaneous biopsy of portal vein thrombus: a new staging technique for hepatocellular carcinoma. *AJR* 1993; **161**: 229-233
23. Buscarini L, Fornari F, Bolondi L *et al.* Ultrasound-guided fine needle biopsy of focal liver lesions: techniques, diagnostic accuracy and complications. A retrospective study on 2091 biopsies. *J Hepatol* 1990; **11**: 344-348
24. Gebel M, Horstkotte H, Kostr C, Brunkhorst R, Brandt M, Atay Z. Ultraschall-geizielte feinnadelpunktion abdomineller organe: indikationen, egebnisse, risiken. *Ultraschall Med* 1986; **7**: 198-202
25. Bret P, Labadie M, Bretagnolle M et al. Hepatocellular carcinoma: diagnosis by percutaneous fine needle biopsy. *Gastrointest Radiol* 1988; **13**: 253-255
26. Weiss H, Weiss A, Scholl A. Todliche komplikation einer feinnadelbiopsie der leber. *Dtsch Med Wochneschr* 1988; **113**: 139-142
27. Nolsoe C, Nielsen L, Torp-Pedersen S, Holm HH. Major complications and deaths due to interventional ultrasonography: a review of 8,000 cases. *J Clin Ultrasound* 1990;**18**: 179-184
28. Onodera H, Oikawa M, Abe M *et al.* Cutaneous seeding of hepatocellular carcinoma after fine needle aspiration biopsy. *J Ultrasound Med* 1987; **6**: 273-275
29. Park YM, Lee CD, Yoon KL *et al.* A case of subcutaneous seeding of hepatocellular carcinoma after fine needle aspiration biopsy. *Korean J Intern Med* 1989; **4**: 96-98
30. Smith EH. Complications of percutaneous abdominal fine needle biopsy. *Radiology* 1991; **178**: 253-258

31. Nakamuta M, Tanabe Y, Ohashi M, Yoshida K, Hiroshige K, Nawata H. Transabdominal seeding of hepatocellular carcinoma after fine needle aspiration biopsy. *J Clin Ultrasound* 1993; **21**: 551-556

32. Livraghi T, Lazzaroni S, Meloni R, Torzilli G, Vettori C. Intralesional ethanol in the treatment of unresectable liver cancer. *World J Surg* 1995; **19**: 801-806

19

Biopsy
Section 2: Cytopathology

G Sangalli

CYTOPATHOLOGY

The diagnosis of HCC from FNB samples is common practice, however, it is not always easy, because the microscopic appearance of HCC is highly variable: for instance, there are problems in distinguishing between well differentiated HCC and benign regenerative lesions and between poorly differentiated HCC and poorly differentiated metastatic carcinomas. We usually classify cases on the basis of differentiation rate: well differentiated HCC, moderately differentiated HCC and poorly differentiated HCC, plus four rare variants: clear cell HCC, fibrolamellar HCC, giant cell HCC and spindle cell HCC. For FNB samples we use a classification based on three degrees of differentiation. In fact, according to four-grade classifications, a diagnosis of grade I HCC is based on clinical behavior (e.g. the evidence of metastases in a formerly diagnosed hepatocellular adenoma), or on surgical specimens, depending on the relationship with surrounding tissue (e.g. vein invasion or association with grade II HCC areas).[1] Moderately differentiated HCCs are the most commonly diagnosed cases, showing the most typical cytological aspects: therefore they will be described first.

MODERATELY DIFFERENTIATED HCC

When a tumour is moderately differentiated the smears are very cellular, chiefly composed of clusters of hepatocytes and trabeculae of variable thickness (Fig. 19.5). The clusters are made up of loosely cohesive malignant hepatocytes crossed by sinusoidal capillaries (Fig. 19.6), sometimes arranged in an "arborescent" manner. The trabeculae consist of plates, variable in number, of malignant hepatocytes firmly joined together and enclosed by endothelial cells (Fig. 19.7,8). Among the clusters and trabeculae naked nuclei of malignant hepatocytes are often scattered. The hepatocytes are readily recognized as malignant: they have central nuclei, roundish or oval, greater in volume than the nuclei of hyperplastic hepatocytes, with fine or coarse irregularly distributed chromatin, and a prominent eosinophilic nucleolus (Fig. 19.9). The cells are polygonal and their cytoplasm contains fine eosinophilic granulations. The naked nuclei, sometimes very numerous, may be isolated or grouped among the clusters and trabeculae and they too present definite signs of malignancy (Fig. 19.10). Other possible features are: multinucleated malignant cells, intranuclear cytoplasmic inclusions (Fig. 19.11), multiple nucleoli, intracytoplasmic bile, intracytoplasmic hyaline globules and an acinar pattern (Fig. 19.12). Here the hepatocytes are arranged around spaces of variable size and sometimes containing bile. The acinar pattern is generally associated with the presence of trabeculae and clusters; in rare cases it is the predominant pattern of aggregation and may simulate a cholangiocarcinoma or a metastatic adenocarcinoma. The cells that form acini nonetheless retain the morphology of hepatocytes and the presence of bile is diagnostic of histotype (Fig. 19.12).

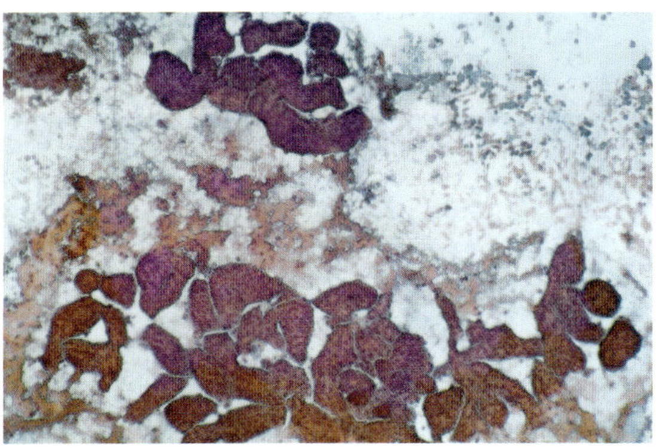

Figure 19.5 – Moderately differentiated HCC. Appearance of smear at low magnification: high cellularity and numerous trabeculae (Papanicolaou x 40)

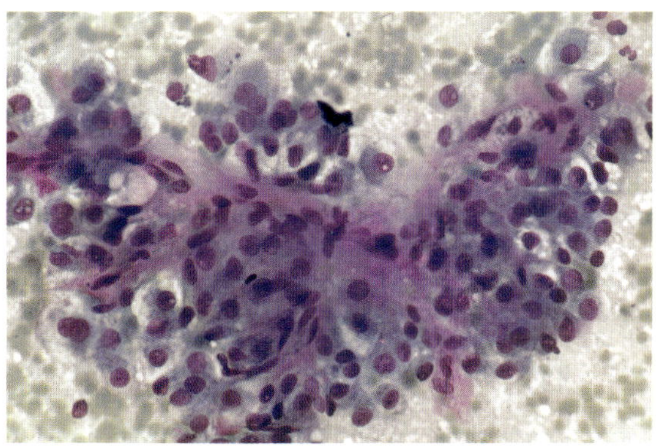

Figure 19.6 – Moderately differentiated HCC. Cluster of malignant hepatocytes crossed by sinusoidal capillaries (May-Grunwald Giemsa x 400).

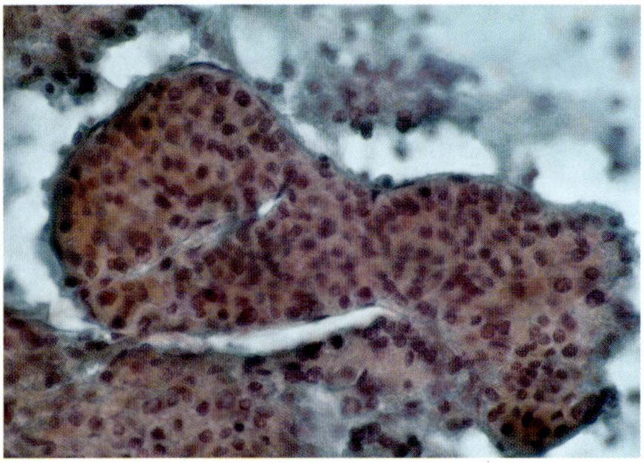

Figure 19.7 - Moderately differentiated HCC. Trabeculae made up of cohesive malignant hepatocytes surrounded by endothelial cells (Papanicolaou x 400).

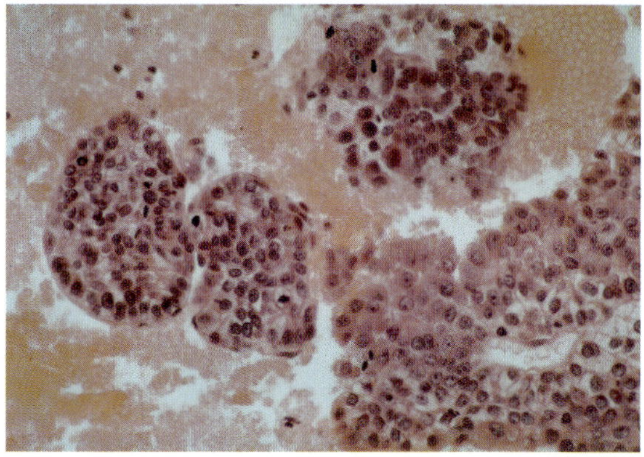

Figure 19.8 - Moderately differentiated HCC. Appearance of the trabeculae on material embedded in paraffin (Hematoxylin-eosin x 250).

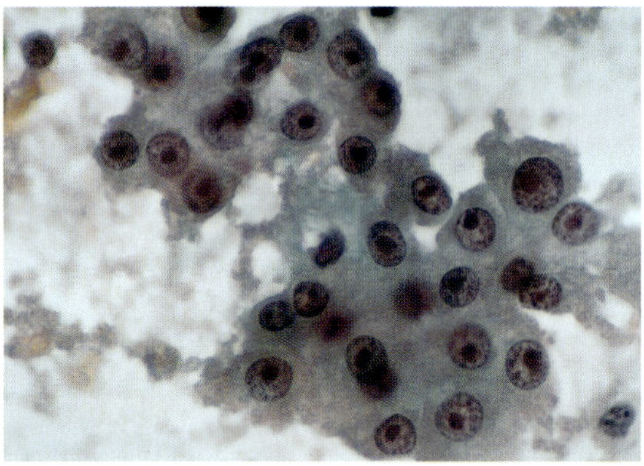

Figure 19.9 – Moderately differentiated HCC. Hepatocytes with nuclear features of malignancy: increased volume irregularly distributed chromatin, single prominent eosinophilic nucleolus (Papanicolaou x 1000).

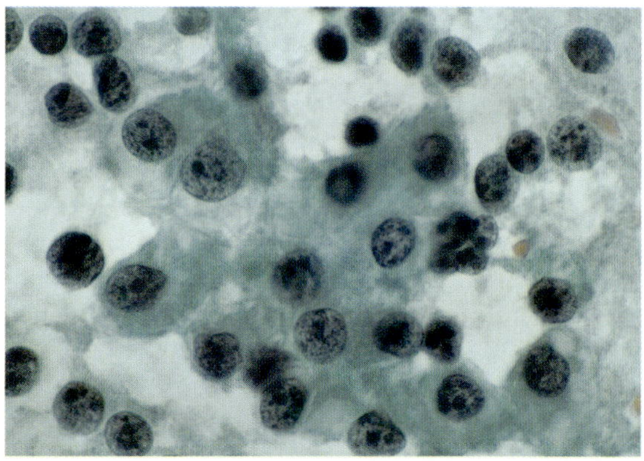

Figure 19.10 – Moderately differentiated HCC. Numerous naked nuclei with malignant features (Papanicolaou x 1000).

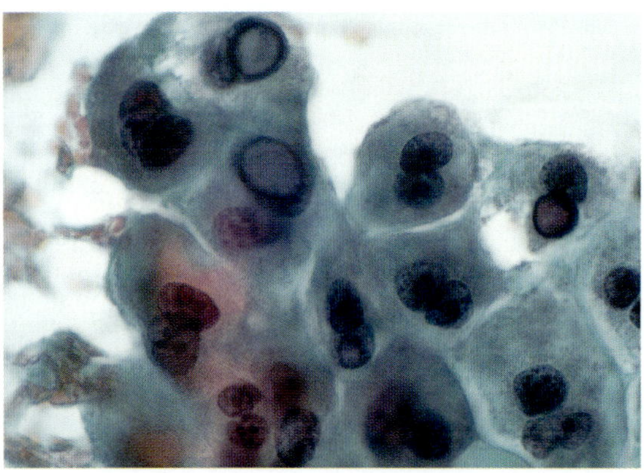

Figure 19.11 – Moderately differentiated HCC. Group of malignant hepatocytes, three of which show intranuclear cytoplasmic inclusions (Papanicolaou x 1000).

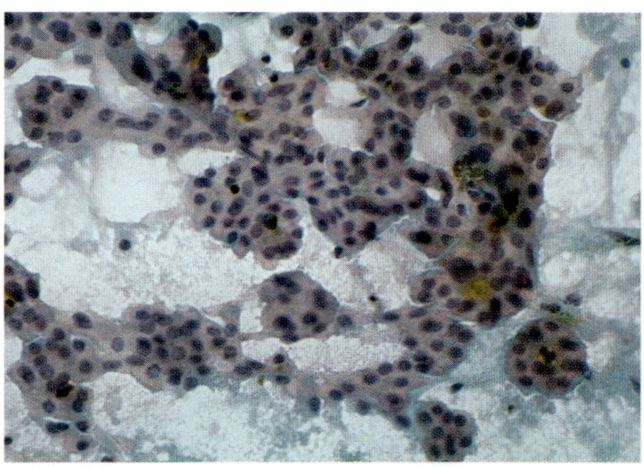

Figure 19.12 – Moderately differentiated HCC. Acinar pattern of the hepatocytes: note bile at the centre of some acini (Papanicolaou x 400).

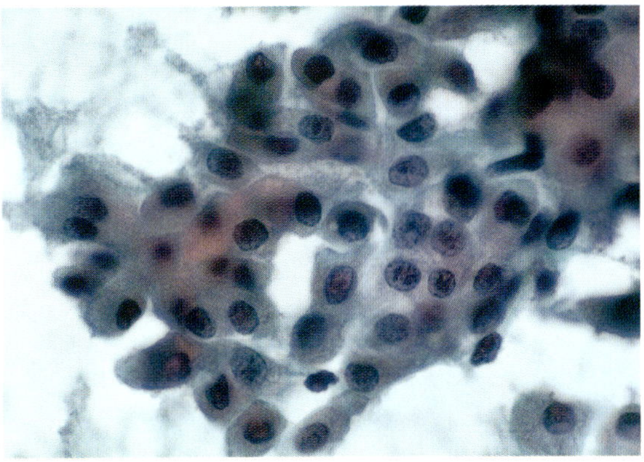

Figure 19.13 – Well differentiated HCC. Hepatocytes with nuclear monomorphism, fine chromatin, no nucleoli and slightly increased nucleocytoplasmic ratio (Papanicolaou x 1000).

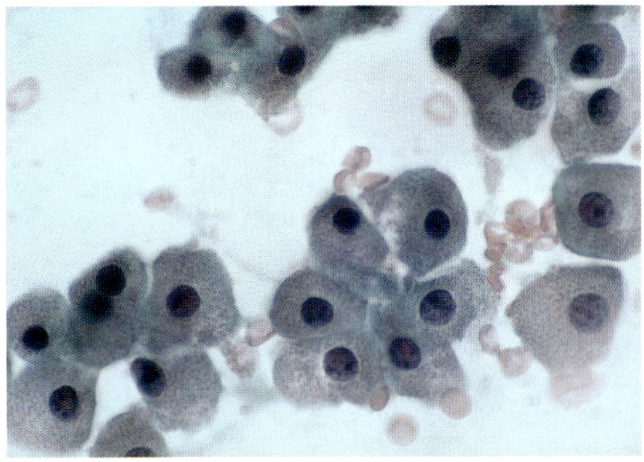

Figure 19.14 – Well differentiated HCC. Isolated hepatocytes with no nuclear signs of malignancy (Papanicolaou x 1000).

WELL DIFFERENTIATED HCC

Greater problems arise in cases of well differentiated HCC: here the differential diagnosis is chiefly from macroregenerative nodules in cirrhosis and, less often, from adenomas and focal nodular hyperplasia. In well differentiated HCC the smear also shows high cellularity, the cells being disposed in clusters crossed by sinusoidal capillaries and, more rarely, trabeculae. The cells are easily identified as hepatocytes, with single nuclei and a slightly increased nucleocytoplasmic ratio, due mainly to the decreased volume of the cytoplasm, one or no nucleoli and finely granular chromatin, sometimes irregularly distributed (Fig.19. 13). Naked nuclei may also be present. Of these cytologic features those recognized as crucial to differential diagnosis from non neoplastic regenerative lesions are: trabecular pattern, increased nucleocytoplasmic ratio and presence of atypical naked nuclei.[2,3]

However, although the presence of atypical naked nuclei is recognized to be of great value in the diagnosis of HCC irrespective of degree of differentiation,[4] it has been considered of little use in the diagnosis of well differentiated HCC by some authors[5,6] and we have found this to be so, since atypical naked nuclei may be absent from cases of well differentiated HCC and present in aspirates of macroregenerative nodules in cirrhotics. In some well differentiated HCC the cells may present none of the nuclear characteristics of malignancy (Fig. 19.14) and the crucial characteristics instead become aggregation of cells into true trabeculae or clusters crossed by sinusoidal capillaries, considered by the majority of authors to be among the principal criteria for diagnosis of well differentiated HCC[2,3,7–10] and by some specific to HCC even if the hepatocytes have a benign appearance.[6] It is thus of great help to have also material embedded in paraffin for histologic evaluation (Fig. 19. 11).[6,11–14] In histologic specimens it is easier to evaluate the relationship of hepatocytes to stroma and hence detect the presence of structures like trabeculae, which in well differentiated HCC are three or more cells thick, whereas in macroregenerative nodules the cell plates are one or two cells thick.[15] Furthermore, nuclear crowding and

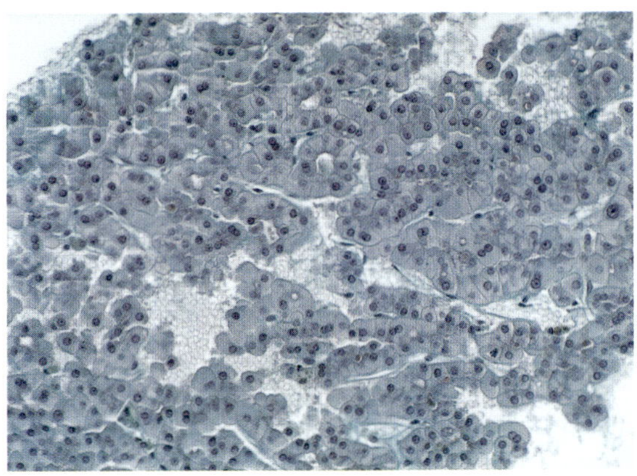

Figure 19.15 – Well differentiated HCC (same case as in Fig. 19.14). Embedded material reveals trabecular and acinar formations (Papanicolaou X 250).

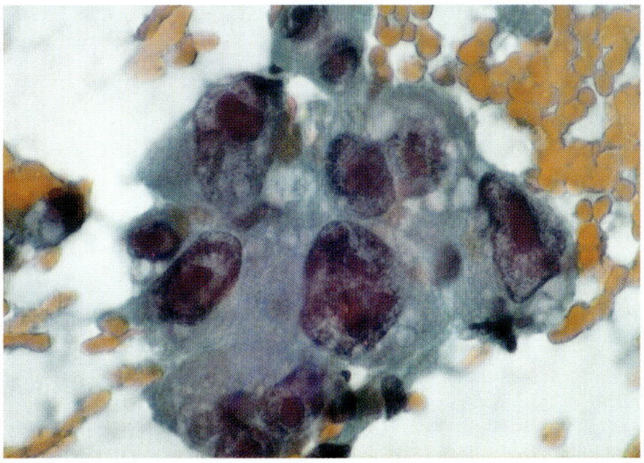

Figure 19.16 – Poorly differentiated HCC. Marked pleomorphism of the nuclei, irregular coarse chromatin, several prominent nucleoli (Papanicolaou x 1000).

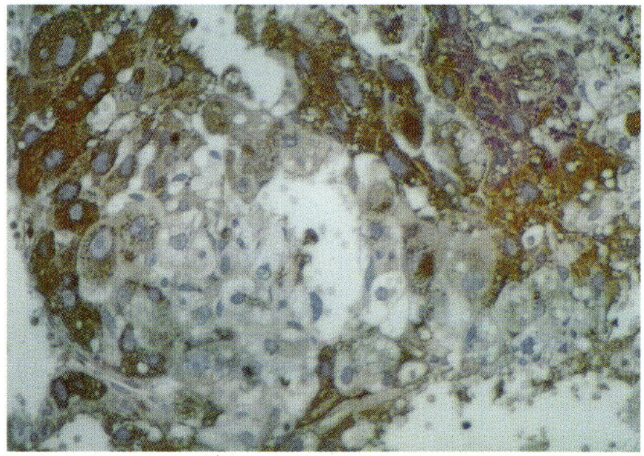

Figure 19.17 – Poorly differentiated HCC. In the embedded material some of the hepatocye cytoplasms are positive for AFP (Immunoperoxidase x 400).

acinar structures are more easily observed: histologic parameters held to be essential to differential diagnosis from macroregenerative nodules.[12] Lastly, it must be remembered that in rare cases even a combination of cytologic and histologic methods cannot distinguish well differentiated HCC from lesions that are classified as borderline on surgical specimens.[15] Other conditions that still more rarely have to be distinguished from HCC are FNH and hepatocellular adenoma. In both cases the clinical history and the imaging data may point to either diagnosis. In FNH the aspirate consists of hepatocytes without any nuclear signs of malignancy, accompanied by epithelial cells of bile ducts[16,17] with no evidence of trabeculae or clusters of hepatocytes crossed by sinusoidal capillaries.[6] In hepatocellular adenoma the smear is cellular with hepatocytes in groups or isolated: the nuclei show no signs of malignancy and the nucleocytoplasmic ratio may be decreased due to an increase in the volume of the cytoplasm, and no bile duct epithelia are present.

POORLY DIFFERENTIATED HCC

In poorly differentiated HCC the cytological specimens are rich in cells, with irregular clusters of weakly cohesive cells and numerous isolated malignant hepatocytes and naked nuclei. Intact trabeculae are rarely found. The nuclei present considerable pleomorphism, a high nucleocytoplasmic ratio, coarsely granular chromatin, irregularly distributed and prominent nucleoli, often multiple; the cytoplasm may be abundant or scanty and contains rare eosinophilic granulations (Fig. 19.16). There may be a background of necrotic material and often cells undergoing mitosis. In some cases large multinucleated cells with clear features of malignancy are present. In poorly differentiated HCC the diagnosis of malignancy is easy, but not the histotype. Indicative of HCC are: presence of trabecular fragments, of eosinophilic granulations and of bile in the cytoplasm, the last being pathognomonic, though rarely found in poorly differentiated tumors. Here again, the availability of material embedded in paraffin for histologic study improves diagnostic

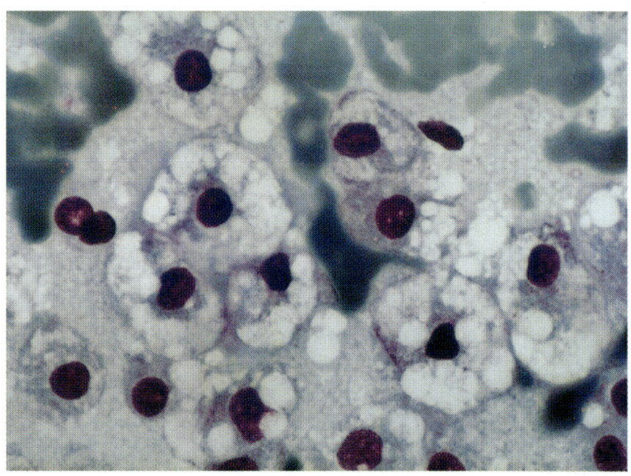

Figure 19.18 – Clear cell HCC. Hepatocytes containing numerous small vacuoles in the cytoplasm (May-Grunwald Giemsa x 1000).

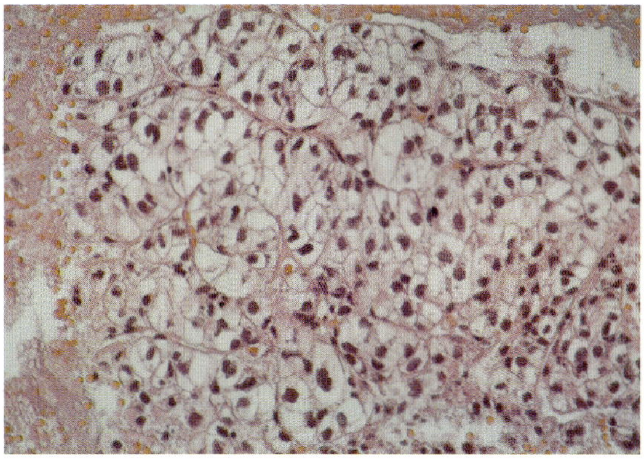

Figure 19.19 – Clear cell HCC. Embedded material allows identification of the trabecular architecture of the HCC (Hematoxylin-eosin x 250).

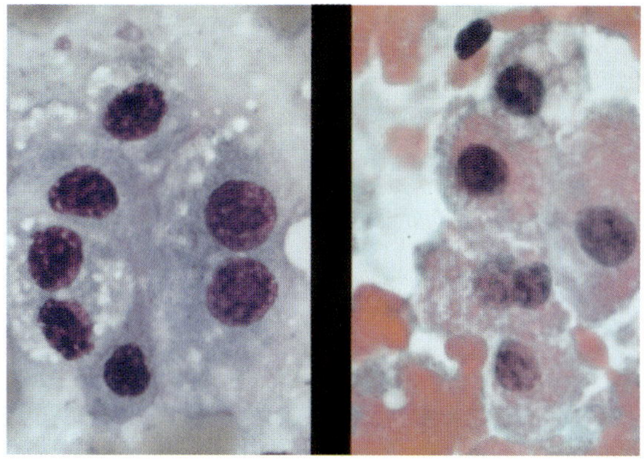

Figure 19.20 – Fibrolamellar HCC. Malignant hepatocytes with large cytoplasm containing eosinophilic granules, more clearly visible with Papanicolaou stain (Papanicolaou x 1000, May-Grunwald Giemsa x 1000).

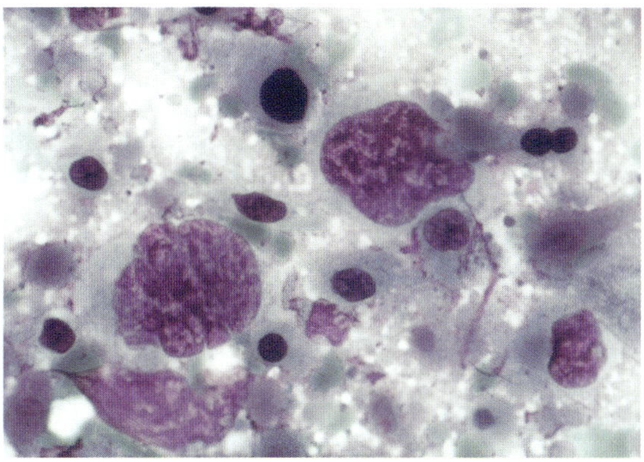

Figure 19.21 – Giant cell HCC. Multinucleated hepatocytes with marked signs of malignancy against a necrotic background (May-Grunwald Giemsa x 1000).

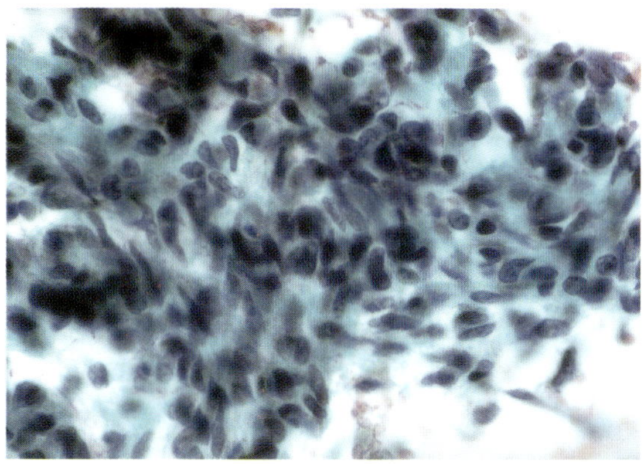

Figure 19.22 – Spindle cell HCC. Cluster of tightly bunched spindle cells without clear signs of malignancy. The presence of classic HCC patterns point to the correct diagnosis (Papanicolaou x 1000).

accuracy.[10,11,14,18,19] For differential diagnosis from metastatic carcinoma immunocytochemical and cytochemical methods may be used, the former being more easily applied to material embedded in paraffin. The antigens sought for confirmation of an HCC diagnosis are: AFP (Fig. 19.17), A1AT, AE1 and AE3 cytokeratins, CEA. AFP is a relatively specific marker, since it is produced by few metastatic neoplasms (e.g. germinal neoplasia), but it is not very sensitive on FNB material, positivity ranging from 44 to 62%.[20,21] A1AT is often expressed by HCC cells, but is not specific, as it is expressed also by metastatic tumors of the colon, pancreas, lung, and breast.[22] AE3 cytokeratins are expressed by the majority of HCC, which are negative for AE1 cytokeratins.[20,21] CEA is expressed by the cells of the majority of HCC in a "canalicular" pattern, which seems to be specific and is not observed in metastatic adenocarcinomas.[21,23] Cytochemical staining for naphtylamidase has been used in rare cases on dried smears for differential diagnosis from metastatic carcinomas.[23,24] But both the canalicular pattern of CEA and naphtylamidase activity are lost in less differentiated HCC and so neither stain is very sensitive. Finally, ultrastructural analysis has been used by some authors in rare cases for confirmation of an HCC diagnosis[21] and differentiation from metastatic adenocarcinoma of the gastrointestinal tract.[25]

VARIANTS

A variant of HCC described some time ago[26] that may pose problems in cytologic differential diagnosis is clear cell HCC. This is a tumor in which some 30 to 100% of the cells have a clear cytoplasm, due to their glycogen and fat content. The smears are very rich in cell clusters and have numerous naked nuclei. The cytoplasm contains a single vacuole occupying the entire cytoplasm or many small clear vacuoles (Fig. 19.18). In some cases the cytoplasm is so fragile that the smear appears to be composed of naked nuclei, single or in groups, against a lacy-like background. Differential diagnosis is between clear cell HCC and metastases from clear cell carcinoma, especially of renal origin. Of great help here is the presence of an HCC component without clear cytoplasm,[27] which presents classic cytologic features, and the availability of embedded samples, in which the architecture of HCC is more easily evaluated (Fig. 19.19). Immunocytochemical staining of embedded material can again confirm the diagnosis.

A second morphologically and biologically distinct variant of HCC is fibrolamellar carcinoma.[28] Smears present low cellularity, with hepatocytes, isolated or in small groups, with oxyphilic granular cytoplasm, nuclei of increased volume with prominent eosinophilic nucleoli and cytoplasmic inclusions in the nucleus (Fig. 19.20). Fragments of fibrous tissue may be observed. In some cases well defined pale bodies like those originally reported in surgical specimens have been seen in the hepatocytes.[29]

Lastly, two rare variants that can be identified cytologically are giant cell HCC and spindle cell HCC. The first is a poorly differentiated tumor in which there are numerous giant cells, which may be multinucleated with abundant cytoplasm and numerous small nuclei (osteoclastoma-like cells) or multinucleated with pleomorphic nuclei, and pronounced signs of malignancy, with several nucleoli, as a rule against a necrotic background (Fig. 19.21). In the two cases of spindle cell HCC that we observed, some smears showed tight clusters of spindle cells with small nuclei, without marked signs of malignancy (Fig. 19.22), while others, evidently representing different areas of the tumor, showed the classic pattern of HCC with trabecular formations. In both cases the patients had a large tumor mass without clinical or radiological evidence of any primary tumor. The presence of mixed, spindle and classic features, led to the correct diagnosis in both cases.

REFERENCES

1. Craig JR, Peters RL, Edmondson HA. *Tumours of the liver and intrahepatic bile ducts. Atlas of Tumour Pathology.* Fascicle 26, second series. Washington DC: Armed Forces Institute of Pathology, 1988
2. Bottles K, Cohen MB. An approach to fine-needle aspiration biopsy diagnosis of hepatic masses. *Diagn Cytopathol* 1991; **7**: 204-210
3. Cohen MB, Haber MM, Holly EA, Ahn DK, Bottles K, Stoloff AC. Cytologic criteria to distinguish hepatocellar carcinoma from non-neoplastic liver. *Am J Clin Pathol* 1991; **95**: 125-130
4. Pedio G, Landolt V, Zobeli L, Gut D. Fine needle aspiration of the liver: significance of hepatic naked nuclei in the diagnosis of hepatocellular carcinoma. *Acta Cytol* 1988; **32**: 437-442
5. Sole' M, Calvet X, Cuberes T, *et al.* Value and limitations of cytologic criteria for the diagnosis of hepatocellular carcinomas by fine needle aspiration biopsy. *Acta Cytol* 1993; **37**: 309-316
6. Pitman MB, Szyfelbein WM. Significance of endothelium in the fine-needle aspiration biopsy diagnosis of hepatocellular carcinoma. *Diagn Cytopathol* 1995; **12**: 208-214
7. Greene C-A, Suen KC. Some cytologic features of hepatocellular carcinoma as seen in fine needle aspirates. *Acta Cytol* 1984; **28**: 713-718
8. Tao L-C, Ho CS, McLoughlin MJ, Evans WK, Donat EE. Cytologic diagnosis of hepatocellular carcinoma by fine needle aspiration biopsy. *Cancer* 1984; **53**: 547-552
9. Wee A, Nilsson B, Chan-Wilde C, Yap I. Fine needle aspiration biopsy of hepatocellular carcinoma: some unusual features. *Acta Cytol* 1991; **35**: 661-670
10. Pitman MB, Szyfelbein WM. Primary malignant liver tumors. In Pitman MB, Szyfelbein WM, eds. *Fine needle aspiration biopsy of the liver.* Boston: Butterworth-Heinemann, 1994: 47-86
11. Noguchi S, Yamamoto R, Tatsuta M, *et al.* Cell features and patterns in fine-needle aspirates of hepatocellular carcinoma. *Cancer* 1986; **58**: 321-328
12. Kondo F, Wada K, Nagato Y, *et al.* Biopsy diagnosis of well-differentiated hepatocellular carcinoma based on new morphologic criteria. *Hepatology* 1989; **9**: 751-755
13. Sangalli G, Livraghi T, Giordano F. Fine needle biopsy of hepatocellular carcinoma: improvement in diagnosis by microhistology. *Gastroenterology* 1989; **96**: 524-526
14. Strachura J, Tomaszewska R, Pietron M, Kulig J. Does microhistology improve the cytological diagnosis of liver and pancreatic tumours? *Cytopathology* 1991; **2**: 39-42
15. Ferrell LD, Crawford JM, Dhillon AP, Scheuer PJ, Nakanuma Y. Proposal for standardized criteria for the diagnosis of benign, borderline, and malignant hepatocellular lesions arising in chronic advanced liver disease. *Am J Surg Pathol* 1993; **17**: 1113-1123
16. Nguyen GK. Fine-needle aspiration biopsy cytology of hepatic tumors in adults *Pathol Annu.* 1986; **21**: 321-349
17. Ruschemburg I, Droese M. Fine needle aspiration cytology of focal nodular hyperplasia of the liver. *Acta Cytol* 1989; **33**: 857-860

18. Kung I, Chan S-K, Fung K-H. Fine-needle aspiration in hepatocellular carcinoma. Combined cytologic and histologic approach. *Cancer* 1991; **67**: 673-680

19. Wee A, Nilsson B, Tan LKA, Yap I. Fine needle aspiration biopsy of hepatocellular carcinoma. Diagnostic dilemma at the ends of the spectrum. *Acta Cytol* 1994; **38**: 347-354

20. Bedrossian CM, Davila RM, Merenda G. Immunocytochemical evaluation of liver fine needle aspirations. *Arch Pathol Lab Med* 1989; **113**: 1225-1230

21. Guindi M, Yazdi HM, Gilliatt MA. Fine needle aspiration biopsy of hepatocellular carcinoma. Value of immunocytochemical and ultrastructural studies. *Acta Cytol* 1994; **38**: 385-391

22. Taylor CR. Lung, pancreas, colon and rectum, stomach, liver. In: Bennington JL ed. *Immunomicroscopy: a diagnostic tool for the surgical pathologist*. Philadelphia: WB Saunders 1986: 238-259

23. Wong MA, Yazdi HM. Hepatocellular carcinoma versus carcinoma metastatic to the liver. Value of stains for carcinoembryonic antigen and naphthylamidase in fine needle aspiration biopsy material. *Acta Cytol* 1990; **34**: 192-196

24. Ekelund P, Wasastjerna C. Cytologic identification of primary hepatic carcinoma cells. *Acta Med Scand* 1971; **189**: 373-375

25. Pinto MM, Avila NA, Heller CI, Criscuolo EM. Fine needle aspiration of the liver. *Acta Cytol* 1988; 32: 15-20

26. Buchanan TF, Huvos AG. Clear- cell carcinoma of the liver: a clinicopathologic study of 13 patients. *Am J Clin Pathol* 1974; 61: 529-539

27. Donat EE, Anderson V, Tao L-C. Cytodiagnosis of clear cell hepatocellular carcinoma. A case report. *Acta Cytol* 1991; **35**: 671-675

28. Craig JR, Peters RL, Edmondson HA, Omata M. Fibrolamellar carcinoma of the liver: a tumor of adolescents and young adults with distinctive clinico-pathologic features. *Cancer* 1980; **46**: 372-379

29. Suen KC, Magee JF, Halparin LS, Chan NH, Greene C-A. Fine needle aspiration cytology of fibrolamellar hepatocellular carcinoma. *Acta Cytol* 1985; **29**: 867-872

20

Diagnostic guidelines

T Livraghi, M Makuuchi and L Buscarini

US is as a rule the most important investigation for the detection and staging of HCC. Whether a patient consults a doctor because he has symptoms or takes part in a screening program because he has chronic hepatitis or cirrhosis, the first evidence of a tumor comes from a US scan and it is US scanning that guides the treatment, often then and there. The low cost, the quasi ubiquity of scanners, the simplicity of execution and high sensitivity, close to that of other procedures (see Chapter 16), all ensure the primacy of US. Furthermore, the US guidance system is the most suitable for piloting FNB (see Chapter 19). US supplies information on the number, size, site, type and degree of infiltration (chiefly in the form of portal thrombosis or satellitosis) of HCC, on its extrahepatic spread and on the grade of cirrhosis, because it shows up any ascites or abdominal varices and permits the Doppler study of portal hypertension.

A very advanced pattern of HCC clearly rules out the need for other diagnostic investigations. The presence of several lesions or of portal thrombosis contraindicates surgery and a very large diameter excludes treatment with conventional PEI. It is equally clear that other, complementary or more sensitive, investigations are needed to confirm that a nodule is single.

Many studies comparing the various procedures have been conducted in order to determine the best flow chart. The highest detection rate is obtained with intraoperative US (IOUS), obviously applicable only in the course of an operation and so not appropriate for pretreatment staging. It is the gold standard for ranking the detection rates of other investigations. CT portography (CTAP), CT with Lipiodol enhancement (LipCT) and US after introduction of CO_2 (CO_2US) proved to be the next most sensitive methods (see Table 20.1).[1-11]

On the basis of these results the most rational flow chart would include one of these procedures immediately after US, omitting conventional CT or MR. In practice, however, since CT or MR may be complementary to US, these two methods are often used as an intermediate step, to spare some patients the next step, which is more invasive and more costly.

Table 20.1 – Detection rate of small HCC with different modalities

Size	Author	US	CT	MR	CTAP	CTA	LIP-CT	DSA	CO_2US	IOUS
≤1 cm	Bartolozzi *et al*[1]	39	29	36			93	57		
	Hayashi *et al*[3] (s)★						67	61		94
	Kudo *et al*[5]						53	33	67	
	Takayasu *et al*[9] (s)	37	42		67	0	83	55		86
	Utsunomiya *et al*[10] (s)★	10	20	10	17			50		
	Winter *et al*[11] (s)		60	40						
1-2 cm	Choi *et al*[2]	52	56				93	74		
	Ikeda *et al*[4] (s)				75			57	72	
	Kudo *et al*[5]						85	75	86	
	Kawasaki *et al*[6] (s)	72	70					56		94
	Merine *et al*[7] (s)★				38		40			
	Utsunomiya *et al*[10] (s)★	54	38	55	57			38		
2-3 cm	Bartolozzi *et al*[1]	91	98	94			98	98		
	Kudo *et al*[5]						97	100	97	
	Ohto *et al*[8]	98	75	79				81		
	Takayasu *et al*[9] (s)	92	91		95	88	96	87		98
	Winter *et al*[11] (s)		100	100						

(s)= in resected patients ★= intrahepatic metastases

Now the new advances made by spiral CT have once again modified the flow chart. With spiral CT the entire organ can be investigated within the time of a single breath hold, which has the dual advantage of not skipping slices of liver and of studying the organ completely during the arterial phase. In one study comparing spiral CT and conventional CT in hypervascularized HCC <2 cm the detection rates were 82% and 24% respectively.[12] In another study comparing spiral CT and US in the same kind of lesion the detection rates were 83% and 55%.[13] Thus both studies demonstrated the definite superiority of spiral CT over both conventional CT and US in the diagnosis of hypervascularized HCC. Since spiral CT seems to have attained the detection rates of investigations using intra-arterial contrast media like CTAP, LipCT and CO_2US, the rational course would appear to be to include it in the diagnostic work-up. Recent technological advances in MR have likewise improved its detection rate in lesions <2 cm. In one study with superparamagnetic iron oxide-enhanced MR imaging with proton-density-weighted or fast low-angle short sequences the investigators visualized 80% of lesions <1 cm, 89% 1-2 cm and 100% 2-3 cm, though there were a few false positives.[14]

There remains the problem of detecting hypovascularized tumors, almost always small and early HCC; in one study in which CT was evaluated in early HCC and in advanced overt HCC, the former less vascularized than the latter, the detection rates were 61% and 80% respectively in tumors of 1-2 cm and 75% and 100% in those of 2-3 cm (29% in early HCC <1 cm).[15] Thus even with the most recent advances many hypovascularized HCC are still missed. In confirmation of this, recent studies checking the true detection rate of imaging on explanted liver[16-18] revealed much lower sensitivity than previously thought. In one of them[18] a lesion-by-lesion analysis yielded a sensitivity of 53% for LipCT (with a mean diameter of 1.6 cm in undetected lesions) compared with 83% in previous studies that checked operative specimens rather than explanted liver.

Although for nonsurgical removal or even for OLT these findings may not suggest substantial changes in patient management, for surgical resection they are of cardinal importance.[18] TAE and PEI are repeatable and so treatment of a new lesion already present but undetected at the baseline and coming to light in the course of follow-up is the rule; for these therapies there will be at most an underestimate of tumor stage and perhaps an error in prognosis. For OLT failure to detect a small lesion is probably also not very serious, that is, unlikely to falsify the prognosis;[18] indeed the mean diameter of undetected nodules is broadly similar to that of nodules found incidentally in patients who have undergone liver explantation because of cirrhosis, since every study has reported long tumor-free survivals (see Chapter 31). These nodules, not being impregnated with Lipiodol, were still hypovascularized and thus had a slow doubling time.[19] But for surgical resection, the principal indication for which is a single tumor, failure to detect a nodule and hence to remove it, will result in certain recurrence, even if reresections are possible. An ideal candidate for resection, that is a patient with a single US-imaged lesion, must therefore undergo all the diagnostic investigations capable of detecting the presence of other lesions. In summary, the work-up must be adapted to the type of therapy one has in mind for the individual patient.

In the event of a lesion too advanced for ablative therapy US may be considered sufficient.

In earlier disease, if the intended treatment is percutaneous ablation, it is sufficient for the next step to be CT (spiral, if possible) or enhanced MR scanning, useful because they are complementary to US and indispensable for evaluation of therapeutic efficacy (see Chapters 25-27).

If the intended treatment is TAE, this presupposes an angiogram and hence the possibility of CTAP (or CO_2US) followed, naturally, by LipCT (see Chapter 24).

If the intention is to perform an OLT, nearly every center requires abdominal and thoracic CT, angiography, LipCT and bone radionuclide scanning (see Chapter 23).

If the option is surgical resection, the second step should be a spiral CT or an enhanced MR. If these investigations reveal no contraindications to surgery, the third step should be one of the procedures with intra-arterial infusion of contrast medium (CTAP, LipCT, CO_2US), the choice depending on the expertise or preference of the individual center.

REFERENCES

1. Bartolozzi C, Lencioni R, Caramella D, Gibilisco G, Cioni R, Vignali C. Stadiazione del carcinoma epatocellulare. *Radiol Med* 1994; **88**: 429-436
2. Choi BI, Park JH, Kim BH, Kim SH, Han MC, Kim CW. Small hepatocellular carcinoma detection with sonography, computed tomography (CT), angiography and Lipiodol-CT. *Br J Radiol* 1989; **62**: 897-903
3. Hayashi N, Yamamoto K, Tamaki N, *et al.* Metastatic nodules of hepatocellular carcinoma: detection with angiography, CT, and *US. Radiology* 1987; **165**: 61-63
4. Ikeda K, Saitoh S, Koida I, Tsubota A, Arase Y, Chayama K, Kumada H. Imaging diagnosis of small hepatocellular carcinoma. *Hepatology* 1994; **20**: 82-87
5. Kudo M, Tomita S, Tochio H, *et al.* Small hepatocellular carcinoma: diagnosis with US angiography with intraarterial CO_2 microbubbles. *Radiology* 1992; **182**: 155-160
6. Kawasaki S, Makuuchi M. Intraoperative ultrasound and other techniques. In: Kawasaki S, Makuuchi M eds. *Novel regional therapies for liver tumors;* Landes Austin 1995; 99-121
7. Merine D, Takayasu K, Wakao F. Detection of hepatocellular carcinoma: comparison of CT during arterial portography with CT after intraaterial injection of iodized oil. *Radiology* 1990; **175**: 707-710
8. Ohto M, Kondo F, Ebara M. Pathology, diagnosis, and treatment for small liver cancer. In: Tobe T, Kameda H, Okudaira M, *et al.* eds. *Primary liver cancer in Japan*; Tokyo: Springer 1992; 129- 138
9. Takayasu K, Moriyama N, Muramatsu Y, Makuuchi M, Hasegawa H, Okazaki N, Hirohashi S. The diagnosis of small hepatocellular carcinomas: efficacy of various imaging procedures in 100 patients. *AJR* 1990; **155**: 49-54
10. Utsunomiya T, Matsumata T, Adachi E, Honda H, Sugimachi K. Limitations of current preoperative liver imaging techniques for intrahepatic metastatic nodules of hepatocellular carcinoma. *Hepatology* 1992; **16**: 694-701
11. Winter TC, Takayasu K, Muramatsu Y, *et al.* Early advanced hepatocellular carcinoma: evalutation of CT and MR appearance with pathologic correlation. *Radiology* 1994; **192**: 379-387
12. Fujita M, Kuroda C, Kumatani T, *et al.* Comparison between conventional and spiral CT in patients with hypervascular hepatocellular carcinoma. *Eur J Radiol* 1994; **18**: 134-136
13. Ueda K, Kitagawa K, Kadoya M, Matsui O, Takashima T, Yamahana T. Detection of hypervascular hepatocellular carcinoma by using spiral volumetric CT: comparison of US and MR imaging. *Abdom Imag* 1995; **20**: 547-553
14. Yamamoto H, Yamashita Y, Yoshimatsu S, *et al.* Hepatocellular carcinoma in cirrhotic livers: detection with unenhanced and iron oxide-enhanced MR imaging. *Radiology* 1995; **195**: 106-112
15. Takayasu K, Furukawa H, Wakao F, *et al.* CT diagnosis early hepatocellular carcinoma: sensibility, findings, and CT- pathologic correlation. *AJR* 1995; **164**: 885-890
16. Selby R, Kadry Z, Carr B, Tzakis A, Madariaga JR, Iwatsuki S. Liver transplantation for hepatocellular carcinoma. *World J Surg* 1995; **19**: 53-58
17. Rizzi PM, Kane PA, Ryder SD, *et al.* Accuracy of radiology in detection of hepatocellular carcinoma before liver transplantation. *Gastroenterology* 1994; **107**: 1425-1429
18. Taourel PG, Pageaux GP, Coste V, *et al.* Small hepatocellular carcinoma in patients undergoing liver transplantation: detection with CT after injection of iodized oil. *Radiology* 1995; **197**: 377-380
19. Tochio H, Tomita S, Kudo M, *et al.* Growth speed of hepatocellular carcinoma. Relationship with arterial vascularity evaluated by US angiography (English abstract). *Acta Hepatol Jpn* 1992; **33**: 758-765

21

Staging

T Livraghi

The first staging scheme was proposed in 1971 following the Kampala symposium[1] and was later modified by Primack *et al*.[2] Those first attempts were little used because they were based on the pattern of the disease in Africa, not comparable with that found elsewhere, and partly because they made no provision for imaging in the evaluation of tumor features.

The classification proposed by Okuda *et al* in 1985, on the other hand, was widely used because of its simplicity and because it took account both of easily available functional parameters (ascites, albumin, bilirubin) and of tumor size.[3] This scheme, which allowed for three stages only, is shown in Table 21.1. It had been validated in a study of the survival of 850 patients, treated and untreated. That study had the merit of underlining the importance for prognostic purposes of the association between cirrhosis and neoplastic disease and of comparing systematically for the first time patients treated in different ways. Because of this, the study signposted the way for many subsequent studies.

Nagasue *et al* also proposed a very simple classification for surgeons, but it was not widely adopted.[4]

Later however, with the discovery of new prognostic factors and the acquisition of increasingly accurate information supplied by imaging and, most importantly, by ultrasound screening programs which made for much earlier diagnosis of HCC, it was felt that more detailed staging schemes had to be designed to meet the new needs. The TNM pathologic staging of UICC[5] was then proposed and later incorporated in the General Rules for the Clinical and Pathological Study of Primary Liver Cancer gradually worked out by the Liver Cancer Study Group of Japan.[6]

The TNM classification (see Table 21.2) is fairly simple and easily applicable, though only to surgical patients. Although its validity was confirmed by some studies,[7,8] the TNM classification was felt by some authors,[9,10] including ourselves, to overplay size and number of lesions and underplay vascular invasion. For instance, a tumor of ≤ 2 cm with vascular invasion and one of 2.1 cm without it are both classified as T2, when portal thrombosis is known to be one of the most important predictive factors. This criticism was vindicated by a study of Izumi *et al* on 104 surgical patients in which multivariate analysis showed that portal invasion was the most important factor.[11] According to their data the difference between stages 1 and 2 and between 3 and 4 was not significant for survival or for disease-free interval, and so these investigators proposed a substantial change to the UICC classification, shown in Table 21.3.

The staging system of the Liver Cancer Study Group of Japan, reproduced here (see Appendix) in its most recent version, is much more comprehensive in that it includes a very detailed pathologic classification and

Table 21.2 – TNM Classification of HCC

Stage	Factor T	Factor N	Factor M
I	T1	N0	M0
II	T2	N0	M0
III	T3	N0	M0
	T1-3	N1	M0
IV-A	T4	N0-1	M0
IV-B	T1-4	N0-1	M1

T1, Solitary, ≤2 cm, without vascular invasion
T2, solitary, ≤2 cm, with vascular invasion; multiple, one lobe, ≤2 cm, without vascular invasion; solitary, 2 cm, without vascular invasion
T3, Solitary >2 cm, with vascular invasion; multiple, one lobe, ≤2 cm, with vascular invasion; multiple, one lobe, >2 cm, with or without vascular invasion
T4, Multiple, more than one lobe; invasion of major branch of portal or hepatice veins
N1, Regional
M1, Distant metastasis, including remote lymph nodal metastasis

Table 21.1 – Staging scheme of HCC by Okuda *et al*[3]

Stage	Tumor size		Ascites		Albumin		Bilirubin	
	>50% (+)	<50% (-)	(+)	(-)	<3g/dl (+)	>3g/dl (-)	>3mg/d (+)	<3mg/dl (-)
I	(-)		(-)		(-)		(-)	
II					1 or 2 (+)			
III					3 or 4 (+)			

+: sign of advanced disease

Table 21.3 – Modified TNM classification and stage grouping of HCC (proposed by Izumi *et al*[11])

Stage 1	T1	N0	M0
Stage 2	T2	N0	M0
Stage 3	T3	N0	M0
	Any T	N1	M0
Stage 4	Any T	Any N	M1

T1, solitary without vascular invasion
T2, solitary or multiple with vascular invasion
T3, solitary or multiple, with invasion of major branch of portal hepatic veins
N1, regional
M1, distant metastasis including remote lymph nodal metastasis

a clinical one too. Its complexity, however, makes it rather difficult to adhere to in its entirety. Furthermore their system is not applicable to nonsurgical therapies like PEI and TAE: hence the pathologic stage of nonsurgical patients, based on imaging alone, is bound to be underestimated.

An interesting classification was proposed by Calvet *et al* in 1990, validated on a study of the survival of 206 patients.[12] By a multivariate survival analysis using clinical, biochemical, ultrasonographic and pathologic data, a prognostic index was constructed allowing division of patients into different groups according to their relative risk of death: RRD=EXP (age x 0.03 + ascites x 0.8281 + blood urea nitrogen x 0.0137 + serum sodium x (-0.0538) + γ-glutamyl-transpeptidase x 0.0019 + bilirubin x 0.0734 + tumor size x 0.33 + toxic syndrome (weight loss >10% premorbid weight, malaise and anorexia) x 0.4965 + metastases x 0.55). In this formula, ascites, toxic syndrome and metastases were introduced as dichotomous variables (present=1, absent=0), tumor size (uninodular ≤5 cm=1, uninodular >5 cm=2, multinodular =3 or diffuse =4) as a semiquantitative variable and the remaining items as continuous variables. According to prognosis, patients were divided into three groups, with RRD<0.025, between 0.025 and 0.085, and >0.085.

At our center in the pretreatment work-up we use a staging card (Fig. 21.1) that contemplates factors on which data are easily obtained and which are at the same time considered relevant to the prognosis. The card is applicable to all patients and yields information sufficiently exhaustive to guide the type of treatment. The card is divided into sections containing the usual information on patient identity, relevant history, data on etiology, stage of liver disease and HCC pattern. The factors considered prognostic are rated from 1 to 3, that is, from most to least favourable, in the appropriate boxes. The card is suitable for computer processing.

The term "associated diseases" means only those likely to affect the choice of therapy or the prognosis, such as a severe heart disease that may impede surgery, or another tumor.

The item "previous therapies" refers to previous HCC therapies, fairly frequent in these patients (see Chapter 30). From this card any intervening changes are evident.

Under "etiology" are recorded B- or C-related viral diseases, the less common ones as "other". In the case of viral diseases it should be stated whether or not the infection is actively replicating, because active liver disease may contraindicate OLT and has a significantly greater risk of intrahepatic recurrences in patients treated with local ablation therapies.[13,14] The possibility of HDV superinfection in HBV carriers is also contemplated, because of its prognostic influence.[15] In the case of other liver diseases, their nature (due to alcohol, hemochromatosis, etc) should be stated in parentheses, if known.

For esophageal varices, we consider at high risk of bleeding in patients with blue varices, red wale marking (+++) and cherry-red spot (+++) of the red color sign category, and esophagitis. Beppu's score may be a more precise method to discriminate bleeders and non bleeders.[16]

For the staging of cirrhosis we use Child's classification, which is easy to apply and universally known.[17] Given the long life expectancy of Child's class A patients, we include chronic liver hepatitis under this heading. Child's classes are one of the factors most relevant to prognosis and to choice of therapy. For instance, class C contraindicates several procedures whereas for the same HCC presentation it may indicate a canditate for OLT.

For grading, that is, classification by cellular atypia, we broadly follow the grading of Edmondson and Steiner[18] but combine their grades I and II under the common heading of well differentiated, in agreement with other workers,[19-21] on the basis that biopsy does

HCC STAGING CARD

Name .... Age .... Sex [M] [F] Date ....

Associated Diseases	....				
Previous Therapies of HCC	....				
Etiology	HBsAg+			anti-HCV+	other
	active	inactive	HDV		(..................................)

	1	2	3
ESOPHAGEAL VARICES	absent	low risk	high risk
CHILD'S CLASS	A	B	C
GRADING	well differentiated	moderately differentiated	poor differentiated
TYPE	nodular	infiltrating	diffuse
NUMBER	1	2-3	> 3 (..........)
SIZE	< 2 cm	2.1 - 5 cm	> 5.1 (..........)
LOCATION	1 segment (...............)	> 1 segment (.................)	bilobar (.................)
TUMOR INVASIVENESS	absent	local	IM
VASCULAR INVASION (P,V,B)	absent	local	diffuse
NM	O	N+	M+
AFP	< 20 (.........)	21-200 (.........)	> 200 (..........)

P = portal veins , V = hepatic veins , B = bile ducts , IM = intrahepatic metastases (satellites)

Note ....

....

....

Figure 21.1 – HCC staging card

not distinguish grade I from non neoplastic tissue; indeed, Edmondson and Steiner themselves acknowledge that grade I can be diagnosed only if it coexists with grade II. Since several grades of differentiation, in addition to adenomatous hyperplasia, may coexist in one tumor, when biopsy reveals this the highest grade is recorded.

With regard to type, we accept the gross classification proposed by Eggel[22]: nodular, or massive (infiltrating) and diffuse. This classification, used by many, including the Liver Cancer Study Group of Japan, ties in pretty well with the imaging rules. "Nodular" means a tumor, single or multiple, in which the boundary between neoplastic and non neoplastic tissue is clearly visible; the term is better suited to imaging than encapsulated form, since it is not always possible to establish whether a capsule is present and intact. "Infiltrating" (or massive) applies to a tumor, single or multiple, whatever the size, in which the boundary between neoplastic and non neoplastic tissue is ill defined. The Liver Cancer Study Group of Japan has had problems in distinguishing a small infiltrating tumor affecting a single segment, and hence similar to a nodular tumor, from the infiltrating variety and have solved the problem for the time being by making some subtypes. On the staging card the various subtypes can be easily described by reference to size, site and invasiveness. A "diffuse" tumor is one that has largely replaced the hepatic parenchyma with innumerable small nodules, a pattern that is often hard to indentify by imaging because it may simulate a pattern of cirrhosis known as "coarse liver". It may be distinguished by a difference in the size and structure of the nodules or by the presence of portal thrombosis.

As to number, the difference in survival between single and multiple tumors is well known. The decision to divide the multiple form into group 2 with 2-3 nodules and group 3 with more than 3 is based on the range of therapies now available at many centers, the cut-off at 3 nodules being held discriminant for OLT or for conventional PEI, for example. The multiplicity of nodules often raises the problem of distinguishing, by imaging procedures but also histologically, between intrahepatic metastases (IM or satellites or daughter nodules) of a main lesion and a multicentric form. On our staging card the term IM denotes small lesions lying around the main lesion, in the same segment or in an adjacent segment, or nodules that after surgery of the main lesion appear in the same segment or in an adjacent segment.

On the score of size, we give the breakdown adopted at most centers, useful because it is practical and because it has some proven prognostic value. Size <2 cm is now the accepted standard for "small" HCC, while 2.1 to 5 cm and over 5 cm are important for many choices of treatment. The diameter of the largest tumor is entered in the box.

With regard to tumor location, the decision to distinguish three types by extent of involvement (a single segment, several segments of one lobe, and both lobes) was based on the proven difference in survival and on the range of choices adopted at many surgical centers. The segment containing the tumor has also been considered by some surgeons resulted relevant to the prognosis.[23] The classic 8 segment division of Couinaud[24] or the 5 segment system adopted by the Liver Cancer Study Group of Japan may be given in parentheses.

Tumor invasiveness refers to peritumoral involvement. It may take the form of clear infiltration of the tumoral border (group 2) or IM (group 3). We do not divide IM according to the number of segments containing them, because this factor is not considered relevant to the prognosis.[25]

Vascular invasion may take the form of portal thrombosis (P), invasion of the hepatic vein (V), or bile duct invasion (B). These various possibilities are stated in parentheses. All have been recognized in every study as having high predictive value and have therefore been categorized by extent, local or diffuse, since the pattern may be crucial to the choice of therapy. Group 2 covers local involvement, that is, for P and V involvement of a distal branch, and for B local dilatation. Group 3 covers diffuse involvement, for P thrombosis of one or more proximal branches, for V invasion of one or more of the hepatic veins or of the inferior vena cava, and for B diffuse dilatation.

As to the presence of lymph node metastases (N) or extrahepatic metastases (M), the former are classified as group 2, being considered less advanced than the latter, classed as group 3. The site of metastases may be cited in parentheses.

With regard to assays for tumor markers, AFP is

included, despite its known lower sensibility in small HCC. However, a high level of AFP has been recognized in many studies as indicating a poor prognosis including a study by the Liver Cancer Study Group of Japan.[26] The proposed levels (20/20-200/200) are accepted as reference standards by most workers. The exact values may be cited in parentheses. Levels of any other complementary markers such as DCP or alphafucosidase may be added in the same box, although their predictive value needs further confirmation.[27]

REFERENCES

1. Vogel CL, Linsell CA. International symposium on hepatocellular carcinoma, Kampala Uganda. *J Natl Cancer Inst* 1971; **48**: 567-571
2. Primack A, Vogel CL, Kyalwazi SK, Ziegler JL, Simon R, Anthony PP. A staging system for hepatocellular carcinoma: prognostic factors in Ugandan patients. *Cancer* 1975; **35**: 1357-1364
3. Okuda K, Ohtsuki T, Obata H, *et al.* Natural history of hepatocellular carcinoma and prognosis in relation to treatment. Study of 850 patients. *Cancer* 1985; **56**: 918-928
4. Nagasue N, Yukaya H, Yuichiro O, Sasaki Y, Chang YC, Niimi K. Clinical experience with 118 hepatic resections for hepatocellular carcinoma. *Surgery* 1986; **99**: 694-702
5. UICC: International Union Against Cancer. In Hermanek P, Sobin LH, eds. *TNM classification of malignant tumor* (4th edn); Berlin: Springer-Verlag 1987; pp 53-55
6. Yamamoto M, Sugahara K. Overview of the general rules for the clinical and pathological study of primary liver cancer in Japan. In Tobe T, *et al* eds. *Primary liver cancer in Japan*; Tokyo: Springer 1992; pp 385-401
7. Ringe B, Pichlmayr R, Wittekind C, Tusch G. Surgical treatment of hepatocellular carcinoma: experience with liver resection and transplantation in 198 patients. *World J Surg* 1991; **15**: 270-285
8. Selby R, Kadry Z, Carr B, Tzakis A, Madariaga JR, Iwatsuki S. Liver transplantation for hepatocellular carcinoma. *World J Surg* 1995; **19**: 53-58
9. Sasaki Y, Imaoka S, Masutani S, Osashi I, Ishikawa O, Koyama H, Iwanaga T. Influence of coexisting cirrhosis on long-term prognosis after surgery in patients with hepatocellular carcinoma. *Surgery* 1992; **112**: 515-521
10. Sugioka A, Tsuzuki T, Kanai T. Postresection prognosis of patients with hepatocellular carcinoma. *Surgery* 1993; **113**: 612-618
11. Izumi R, Shimizu K, II T, Yagi M, Matsui O, Nonomura A, Miyazaki I. Prognostic factors of hepatocellular carcinoma in patients undergoing hepatic resection. *Gastroenterology* 1994; **106**: 720-727
12. Calvet X, Bruix J, Ginés P, Bru C, Solé M, Vilana R, Rodes J. Prognostic factors of hepatocellular carcinoma in the West: a multivariate analysis in 206 patients. *Hepatology* 1990; **12**: 753-760
13. Adachi E, Maeda T, Matsumata T, Shirabe K, Kinukawa N, Sugimachi K, Tsuneyoshi M. Risk factors for intrahepatic recurrence in human small hepatocellular carcinoma. *Gastroenterology* 1995; **108**: 768-775
14. Benvegnù L, Fattovich G, Noventa F, *et al.* Concurrent hepatitis B and C virus infection and risk of hepatocellular carcinoma in cirrhosis. *Cancer* 1994; **74**: 2442-2448
15. Verme G, Brunetto MR, Oliveri F, *et al.* Role of hepatitis delta virus infection in hepatocellular carcinoma. *Dig Dis Sci* 1991; **36**: 1134-1136
16. Beppu K, Inokuchi K, Koyanagi N, Nakayama S, Sakata H, Kitano S, Kobayashi M. Prediction of variceal hemorrhage by esophageal endoscopy. *Gastrointest Endosc* 1981; **27**: 213-218
17. Child CG, Turcotte JG. Surgery in portal hypertension. In Child CG, editor. *Major problems in clinical surgery: the liver and portal hypertension*; Philadelphia: WB Saunders 1964; pp 1-85
18. Edmondson HA, Steiner PE. Primary carcinoma of the liver. A study among 48900 necropsies. *Cancer* 1954; **7**: 462-503
19. Kondo F, Wada K, Nagato Y, *et al.* Biopsy diagnosis of well-differentiated hepatocellular carcinoma based on new morphologic criteria. *Hepatology* 1989; **9**: 751-755
20. Sato M, Watanabe Y, Lee T, *et al.* Well-differentiated hepatocellular carcinoma: clinicopathological features and results of hepatic resection. *Am J Gastroinest* 1995; **90**: 112-116
21. Calvet X, Bruix J, Bru C, *et al.* Natural history of hepatocellular carcinoma in Spain: a five year experience in 249 cases. *J Hepatol* 1990; **10**: 311-331
22. Eggel H. Ueber das primare carcinoma der leber. *Beitr Path Anat* 1901; **30**: 506-604
23. Wu CC, Ho YZ, Ho LZ, Wu TC, Liu TJ, P'eng FK. Preoperative transcatheter arterial chemoembolization for resectable large hepatocellular carcinoma: a reappraisal. *Br J Surg* 1995; **82**: 122-126
24. Couinaud C. Lobes et segments hépatiques; notes sur l'architecture anatomique et chirurgicale du foie. *Presse Med* 1954; **62**: 709-712
25. Monden M, Sakon M, Gotoh M, *et al.* Selection of therapeutic modalities for hepatocellular carcinoma in patients with multiple hepatic lesions. *Cancer Chemother Pharmacol* 1992; **31**: 38-44
26. The Liver Cancer Study Group of Japan. Predictive factors for long-term prognosis after partial hepatectomy for patients with hepatocellular carcinoma in Japan. *Cancer* 1994; **74**: 2772-2780
27. Suehiro T, Matsumata T, Itasaka H, Taketomi A, Yamamoto K, Sugimachi K. Des-gamma-carboxy prothrombin and proliferative activity of hepatocellular. *Surgery* 1995; **117**: 682-691

APPENDIX

The following are general rules for the clinical and pathologic study of primary liver cancer.

1. ANATOMY

Liver lobes and segments

The right and left lobes, which are divided by Cantlie's line, are each divided into two segments, and together with the caudate lobe, there are five segments. Each segment is divided into upper and lower subsegments except for the caudate lobe.

Lymph node

Lymph node metastasis in liver cancer awaits further study, but for the time being, descriptions should be made in accordance with the general rules for cancer in other organs.

1. *Group 1 lymph nodes*
    a) Subdiaphragmatic lymph nodes of the upper region of the liver
    b) Lymph nodes in the hepatic porta
2. *Group 2 lymph nodes*
    a) Lymph nodes in the hepatoduodenal ligament
3. *Group 3 lymph nodes*
    a) Lymph nodes around the vena cava above the diaphragm
    b) Lymph nodes at the posterior aspect of the pancreas
    c) Lymph nodes along the common hepatic artery
    d) Lymph nodes around the celiac artery
    e) Low thoracic paraesophageal lymph nodes

2. DESCRIPTIVE METHODS OF STATE OF TUMOR BY IMAGING DIAGNOSIS

Location of tumor

The site of a liver tumor should be indicated, according to (4) below. Descriptive methods of operative findings and resected specimens of liver cancer, using the abbreviation for the liver segments (P, A, M, L, C) as described in Fig. 21.2, and adding St for single, Mt for multiple, or Dt for not-countable diffuse tumors.

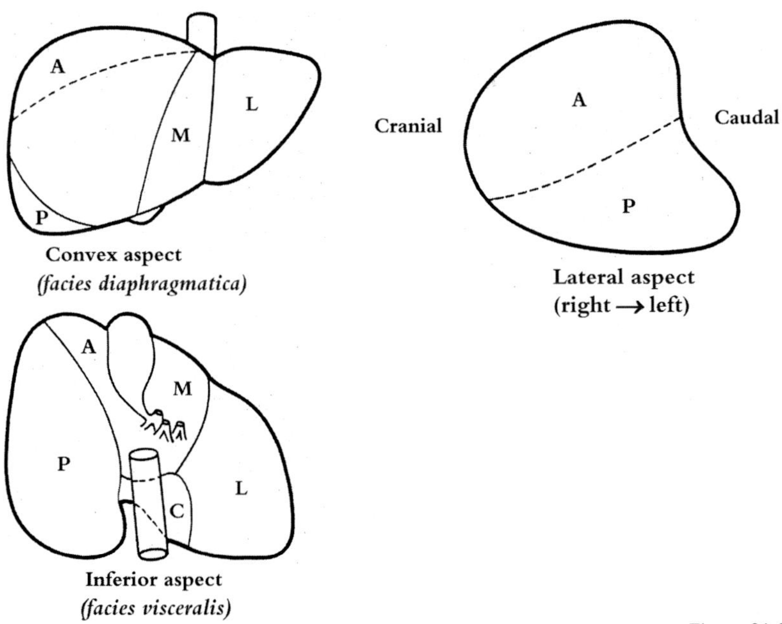

Figure 21.2

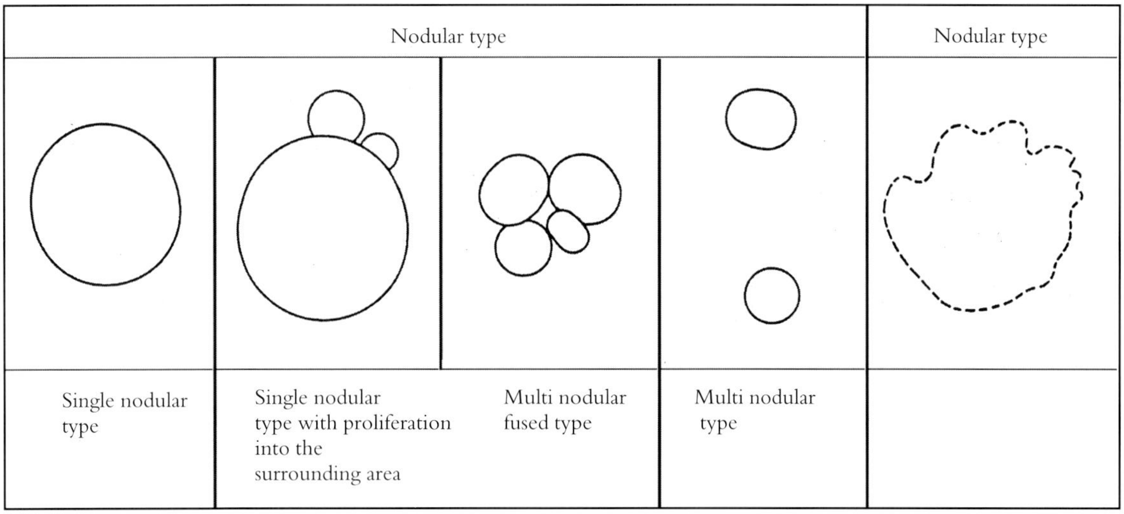

Figure 21.3

Size

The size of a tumor should be measured as long diameter (cm) x short diameter (cm). If this is not possible, the longest diameter should be entered.

State of tumor border

1. *PD. Poorly demarcated*
2. *WD. Well demarcated*
    a) Fc(+). Clear capsule formation
    b) Fc(-). No clear capsule formation

If a macroscopic type of tumor can be determined by imaging diagnosis according to (3) below, macroscopic classification of the liver cancer, should be so indicated.

State of internal tumor structure

1. *Solid*
    a) Nc (+). Necrotized in some parts; the Nc% (necrotized percent) should be calculated
    b) Nc (-). No necrosis
2. *Cystic*

Practices of transcatheter arterial embolization (TAE) or ethanol injection should be indicated. If Lipiodol or an anti-cancer drug was used at the same time as TAE, it should be so indicated.

Vascular invasion

Vascular invasion should be examined by imaging techniques, and it should be described according to (4) below.

Distant organ metastasis (DM)

Metastasis of liver cancer to a distant organ is expressed as DM. The metastasized organ as identified from X-rays, scintigraphy, ultrasonography, computed tomography, magnetic resonance imaging or clinical findings, should be indicated in parentheses.

1. DM_0. No metastasis to distant organs
2. DM_1. Metastasis to distant organs

3. MACROSCOPIC CLASSIFICATION OF LIVER CANCER

The macroscopic findings of liver cancer are divided into the nodular, massive, and diffuse type (Fig. 21.3).

1. *Nodular type.* In this type of cancer, a clear border can be seen between the cancerous and noncancerous portions, and it can be divided into three basic subtypes: *1)* the single nodular type, *2)* the single nodular type with proliferation into the surrounding tissues, and *3)* the multinodular fused type.

When multiple tumors of the nodular type exist in the liver, it is called the multinodular form, and the subtype of each nodule should be described.

A small tumor located within one segment with an unclear and irregular border between the cancerous and non-cancerous portions is treated provisionally as a subdivision of the nodular type, the infiltrative form, and this is indicated in parentheses.

2. *Massive type*. Large liver cancers occupy more than one segment of the liver, and the borders between the cancerous and non-cancerous portions are unclear and irregular. This definition conforms with Eggel's classification[22] of the massive type.

3. *Diffuse type*. The liver as a whole is replaced by a great number of small, disseminated tumor nodules. It is often difficult, when examining the liver surface macroscopically, to distinguish between this type of cancer and cirrhosis of the liver.

4. DESCRIPTIVE METHODS OF OPERATIVE FINDINGS AND RESECTED SPECIMENS OF LIVER CANCER

Operative findings should be recorded for all cases having undergone laparotomy. When the size of the tumor, macroscopic findings, infiltration of the surrounding tissues, lymph node metastasis, and so on, are unconfirmed because a case was inoperable, the entry should be made in parentheses. When an item is unclear or unknown, "unclear" or "unknown" should be entered.

Location of cancer

1. The *site* of liver cancer should be indicated using the abbreviations for the liver segments (P, A, M, L, C) as described previously and adding St for single or Mt for multiple tumors.

2. When liver cancer is present in two segments, the segment containing most cancer should be entered first.

3. When the liver cancer is present in more than two segments, the segments should be entered in the order of the amount of cancer present in each segment. For example, single liver cancer in which the majority of the neoplasm is located in the posterior segment, but part of it is also located in the anterior segment should be indicated as St-PA. Moreover if the liver cancer has spread from the medial segment to the lateral segment, and there are also two tumors in the anterior segment, the entry should be indicated as Mt-MLA.

Size and surroundings (H)

The size of the cancer in each segment should be measured, and the length (long diameter), width (short diameter) and thickness (height) entered in cm. The following symbols should also be employed:

1. H_0. Liver cancer is T1 and is present only in one subsegment
2. H_S. Liver cancer is present only in one subsegment
3. H_1. Liver cancer is present in only one segment
4. H_2. Liver cancer is present in two segments
5. H_3. Liver cancer is present in three segments
6. H_4. Liver cancer is present in more than three segments

Macroscopic findings of liver cancer

The macroscopic findings of liver cancer at resection or autopsy are classified into three main types (nodular, massive, and diffuse) and then into the subtypes as specified in (3) above. Since it is often difficult to distinguish between the nodular and massive types in inoperable cases, however, entries should be based on local findings, imaging findings, and so on, and should be made in parentheses.

The macroscopic conditions, such as the border between the cancerous and non-cancerous portions, are expressed as follows:

1. *Growth type*
   a) Expansive growth (Eg). The border between cancerous and non-cancerous tissue is clear.
   b) Infiltrative growth (Ig). The border between cancerous and non-cancerous tissue is not clear.

2. *Capsule formation (Fc)*
   a) Fc(-). No clear connective tissue capsule is formed around the cancer.
   b) Fc(+). A clear connective tissue capsule is formed around the cancer.

3. Capsule infiltration (Fc-Inf)

a) Fc-Inf(-). There is no apparent cancer infiltration into the cancer capsule.

b) Fc-Inf(+). There is cancer infiltration into the cancer capsule and/or outside the capsule.

4. Septal formation (Sf)

a) Sf(-). No formation of fibrous septa can be seen within the cancer.

b) Sf(+). Formation of fibrous septa can be seen within the cancer and there is clear lobe formation.

5. Serosal infiltration (Si)

Serosal infiltration should be classified under the following four headings on the basis of macroscopic expansion:

a) S0. No cancer tissue in the serosa.

b) S1. Cancer tissue in the serosa.

c) S2. Cancer tissue infiltration to other organs. The name of the infiltrated organ should be noted.

d) S3. Ruptured cancer tissue, accompanied by intraperitoneal hemorrhage.

Lymph node metastasis (N)

1. N_0(-). No apparent lymph node metastasis
2. N_1(+). Metastasis to Group 1 lymph nodes
3. N_2(+). Metastasis to Group 2 lymph nodes
4. N_3(+). Metastasis to Group 3 or more distant lymph nodes
5. N_1(-). No metastasis to Group 1 lymph nodes
6. N_2(-). No metastasis to Group 2 lymph nodes
7. N_3(-). No metastasis to Group 3 or more distant lymph nodes

Determination of N_3 metastasis is often difficult in operative cases, N_2(+), N_3(+) are treated as M1 (see (6) below).

Vascular invasion (V)

1. Vp_0. No tumor embolus in the portal vein
2. Vp_1. Tumor embolus distal to the second branch of the left or right portal veins (not including second branches)
3. Vp_2. Tumor embolus in the second branch of the portal vein.
4. Vp_3. Tumor embolus in the first branch, or trunk of the portal vein, or in a branch on the opposite side
5. Vv_0. No tumor embolus in the hepatic vein
6. Vv_1. Tumor embolus in a branch of the hepatic vein
7. Vv_2. Tumor embolus in the right, middle or left hepatic vein trunk, posterior inferior hepatic venous trunk or short hepatic vein
8. Vv_3. Tumor embolus in the inferior vena cava

The first branch of the portal vein consists of a common trunk on the right side and the transverse portion on the left side. The second branch consists of the segment branch trunk on the right side and the umbilical portion on the left side.

Bile duct invasion (B)

1. B_0. No expansion into the intrahepatic bile ducts
2. B_1. Expansion into the intrahepatic bile ducts
3. B_2. Expansion into the intrahepatic bile ducts and further into the extrahepatic bile ducts

Intrahepatic metastasis (IM)

1. IM_0. No intrahepatic metastasis
2. IM_1. Intrahepatic metastasis only in the same segment as the main tumor
3. IM_2. Intrahepatic metastasis in two segments
4. IM_3. Intrahepatic metastasis in three or more segments

The liver segment containing the intrahepatic metastasis should be indicated in parentheses. For example, when the main tumor is present in the posterior segment and another tumor, considered to be metastatic, is found in the posterior segment, the entry should be IM_1 (P). When metastasis is also found in the lateral segment, it should be IM_2 (PL).

Peritoneal dissemination (P)

The degrees of peritoneal disseminating metastasis fall into the following three categories:

1. P_0. No disseminating metastasis in the serosal surface of the entire peritoneal cavity
2. P_1. Disseminating metastasis in the adjacent peritoneum (cranial to the transverse colon, but including the greater omentum), but no metastasis in the distant peritoneum
3. P_2. Disseminating metastasis in the distant peritoneum

Findings from histologic examinations above should be written in small letters, such as eg, ig, fc(+), fc-inf(+), sf(+), s_2, n_1, vp_1, b_1, im_2, or p_1.

Evalutation of the cancer infiltration of the resected liver surface

Cancerous infiltration of the resected liver specimens should be evaluated macroscopically and histologically.

1. *Macroscopic classification (TW)*
   a) TW(-). No macroscopic cancerous infiltration within 10 mm from the cut liver surface in freshly excised specimens
   b) TW(+). Macroscopic cancerous infiltration within 10 mm from the cut liver surface in freshly excised specimens
2. *Histologic classification (tw)*
   a) tw(-). No cancer cells observed histologically within 5 mm from the cut liver surface in fixed specimens
   b) tw(+). Cancer cells observed histologically within 5 mm from the cut liver surface in fixed specimens

In TW(-) cases, when tumor emboli are found in the intrahepatic vasculature and bile ducts by means of pre- and intraoperative imaging diagnosis, removal of the tumor emboli is required.

Description of tumors remaining in the remnant liver

In cases of reduction surgery, where tumors remaining in the remnant liver are determined macroscopically or by image diagnosis on liver resection, the state of the tumors should be examined using ultrasonography and described according to (2) above.

Concomitant liver cirrhosis (Z)

1. Z0. Normal liver
2. Z1. Accompanying fibrosis but not defined as liver cirrhosis
3. Z2. Liver cirrhosis

5. CLINICAL STATUS OF THE HOST

Clinical stage (Table 21.4)

There are three clinical stages of hepatocellular carcinoma which are classified according to clinical and laboratory findings. The degree of progress is obtained by evaluating the patient's condition for each item, and when at least two items within any stage are found to apply, that stage is then assigned.

Table 21.4 – Clinical stage

Findings	Stage I	Stage II	Stage III
Ascites	None	Treatment effective	Treatment ineffective
Serum bilirubin (mg/dl)	Below 2.0	2.0-3.0	Over 3.0
Serum albumin (g/dl)	Over 3.5	3.0-3.5	Below 3.0
ICG R_{15} (%)	Below 15	15-40	Over 40
Prothrombin activity value (%)	Over 80	50-80	Below 50

Endoscopic findings of esophageal varices (EV)

1. EV(-). No concomitant esophageal varices
2. EV(+). Concomitant esophageal varices

6. MACROSCOPIC STAGING

(Table 21.5)

In macroscopic staging, the stage for each item is determined and the highest value selected.

The degree of macroscopic progress is classified into four stages, as follows:

1. *T factor.* This depends on three items: cancer size, whether it is single or multiple, and vascular inva-

Table 21.5 – Macroscopic stage

Stage 1	T1	N0	M0
Stage 2	T2	N0	M0
Stage 3	T1	N10	M0
	T2	N1	M0
	T3	N0, N1	M0
Stage 4A	T3	N0, N1	M0
Stage 4B	Any-T	Any N	M1

T1, Solitary, ≤2 cm, without vascular invasion
T2, solitary, ≤2 cm, with vascular invasion; multiple, one lobe, ≤2 cm, without vascular invasion; solitary, 2 cm, without vascular invasion
T3, Solitary >2 cm, with vascular invasion; multiple, one lobe, ≤2 cm, with vascular invasion; multiple, one lobe, >2 cm, with or without vascular invasion
T4, Multiple, more than one lobe; invasion of major branch of portal or hepatice veins
N1, Regional
M1, Distant metastasis, including remote lymph nodal metastasis

sion. Multiple tumors can be either multicentric tumors or intrahepatic metastatic tumors.

a) T1. A single tumor of 2 cm or less in its greatest dimension without vascular invasion
b) T2. A single tumor of 2 cm or less in its greatest dimension with vascular invasion
   i) Multiple tumors with maximum tumor diameter of 2 cm or less confined to one lobe
   ii) A single tumor with diameter exceeding 2 cm, without vascular invasion
c) T3. A single tumor with a diameter exceeding 2 cm, with vascular invasion
   i) Multiple tumors with diameters exceeding 2 cm confined to one lobe
d) T4. Multiple tumors in more than one lobe
   i) Associated vascular invasion in the first branch of the portal or hepatic veins

2. *N factors*.
   a) N_0. No metastasis in the Group 1 lymph nodes
   b) N_1. Metastasis in at least the Group 1 lymph nodes
3. *M factors*.
   a) M_0. No distant metastasis
   b) M_1. Distant metastasis

In the classification of lymph node metastasis (N) above, $N_2(+)$ and $N_3(+)$ are included for convenience under M1 of M factors. For cases of ruptured liver cancer, there are no special items and the stage is decided from the above T, N and M classification.

The degree of macroscopic advance is considered to be the same as the TNM classification of the UICC. In the same patient, the stage is almost the same as that given by the stage classification of the former general rules.

7. TYPES OF HEPATIC RESECTION (HR)

Extent of resection

The methods are classified as follows according to the extent of resection.

1. Hr0. Resection of less than one subsegment
2. HrS. Resection of one subsegment
3. Hr1. Resection of one segment
4. Hr2. Resection of two segments
5. Hr3. Resection of three segments
6. Hr4. Resection of four segments

Resected segments

The names of the resected segments should be shown in parentheses. In cases where resections exceed the range concerned, the segment partially resected should be added as + and lower case first letter of the segment.

In cases where concomitant resections or additional operations are performed, this fact should be noted. For example, when a splenectomy and a transabdominal esophageal transection are performed at the same time as a lateral segmentectomy, the entry should be: H_21(L), splenectomy, transabdominal esophageal transection.

Abbreviations for common hepatic resections are as follows:

1. Left lobectomy: Hr2(L, M)
2. Right lobectomy: Hr2(P, A)
3. Lateral segmentectomy: Hr1(L)
4. Extended left lobectomy: Hr2+(L, M, a)
5. Left lobectomy with partial resection of caudate lobe: Hr2+(L, M, c)
6. Extended right lobectomy: Hr2+(P, A, m)
7. Posterior segmentectomy: Hr1(P)
8. Subsegmentectomy: for example of the anterior segment, HrS(A)
9. Subsegmentectomy in two areas: for example of the anterior and posterior segments; HrS(A)+HrS(P)
10. Trisegmentectomy: trisegmentectomy from the right, Hr3(P, A, M); trisegmentectomy from the left, Hr3(L, M, A); left lobectomy with simultaneous resection of caudal lobe, Hr3(L, M, C)
11. Wedge resection, enucleation, partial resection: for example wedge resection of the posterior segment, Hr0(P)

In the case of reduction surgery, for example, where tumors remain in the medial and lateral segments after right lobectomy: Red(L, M) Hr2(P, A)

Extent of lymph node dissection (R)

Resection according to the extent of lymph node dissection is classified in the following three stages:

1. R0. Liver resection with no dissection or incomplete dissection of the Group 1 lymph nodes
2. R1. Liver resection with dissection of the Group 1 lymph nodes
3. R2. Liver resection with dissection of the Group 1 and confirmed Group 2 lymph nodes

8. CURATIVE AND NON-CURATIVE RESECTION

1. *Curative resection*
   a) Absolute curative resection
      i) Liver resection TW(-) in Stage I
   b) Relative curative resection
      i) Liver resection TW(+) but with tumor tissue removed in Stage I
      ii) Liver resection Hr≥H, R≥N, TW(-) in Stage II or III
      iii) Liver resection Hr≥H, R≥N, TW(+) but with tumor tissue removed, and tumor diameter 5 cm or less in Stage II or III

   In either case, no tumor emboli must remain in the portal vein or bile duct in images of the remnant liver.
2. *Non-curative resection*
   a) Relative non-curative resection.

      Any liver resection other than a curative resection in which all the macroscopic tumor tissue is removed.
   b) Absolute non-curative resection

      Liver resection with part of the macroscopic tumor tissue remaining.

9. RECORD OF RECURRENT TUMOR

In cases where patients have undergone a liver resection other than absolute non-curative resection and no remnant tumors were identified by image diagnosis during operation, when recurrence of liver cancer is recognized, duration after the first operation, method of diagnosis of recurrence, and changes in tumor-markers as well as state of tumor according to (2) above should be described.

PART IV
TREATMENT

22

Surgical resection

T Takayama and M Makuuchi

Among the various therapeutic options available for the treatment of hepatocellular carcinoma (HCC), surgery is the leading form of treatment because it offers the chance of long-term cure.[1] In the 1970s Western surgeons instituted major hepatectomy procedures for patients with large tumors,[2] while Eastern surgeons treating patients with HCC which arises frequently in cirrhotic livers have had the dilemma of how to balance the risks of the surgical procedure with preservation of postoperative hepatic function. In patients with cirrhosis, the major cause of operative mortality and morbidity is liver failure, and the risk rises with the volume of functional parenchyma resected. One impressive Eastern report showed that postoperative liver failure occurred in 64% of cirrhotic patients who underwent right hepatectomy, and in 28% of those having a left hepatectomy.[3] This experience suggests that major hepatectomy would be suboptimal as a procedure of choice in patients with HCC and cirrhosis. To overcome this dilemma, minor but anatomic types of hepatectomy procedure such as segmentectomy[4] and subsegmentectomy[5] were devised in the 1980s by the use of intraoperative ultrasonography (IOUS).[6,7] More recently, modified hepatectomy procedures based on transplantation techniques may possibly improve resectability in some patients with far-advanced HCC. In this chapter, we review the recent progress in operative techniques and outcome of liver surgery for patients with HCC and chronic liver disease.

OPERATIVE INDICATIONS

The operative indications for hepatectomy in patients with HCC depend mainly on two factors: the degree of extension of the tumor, and hepatic functional reserve. Several criteria have been proposed, but they all eventually seem to rely on the policy and expertise of each surgical team. However, the exclusion criteria for surgery which include bilobar dissemination of HCC, or serious hepatic dysfunction appear consistently among the different criteria.

To comprehensively evaluate tumor status, a staging system for HCC according to the clinical tumor, node, and metastasis (TNM) classification of the UICC is available (see Chapter 21).[8] The level for each of these three items is determined and the highest values are selected. The T factor is crucial and comprises tumor size (less or more than 2 cm) and number (single or multiple), and the presence of vascular invasion. The stage indicates the degree of extension of the HCC and should reflect the prognosis. Despite numerous options which are available for the treatment of HCC, patients with clinical stage I or II tumors can usually be considered to be candidates for surgery unless their hepatic function is extremely poor.

The other limiting factor is the determination of the hepatic functional reserve for each patient. For patients with chronic liver disease, we have defined criteria for surgical indication using three parameters (Fig. 22.1): the presence or absence of ascites, the level

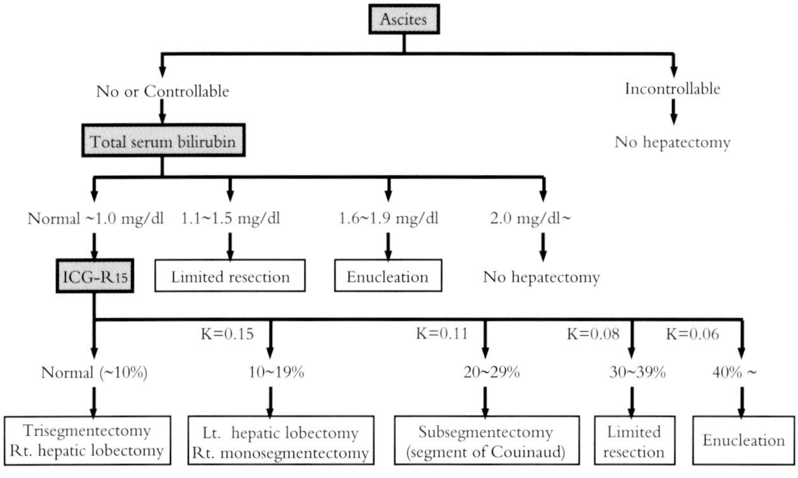

Figure 22.1 – Decision-tree of hepatectomy and its procedure for patients with HCC (from Ref.[9] with permission).

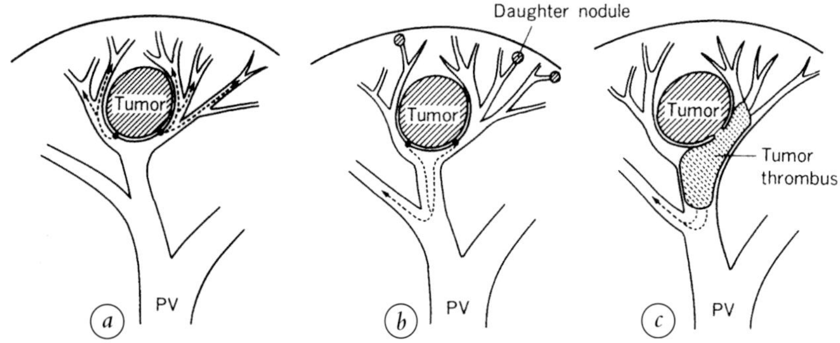

Figure 22.2 – A possible form of intrahepatic extension of HCC (from Ref. [5] with permission).

a) An HCC invades nearby portal venous branches and tumor cells are carried to the periphery,

b) these cells form microscopic tumor thrombi and then intrahepatic metastases,

c) tumor thrombi are a source of wider spread. PV:portal venous branch.

of total serum bilirubin and the indocyanine green retention rate at 15 minutes ($ICG\text{-}R_{15}$).[9] Briefly, patients without ascites and a normal bilirubin level (less than 1.0 mg/dl) are considered to be good candidates, and are then classified according to their $ICG\text{-}R_{15}$ value; trisegmentectomy or right hepatic lobectomy (removing about two thirds of the total hepatic parenchyma) is possible when the patient has an $ICG\text{-}R_{15}$ value less than 10%; left hepatic lobectomy or right monosegmentectomy (removing one-third) at 19% or less; subsegmentectomy (resection of Couinaud's segment) at 29% or less; and limited or local resection over 30%. Our policy originated from the need for radical, but safe, resection of HCC since the majority of the patients may have hepatic functional impairment but are usually asymptomatic. In our recent series, these criteria have allowed us to decrease operative mortality to around 1%, even in patients with chronic liver disease.[10]

To minimize the risk of postoperative hepatic failure, three methods that we have devised are routinely used. Vascular occlusion techniques, such as hemihepatic vascular occlusion or Pringle's maneuver, are applied during transection of hepatic parenchyma to decrease operative blood loss.[11] Fresh frozen plasma is transfused to replace the intraoperative blood loss up to 1,500 ml; such replacement also reduces the increase in serum bilirubin.[12] Preoperative portal vein embolization is used in cases who need to undergo major lobectomy for curative resection of an HCC invading the major trunk of the portal vein, in order to compensate for the postoperative hepatic deficit.[13] Recently, Fan *et al.*[14] have proposed the use of perioperative nutritional support to reduce complications after hepatectomy in these patients.

STANDARD HEPATECTOMY PROCEDURES

In the 1970s, six major hepatectomy procedures were established for patients with relatively large HCC who did not have impaired liver function. These include right or left trisegmentectomy, right or left hepatectomy, central bisegmentectomy, and left lateral segmentectomy.[2] For patients with HCC and cirrhosis, however, these standard hepatectomies would not be feasible because of the high risk of postoperative liver failure.[3] As an alternative, minor hepatectomy procedures such as limited or local resection could be procedures of choice in these patients. However, our clinicopathologic study of HCC demonstrated that the frequency of tumor thrombi and intrahepatic metastases in the resected specimens was 41% and 31%, respectively.[5] This finding led to speculation that HCC infiltrates a nearby portal vein and then forms intrahepatic metastases in the regional area (Fig. 22.2). For this reason, limited resection seemed inadequate for the removal of all possible tumor lesions. Therefore, the HCC-related portal venous branch should be ligated as far from the tumor as the hepatic function permits, and regional liver parenchyma harboring the HCC should be removed completely. Systematic subsegmentectomy was thus devised to meet such a requirement.[5]

In 1981, the concept of subsegmentectomy became possible as a result of the introduction of IOUS in

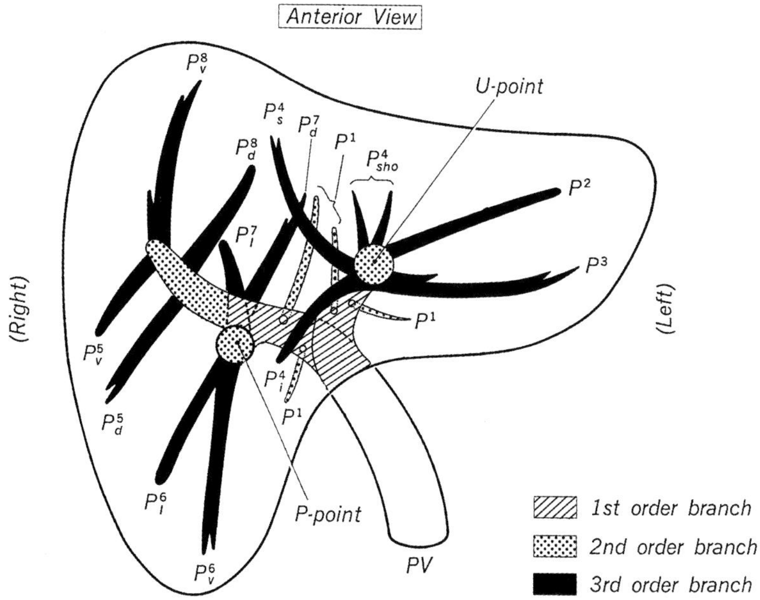

Figure 22.3 – Map of intrahepatic portal venous branches (from Ref.[15] with permission). Superscripts refer to the eight hepatic subsegments, and subscripts to the subsegmental branches of the portal vein *(P)* which are named after the major feeding area in each subsegment: *v*= ventral area; *d*= dorsal area; *l*= lateral area; *s*= superior area; *i*= inferior area; *sho* = short branches. *U-point* = umbilical point; *P-point* = posterior point.

liver surgery.[6] Each subsegmental border can be visualized by an IOUS-guided staining method. Systematic subsegmentectomy has now become a standard procedure for removing small HCC associated with chronic hepatitis or cirrhosis. This procedure allows complete removal of the HCC confined to a subsegment with full preservation of the other segments. Candidates would need to fulfil the following criteria: tumors limited to within a subsegmental domain, a bilirubin below 1.0 mg/dl, and the ICG-R_{15} less than 30%. This procedure requires precise identification of tumor-oriented intrahepatic vascular anatomy. Before carrying out such surgery, the surgeon should have knowledge of the approximate intrahepatic vascular anatomy which is usually provided by a series of preoperative imaging procedures. Of the hepatic vascular systems, the portal venous system is the most easily identifiable on images and, therefore, is a good surgical landmark. As shown in Figure 22.3, the first order branches of the portal vein include the right and left lobal branches, the second order includes the right anterior and posterior segmental branches, the left umbilical portion and caudate (segment 1) veins, and the third order includes the subsegmental (segments 2-8) branches.[15] We have named each third order branch after its major feeding area in the subsegmental domain. During IOUS scanning, such a map facilitates surgeons' understanding of the anatomical layout in each patient. All portal venous branches and hepatic veins can thus be traced by referring to the map.

Figure 22.4 illustrates the operative steps of Makuuchi's procedure.[5] First, IOUS is performed to confirm the location of the HCC-bearing subsegment and the third order portal venous branches that feed it. Next, IOUS-guided staining is performed to identify the subsegmental domain to be resected, and the domain is marked by electrocautery. This is followed by the tattooing technique in order to facilitate recognition of the relevant branch during the subsequent transection. Finally, under hemihepatic vascular occlusion,[11] hepatic parenchymal division is carried out along the external and internal landmarks using the forceps fracture method. On completion of the subsegmentectomy, the major hepatic venous trunks that run between the subsegments are exposed on the raw surface.

As a representative example of this operation, resection of segment 8 is described in brief.[5,7] The abdominal cavity is entered through an L-shaped incision and a right thoracotomy performed through the 9th intercostal space. After cholecystectomy, the common bile duct, hepatic arteries and portal veins

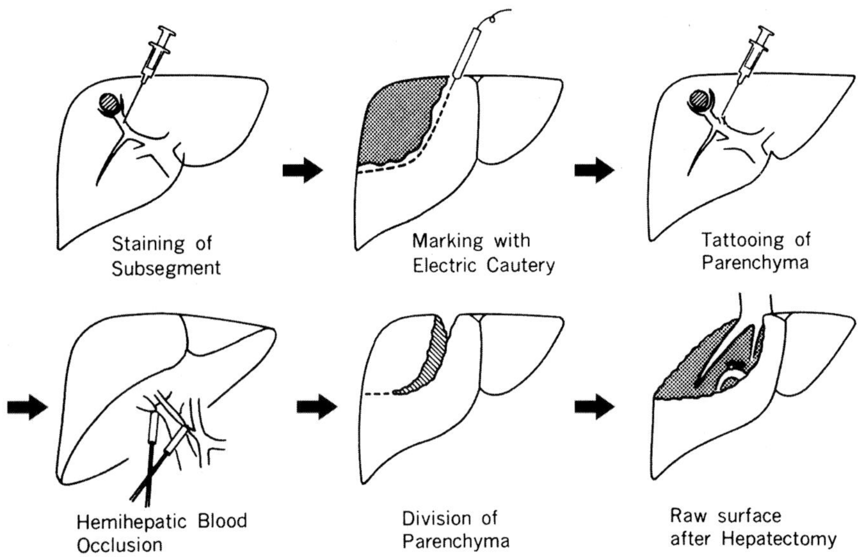

Figure 22.4 – Operative procedure for systematic subsegmentectomy of the liver (from Ref.[5] with permission). The procedure involves staining the subsegment to be resected, marking the domain with electric cautery, tattooing the parenchyma around the relevant portal venous root, hemihepatic vascular occlusion, dividing the hepatic parenchyma, and complete exposure of the partition veins on the raw surface.

are dissected and taped at the hepatic hilum. Segment 8 usually has two major subsegmental branches (P^8-ventral (v.) and P^8-dorsal (d.)) and, therefore, the staining technique must be performed twice to identify the whole domain. Division of the hepatic parenchyma is started about 1 cm to the left of Cantlie's line under hemihepatic vascular occlusion of the left lobe, and continued until the middle hepatic vein and its confluence with the inferior vena cava are exposed. Then, using right-sided occlusion, the parenchyma is divided between segments 8 and 5. Deep in the parenchyma, the roots of P^8-v. and P^8-d. can be exposed, ligated and divided in accordance with their tattoos. The next step is exposure of the right hepatic vein, which is usually situated about 2 cm dorsolateral to the P^8 branches. Further divisions expose this vein from its caudal to its cranial aspect. The final division is directed toward the demarcation line on the cranial surface of the liver. Complete resection of segment 8 reveals the trunks of the middle and right hepatic veins, and the stumps of the P^8 branches on the raw surface (Fig. 22.5). The operative procedures for the other subsegments are described elsewhere.[7]

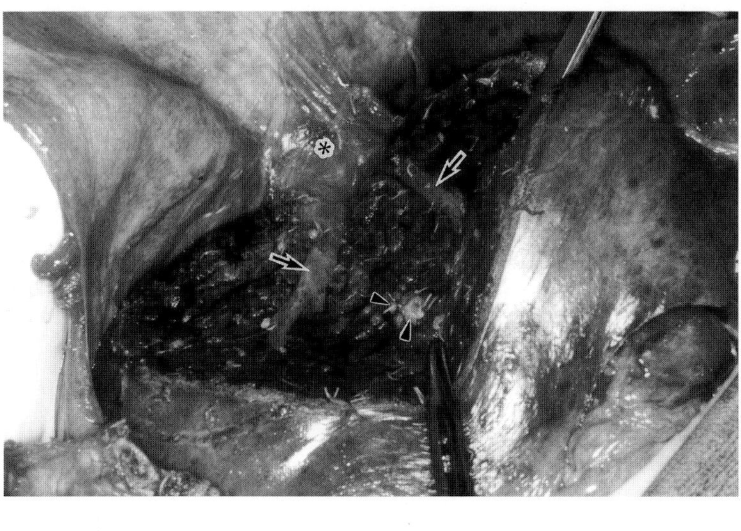

Figure 22.5 – Raw surface after systematic resection of segment 8. The trunks of the middle and right (arrows) hepatic veins, the stumps of the P^8 branch (arrow heads) and suprahepatic inferior vena cava (*) are exposed.

MODIFIED HEPATECTOMY PROCEDURES

Besides the standard procedures, modified hepatectomy procedures which have the potential to improve the resectability of HCC that were previously deemed unresectable have been devised. The criteria for excluding patients from surgery include serious hepatic impairment, bilobar tumor dissemination, and tumor involvement of the great vessels. The latter criterion can now be considered to be a relative contraindication since new methods for the removal of the HCC and the involved portions of these vessels are being sought while at the same time preserving remnant liver function.

In cirrhotic patients, radical resection of an HCC which involves the root of the right hepatic vein is less practicable since right hepatic lobectomy may cause postoperative liver failure. As an alternative, Makuuchi *et al.*[16] have proposed the resection of segments 7 and 8 including the right hepatic vein, while preserving segment 6 which could be drained by the inferior right hepatic vein.[17] Besides this, three new procedures based on the same policy have also been introduced (Fig. 22.6). The most extensive procedure proposed is subtotal hepatectomy leaving only one segment.[16,18,19] In a case without this accessory vein, we recently performed subtotal hepatectomy with reconstruction of the single remnant right hepatic vein with an autovein graft to save segment 6 (Fig. 22.7).[20] Patients in both series had an uneventful postoperative course. The inferior vena cava may be involved most frequently by HCC that originates in the caudate lobe, and surgery is seldom indicated in this situation. Successful resection of caudate tumors that involve the vena cava has been demonstrated using combined right or left and caudate lobectomies with or without resection of the vena cava (Fig. 22.8).[21,22] Recently, Sauvanet *et al.*[23] reported *ex situ* resection of a caudate tumor with prosthetic caval replacement and reimplantation of the three hepatic veins. In these cases, the absence of cirrhosis allowed hepatic lobectomy to be performed which greatly facilitated the radical resection. For cirrhotics, however, the authors have reported various procedures which are smaller than lobectomy and allow safe resection of caudate tumors, whilst preserving sufficient functional parenchyma (Fig. 22.9).[24] For isolated total caudate lobectomy,

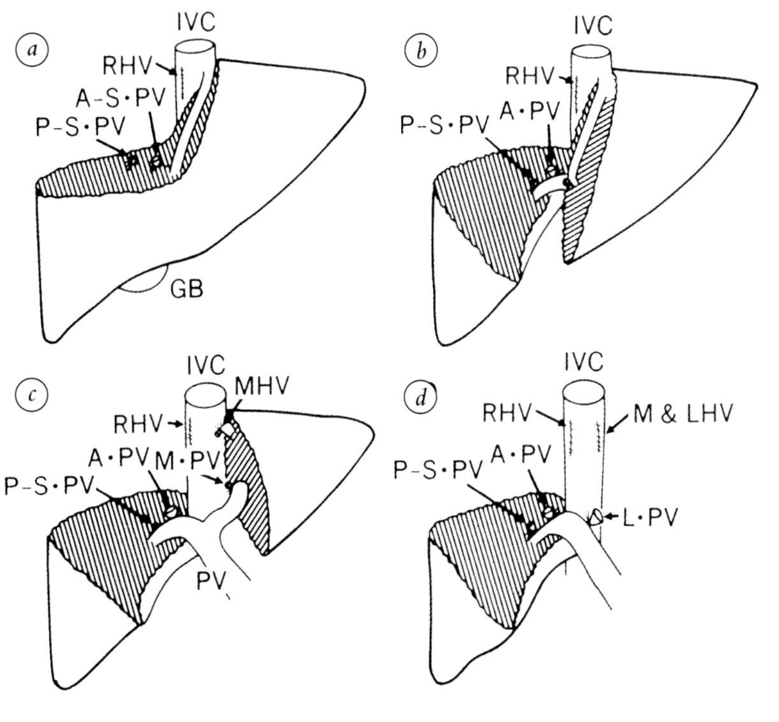

Figure 22.6 – Four hepatectomy procedures preserving the inferior right hepatic vein (from Ref.[16] with permission).
a) Resection of segments 8 and 7.
b) Resection of anterior segment and segment 7.
c) Resection of central bisegments and segment 7.
d) Extended left trisegmentectomy. IVC: Inferior vena cava; RHV: right hepatic vein; MHV: middle hepatic vein; LHV: left hepatic vein; PV: portal vein; A: anterior; P: posterior; S: superior; M: middle; L: left; GB: gallbladder.

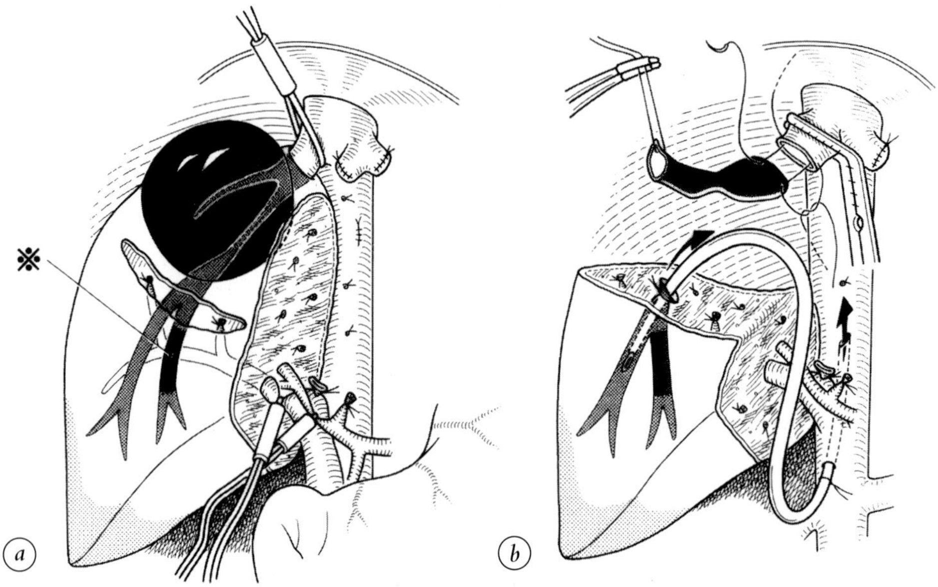

Figure 22.7 – Re-reconstruction of the right hepatic vein during repeat hepatectomy (from Ref.[20] with permission).
a) Hepatic transection under inflow and occasional outflow occlusion (asterisk indicates the first reconstruction).
b) venovenous bypass formation and the second reconstruction using the common iliac vein graft.

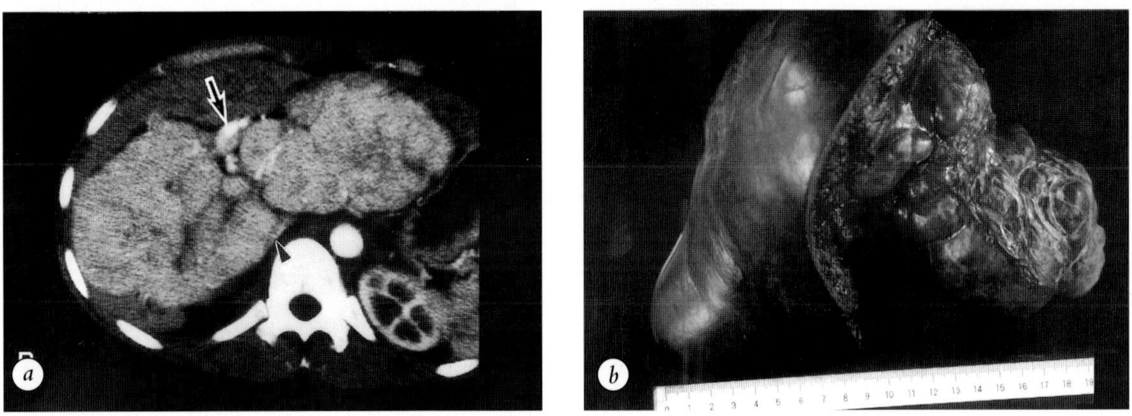

Figure 22.8 – Total caudate lobectomy combined with right hepatectomy (from Ref.[24] with permission).

a) A dynamic computed tomogram showing a dumbbell shaped enhanced tumor (21 cm in diameter) located between the hepatic hilum (arrow) and the inferior vena cava (arrow heads).

b) Resected specimen (1,130 g) of the right lobe and the caudate tumor, pathologically diagnosed as focal nodular hyperplasia.

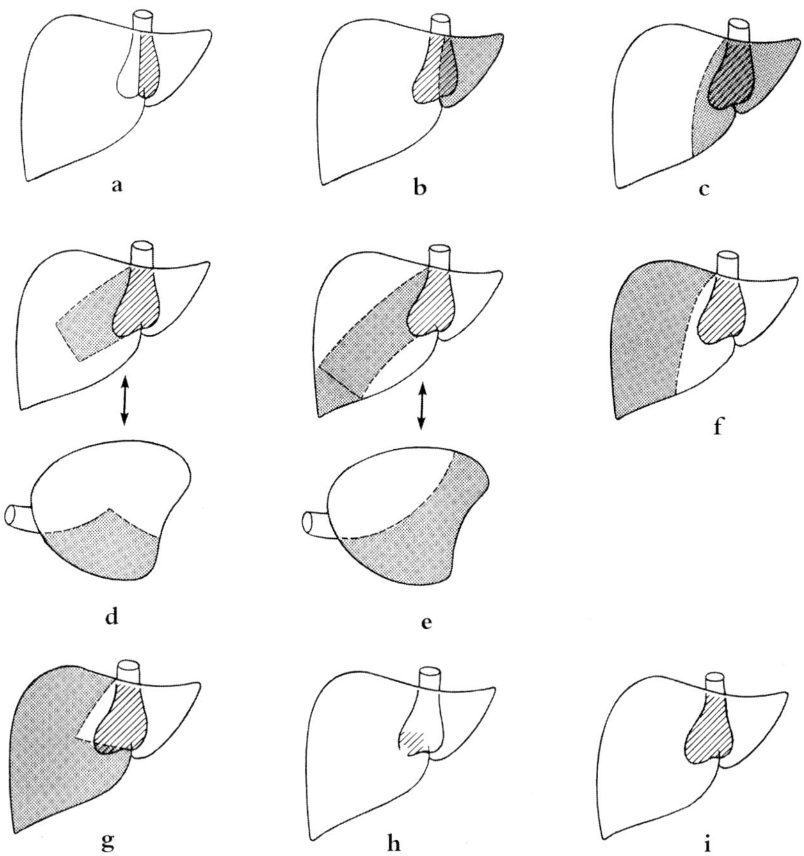

Figure 22.9 – Anatomic resection of the caudate lobe of the liver (from Ref.[24] with permission)

a) Resection of the left caudate lobe;

b) Total caudate lobectomy (TCL) with lateral segment;

c) TCL with the left lobe;

d) TCL with segment 7;

e) TCL with posterior segment;

f) TCL with the right lobe;

g) TCL with the right lobe and the inferior part of segment 4;

h) Resection of the caudate process:

i) Isolated TCL. The resection area of the caudate lobe is indicated by oblique lines, and the part of the liver to be resected in combination is shown by dots.

high dorsal resection (Fig. 22.10)[25] or transhepatic resection[26] have been devised. The presence of tumor thrombus of HCC in the portal vein trunk seems a contraindication to operation especially in patients with cirrhosis. However, Kumada *et al*[27] and ourselves[28] have reported a series of aggressive procedures by which more than one segment with a primary HCC tumor and concomitant thrombi in the portal trunk were removed; about half of the patients had a cirrhotic liver. With transplantation techniques, Pichlmayr *et al.*[29] described a new technique of *ex vivo* hepatic operation, which was applied to patients with tumors which were otherwise deemed to be unresectable by conventional procedure. Extracorporeal tumor resection on the back table was undertaken using hypothermic preservation, and was followed by autotransplantation of the remnant part of the liver. It was stated that hepatic tumors which did not compromise global hepatic function or caused cholestasis would be suitable for such a procedure. The assessment of its final therapeutic value, however, requires further clinical evaluation.

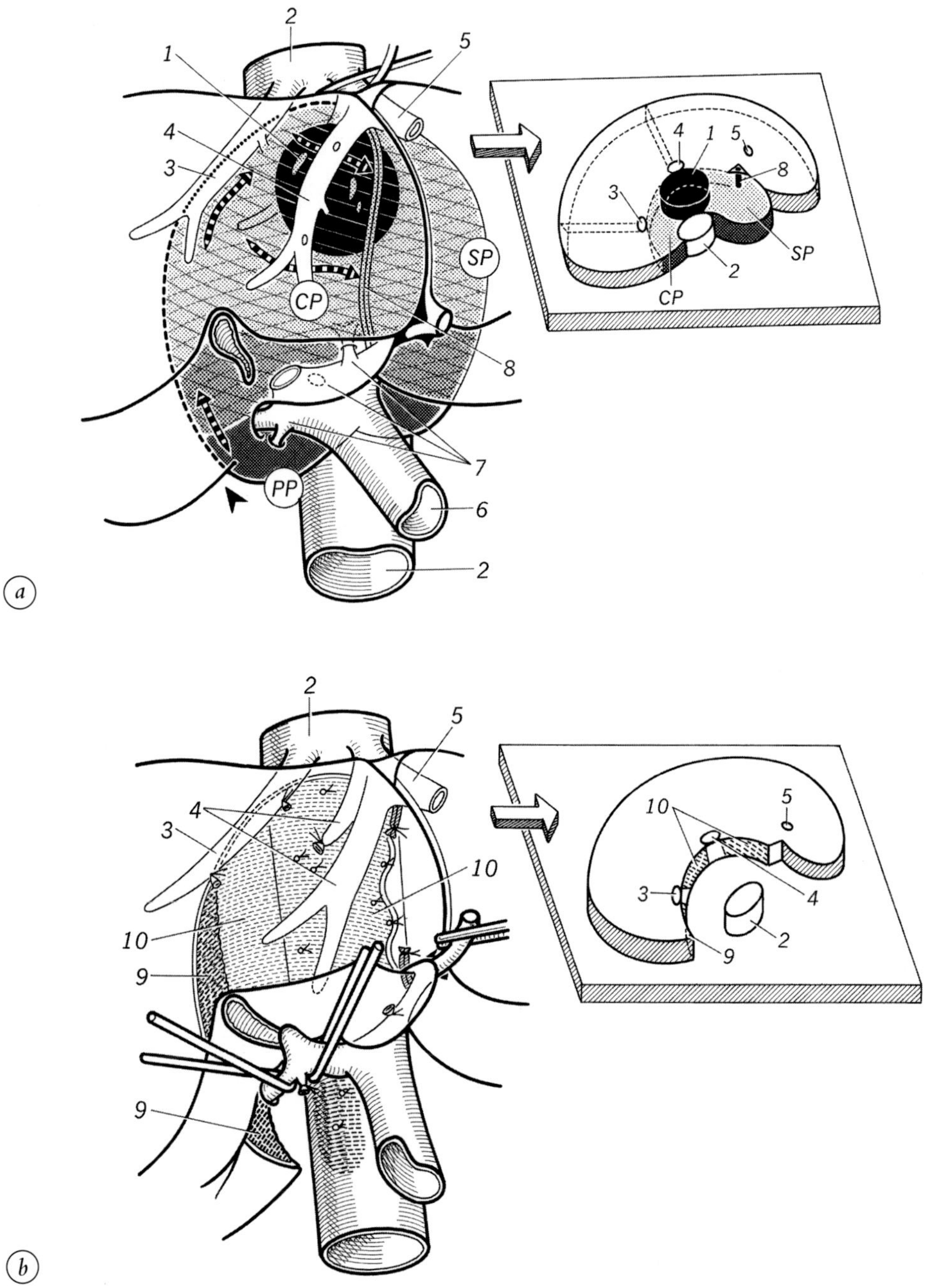

Figure 22.10 – High dorsal resection as a procedure of isolated total caudate lobectomy of the liver (from Ref.[25] with permission)

*a)*The entire caudate lobe comprises the Spiegel portion (SP), the process portion (PP) and the caval portion (CP). An HCC is mainly located in the upper one-half of the CP. The right margin of the caudate lobe (arrowhead) and the transection sequence (broken arrows) are shown.

b) Raw surface of the liver (shaded plane) appears after total caudate lobectomy. Each inset demonstrates a horizontal plane through the HCC. 1: HCC; 2: inferior vena cava; 3: right hepatic vein; 4: middle hepatic vein; 5: left hepatic vein; 6: portal vein; 7: caudate branches; 8: Arantius' ligament; 9: cut surface of the posterior segment; 10: cut surface of the anterior and medial segment.

Table 22.1 – Overall survival rate after resection of HCC

Author	Country	Year	Cases resected	With cirrhosis (%)	Operative mortality (%)	Survival rate (%)		
						1 year	3 years	5 years
Iwatsuki & Starz[30]	USA	1988	67	–	7	76	49	25
Chen *et al*[31]	Taiwan	1989	120	46	4	56	–	26
LCSGJ *et al*[32] ⋆	Japan	1990	2174	74	4	67	40	29
Yamanaka *et al*[33]	Japan	1990	295	80	-	76	44	31
Tsuzuki *et al*[34]	Japan	1990	119	67	9	–	47	39
Kosuge *et al*[35]	Japan	1993	480	63	2	87	63	44
Tang *et al*[36]	China	1993	314	–	–	86	68	61
Nagasue *et al*[37]	Japan	1993	229	77	7	80	51	36
Gozzetti *et al*[38]	Italy	1993	168	69	8	–	57	26
Bismuth *et al*[39]	France	1993	60	100	10	90	52	–
Izumi *et al*[40]	Japan	1994	104	71	7	–	65	59
Fuster *et al*[41]	Spain	1996	48	100	4	79	64	–

⋆ The Liver Cancer Study Group of Japan

FOLLOW-UP AFTER HEPATECTOMY

The survival rates after hepatic resection for HCC[30-41] and for small HCC of less than 5 cm[9,42-48] are summarized in Tables 22.1 and 22.2, respectively. Most recent series after the late 1980s have reported a 1-year survival rate of between 56% and 90%, a 3-year survival rate of between 40% and 68%, and a 5-year survival rate of between 25% and 61%. A national study based in Japan demonstrated 1-, 3-, and 5-year survival rates of 67%, 40%, and 29%, respectively, in 2,174 consecutively resected cases.[32] Cirrhosis was the most common background condition, being present in over half of these patients. A perioperative mortality of 10% or less was achieved by all the teams. Although the results vary among different surgeons, it is obvious that the survival rate is much better for small HCC less than 5 cm in diameter. The 1-year survival exceeds 80% in all of the six reports from the East, and 5-year survival is over 40% in most reports, and 60% in two reports from China. Patients with HCC less than 2 cm in diameter had a better postoperative prognosis.[49] These excellent outcomes for small HCC emphasize the importance of early detection of small lesions, and of precise and safe resection.

The optimal procedure to achieve a better prognosis in cirrhotic patients with small HCC is an important matter for concern. Table 22.2 demonstrates two series in which survival rates achieved by different operative procedures were compared. Kanematsu *et al.*[42] failed to show any difference between standard and limited resection, while our series[47] show that the outcome is superior after subsegmentectomy than after limited resection. Our recent series which includes patients up to 1995 has revealed a significantly better long-term outcome in patients who underwent systematic subsegmentectomy (Fig. 22.11). The prognostic factors after hepatic resection for HCC, such as tumor size, capsular infiltration, portal vein invasion, and intrahepatic metastasis are widely accepted as being significant.[9] Others factors which include tumor number, surgical procedure, and surgical margin, however, remain controversial.

For patients with small HCC, selection of the most appropriate therapeutic modality remains controversial. Recently, several investigators have reported that the long-term outcome after percutaneous ethanol injection (PEI) therapy is comparible to that after hepatic resections in selected patients with small HCC.[50,51] In order to assess this issue, a retrospective study of 3,000 patients who recently underwent initial treatment in 10 institutes in Japan was undertaken. Figure 22.12 shows the survival curves of 759 patients with HCCs no larger than 3 cm in diameter, and with no more than three nodules, after undergo-

Table 22.2 –Survival rate after resection of HCC smaller than 5cm

Author	Country	Year	Cases resected	With cirrhosis (%)	Operative mortality (%)	Survival rate (%)		
						1 year	3 years	5 years
Kanematsu *et al*[42]	Japan	1984						
standard*			13	–	15	79	–	23
limited			37	–	11	80	–	33
Wu *et al*[43]	China	1986	65	78	4	83	74	64
Li *et al*[44]	China	1986	23	79	9	90	71	41
Tang *et al*[45]	China	1989	132	90	2	92	76	63
Franco *et al*[46]	France	1990	50	–	–	67	42	–
Makuuchi *et al*[47]	Japan	1991						
subseg*			87	–	0.8	86	61	45
limited			168	–	0.8	89	58	30
Paquet *et al*[48]	Germany	1991	23	100	13	77	–	49
Makuuchi *et al*[9]	Japan	1993	349	74	2	90	66	44

* represents hepatectomy procedures: standard resection, limited resection, and subsegmentectomy.

ing hepatic resection, transcatheter hepatic arterial embolization (TAE), or PEI.[52] During the first 3 years, PEI yielded better survival rates than surgery, while after 3 years, the survival curve for PEI declined rapidly and showed a tendency similar to that observed with TAE. However, it is important to note that the tumors treated by PEI tended to be smaller, fewer and better differentiated than those treated by the other modalities. It is thus likely that these factors are responsible for the better early survival observed with PEI compared with surgery. Moreover, another study has shown that in patients with early (very well-differentiated) HCC, the 5-year survival rate after surgery was significanltly better than that after PEI (90% *vs* 72%, $p<0.05$), and the difference was even more significant in recurrence-free survival rates (48% *vs* 28%, $p<0.01$).[53] Because of improved outcome, it can be recommended that surgery is

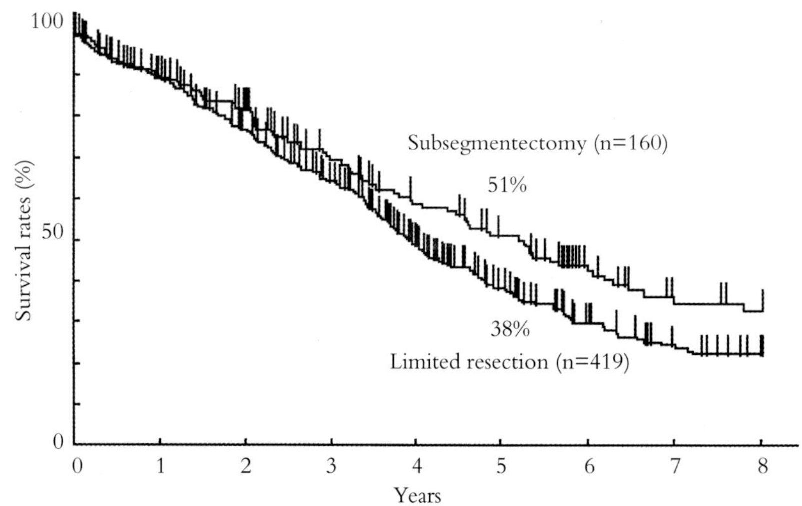

Figure 22.11 – Survival rates after systematic subsegmentectomy and limited resection in patients with HCC. The 5-year rate is significantly better in patients after subsegmentectomy than in those after limited resection (51% vs 38%, $p<0.05$).

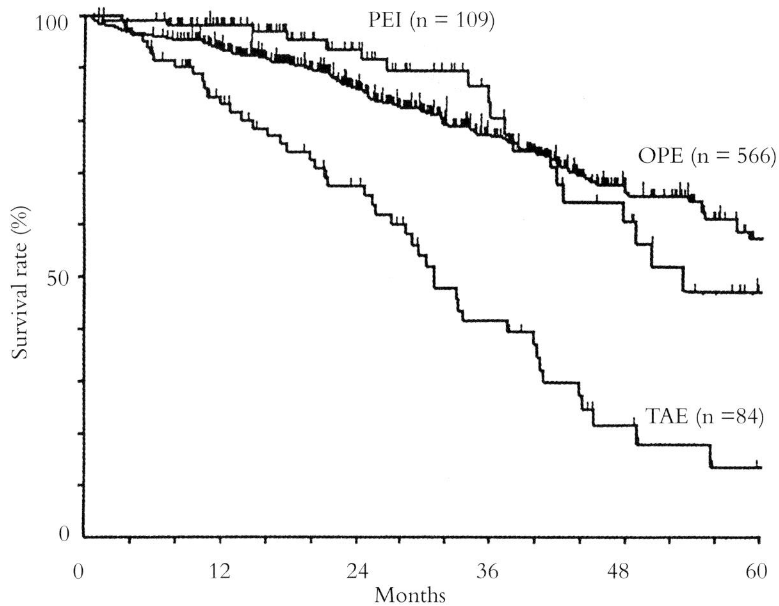

Figure 22.12 – Difference between survival rates of patients with HCC by three therapeutic methods (from Ref.[52] with permission). The patients who had HCC 1 to 3 cm in diameter and no more than 3 nodules were treated by hepatic resection (OPE), transcatheter hepatic arterial embolization (TAE), and percutaneous ethanol injection (PEI) therapy , respectively.

the treatment of choice even for small, early HCC, and the indication for PEI has to be limited. It remains to be clarified by prospective, randomized trials what modality can best improve the survival of these patients.

CONCLUSION

Surgery has played a leading role among several options which are available for the treatment of patients with HCC. Technical innovations have led to an increase in the resectability rate, a decrease in operative mortality, and improved long-term survival. In the 1980s, surgeons in the East devised criteria for resection of HCC associated with cirrhosis. These criteria are designed to select suitable patients for surgery so as to minimize the risk of fatal liver failure after hepatectomy. Our evidence of the superior efficacy of ultrasonically guided subsegmentectomy compared with limited resection has underlined the importance of anatomic resection of the relevant portal domain in the removal of small HCC. Other methods of resecting currently unresectable tumors are being evaluated, but are only likely to be of benefit in a minority of pateints. Recently, surgeons in the West have demonstrated that liver transplantation is a rational form of treatment for some patients, but its role still remains limited. We therefore recommend early diagnosis and anatomic resection of small HCC as the most reasonable management strategy for patients with cirrhosis, until controlled prospective studies provide objective information.

REFERENCES

1. Okuda K, Obata H, Nakajima Y *et al.* Prognosis of primary hepatocellular carcinoma. *Hepatology* 1984; **4** (suppl): 3-6
2. Fortner JG, Maclean BJ, Kim DK *et al.* The seventies evolution in liver surgery for cancer. *Cancer* 1981; **47**: 2162-2166
3. Lin TY. Resectional therapy for primary malignant hepatic tumors. In: Murphy GP, ed. *International Advances in Surgical Oncology.* New York: Alan R Liss, 1979: p 25-54
4. Makuuchi M, Hashikura Y, Kawasaki S, Tan D, Kosuge T, Takayama T. Personal experience of right anterior segmentectomy (segments V and VIII) for hepatic malignancies. *Surgery* 1993; **114**: 52-58
5. Makuuchi M, Hasegawa H, Yamazaki S. Ultrasonically guided subsegmentectomy. *Surg Gynecol Obstet* 1985; **161**: 346-50
6. Makuuchi M, Hasegawa H, Yamazaki S. Intraoperative ultrasonic examination for hepatectomy. *Jpn J Clin Oncol* 1981; **11**: 367-90
7. Makuuchi M. Application of intraoperative ultrasonography to hepatectomy. In: Makuuchi M, ed. *Abdominal Intraoperative Ultrasonography.* Tokyo: Igaku-shoin, 1987: p 89-123

8. UICC International Union against Cancer. Digestive system tumours, Liver. In: Hermanek P, Sobin LH, eds. *TNM Classification of Malignant Tumours* (4th edn). Berlin: Springer-Verlag, 1987: p 53-55

9. Makuuchi M, Kosuge T, Takayama T *et al.* Surgery for small liver cancers. *Sem Surg Oncol* 1993; **9**: 298-304

10. Miyagawa S, Makuuchi M, Kawasaki S, Kakazu T. Criteria for safe hepatic resection. *Am J Surg* 1995; **169**: 589-594

11. Makuuchi M, Mori T, Gunven P, Yamazaki S, Hasegawa H. Safety of hemihepatic vascular occlusion during resection of the liver. *Surg Gynecol Obstet* 1987; **64**: 155-158

12. Makuuchi M, Takayama T, Gunven P, Kosuge T, Yamasaki S, Hasegawa H. Restrictive vesus liberal blood transfusion policy for hepatectomies in cirrhotic patients. *World J Surg* 1989; **13**: 644-648

13. Makuuchi M, Thai BL, Takayasu K *et al.* Preoperative portal embolization to increase safety of major hepatectomy for hilar bile duct carcinoma: a preliminary report. *Surgery* 1990; **107**: 521-527

14. Fan ST, Lo CM, Lai ECS, Chu KM, Liu CL, Wong J. Perioperative nutritional support in patients undergoing hepatectomy for hepatocellular carcinoma. *N Engl J Med* 1994; **331**: 1547-1552

15. Takayasu K, Moriyama N, Muramatsu Y *et al.* Intrahepatic portal vein branches studied by percutaneous transhepatic portography. *Radiology* 1985; **154**: 31-36

16. Makuuchi M, Hasegawa H, Yamazaki S, Takayasu K. Four new hepatectomy procedures for resection of the right hepatic vein and preservation of the inferior right hepatic vein. *Surg Gynecol Obstet* 1987; **164**: 68-72

17. Makuuchi M, Hasegawa H, Yamazaki S *et al.* The inferior right hepatic vein: ultrasonic demonstration. *Radiology* 1983; **148**: 213-217

18. Baer HU, Dennison AR, Maddern GJ, Blumgart LH. Subtotal hepatectomy: a new procedure based on the inferior right hepatic vein. *Br J Surg* 1991; **78**: 1221-1222

19. Ozeki Y, Uchiyama T, Katayama M, Sugiyama A, Kokubo M, Matsubara N. Extended left hepatic trisegmentectomy with resection of main right hepatic vein and preservation of middle and inferior right hepatic veins. *Surgery* 1995; **117**: 715-717

20. Takayama T, Nakatsuka T, Makuuchi M *et al.* Re-reconstruction of a single remnant hepatic vein. *Br J Surg* 1996; **83**: 762-763

21. Takayama T, Makuuchi M, Takayasu K *et al.* Resection after intraarterial chemotherapy of a hepatoblastoma originating in the caudate lobe. *Surgery* 1990; **107**: 231-235

22. Takayama T, Makuuchi M, Kosuge T *et al.* A hepatoblastoma originating in the caudate lobe radically resected with the inferior vena cava. *Surgery* 1991; **109**: 208-213

23. Sauvanet A, Dousset B, Belghiti J. A simplified technique of ex situ hepatic surgical treatment. *J Am Coll Surg* 1994; **178**: 79-81

24. Makuuchi M, Kawasaki S, Takayama T, Kumon M. Caudate lobectomy. In: Lygidakis NJ, Makuuchi M, eds. *Pitfalls and Complications in the Diagnosis and Management of Hepatobiliary and Pancreatic Diseases*. Stuttgart: Thieme, 1993: p 124-132

25. Takayama T, Tanaka T, Higaki T, Katou K, Teshima Y, Makuuchi M. High dorsal resection of the liver. *J Am Coll Surg* 1994; **179**: 72-75

26. Yamamoto J, Takayama T, Kosuge T *et al.* An isolated caudate lobectomy by the transhepatic approach for hepatocellular carcinoma in cirrhotic liver. *Surgery* 1992; **111**: 699-702

27. Kumada K, Ozawa K, Okamoto R *et al.* Hepatic resection for advanced hepatocellular carcinoma with removal of portal vein tumor thrombi. *Surgery* 1990; **108**: 821-827

28. Takayama T, Nakatsuka T, Makuuchi M *et al.* Function-preserving segmentectomy of the cirrhotic liver. *Hepato-Gastroenterol* 1995; **42**: 415-417

29. Pichlmayr R, Grosse H, Hauss J, Gubernatis G, Lamesch P, Bretschneider HJ. Technique and preliminary results of extracorporeal liver surgery (bench procedure) and of surgery on the in situ perfused liver. *Br J Surg* 1990; **77**: 21-26

30. Iwatsuki S, Starzl TE. Personal experience with 411 hepatic resections. *Ann Surg* 1988; **208**: 421-434

31. Chen MF, Hwang TL, Jeng LBB, Jan YY, Wang CS, Chou FF. Hepatic resection in 120 patients with hepatocellular carcinoma. *Arch Surg* 1989; **124**: 1025-1028

32. The Liver Cancer Study Group of Japan. Primary liver cancer in Japan: clinicopathologic features and results of surgical treatment. *Ann Surg* 1990; **211**: 277-287

33. Yamanaka N, Okamoto E, Toyosaka A *et al.* Prognostic factors after hepatectomy for hepatocellular carcinomas: a univariate and multivariate analysis. *Cancer* 1990; **65**: 1104-1110

34. Tsuzuki T, Sugioka A, Ueda M *et al.* Hepatic resection for hepatocellular carcinoma. *Surgery* 1990; **107**: 511-520

35. Kosuge T, Makuuchi M, Takayama T, Yamamoto J, Shimada K, Yamasaki S. Long-term results after resection of hepatocellular carcinoma: experience of 480 cases. *Hepato-Gastroenterol* 1993; **40**: 328-332

36. Tang ZY, Yu YQ, Zhou XD, Yang BH, Ma ZC, Lin ZY. Subclinical hepatocellular carcinoma: an analysis of 391 patients. *J Surg Oncol* 1993; **3** (suppl): 55-58

37. Nagasue N, Kohno H, Chang YC *et al.* Liver resection for hepatocellular carcinoma: results of 229 consecutive patients during 11 years. *Ann Surg* 1993; **217**: 375-384

38. Gozzetti G, Mazziotti A, Luca Grazi G. Surgical experience with 168 primary liver cell carcinomas treated with hepatic resection. *J Surg Oncol* 1993; **3** (suppl): 59-61

39. Bismuth H, Chiche L, Adam R, Castaing D, Diamond T, Dennison A. Liver resection versus transplantation for hepatocellular carcinoma in cirrhotic patients. *Ann Surg* 1993; **218**: 145-151

40. Izumi R, Shimizu K, Ii T, *et al.* Prognostic factors of hepatocellular carcinoma in patients undergoing hepatic resection. *Gastroenterology* 1994; **106**: 720-727

41. Fuster J, Garcia-Valdecasea CJ, Grande L, *et al.* Hepatocellular carcinoma and cirrhosis: results of surgical treatment in a European series. *Ann Surg* 1996; **223**: 297-302

42. Kanematsu T, Takenaka K, Matsumata T, Furuta T, Sugimachi K, Inokuchi K. Limited hepatic resection effective for selected cirrhotic patients with primary liver cancer. *Ann Surg* 1984; **199**: 51-56

43. Wu MC, Zhang XH, Chen H. Hepatic resection for primary liver cancer. *Chin Med J* 1986; **99**: 175-180

44. Li GH, Li JQ, Zhou YQ. Surgical treatment of small primary liver carcinoma. *Chin Med J* 1986; **99**: 827-828

45. Tang ZY, Yu YQ, Zhou XD *et al.* Surgery of small hepatocellular carcinoma: analysis of 144 cases. *Cancer* 1989; **64**: 536-

46. Franco D, Capussotti L, Smadja C *et al*. Resection of hepatocellular carcinomas: results in 72 European patients with cirrhosis. *Gastroenterology* 1990; **98**: 733-738

47. Makuuchi M, Takayama T, Kosuge T, *et al*. The value of ultrasonography for hepatic surgery. *Hepato-Gastroenterol* 1991; **38**: 64-70

48. Paquet KJ, Koussouris P, Mercado MA, Kalk JFr, Ming D, Rambach W. Limited hepatic resection for selected cirrhotic patients with hepatocellular or cholangiocellular carcinoma: a prospective study. *Br J Surg* 1991; **78**: 459-462

49. Nagashima I, Hamada C, Naruse K, *et al*. Surgical resection for small hepatocellular carcimona. *Surgery* 1996; **119**: 40-45

50. Livraghi T, Bolondi L, Lazzaroni S, *et al*. Percutaneous ethanol injection in the treatment of hepatocellular carcinoma in cirrhosis: a study in 207 patients. *Cancer* 1992; **69**: 925-929

51. Castells A, Bruix J, Bru C, *et al*. Treatment of small hepatocellular carcinoma in cirrhotic patients: a cohort study comparing surgical resection and percutaneous ethanol injection. *Hepatology* 1993; **18**: 1121-1125

52. Ryu M. Treatment strategy for hepatocellular carcinoma. In: Terada M,cd. *Reports on projects of the comprehensive ten-year strategy of cancer control supported by the Ministry of Health and Welfare of Japan*. Tokyo. National Cancer Center Research Institute, 1993: p176-181

53. Sakamoto M. Personal communication with permission, data from the study group on small HCC supported by the Ministry of Health and Welfare of Japan, 1995

23

Orthotopic liver transplantation

BI Carr

Human hepatocellular carcinoma (HCC) presents predominantly on the basis of cirrhosis. The incidence of cirrhosis varies with population, but overall an excess of 70% of HCC patients in the Orient and in the West have an associated chronic hepatitis and/or cirrhosis. The cirrhosis may be due to causes other than hepatitis, including hemochromatosis, porphyria, glycogenoses, alpha-1 antitrypsin deficiency, Alagille's syndrome, ethanol consumption, auto-immune chronic hepatitis, hereditary tyrosinemia and Wilson's disease. In Africa by contrast, HCC can present without any obvious underlying cirrhosis and is often advanced and aggressive at time of presentation. The background liver of non-African HCC is thus usually diseased, most commonly by chronic hepatitis B or C or a combination of chronic hepatitis and ethanol consumption. This makes HCC in the liver quite different to deal with from metastatic tumors to the liver and from other primary tumors, since most HCC patients thus have two diseases, and not one; they have the HCC and cirrhosis.[1,2] The majority of patients in countries where there is not a surveillance program for HCC present with advanced stage HCC. This is in contrast to countries such as Japan, where because of the high background incidence of chronic hepatitis, an active surveillance program is in place and patients are regularly screened. As a consequence, in such countries, HCCs tend to be diagnosed at a smaller size. This has a strong influence on the ability to resect or perform local therapies such as ethanol injection, and in addition has an influence on long-term survival. The majority of patients in most countries, however, present with advanced stages of HCC. Two factors impact most profoundly on the technical feasibility of resection for HCC. These are *advanced stage* of HCC, and the *presence and degree of cirrhosis*. Various indices have been used to assess the ability of the liver to regenerate and survive various levels of resection, and these include the standard biochemical liver function tests, Indocyanine Green (ICG) clearance and Megx clearance. None of them is too precise in giving estimates of the likelihood of hepatic survival after various degrees of hepatic resection however. The type and degree of chronic hepatitis is also crucially important for orthotopic liver transplantation (OLT). Not only can there be recurrence of HCC after OLT, but also recurrence of the underlying chronic hepatitis leading to liver failure in the newly transplanted liver.[3] Attempts have been made to try and define which categories of patient are at most risk from this. Specifically, it is clear that in patients with hepatitis B E-antigen positivity and circulating hepatitis B virus, DNA levels are at highest risk from recurrence, and most centers have now abandoned transplanting such patients unless they are part of a protocol that has induced a response to these features of their hepatitis infection prior to liver transplantation. For hepatitis C infection, the diagnostic sub groups of patients that are at greatest risk for recurrence are still in the process of being defined.

SPREAD OF HCC

Hepatic spread. Multiple nodules of HCC have an adverse impact both on the ability to resect them as well as on the prognosis of resected HCC and on the prognosis of HCC after OLT. Multiple nodules of HCC within the liver can result from two causes. These are spread of the HCC within the liver, as well as development of multiple primaries from different cirrhotic nodules, which are all putatively premalignant. The latter is an important point to consider in the follow-up and general management of patients who may have had local treatment, since patients with cirrhosis who live long enough have a high probability of developing HCC from one or more cirrhotic nodules. Recent papers from the follow-up of patients with chronic HBV or chronic HCV infection show that there is between a 3 and 6% likelihood per annum, of developing HCC.[4] This means that for a patient to be followed for 10 years, there is between a 30 and 60% chance of HCC developing in the liver. Several studies have also examined the clonality of multiple HCC masses, and there is considerable evidence for heterogeneity and multiclonality, indicating separate development of multiple primary lesions from individual cirrhotic nodules. However, by far the most important cause of multiple HCC nodules in the liver is spread of the primary HCC within the liver parenchyma. The exact mechanisms are unclear. The diffuse type of non-encapsulated HCC probably spreads by direct extension within and across the trabecular plates. However, this is not the commonest type of spread. HCC has a characteristic predilection for invading the portal veins.[39] This is manifested as a portal vein thrombus by CT scan or US, most characteristically in association with an expansion of the portal vein diameter at the site of the thrombus. The latter is a tell-tale sign that most usefully distinguishes benign from malignant thrombus. The invasion of the portal vein with associated thrombus is probably the most significant adverse prognostic feature for HCC transplantation and resection. It is also currently the second most important exclusion criterion for OLT after proven metastatic disease. As a consequence, some effort has been made to establish the diagnosis of malignant portal venous thrombosis definitively. Several articles have recently showed the usefulness and safety of percutaneous needle ultrasound guided biopsy of portal vein thrombosis, in order to provide proof of the presence of malignant cells.[5,6] Portal venous invasion probably occurs quite early in the development of HCC, with approximately 20% of HCC nodules of less than 2 cm diameter having associated portal venous microscopic invasion, and more than 90% of HCC nodules of greater than 5 cm diameter having this association.

Extra-hepatic spread. Almost any organ can be involved with metastatic HCC. However, the commonest sites are the abdominal lymph nodes and the lungs. Other sites commonly associated with metastatic disease include the peritoneum, bones, adrenals, and mediastinal lymph nodes. Although HCC skin nodules have been reported in the older literature from 'tracking' associated with liver biopsy at the time of diagnosis, we have seen this in only two cases out of our last 550 core needle biopsies. We thus believe this to be a rare event and should not be taken into account as a factor in making a decision to biopsy, since it is more important to make the correct diagnosis than to avoid a biopsy because of the possibility of a rare event. The relatively high incidence of metastatic recurrence after OLT for advanced stage HCC, despite an apparently negative pre-transplant clinical search for extra hepatic disease, has led to the idea that HCC may be a microscopic metastatic disease, as has been proposed for breast cancer and many other types of tumor. The thinking is that there must be microscopic HCC cells that are below the limits of deductibility by current clinical and radiologic means. To account for the presence of extrahepatic HCC in distant organs, it is suggested that HCC must disseminate within the bloodstream. In an attempt to identify patients who may have microscopic hematogenous metastases, and thus be at high risk from recurrence after OLT, assays have recently been developed to try and identify liver-specific gene products in the circulating blood. So far, these have been based upon the measurement by the polymerase chain reaction (PCR) of mRNA for albumin and AFP.[7-10] While several reports have all shown the feasibility and usefulness of this assay, some investigators have found the presence of these gene products even in patients without HCC. This is probably due to the high sensitivity of the assay. The problem of false positives may well be resolved once a standard range of liver-specific gene products is established in the blood of patients with cirrhosis and for those with HCC, since almost all cancer tests so far can be positive in noncancer patients, if their level of sensitivity is set too high. At the very least, these new assays show that HCC is probably a microscopic metastatic disease that spreads through the bloodstream.

PRE-TRANSPLANT CLINICAL EVALUATION

The evaluation centers on two categories of test. The first deals with transplant-specific and liver-specific factors and the second deals with the tumor size and extent of spread. For transplant evaluation in general, blood liver function tests, hepatitis profiles and HBV quantitative DNA or HCV quantitative RNA and blood type are measured, as are the volume of the liver by CT scan. The patient's history is evaluated as well, including current use of intravenous addictive drugs or ethanol consumption. The tumor-specific evaluation includes a helical (or spiral) CT scan of the liver, with and without contrast medium and a CT scan of the chest. A bone scan is also performed in all patients. We no longer perform routine brain CT scans because of the low positive yield in patients without specific symptoms. The purpose of the CT scan of the liver is to define the maximum diameter, location and number of tumor nodules, the involvement of the portal vein; the presence of cirrhosis and the stigmata of portal hypertension, including varices in the esophagus, stomach, and intestine, the presence of ascites and splenomegaly. Some tumor nodules appear best on the non-contrast CT scan, others on the contrast CT scan, portal venous phase or arterial phase, depending upon the extent of the neovasculature. CT-portography or CT-arteriography (in the presence of cirrhosis) is an important component of current radiologic evaluation because of the greater sensitivity of this modality and the increased likelihood of obtaining evidence for bilobar disease, which is an important prognostic consideration.[11-16] For unclear reasons, occasional HCCs are best visualized on theUS or MRI. A core biopsy is always obtained at our institution from any hepatic mass. Fine needle aspiration (FNA) is usually insufficient for tumor architecture and can normally only be used for detecting the presence or absence of malignant cells but not always for identifying the tumor type. In addition, cutting biopsies also provide tissue to do other special stains in case of diagnostic doubt. We also obtain a biopsy of the underlying liver from a site different from the tumor as a routine, to assess the underlying cirrhosis.

PROCEDURE

The idea behind OLT for HCC was to extend the limits of surgical resection. This was done with two aims: firstly to remove tumors that were more advanced than could be technically resected; secondly, to treat those HCCs of whatever size in which there was a severe degree of cirrhosis, limiting the ability of the surgeon to safely resect liver tissue and still be left with adequate functional hepatic reserve.

RESULTS

Initially reported results of survival after OLT for HCC were discouraging.[18-26] Patients of all categories of TNM classification were lumped together for reporting purposes in several early series, and particularly were weighted in favor of patients with extensive tumors that could not be resected by standard means. Early reports reserved OLT mainly for advanced tumors. As a consequence, initial reports showed poor patient survival in either absolute terms or with respect to tumor-free survival. This led to a general disillusion with liver transplantation as a tool for HCC management. However, more careful analysis of more carefully selected and evaluated patients with HCC have led to a more optimistic re-evaluation.[27,30,36,38] In particular, patients with limited TNM stages I and II tumors with cirrhosis appear to do at least as well as those patients treated by resection and maybe better, since the resection is no longer limited by the severity of the underlying cirrhosis when patients receive a liver transplant. These patients are thus cured both of their HCC and of their cirrhosis.[29,30] Their likelihood of recurrence is thus less than after resection, since they no longer have additional cirrhotic pre-malignant nodules in their liver.[18,30] Thus, one of the main aims of liver transplantation for HCC has been achieved, namely the ability to treat the underlying cirrhosis as well as the HCC. It has become increasingly clear from several centers that limited TNM stage I and II tumors, confined to one lobe of the liver and without vascular invasion, appear to have excellent long-term survival after OLT[36] (Table 23.1). For patients with advanced-stage TNM IVa disease with bilobar masses and particularly in patients with portal venous invasion (stages III and IVa disease) the results are mixed. It is clear that OLT alone does not cause prolonged tumor-free survival for patients with stage IVa disease as a sole modality of treatment. However, several centers have recently offered preliminary evidence indicating that even stage IVa tumors can be treated with encouraging longer term survival when OLT is coupled with some form of chemotherapy. Adverse prognostic factors (Table 23.2), include extra-hepatic disease, macroscopic and to a lesser extent microscopic vascular invasion in the liver, bilober and multiple tumors. Large size may be a factor in stage II disease,[30,37] but probably not when a single tumor is involved (stage II). Attempts to extend the surgical procedure, as in upper abdominal

Table 23.1 – Survival after liver transplantation for hepatocellular carcinoma.[17,18]

	1year	2 years	3 years	4 years
TNM				
Stage I	80	75	75	75
Stage II	80	70	60	60
Stage III	55	30	30	30
Stage IVa	50	30	15	10

Table 23.2 – Adverse prognostic factors for liver transplantation of HCC.[17,18,30]

Positive resection margin
Lymph node metastasis
Vascular invasion of portal vessels
Bilobar hepatic tumor involvement
More than 3 tumor nodules
(Tumors >5 cm diameter)

exenteration, have predictably produced disappointing results,[42] probably because this approach has been used for advanced stage tumors, which are like metastatic ones prior to treatment.

The relatively high recurrence rates of chronic HBV and HCV infection in the majority of patients with HCC who have underlying hepatitis also has an impact on survival, since recurrent hepatitis has a major impact on patient survival, even though survival may not be diminished by tumor growth. Analysis of the published data needs to carefully dissect out the cause of death of patients with HCC and distinguish the cause due to recurrent tumor from other factors. In general, exclusion criteria for OLT include HCC that is growing during the waiting period for OLT patients with lymph node involvement or macroscopic portal venous trunk involvement as seen by CT scan and patients with detectable extra-hepatic tumor metastases. Figure 23.1 shows the results of recent University of Pittsburgh liver transplant patients with TNM stages III and IVa HCC who had pre-operative neo-adjuvant chemotherapy. Median survival is currently 46 months. Pre-operative chemotherapy doses of doxorubicin and cisplatin were given from 2-12 times prior to transplant.

General surgical considerations

In order for the reader to better assess the "special surgical considerations" (see below), a general understanding of the OLT procedure, especially as it relates to OLT for HCC, will be summarized.

The OLT procedure requires broad access to the upper abdominal organs. Specifically, a bilateral subcostal incision with an upper midline extension is generally preferred. This will allow generous mobilization of the liver and sampling of the lymph nodes, as well as access to the portal vein and aorta, should the need for alternative revascularization routes be required.

Generally, after any previous adhesions are taken down, inspection of the hepatoduodenal ligament commences. This requires dissection of the bile duct, hepatic artery, and portal vein. At this level, numerous lymph nodes are encountered, and generous lymph node samples should be taken for immediate frozen section. The portal vein should be carefully inspected for evidence of thrombosis. In cases where portal vein thrombosis cannot be assessed pre-operatively as to the presence or absence of tumor thrombosis, an intra-operative True-cut needle biopsy can be performed.

Following skeletonization of the hilar structures, the ligamentous attachments of the liver are taken down. Veno-venous bypass is then initiated, which allows

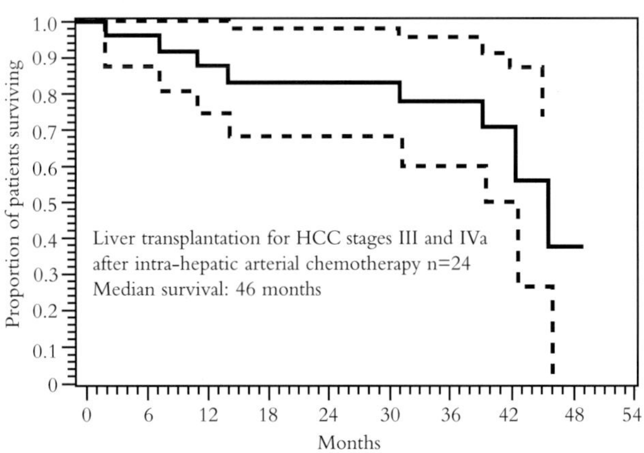

Figure 23.1– Patient survival after intrahepatic arterial chemotherapy and OLT in stages III and IVa

Table 23.3 – Common patterns of HCC recurrence after liver transplantation[17,18,40]

Transplanted liver (50%)
Lung
Bone
Brain
Adrenals

decompression of the splanchnic circulation, as well as the lower systemic venous circulation. This also allows intraoperative hemodynamic stability to be achieved during the anhepatic phase, in which the vena caval flow is interrupted.

After veno-venous bypass is established, the supra-hepatic and intraheptic vena cava are isolated and clamped. The liver is then removed. The new liver is brought onto the operating room table, and the major vascular structures are reconstructed, starting with the vena cava, proceeding next to the portal vein, and finally to the hepatic artery. After flow is reestablished, veno-venous bypass is discontinued and after hemostasis is assured, the bile duct is then reconstructed.

Deviations from this standard operation include the use of "jump" grafts. In situations where the hepatic artery is tenuous, or has been subjected to insults (such as intraarterial chemotherapy or radiation), an infra-renal "jump" graft is utilized. This is a long segment of iliac artery taken from the donor and connected to the aorta of the recipient and utilized as inflow for the newly transplanted liver. In situations where the portal vein may atretic, or in cases where it is thrombosed and the thrombus is proven to be not tumorous, then the superior mesenteric vein is isolated and a donor iliac vein is connected to the superior mesenteric vein and used as in-flow to the portal vein of the new transplanted liver.

Special surgical considerations

Prior to removal of the native liver containing an HCC, an extensive effort is made at the surgical staging of the tumor. This involves examination of the surrounding abdominal wall and abdominal organs for evidence of local tumor spread, evaluation of the hepatic hilar lymph nodes and examination of the portal vein, inferior vena cava and retro-hepatic inferior vena cava for evidence of direct invasion by tumor thrombus. Another major consideration in the liver transplant procedure for patients with HCC, is an evaluation of the hepatic artery that will be used for re-vascularizing the new liver, since intimal injury can be produced by preliver transplant intra-hepatic arterial chemotherapy. If there is any evidence for acute or chronic damage in the form of intimal hyperplasia in the resected hepatic artery, or thickening or a sclerotic reaction of the adventitia of the artery, then an arterial graft is placed to the infra-renal aorta. The blood flow in the hepatic artery is also checked by removing the clamps and directly visualizing the arterial pulsatile flow from the stump of the artery. If this is inadequate, then it suggests a stenosing lesion more proximal to the stump and for this reason also an arterial graft is placed.

HCC RECURRENCE POST OLT

The high incidence of HCC recurrences (Tables 23.1, 3), especially for patients with TNM stages III and IVa tumors, in the new liver and in extra-hepatic sites such as the lungs, strongly suggests the presence of microscopic tumor metastases prior to the OLT procedure for these advanced stage HCC patients. Evidence in support of this hypothesis comes from recent work in human HCC in which the signal for liver-specific genes has been found in the peripheral blood cells of patients[9,10] with advanced stage HCC (see above). Several possible mechanisms might explain the growth and development of microscopic blood-borne metastases. Probably the most important is the characteristic propensity of HCCs to invade the portal vein within the native patient liver, providing a mechanism for more general invasion and spread of the tumor. Several factors could influence the growth of HCC microscopic metastases once they have occurred. These include the growth of the engrafted liver, which almost certainly secretes hepatotrophic factors. Donor livers that are smaller than the resected livers have clearly been shown to grow in the weeks after liver transplantation in the recipient. Such hepatotrophic factors almost certainly affect the growth of microscopic seeded tumor cells. In addition, the immunosuppressive drugs cyclosporin and FK506 have been shown experimentally to enhance the process of hepatocarcinogenesis in rodents. Besides the direct effect of these two drugs on stimulating hepatocarcinogenesis, it is likely that the immunosuppressed state will also be associated with the enhanced ability of microscopic tumor cells to grow. Although it is usually believed that HCCs take upwards of 10 years to evolve, it cannot be excluded that new HCCs could develop in the environment of the immunosuppressed transplanted liver. In particular, in the presence of recurrent HBV or HCV infection, plus immunosuppression, the usual carcinogenic processes could be accelerated. Finally, as a consequence of OLT, many patients live longer than they otherwise would have done. This gives dormant microscopic HCCs in extra-hepatic sites an opportunity to grow, whereas previously without transplantation such patients would have died without clinically detectable metastases.

ADJUVANT AND NEO-ADJUVANT THERAPY

The OLT is capable of removing bulk tumor, but cannot deal with microscopic disease outside the confines of the liver or in association with the extra-hepatic tumor vasculature. Chemotherapy, by contrast, has the potential to eradicate microscopic tumor cells both in extensions of the liver vasculature as well as in the systemic circulation. Given the excellent long-term survival and disease-free survival of patients with TNM stages I and II disease (tumors less than 2 cm or multiple tumors of any size confined to a single lobe of the liver without vascular invasion), the potential benefits of added chemotherapy would most likely be seen for advanced-stage HCC patients with TNM stages III or IVa disease who are being treated with OLT. The choices lie between giving the chemotherapy before or after the OLT. Factors in favor of pre-transplant chemotherapy include the ability to evaluate whether the chemotherapy is useful (CT scan evidence of tumor shrinkage), and the availability of a hepatic artery that can be safely cannulated for the delivery of the chemotherapy. In general, (see Chapter 28), the chemotherapeutic agents currently available have only been shown to be useful in the management of HCC when delivered into the hepatic artery and not when administered systemically by intravenous injection. Pre-transplant chemotherapy can be continued during the months while the patient is awaiting a liver transplant, in order to prevent the tumor from progressing and hopefully from spreading. By contrast, chemotherapy when given in the post-transplant period can be given to a relatively better functioning liver. However, since no tumor is visible, the effects of the chemotherapy cannot be assessed and it may be given unnecessarily. In addition, in the post-transplant period, patients may often be in a fragile state as a result of their surgery or the consequences of their immunosuppressant therapy, which include changes in their renal function and bone marrow activity. These may limit the ability to deliver tumoricidal doses of chemotherapy. Furthermore, the dependence of the liver graft on the hepatic artery in the post-transplant period results in major risks in using the hepatic artery for chemotherapy in this situation. For safety, one may be limited to intravenous administration of chemotherapy, which has not so far been found to be of proven benefit, in contrast to the intra-hepatic artery route. On balance therefore, the use of neo-adjuvant intra-hepatic arterial chemotherapy prior to the OLT would seem to be preferable (Table 23.2). In addition, the necessary wait for the arrival of a donor organ and the requirement for a minimum of three cycles of chemotherapy, may well permit diagnosis of patients with rapidly metastasizing HCCs and prevent them from receiving an unnecessary OLT. However, patients with end-stage liver disease, with blood levels of bilirubin greater than 3.0 mg/dl cannot normally tolerate intra-hepatic arterial chemotherapy with the currently available drugs at meaningful doses. The impaired liver can easily be tipped into complete failure in this circumstance. Thus, patients with advanced stage HCC whose underlying liver function cannot tolerate intra-hepatic arterial chemotherapy, may not be candidates for OLT at the present time. The most useful agents for intra-hepatic arterial chemotherapy at present include cisplatinum (Platinol), doxorubicin (Adriamycin), and mitomycin C (Mitamycin). Several recent preliminary reports suggest that even advanced stage HCC patients can have prolonged survival when liver transplant is coupled with aggressive chemotherapy.[31-35,41,43] Randomized studies are now needed to evaluate the actual benefit of multimodal therapy compared to transplant alone.

ALGORITHM FOR THE MANAGEMENT OF THE HCC PATIENT FOR OLT

A. Clinical evaluation of the patient includes routine blood hematology, liver profile and electrolytes; measurement of blood tumor markers, alpha-fetoprotein and PIVKA-2 (des-gamma carboxy prothrombin); assessment of hepatitis status. Evaluation of liver size by CT scanning; evaluation of tumor size and extent and portal venous invasion and tumor spread by helical (spiral) CT scan of the abdomen and chest and a bone scan. For apparently unilateral hepatic tumors, a CT-portogram or CT-arteriogram needs to be performed. A core needle biopsy needs to be obtained in all patients with suspected HCC.

B. Patients with well encapsulated tumors confined to one lobe of the liver and without vascular invasion proceed directly to the liver donor waiting list without further therapy.

C. The presence of impairment of portal vein blood flow and particularly signs of portal vein thrombus requires careful work-up including portal vein percutaneous biopsy. Cytologic evidence of malignant cells is currently an exclusion criterion for OLT, as is the presence of nodal or other extra-hepatic tumor involvement.

D. Patients with vascular invasion or bilobar HCC (probably also patients with multiple unilobar lesions, stage III) are currently best treated with aggressive intra-hepatic arterial chemotherapy and a decision for transplantation made after a major objective tumor response to the chemotherapy has been obtained.

E. Patients with stages III or IVa disease who have hepatic insufficiency with livers that cannot tolerate chemotherapy are probably not candidates for OLT at the present time.

F. All patients destined for OLT and who are waiting for a OLT should have repeated CT scans of the chest and abdomen every 3 months to exclude newly appearing extra-hepatic disease or progressive disease.

CONCLUSION

Liver transplantation in the presence of HCC has fulfilled the major objective of extending the resectability of tumors which arise in the presence of varying degrees of cirrhosis.[28,29] This has the potential for curing both the tumor and the cirrhosis in one maneuver. Using liver transplantation, cirrhosis is thus no longer a limiting factor in the treatment of HCC. Liver transplantation has produced excellent long-term survival for patients with any degree of cirrhosis and TNM stages I and II tumors, confined to one lobe of the liver and without vascular invasion. For TNM stages IVa and possibly III HCC, the uses of liver transplantation are currently unclear. Efforts are now underway to determine whether neo-adjuvant chemotherapy in addition to liver transplantation can cause longer term survival in these patients with advanced-stage HCC and relatively good liver function prior to their transplant. Preliminary results from several centers are encouraging for this multiple modality therapy. However, the presence of two diseases, namely cirrhosis and HCC in the majority of patients with HCC, means that the underlying cirrhosis cannot be ignored and is often the major determinant of survival, not just the tumor. The future will therefore bring renewed efforts to control the growth of advanced HCCs prior to liver transplantation, so that both the tumor and the underlying liver disease can be treated concomitantly. Although there is a shortage of suitable donor organ livers in those countries where liver transplantation is currently available, this problem may be resolved, with advances in liver splitting, so that one donor can provide liver tissue for several recipients, and advances in xenobiotic transplantation, so that animal organs may also be used for liver transplantation.

REFERENCES

1. Carr BI, Flickinger JC, Lotze MT. Hepatic neoplasms. In: Devita, VT, Hellman S, Rosenberg SA (eds). *Cancer: Principles and Practice of Oncology.* Lippincott, New York, Fifth edition. 1996. (in press)
2. Carr BI, Michaelopoulos GK. The biology of human hepatocellular carcinoma in primary liver cancer: etiological and progression factors in: Ed Brechot C (ed). CRC Press, Inc., Fl. 1994; 249-267.

3. Wong PYN, McPeake JR, Portmann B *et al.* Clinical course and survival after liver transplantation for hepatitis B virus infection complicated by hepatocellular carcinoma. *Am J Gastroenterol.* 1995; **90:** 29-34.

4. Shiratori Y, Shina S, Imamura M, *et al.* Characteristic difference of hepatocellular carcinoma between hepatitis B- and C-viral infection in Japan. *Hepatology* 1995; **22:** 1027-1033.

5. Duesenbery D, Ferris JV, Thaete FL, Carr BI. Percutaneous ultrasound-guided needle biopsy of hepatic mass lesions using a cytohistologic approach. *J Clin Pathol* 1995; **104:** 583-587.

6. Dodd GD, Carr BI. Percutaneous biopsy of portal vein thrombus: A new staging technique for hepatocellular carcinoma. *Am J Radiology* 1993; **161:** 229-233.

7. Carr BI, Kar S. An assay for hepatoma micrometastasis; Albumin gene expression in peripheral blood from patients with advanced hepatocellular carcinoma. *Hepatology* 1991; **14:** A242.

8. Matsumura M, Niwa Y, Kato N *et al.* Detection of alpha-fetoprotein mRNA, an indicator of hematogenous spreading hepatocellular carcinoma in the circulation: a possible predictor of metastatic hepatocellular carcinoma. *Hepatology* 1994; **20:** 1418-1425.

9. Kar S, Carr BI. Detection of liver cells in peripheral blood of patients with advanced stage hepatocellular carcinoma. *Hepatology* 1995; **21:** 403-407.

10. Hillaire S, Barbu V, Boucher E *et al.* Albumin mRNA as a marker of circulating hepatocytes in hepatocellular carcinoma. *Gastroenterology* 1994; **106**: 239-242.

11. Merine D, Takayasu K, Wakao F. Detection of hepatocellular carcinoma: comparison of CT during arterial portography with CT after intraarterial injection of iodized oil. *Radiology* 1990; **175:** 707-710.

12. Nelson RC, Chezmar JL, Sugarbaker PH, Bernardino ME. Hepatic tumors: comparison of CT during arterial portography, delayed CT, and MR imaging for preoperative evaluation. *Radiology* 1989; **172:** 27-34.

13. Baron RL, Oliver JH, Dodd GD, Nalesnik M, Holbert BL, Carr BI. Hepatocellular carcinoma: evaluation with helical biphasic contrast enhanced CT. *Radiology* 1996; **199:** 505-511.

14. Matsui O, Takashima T, Kadoya M *et al.* Dynamic computed tomography during arterial portography: the most sensitive examination for small hepatocellular carcinomas. *J Comput Assisted Tomogr* 1985; **9(1)**:19-24.

15. Baron RL. Understanding and optimizing use of contrast material for CT of the liver. *Am J Roentgenol* 1994; **163:** 3323-331.

16. Miller WJ, Baron RL, Dodd GD, Federle MP. Malignancies in patients with cirrhosis: CT sensitivity and specificity in 200 consecutive transplant patients. *Radiology* 1994; **193:** 645-650.

17. Ringe B, Pichlmayr R, Wittekind C, Tusch G. Surgical treatment of hepatocellular carcinoma: experience with liver resection and transplantation in 198 patients. *World J Surg* 1991; **15:** 270-285.

18. Iwatsuki S, Starzl TE, Sheahan DA *et al.* Hepatic resection versus transplantation for hepatocellular carcinoma. *Ann Surg* 1991; **214:** 221-229.

19. Penn I. Hepatic transplantation for primary and metastatic cancer of the liver. *Surgery* 1991; **110 (4)**: 726-735.

20. O'Grady JG, Paulson RJ, Rolles K *et al.* Liver transplantation for malignant disease. *Ann Surg* 1988; **207:** 373-379.

21. Ringe B, Wittekind C, Beckstein WO *et al.* The role of liver transplantation in hepatobiliary malignancy. *Ann Surg* 1989; **209:** 88-98.

22. Ringe B, Pichlmayr R, Wittekind C, Tusch G. Surgical treatment of hepatocellular carcinoma: Experience with liver resection and transplantation in 198 patients. *World J Surg* 1991; **15:** 270-285.

23. Van Thiel DH, Carr BI, Iwatsuki S *et al.* Liver transplantation for alcoholic liver disease, viral hepatitis and hepatic neoplasms. *Transplant Proc* 1991; **23:** 1917-1921.

24. Van Thiel DH, Carr BI, Yokoyama I *et al.* Liver transplantation as a treatment for hepatocellular carcinoma. In: *Etiology, Pathology, and Treatment of Hepatocellular Carcinoma in North America.* Tabor E *et al.*(eds) Gulf Publishers, Houston, 1991, pp 309-315.

25. Haug CE, Jenkins RL, Rohrer RJ *et al.* Liver transplantation for primary hepatic cancer. *Transplantation* 1992; **53:** 376-382.

26. Ismail T, Angrisani L, Junson BK *et al.* Primary hepatic malignancy: The role of liver transplantation. *Br J Surg* 1990; **77:** 983-987.

27. Pichlmayr R, Weimann A, Ringer B. Indications for liver transplantation in hepatobiliary malignancy. A consensus conference on indications of liver transplantation. *Hepatology* 1994; **20:**(Supp) 33s-40s.

28. Stone MJ. Transplantation for primary hepatic malignancy. In: Busuttil RW, Klintmalm GB (eds) *Transplantation of the liver* W.B. Saunders Co., Philadelphia. 1996; pp 120-129.

29. Gennari L, Mazzaferro V, Regalla E,*et al.* Reappraisal of the role of liver transplantation in the treatment of hepatocellular carcinoma arising in cirrhosis. *J Surg Oncol* 1993; **3**(Suppl): 83-86.

30. Bismuth H, Chiche L, Adam R *et al.* Liver resection versus transplantation for hepatocellular carcinoma in cirrhotic patients. *Ann Surg* 1993; **218:** 145-151.

31. Vernook AP, Ferrell LD, Roberts JP *et al.* Liver transplantation for hepatocellular carcinoma: Results with preoperative chemoembolization. *Liver Transplant Surg* 1995; **1:** 242-248.

32. Cherqui D, Piedbois P, Pierga J-Y *et al.* Multimodal adjuvant treatment and liver transplantation for advanced hepatocellular carcinoma. *Cancer* 1994; **73:** 2721-2726.

33. Carr BI, Selby R, Madariaga J, Iwatsuki S, Starzl TE. Prolonged survival after liver transplantation and cancer chemotherapy for advanced-stage hepatocellular carcinoma. *Transplant Proc.* 1993; **25:** 1128-1129.

34. Stone MJ, Klintmalm G, Polter D *et al.* Neoadjuvant chemotherapy and liver transplantation for hepatocellular carcinoma: A pilot study in 20 patients. *Gastroenterology* 1993; **104:** 196-202.

35. Olthoff KM, Rosove MH, Shackleton CR,*et al.*. Adjuvant chemotherapy improves survival after liver transplantation for hepatocellular carcinoma. *Ann Surg* 1995; **221:** 734-743.

36. Mazzaferro V, Regalla E, Doci R *et al.* Liver transplantation for the treatment of small hepatocellular carcinomas in patients with cirrhosis. *N Engl J Med* 1996; **334:** 693-699.

37. McPeake JR, O'Grady JG, Zaman S *et al.* Liver transplantation for primary hepatocellular carcinoma: Tumor size and number determine outcome. *J Hepatol* 1993; **18:** 226-234.

38. Selby R, Kadry Z, Carr BI *et al.* Liver transplantation for hepatocellular carcinoma. *World J Surg* 1995; **19:** 53-58

39. Ohto M, Kondo F, Ebara M. Pathology diagnosis and treatment for small liver cancer. In: Tobe T *et al.*(eds) *Primary Liver Cancer in Japan* 1992; Springer-Verlag, Tokyo and New York pp. 365-373.

40. Regalia E, Sansalone C, Mazzaferro V *et al.* Pattern of recurrence of hepatocellular carcinoma after liver transplantation: Milan multicenter experience. *Trans Proc* 1994; **26:** 3579-80.

41. Spreafico C, Marchiano A, Regalia E *et al.* Chemoembolization of hepatocellular carcinoma in patients who undergo liver transplantation. *Radiology* 1994; **192:** 687-90.

42. Alessiani M, Tzakis A, Todo S *et al.* Assessment of five-year experience with abdominal organ cluster transplantation. *J Am Coll Surg* 1995; **180:** 1-9.

43. Farmer DG, Rosove MH, Shaked A *et al.* Current treatment modalities for hepatocellular carcinoma. *Ann Surg* 1994; **236:** 1994.

24

Chemoembolization

M Okazaki, H Higashihara and H Shijo

Primary liver cancer is one of the most common causes of cancer death in Japan. Approximately 23,000 patients died of this cancer in 1989. Moreover, the number of deaths due to primary liver cancer is increasing markedly every year.[1] HCC accounts for 90% of primary liver cancer in Japan, and 80 to 90% of HCC is associated with liver cirrhosis. Poor hepatic functional reserve due to underlying cirrhosis is the primary factor which limits extended surgical resection in many cases.[2] It is extremely important to detect HCC at an early stage for curative treatment. With recent advances in imaging modalities, particularly US, it is possible to easily detect small HCCs less than 2 cm in diameter and the criteria of histologic diagnosis for HCC have been changed.[3]

Based on the recent pathomorphologic study of resected hepatocellular carcinomas (HCCs) of various sizes and biopsied materials of small HCCs in the early stage, well-differentiated (early HCC) is characterized by increased cell density with nuclear/cytoplasmic ratio, increased cytoplasmic eosinophilia, and irregular pattern, with occasional pseudoglandular pattern. Almost all advanced HCCs are moderately to poorly differentiated.[4] Portal tracts are retained within the early HCC and there is a "replacing growth pattern" at the tumor/non-tumor boundary.[3-5] Furthermore, the study of resected tumors of various sizes consisting of mixtures of different histologic grades has clarified that when the small well-differentiated HCCs increase in size, foci of less well-differentiated cancerous tissues arise in them (early-advanced HCC) and increase their areas until they totally replace the well-differentiated HCC tissues (advanced HCC).[3-5] This morphologic evidence suggests the presence of a close relationship between tumor dedifferentiation and proliferation in HCC.

Indeed, such small HCCs now comprise approximately 10% of the total cases in Japan.[6] However, because of associated liver cirrhosis and occasional multicentricity, about 70-80% of cases are inoperable.[5] Therefore, transcatheter hepatic arterial chemoembolization (TACE) plays an important role even in the treatment of small HCCs. TACE has the dual aim of producing tumor ischemia by embolization of the arterial supply to the tumor and by increasing the time that chemotherapeutic agents act on the target area.[7]

Transcatheter management of hepatic neoplasms is based on the principle that most hepatic neoplasms receive their blood supply almost exclusively from the hepatic artery.[8] Approximately 75% of the blood flow to normal liver parenchyma is from the portal vein, with the remaining 25% from the hepatic artery. Thus, treatment involving the hepatic artery predominantly affects neoplasms.[9,10]

However, it is almost impossible to achieve complete necrosis of the cancerous tissue even in advanced HCC, especially in the cancerous tissues that are located in the capsule, extracapsular area and satellite nodule, by conventional TACE alone.[11-13] These tumors are supplied by both the hepatic artery and the portal vein.[11-13] Furthermore, repeat TACE may have an adverse effect on liver function. To achieve a more complete necrosis of the foci of the residual viable cells, Uchida *et al.*[14] introduced segmental or subsegmental TACE. In this chapter, we describe the efficacy and pitfalls of conventional TACE and subsegmental TACE. Furthermore, we describe our initial experiences with a newly devised subsegmental TACE under balloon occlusion of the corresponding hepatic vein (NDS-TACE)[15] which may allow us to achieve the simultaneous embolization of both the hepatic artery and the portal vein.[15,16]

ELECTIVE TACE

Technique

We define conventional TACE as that which is performed from the proximal hepatic artery, such as the proper hepatic artery, the right hepatic artery or the left hepatic artery, rather than from the segmental artery or a more peripheral artery.[9]

Initial diagnostic angiography is performed in all patients with a 5.0 or 6.5 French torque-control pre-shaped catheter using the Seldinger technique. In older patients with more tortuous arteries, a 6.5 Fr. catheter with its improved torque control and radiopacity is preferable. In principle, all of the arteries which feed the HCCs must be identified, and the extent of tumor, including portal vein tumor thrombus (PVTT) or hepatic vein tumor thrombus, and arterio-portal shunt must be evaluated before TACE is begun. In all cases, hepatic arteriography was performed following vasodilator-assisted superior

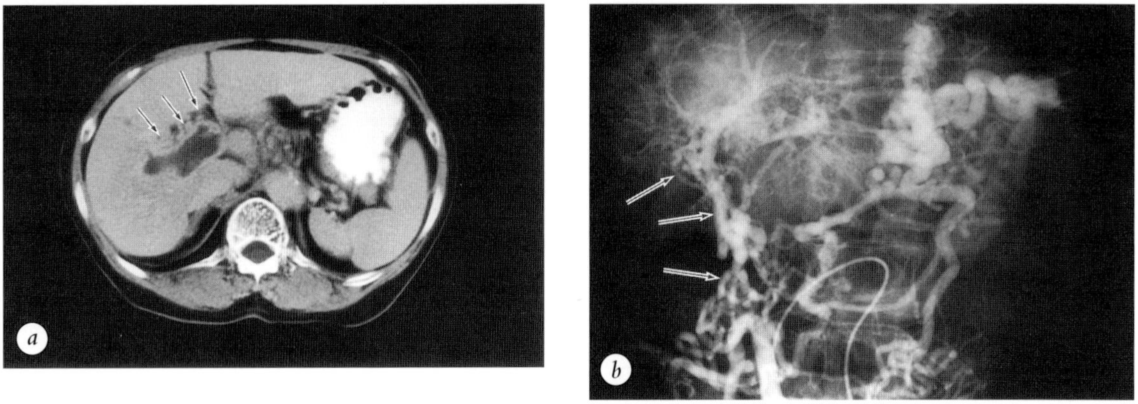

Figure 24.1 – Portal vein tumor thrombus in the portal trunk with cavernous transformation.

a) CT scan at the level of liver hilum reveals non-enhanced tumor thrombus of the right portal vein and cavernous transformation (arrows).

b) Trans-superior mesenteric arterial portogram shows numerous collateral veins such as esophageal varices & spleno-renal shunt and cavernous transformation (arrows). The main portal trunk is not visualized and the intrahepatic portal vein is visualized via cavernous transformation.

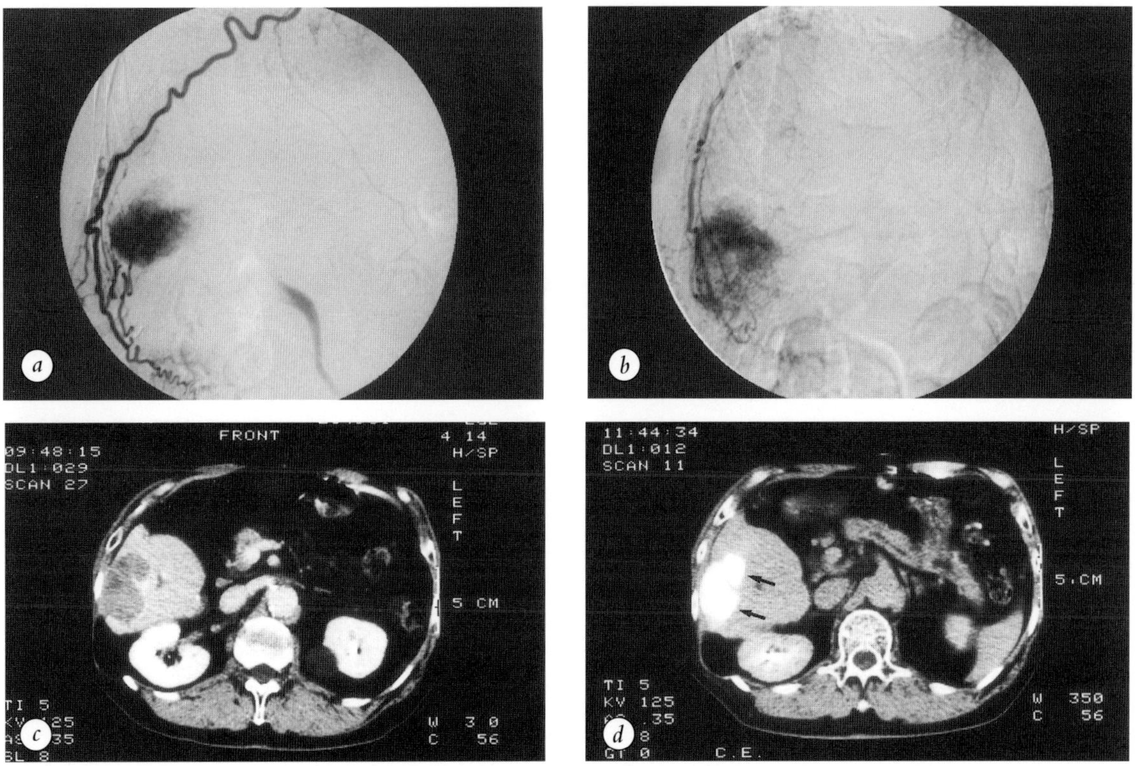

Figure 24.2 – One of several recurrent HCCs in the residual liver 3 years 9 months after hepatectomy, fed by the right intercostal artery.

a) XI intercostal arteriogram reveals tumor stain in the segment 6.

b) X intercostal arteriogram reveals tumor stain at the cranial side of HCC in the segment 6.

c) CT scan obtained before TACE reveals dumbbell shaped low density area in the segment 6.

d) CT scan 1 month after TACE under superselective catheterization into the X and XI intercostal artery branches using coaxial catheter reveals good Lipiodol accumulation in the tumor.

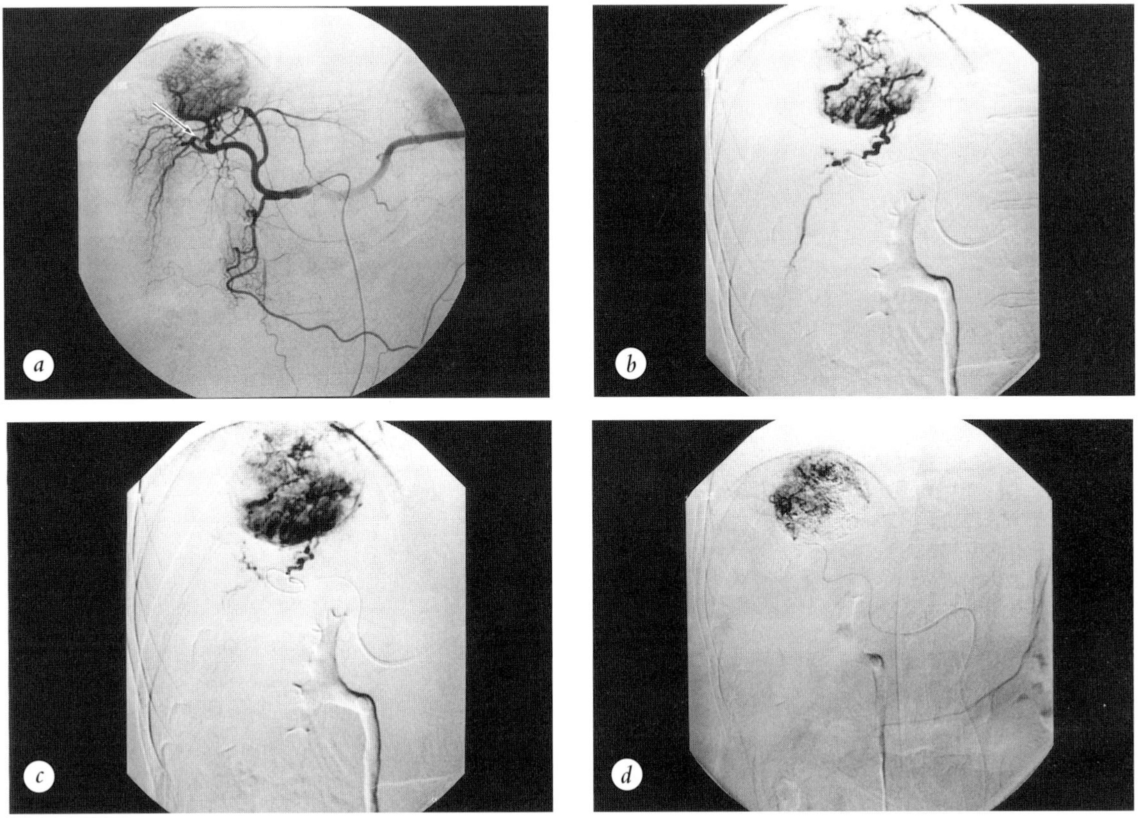

Figure 24.3 – Superselective TACE using coaxial catheter.

a) Common hepatic arteriogram reveals tumor stain in the segment 8 and 7. Arrow indicates the site of catheter tip in the Figure 24.3c.

b) Right superior posterior hepatic (A7) arteriogram tumor blushes at the ventro-caudal side of tumor.

c) The late phase of superselective hepatic arteriogram reveals tumor stain at the caudal side of tumor.

d) Superselective right superior anterior hepatic (A8) arteriogram reveals tumor stain at the cranio-dorsal site of tumor.

mesenteric arterial portography to determine the presence of PVTT and collateral veins such as esophago-cardiac varices and splenorenal shunt (Fig. 24.1).

In some cases with HCC located on the surface of the liver, extrahepatic parasitic arteriogram, such as inferior phrenic arteriogram, middle adrenal arteriogram, inferior adrenal arteriogram and intercostal arteriogram (Fig. 24.2), was performed.[17,18]

Immediately after diagnostic angiography, a catheter is advanced into hepatic arteries (right, left or proper hepatic artery) and/or the extrahepatic parasitic artery. In our early experience (1983-1989), since the smallest catheter available was a 6.5 Fr. or 5.0 Fr., the tip of the catheter was advanced just into the proximal right hepatic artery beyond the confluence of the cystic and/or left hepatic artery. Conventional TACE is performed from this point.

When small coaxial catheters became available (1990), a 3.0 Fr. microcatheter was used as the inner coaxial catheter.[18] This new commercially available 3.0 Fr. coaxial catheter and a tapered 0.41-mm platinum-tipped steerable guidewire or a hydrophilic polymer-coated guidewire can be used to successfully catheterize and embolize a small artery (Fig. 24.3). The flexible polyethylene tip and the semirigid proximal portion of the microcatheter allow us some control of torque, so that it can be advanced past the tip of the introducing catheter without a guidewire and directly into a small branch without accompanying trauma.[18] Alternatively, the catheter can be advanced over a microcatheter-guidewire (a 0.41 mm steerable guidewire or a hydrophilic polymer-coated guide-wire) into a superselective position. Occasionally, the catheter or guidewire cannot be threaded into the targeted small artery. In such cases, to control the direction of the catheter, we use a curved steerable guidewire and/or microcatheter which have been bent by hand and steam respectively. This guidewire system almost always makes it possible to insert a catheter into targeted small arteries.[18] The platinum tip on the steerable guidewire, the golden tip on the hydrophilic polymer-coated guidewire and the platinum coil in the catheter tip allow easy fluoroscopic visualization of the position of the wire and catheter. Furthermore, Gelfoam particles, as well as a variety of small permanent embolic agents, such as iodized oil emulsion and microcoils, can be injected through the catheter. In our series, we were able to introduce the catheter into almost all of the targeted small branches superselectively, without subintimal injury or spasms.

In patients with marked arterioportal shunt, or arteriovenous shunt, TACE must be performed after occlusion of the shunt by microcoil embolization or temporary occlusion of hepatic vein by balloon catheter, to prevent the massive migration of embolic materials into the portal vein or the hepatic vein and lung. Iodized oil (Lipiodol: André Guerbet, France) mixed with various anticancer agents, such as mitomycin (Mitomycin-C: Kyowa Hakko Kogyo, Tokyo, Japan), doxorubicin hydrochloride (Adriamycin: Adria, Dublin, Ohio, USA), anthracycline 4-epidoxorubicin (Epirubicin: Pharmacia, Milan, Italy), Gelfoam particles (Gelfoam: Upjohn, Kalamazoo, Mich), are used for conventional TACE.[10,19]

In our institution, the embolic materials used in conventional TACE, subsegmental TACE and NDS-TACE are prepared as follows. An oil suspension is prepared by mixing 3-10 ml iodized oil and anticancer agents dissolved in contrast medium (iopamidol) at half the volume of the Lipiodol, and shaking the mixture for a few minutes. The anticancer drugs include 10 to 20 mg doxorubicin hydrochloride or 10 to 20 mg anthracycline 4-epidoxorubicin and/or the same dose of mitomycin. About 5 to 10 ml of the Lipiodol suspension is then injected into the hepatic arteries and/or extrahepatic parasitic feeding arteries until all parts of the tumor are filled. After the Lipiodol suspension is injected, the feeding arteries are embolized with gelatin sponge particles that had been soaked in contrast medium mixed with anticancer drugs, until blood flow from the feeding artery to the main tumor (the right or left hepatic artery) is almost stopped.

EFFICACY, SIDE EFFECTS AND PITFALLS

Encapsulated HCCs are highly susceptible to conventional TACE because these tumors are completely fed by hepatic arterial blood.[11-13] However, not all HCCs can be successfully treated by conventional TACE alone: in some HCCs, such as well-differentiated HCC, part of the capsular and/or extracapsular invasion of tumor cells and intrahepatic metastasis is supplied by both the hepatic artery and the portal vein.[11-13] Furthermore, either capsular or extracapsular invasion of tumor cells can occur even in small encapsulated HCCs.[11-13]

In our previous study of 39 patients with encapsulated HCCs (maximum diameter < 30 mm) who were treated by hepatectomy following conventional TACE, no viable cells were found in the tumor by histologic analysis in 33 cases (85%), while viable tumor cells were found in the extracapsular area in 12 cases (31%) and in the intracapsular area in 4 cases (10%).[12] Histopathologic studies have indicated that cancer cells at the front of the extracapsular area show well-differentiated HCC with replacing growth, which may be nourished by blood from both the artery and portal vein.[4,12,23] Thus, even if the artery is successfully embolized, some HCCs, such as extracapsular tumor cells,[11-13] can survive. These factors often lead to tumor recurrence after conventional TACE. As a result, it is often necessary to perform TACE repeatedly, even in patients with small encapsulated HCCs.

Nakamura *et al.*[19] reported that when an excessive amount of Lipiodol was administered into the hepatic artery for HCC, peripheral portal branches became visible in many cases, regardless of the presence or absence of an arterioportal shunt angiographically, and induced not only massive necrosis of the tumor but also atrophy of the surrounding liver parenchyma. However, Chung *et al.*[24] reported that overt pulmonary oil embolism developed in 6 of 14 patients in whom more than 20 ml of Lipiodol had been used for TACE of HCC. As a result, either segmental or subsegmental administration was used to increase its efficacy and avoid any potential liver failure.

Uchida *et al.*[14] introduced segmental TACE and reported good results. Matsui *et al.*[25] performed subsegmental TACE on 100 patients with 124 nodular-type HCCs measuring less than 4 cm in diameter (average, 2.3 cm) by injecting either a mixture of Lipiodol and anticancer drugs followed by gelatin sponge particles, or a mixture of Lipiodol and absolute ethanol. Park *et al.*[26] performed subsegmental embolization on 14 patients with HCC measuring less than 5 cm in diameter by injecting 75% ethanol mixed with Lipiodol. Complete necrosis was reported based on histologic findings in 7 of 11 resected lesions following subsegmental TACE by Matsui *et al.*,[25] in 10 of 12 resected main tumors (80%) following segmental or subsegmental TACE by Matsuo *et al.*[27] and in 3 of 5 resected main tumors following subsegmental TACE by Park *et al.*[26]

Subsegmental TACE has potential drawbacks under certain circumstances. For example, if the dose is insufficient due to either poor estimation of volume or vascular spasm, the chances of recurrence are high. Even if Lidocaine were injected intraarterially through the microcatheter to prevent vasospasm, some volume of Lipiodol emulsion cannot enter the portal vein, and the emulsion regurgitates into the proximal hepatic artery. This phenomenon is not rare.

Side-effects most commonly observed after TACE are upper abdominal pain, nausea and fever. The pain probably results from ischemia of HCCs, liver and gall bladder, tension of the liver capsule due to transient swelling of the liver and peritoneal irritation. Absorption fever associated with necrosis of tumor tissue may also be involved. The severity of these symptoms increases with the extent of HCCs and the volume of the liver embolized. Therefore, these symptoms are more severe in patients with PVTT than in patients without PVTT. It is not uncommon for high fever and pain to persist for 7 to 14 days, or at times up to 4 weeks. These postembolization syndromes are treated conservatively.

TACE IN EMERGENCY

According to the 11th report of the Liver Cancer Study Group of Japan (covering the years 1990 through 1991),[6] 9,868 patients had HCC and 3,092 of them died during the period. Intraperitoneal hemorrhage due to spontaneous rupture of HCC was the cause of death in 7.7% of them. Spontaneous rupture of HCC usually constitutes a critical and life-threatening condition because of hypovolemic shock due to massive blood loss into the peritoneal cavity, underlying liver cirrhosis, and extensive tumor growth.[17,20]

In this chapter, we describe our experience and approach to emergency embolization for spontaneous rupture of HCC.[17]

Review of spontaneous rupture of HCC treated by emergency embolization

From February 1982 to June 1995, 1,393 patients with HCC underwent embolization at Fukuoka University Hospital. Among these 59 patients with spontaneous rupture of HCC underwent emergency embolization (51 male, 8 female: age 34-87 years). The patients were divided into two groups. Group A consisted of 41 patients who had a serum total bilirubin value equal to or less than 3.0 mg/dl, and Group B consisted of 18 patients who had hyperbilirubinemia with a value of more than 3.0 mg/dl (normal value, < 1.2 mg/dl).

After the clinical diagnosis of spontaneous hemorrhage from HCC, hepatic angiography was performed, followed by embolization with or without administration of anti-cancer drug and iodized oil. First, arterial portograms were obtained via the superior mesenteric artery to evaluate the presence of a tumor thrombus in the portal vein (PVTT). Then hepatic arteriography and embolization were performed. Selection of embolization procedure with or without anti-cancer agents and iodized oil was rather arbitrary in the earlier cases. In the later cases, however, chemoembolization was preferred for patients without hyperbilirubinemia, while embolization with particles of absorbable gelatin sponge or stainless-steel coil (Cook, Bloomington, Ind) alone was selected for patients with extensive tumors or occlusion of the celiac trunk.

Clinical symptoms and diagnosis

All patients had a sudden onset of abdominal pain, abdominal distention and anemia.

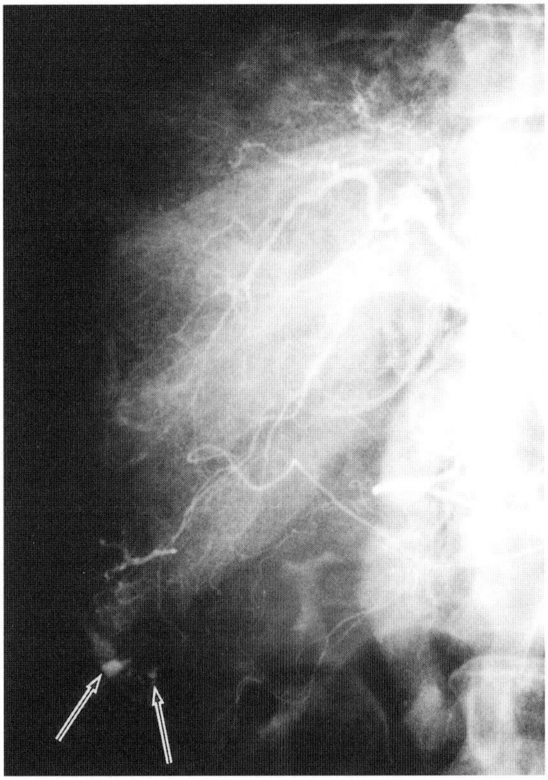

Figure 24.4 – Extravasation of contrast material. Emergency hepatic arteriogram reveals extravasation of contrast material (arrows) in the patient without PVTT.

To obtain an accurate diagnosis of hemorrhage, it is most important to know the history of HCC by verifying the presence of bloody ascites with abdominal paracentesis and demonstrating hypervascular tumors and extravasation of the contrast medium from HCC with angiography.[17] The prevalence of extravasation has been reported to be 0%, 10%, and 23.5% in previous reports.[20-22] The prevalence was only 14% (8 patients) in our series (Fig. 24.4). We believe that using angiographic evidence of extravasation is not reliable because (a) great amounts of ascites dilute the contrast medium, preventing any enhancement of extravasation, and (b) it is difficult to make a differential diagnosis between tumor stain and extravasation from an anteroposterior view.

US is the most useful modality for diagnosing ruptured HCC because it can be used to easily detect not only fluid collection but also liver tumor under these emergency conditions.[17] Furthermore, US-guided abdominal paracentesis that reveals bloody ascites confirms the diagnosis.

Extent of tumor

Arterial portography revealed PVTT in 32 patients. The PVTT extended the main trunk of the portal vein (Vp4) in 13 patients, right or left portal vein (first-order branch; Vp3) in 15 patients, and more peripheral branches (second-order branch; Vp2) in 4 patients.

At hepatic arteriography, only 6 patients without PVTT had HCC of the solitary nodular type in the surface of the liver. Twenty had multinodular HCCs, 23 a massive tumor, which was not well demarcated and was frequently accompanied by small intrahepatic metastatic nodules due to PVTT, and the remaining 10 had diffuse tumors, ie numerous small foci throughout the liver.

Hemorrhagic site of tumor

It is very difficult to detect the hemorrhagic site in a patient with spontaneous rupture of HCC by an imaging modality because out of 59 patients in our series, extravasation of contrast material from the tumor was demonstrated in only 8 patients as described before, and hypervascular tumor stains were the only evidence of ruptured HCC in the other 51.

To clarify these results, we analyzed clinicoroentogenological findings in 30 patients in whom follow-up CT findings after emergency TACE could be estimated satisfactorily.

All of the solitary and massive HCCs were located on the surface of the liver. Furthermore, in all of the patients with multinodular and diffuse HCCs, at least one tumor was located on the surface of the liver (Fig. 24.5).

The liver is covered by a thin but strong connective tissue capsule called Glisson's capsule. This capsule is covered by visceral peritoneum, except in the subdiaphragmatic bare area of the liver. Therefore, intraperitoneal hemorrhage cannot develop without the rupture of liver capsule. Irregular lines in the liver capsule at the site of the tumor were found in 84% on follow-up CT (Fig. 24.6). Our data suggest that the hemorrhagic site in patients with ruptured HCC coincides with the irregular line in the liver capsule at the site of the tumor.

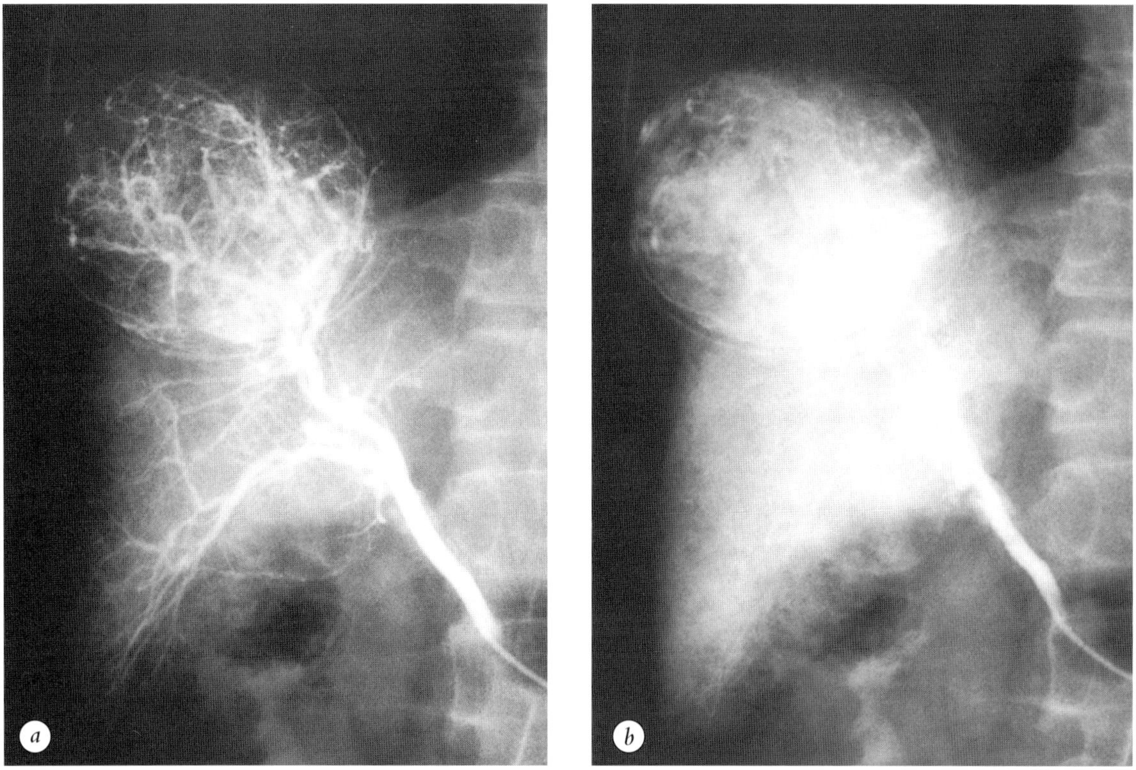

Figure 24.5 – Ruptured pedunculated HCC without PVTT. *a)* Right hepatic arteriogram reveals tumor blushes in S8.

b) The late phase of Fig.5A reveals tumor stain which proliferates extrahepatically. This type of HCC is included in the category of pedunculated HCC.

Embolization procedure

The iodized oil suspension as mentioned before was injected into hepatic arteries or extrahepatic collateral arteries such as the right inferior phrenic artery, until all parts of the tumor were filled with it (about 2-10 ml). Gelatin sponge particles, approximately 500 μm to 1 mm in size, were introduced until the arterial blood supply to the tumor was completely stopped. This procedure was used in 48 patients.

Embolization was performed in 4 patients with a stainless-steel coil only and in 7 patients with gelatin sponge particles not soaked in anticancer drugs and iodized oil. Our goal in emergency embolization was to embolize as rapidly as possible, yet selectively if possible, to stop bleeding completely and to reduce hepatic damage caused by embolization.[17]

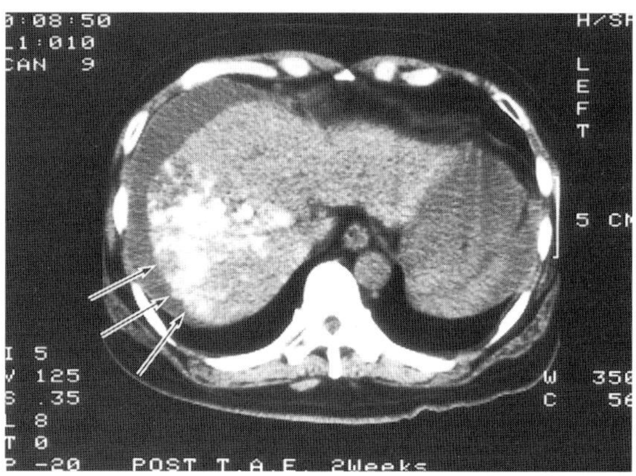

Figure 24.6 – Follow-up CT 2 weeks after emergency TACE for the ruptured HCC with PVTT reveals massive ascites, irregular line in the liver capsule (arrows) and Lipiodol accumulation in massive type HCC. Lipiodol accumulation in the tumor is scanty in the surface of the liver.

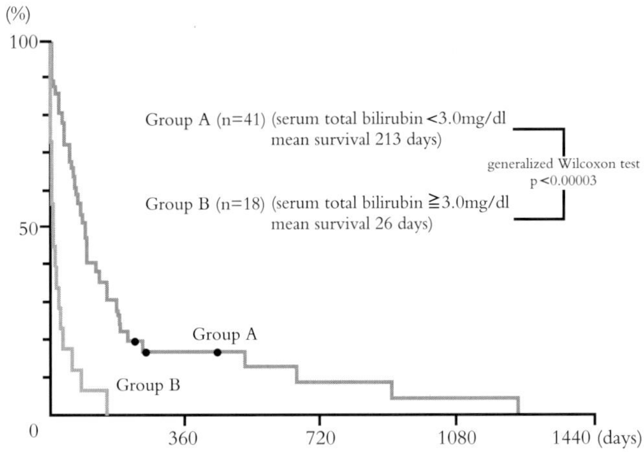

Figure 24.7 – Cumulative survival rates for patients with and without hyper bilirubinemia

Hemostasis and outcome

Hemorrhage was stopped immediately after embolization in all patients, as confirmed by the occlusion of feeding arteries of tumors and/or disappearance of extravasation, elevated blood pressure, and increased hemoglobin values, Progressive jaundice developed in 14 patients who died of hepatic failure and repeated bleeding within 10 days after emergency embolization. Repeated hepatic arteriography was not performed in these 14 patients because of severe hepatic failure; thus, the site of bleeding could not be estimated. Of these 14 patients, 9 had hyperbilirubinemia (group B) and 1 had renal failure before embolization.

The prevalence and severity of the postembolization syndrome, such as fever and pain, in these patients were similar to those previously described in patients who had undergone conventional elective hepatic arterial chemoembolization or embolization.[9]

The relationship between the prognosis of these patients, the serum total bilirubin level and the presence of PVTT as determined before emergency chemoembolization or embolization was examined. The cumulative survival rates of the 41 patients in group A including 3 patients treated by emergency TACE followed by hepatic resection and the 18 patients in group B are shown in Figure 24.7. Eight (20%) of 41 patients in group A and 14 (78%) of 18 patients in group B died within 1 month. Furthermore, 23 (56%) of 41 patients in group A survived more than 3 months. Two (11%) of 18 patients in Group B survived more than 3 months. A significant correlation between the serum total bilirubin level

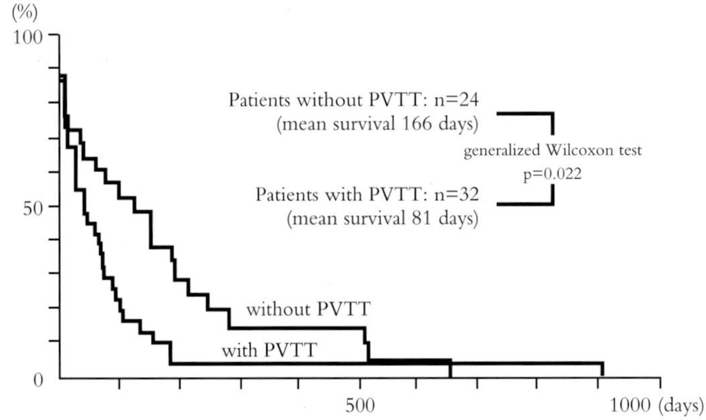

Figure 24.8 – Cumulative survival rates for patients with and without PVTT treated by emergency TACE alone

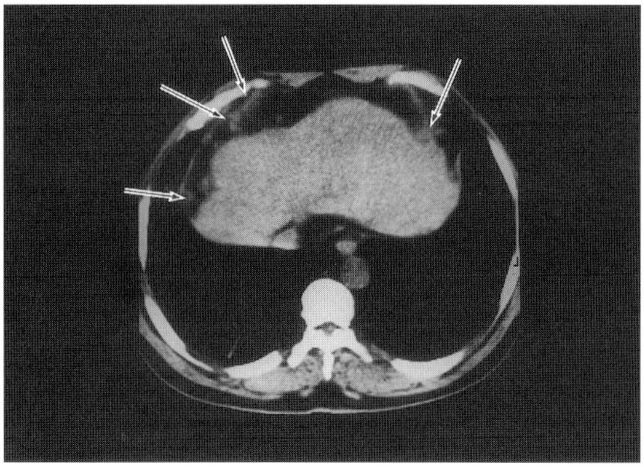

Figure. 24.9 – Intraperitoneal seeding. Follow-up CT obtained 2 months after emergency embolization reveals newly developed soft-tissue masses around the liver (arrows). Exploratory laparatomy was performed after the patient's condition stabilized. Intraperitoneal dissemination was verified at histological examination, and hepatectomy was not carried out. The patient died of peritonitis carcinomatosa 153 days after embolization.

and prognosis was obtained with rigid analysis ($p < 0.00003$). The median duration of survival was 213 days for group A (165 days: excluding 3 patients treated by emergency TACE followed by hepatic resection) and 26 days for group B.

The cumulative survival rates of patients with PVTT and those without PVTT are shown in Figure 24.8. Among the 32 patients with PVTT, 15 (47%) died within 1 month and 9 (28%) survived more than 3 months. Seven (26%) of the 27 patients without PVTT died within 1 month, and 16 (59%) survived more than 3 months. The median survival was 81 days for patients with PVTT and 166 days for those without PVTT treated by emergency embolization alone ($p=0.02$).

In 8 (33%) of 24 patients, newly developed intraperitoneal soft tissue masses (Fig. 24.9) were found at the follow-up CT obtained 3 months or more after emergency TACE. In 4 of the eight, confirmation of intraperitoneal disseminations was made by means of histologic examination of biopsy or autopsy specimens.

Intraperitoneal dissemination was uncommon in the patients with unruptured HCC, and the prevalence of peritoneal dissemination by autopsy was 15.7%.[6] On the other hand, a high prevalence of dissemination (33%) was suggested in our series of patients with ruptured HCC who survived more than 3 months. Peritoneal dissemination might be one of the important factors that make the prognosis of hemorrhage from HCC poor.

The risk and prognostic factors of emergency chemoembolization or embolization have not been analyzed previously. In our series, there was no correlation between the total amount of blood loss, as measured by means of transfusion requirements, and length of survival. The median survival durations in group A (n=41) and B (n=18) were 213 days and 26 days, respectively. The latter duration of survival was the same as the prognosis for patients who underwent supportive care, as previously reported.[22] Furthermore, 20% of patients in group A (including 13 patients with PVTT) and 78% of patients in group B (including 9 patients with PVTT) died within 1 month.

These data suggest that patients in group B would probably have less hepatic reserve for ischemia than those in group A and may not tolerate chemoembolization or embolization.

Our data suggest that emergency chemoembolization or embolization for ruptured HCC is contraindicated in patients with hyperbilirubinemia (> 3.0 mg/dl).[17]

SUBSEGMENTAL TRANSCATHETER HEPATIC ARTERIAL CHEMOEMBOLIZATION (NDS-TACE)

To overcome these shortcomings, we introduced a newly devised subsegmental TACE (NDS-TACE), in which the hepatic vein which drains the tumor-bearing segment is occluded with a balloon catheter. This procedure was based on the experimental reports of Rousselot *et al*[16] and Kanazawa *et al*[28] and on our previous experience in treating a case of HCC complicated by a severe arteriovenous shunt.

Approximately 30 years ago, Rousselot *et al*,[16] in an attempt to improve the delivery of therapeutic agents to hepatic tumors, performed experimental hepatic arteriography and arterial infusion chemotherapy in dogs during temporary total hepatic venous occlusion. This procedure produced a high concentration

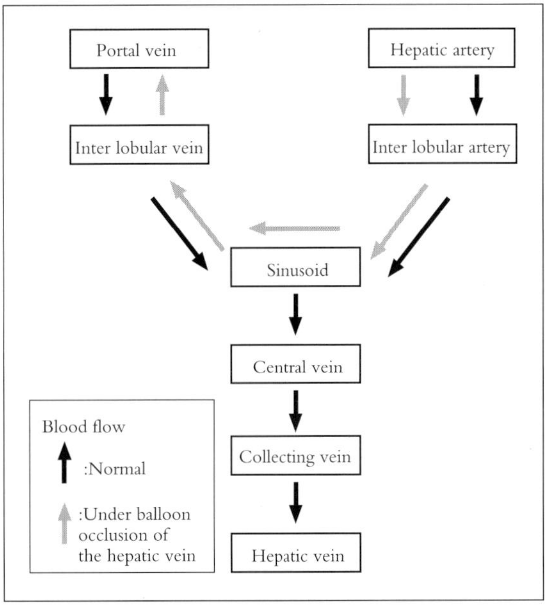

Figure 24.10 – Hepatic blood flow

of drug in the hepatic vein and liver parenchyma, and has been subsequently used to treat 1 patient with liver metastasis from colon cancer, but no objective results were obtained. Kanazawa *et al*[28] reported that temporary segmental hepatic vein occlusion is safe for up to 60 minutes and may be used clinically as a means of improving the therapeutic index of agents within the liver when they are administered via concomitant hepatic arterial infusion. These procedures involve chemoinfusion therapy using anticancer drugs alone. In contrast, NDS-TACE involves chemoembolization therapy using anticancer drugs in Lipiodol suspension and embolic materials. In our HCC case with arteriovenous shunt, a hepatic arteriogram under occlusion of the hepatic vein with a balloon catheter demonstrated disappearance of the arteriovenous shunt, a dense hepatogram, numerous portal vein branches and tumor staining in the occluded lobe, while a hepatic arteriography without hepatic vein occlusion did not reveal such findings. In our series, we found that the degree of visualization of the subsegmental portal vein and the sinusoidgram in a subsegmental arteriogram were much better with balloon occlusion than without. The changes in hepatic blood flow induced by the balloon occlusion are summarized in Figure 24.10.

Technique

(Fig. 24.11)

NDS-TACE was performed as follows:[15] After performing diagnostic hepatic angiography using either a 5.0 or 6.5-Fr. catheter, a microcatheter was introduced into the subsegmental feeding artery. Thereafter, a 7.0 Fr. occlusion balloon catheter (Medi-Tech, Boston Scientific Corperation, MA) was introduced into the corresponding hepatic vein that drained from the tumor-bearing subsegment through the femoral vein. After the catheter tip was seated in the proximal part of the corresponding hepatic vein, the balloon was inflated with up to 1 cm^3 of saline to occlude the hepatic blood outflow, and resulted in a sudden increase in the transsinusoidal and transtumoral arterioportal communication only in the tumor-bearing subsegment. NDS-TACE was then performed through the microcatheter by injecting the embolic materials which were the same as those normally used in conventional and subsegmental TACE.

Results

From August 1992 to July 1995, this NDS-TACE technique was performed in 20 patients with 23 small nodular-type HCCs which measured less than 7 cm in diameter (average 3.4 cm) and were limited to a single subsegment. Except for 1 patient who demonstrated three lesions, all of the patients had only one tumor.

During NDS-TACE, we fluoroscopically observed that the Lipiodol emulsion flowed into the tumor(s) and portal vein branches around each tumor in all cases (Fig. 24.12a,b). Choi *et al*[29] reported that the concentration of Lipiodol in the liver tissue which surrounds the tumor tends to coincide with the degree of necrosis of the tumor. Thus, a lack of retention of Lipiodol in the surrounding liver is associated with incomplete necrosis. In all of our cases, dense retention of Lipiodol in both the tumor(s) and the surrounding liver, including the portal vein branches, was recognized in both the follow-up CT and plain radiograms following NDS-TACE (Fig. 24.12b). Furthermore, a subsegmental atrophy-like infarction (Fig. 24.12c), was encountered in 13 out of 15 patients on the follow-up CT obtained 6 months or more after NDS-TACE. Matsui *et al*[25] also reported favorable local recurrence rates for 113 unresected lesions after conventional

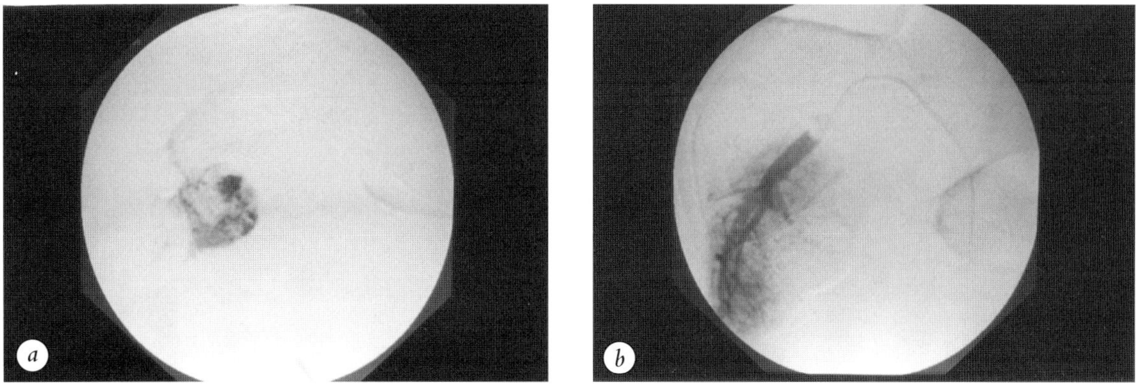

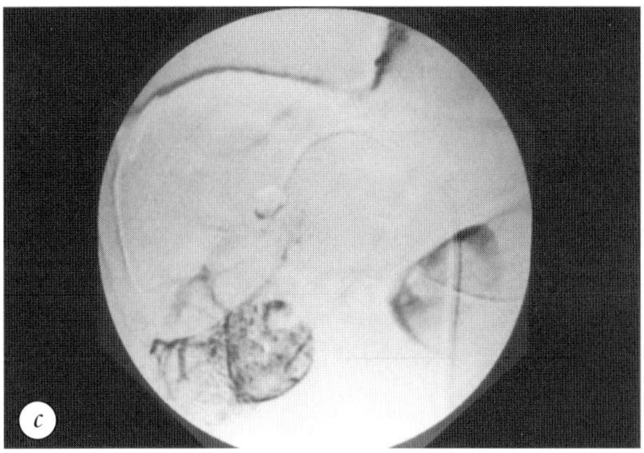

Figure 24.11 – Subsegmental TACE under balloon occlusion of the corresponding hepatic vein.

a) Superselective right inferior posterior hepatic (A6) arteriogram without balloon occlusion of the right hepatic vein reveals tumor stain and draining hepatic vein.

b) Right hepatic venogram under balloon occlusion reveals hepatic vein branches and liver parenchyma.

c) A6 arteriogram under balloon occlusion reveals not only the tumor stain in the segment 6, but also the subsegmental portal veins. Under these condition, NDS-TACE is performed.

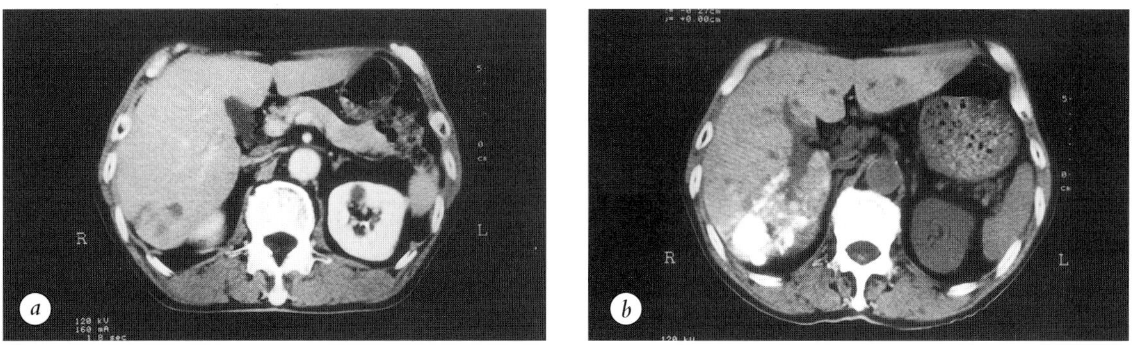

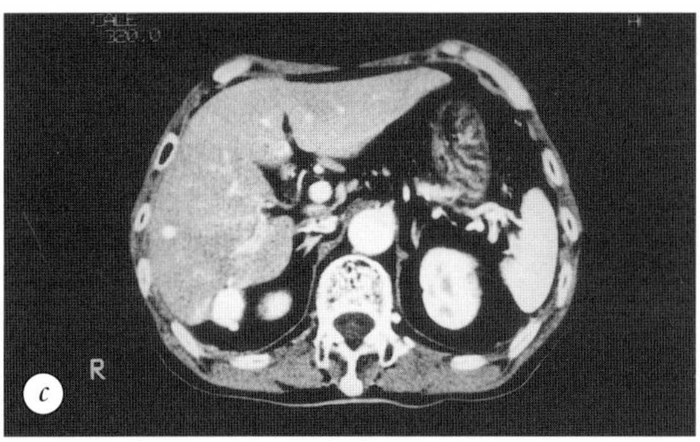

Figure 24.12 – Changes of liver including HCC after NDS-TACE.

a) CT scan before NDS-TACE reveals low density area in S6 the segment 6.

b) CT scan 2 weeks after NDS-TACE reveals Lipiodol accumulation in not only the tumor but also subsegmental portal veins.

c) CT scan 1 year after NDS-TACE reveals subsegmental atrophy-like infarction including shrunken tumor.

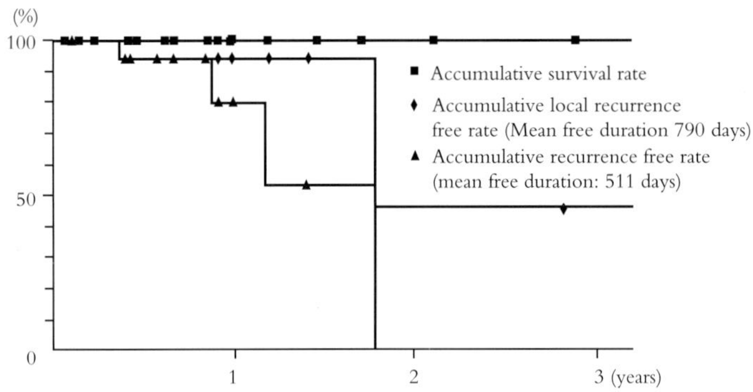

Figure 24.13 – Accumulative recurrence free rate

subsegmental TACE (the 1- and 4-year local recurrence rates were 18% and 33%, respectively).

The outcome and the accumulative recurrence free rate in the 20 patients treated by NDS-TACE are shown in Figure 24.13. The follow-up period ranged from 4 to 40 months (mean 16 months, 12 cases have been followed for more than a year after NDS-TACE). All 20 patients treated by this method are still alive. Recurrent lesions were found in 4 of the 20 patients. Local recurrent lesions were found in two. In addition, newly developed lesions outside of the embolized subsegment were found in 4 patients including 2 patients with local recurrence.

These data suggest that this procedure makes it possible to easily embolize both the hepatic artery and the portal vein branch in only the tumor-bearing subsegment. This procedure can also be used to treat extracapsularly infiltrated HCC and satellite nodules nourished by a portal vein.

In all of our cases, each tumor was drained by only a single vein; however, some tumors, such as those in subsegment 8 and near subsegment 4, may be drained by more than one segmental hepatic vein. Further study of the hepatic vein which corresponds to the tumor is required.

NDS-TACE is thought to cause much more damage to the non-cancerous area than conventional subsegmental TACE. However, no definite deterioration of the physical condition attributable to NDS-TACE was detected in any of the patients.

Until we can learn more from additional case studies, we recommend that NDS-TACE should be performed only in cases in which HCCs are limited to a single subsegment.

In conclusion, this newly devised TACE method was found to be effective and technically straightforward, and may therefore be a viable alternative to subsegmentectomy for the treatment of HCC.

ELECTIVE TACE FOR PATIENTS WITH PVTT

HCC commonly involves the portal vein, and produces PVTT.[4,30] HCC with PVTT is the most advanced condition: it has a poor prognosis and is typically inoperable.[30] Although there is much clinical experience with TACE for HCC in Japan, the indications for TACE for HCC patients with PVTT are still unclear.[9,31] Several authors have reported that TACE is contraindicated in patients with PVTT due to the high mortality associated with TACE.[9,31] We performed TACE in HCC patients with PVTT according to our selection criteria under pre-, intra-

Table 24.1 – Pre-, intra- and post-embolization intensive care

1. Urine volume and electrolyte: Aldosterone antagonist and/or diuretics
2. Liver dysfunction: fresh frozen plasma
3. Respiratory disturbance: blood gas check and O_2 inhalation
4. Pain and fever: analgesic and antibiotics
5. Gastrointestinal bleeding: H_2 blocker

Table 24.2 – Profiles of the patients with portal vein tumour thrombus treated by TACE

PVTT	No. of cases	Sex		Age	Clinical stage	No. of cases with
		M	F	(mean)		distant metastasis (+)
Vp2	78	68	10	40-81 (52.5)	I 34 II 21 III 16	11
Vp3	68	56	12	30-78 (58.9)	I 24 II 26 III 16	5
Vp4	82	73	9	36-82 (57.6)	I 27 II 39 III 13	11
Total	228	197	31	30-81 (56.2)	I 85 II 86 III 45	27

TACE: Transcatheter hepatic arterial chemoembolization, PVTT: Portal vein tumor thrombus, M: Male, F: Female, meta: Metastasis

and post-TACE intensive care (Table 24.1), which has reduced the mortality associated with TACE in these patients.[32] In this chapter, we describe our experience and approach to TACE for HCC patients with PVTT.

Review of cases

From February 1982 to June 1995, 1,393 patients with HCC underwent chemoembolization at Fukuoka University Hospital. Among these patients, 228 with PVTT underwent elective TACE (197 male, 31 female; age 30-81 years). Profiles of the patients with PVTT treated by elective TACE are summarized in Tables 24.2 and 24.3.

At the time of the initial TACE, distant metastasis, such as lung, adrenal gland or bone metastasis, was found in 27 of the 228 patients. Two patients with Vp2 underwent hepatectomy following TACE.

Indications for TACE for 110 patients with PVTT were rather arbitrary in our earlier experience (June 1983-May 1988). More recently, however, TACE was the preferred treatment option for 118 patients with PVTT according to our patient selection criteria.[32]

Patient selection criteria

Mortality and morbidity associated with TACE for patients with PVTT are primarily based on whether the patient has sufficient hepatic functional reserve to tolerate this procedure. Thus, we do not perform TACE if the patient meets even one of the following five selection criteria.[32]

Table 24.3 – HCC with PVTT died within 1 month after elective TACE

	Early cases (1983.6-1988.5)	Late cases (1988.6-1995.6)	Total
Vp2	3/38 (7.9%)	2*1/40 (5.0%)	5*1/78 (6.4%)
Vp3	3/34 (8.8%)	1/34 (2.9%)	4/68 (5.9%)
Vp4	3/38 (7.9%)	0/44 (0%)	3/82 (3.7%)
Total	9/110 (8.2%)	3*1/118 (2.5%)	12*1/228 (5.3%)

* 1 case died of cerebral hemorrhage

i) Persistent hyperbilirubinemia above 2.0 mg/dl (normal value < 1.2 mg/dl)

If a patient with PVTT has a persistently elevated serum bilirubin level of more than 2.0 mg/dl, we are reluctant to perform TACE and other types of angiographic management, such as hepatic arterial chemoinfusion, would be indicated.

ii) Vp4 without cavernous transformation

Approximately 75% of the blood flow to non-cancerous liver parenchyma is from the portal vein.[8] Cavernous transformation is an essential pathway of portal vein blood flow into non-cancerous liver parenchyma in the main tumor-bearing segment or lobe (Fig. 24.1).[32] When arterial blood flow is stopped or diminished by TACE, the volume of portal vein blood flow may increase through cavernous transformation to prevent ischemia of non-cancerous liver parenchyma in the embolized segment or lobe. On the other hand, in patients with Vp4 without cavernous transformation, TACE could produce necrosis of not only HCCs, but also non-cancerous liver parenchyma.

iii) Performance status [4]

iv) Uncontrollable ascites and pleural effusion

The presence of ascites and/or pleural effusion is a clinical manifestation of poor hepatic functional reserve.[33] TACE is contraindicated if ascites and/or pleural effusion are not controlled with diuretics, aldosterone antagonist and fresh frozen plasma beforehand, since portal pressure tends to be elevated following TACE, which would, in turn, cause a further increase in ascites and/or pleural effusion. These increased ascites and/or pleural effusion disrupt the pulmonary gas exchange, which prevents liver cell regeneration and leads to hepatic failure. We used to administer these drugs and fresh frozen plasma to patients with a history of hypoproteinemia, ascites and pleural effusion 2-3 days before TACE.[32]

v) Uncontrolled esophagocardiac varices

Since portal pressure tends to be elevated after TACE, endoscopic sclerotherapy has to be performed before TACE in HCC patients with esophageal varices at risk for hemorrhage.

Technique

In patients with PVTT, it is important to determine whether or not cavernous transformation is present in the liver hilus.[32] As mentioned above, cavernous transformation is an important pathway of portal vein blood flow to non-cancerous liver cells located in the main tumor-bearing segment or lobe.[32,34]

In some cases with HCC located on the surface of the liver, extrahepatic parasitic arteriogram, such as inferior phrenic arteriogram, inferior adrenal arteriogram or intercostal arteriogram, was performed.[17,31]

Mortality after TACE

The incidence of mortality and clinical profiles of 12 patients who died within 1 month following TACE are summarized in Tables 24.3 and 24.4. In our earlier series of 110 patients with PVTT (38 Vp2, 34 Vp3 and 38 Vp4), 9 (8.2%) died within 1 month after TACE. Of these, 7 patients (2 Vp2, 3 Vp3 and 2 Vp4) died of hepatic failure and 2 died of esophagogastric variceal hemorrhage. Among the 7 patients who died of hepatic failure, 4 had hyperbilirubinemia. On the other hand, in the most recent series of 118 cases with PVTT (from 1988 to 1995, 40 Vp2, 34 Vp3 and 44 Vp4), in which we applied our patient selection criteria for TACE for HCC with PVTT, only 3 patients (2.5%) died within 1 month. Among them, 2 patients (Vp3 and Vp2) died of hepatic failure and the remaining 1 died of cerebral hemorrhage. After TACE, newly developed ascites and pleural effusion were found in all of the 8 patients who died of hepatic failure. An inverse correlation was observed between mortality and hepatic functional reserve, as reflected by Child's criteria and clinical stage according to the general

Table 24.4 – Clinical data of 12 cases with PVTT who died within 1 month after TACE

	No. of cases
Total bilirubin level (mg/dl)	
— 1.5	7
2.0 — 3.9	3
4.0 — 4.4	2
Child's classification	
B	5
C	7

Table 24.5 – Cumulative survival rates in patients with PVTT treated by TACE alone

PVTT	Years							
	1	2	3	4	5	6	7	8
Vp2(n=78)	26.9	18.6	9.9	9.9	9.9	9.9	9.9	5.0
Vp3(n=68)	17.5	6.4	6.4	6.4	4.2	4.2	—	—
Vp4(n=82)	20.3	10.8	8.1	8.1	6.1	6.1	6.1	6.1

PVTT: Portal vein tumor thrombus

rules of the Liver Cancer Study Group of Japan.[2]

There was no difference in mortality among patients with Vp2, Vp3 and Vp4.

Results

Cumulative survival rates in the 226 HCC patients with PVTT who were treated by TACE alone, excluding 2 patients treated by TACE following hepatectomy, are shown in Table 24.5. The 5-year-survival rates in patients with Vp2, Vp3 and Vp4 were 9.9%, 4.2% and 6.1%, respectively. Mean survival duration in Vp2, Vp3 and Vp4 was 410 days, 313 days and 401 days, respectively. There were no significant differences in cumulative survival rates among patients with Vp2, Vp3 and Vp4.

Among patients with PVTT, 16 survived more than 3 years after initial TACE. Eight of these 16 patients survived more than 5 years after the initial TACE, as shown in Table 24.6. Five patients are still alive and 3 (1 Vp4, 1 Vp3 and 1 Vp2) died of tumor growth including distant metastasis such as adrenal metastasis, lung metastasis and bone metastasis, 8 years 9 months and 6 years 8 months after the initial TACE (Fig. 24.14). Repeated TACEs were necessary to achieve a long-term survival of more than 5 years in all of the patients except 1 (Case 3), who has thus far been tumor-free for 9 years and 2 months after the initial TACE. None of the patients with poor hepatic functional reserve (Child's C and clinical stage 3) survived more than 5 years.

Characteristic clinicoroentgenologic findings in patients with PVTT who showed long-term survival after TACE are as follows:

i) Segmental or lobar atrophy due to infarction:

Almost all of the HCCs with PVTT used to consist of a huge HCC with extracapsular invasion and intrahepatic metastasis. Therefore, HCC with PVTT may be resistant to TACE.

Table 24.6 – Summary of 8 patients with PVTT surviving more than 5 years after TACE

Case/Age/Sex	Type	Stage	Clinical Stage	PVTT	TACE frequency	AFP levels pre-TACE	Catheter tip	Survival (years-months)
1/62/M	M	IV	II	4	4	—	RHA	8-9
2/56/M	M	IV	I	3	8*3	25,600	RHA	6-8
3/54/M	S	IV	I	2	1	3,200	RHA	9-2#
4/54/F	M	IV	I	2	6*3	220,000	RHA, RIPA	7-8
5/57/M	D	IV	II	4	2	1,900	RHA	7-11#
6/62/M	S	III	I	2	3*1	1,310,720	PHA, RIPA	7-11#
7/68/M	M	IV	II	4	1	98	RHA	6-4#
8/57/F	S	IV	I	3	2*1	900	RHA	6-0#

PVTT: Portal vein tumor thrombus, M: Massive, S: Solitary, D: Diffuse, *: Collateral TACE,

RHA: Right hepatic artery, RIPA: Right inferior phrenic artery, PHA: Proper hepatic artery, #:Alive.

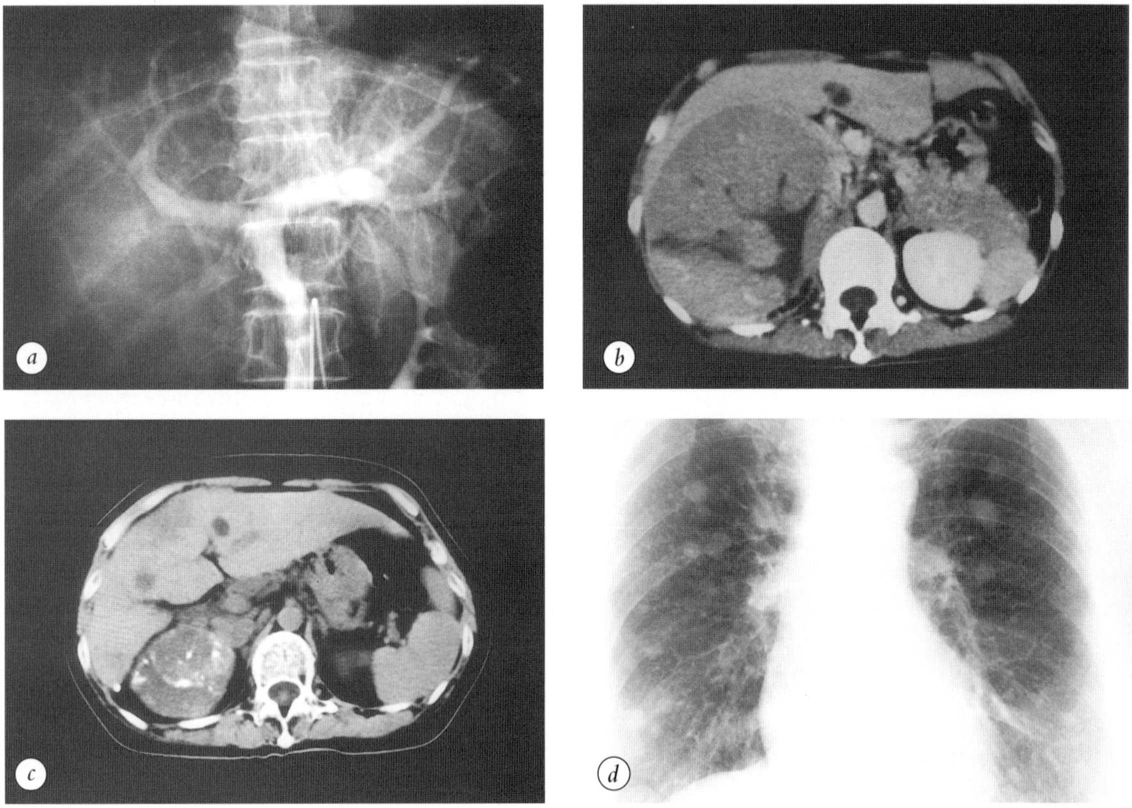

Figure 24.14 – Long-surviving HCC patients with PVTT. (Case 4 in the Table 24.6)

a) Trans-superior mesenteric arterial portogram does not demonstrate the right posterior portal vein branch.

b) CT scan before TACE reveals a huge tumor in the right lobe.

c) Follow-up CT 6 years and 8 months after the initial TACE reveals right lobar atrophy including tumor and intrahepatic metastasis in the compensatory hypertrophied left lobe.

d) Chest X-ray film 7 years 2 months after the initial TACE reveals multiple metastatic tumors in bilateral lung.

In some patients with PVTT, infarction-like segmental or lobar atrophy including the main tumor, intrahepatic metastasis and non-cancerous liver parenchyma (Fig. 24.14c) occurred gradually due to both the blockade of arterial blood flow by TACE and diminished portal blood flow caused by PVTT. Segmental or lobar atrophy requires at least 3 months to develop.

ii) Compensatory hypertrophy of the opposite lobe:

As segmental or lobar atrophy develops, the opposite lobe or non-embolized segment begins to develop compensatory hypertrophy, which may maintain a good hepatic functional reserve. These characteristic findings after TACE are very similar to those associated with surgical segmentectomy or lobectomy (medical lobectomy).

iii) Lipiodol accumulation in the PVTT and/or disappearance of the PVTT:

Intrahepatic metastasis through the PVTT occurs in the early stage. Intrahepatic infiltrates and metastases have been observed to form around branches of the portal vein. Therefore, to prevent intrahepatic metastasis, it is important to kill the PVTT itself.

Lipiodol accumulation in the PVTT was found in only about 30% of patients with PVTT after TACE (Fig. 24.15). Lipiodol accumulation in the PVTT was excellent in patients in whom hepatic arteriography revealed the thread and streaks sign.[35] As the main tumor decreased in size by TACE, the PVTT decreased in size or disappeared altogether in some patients.

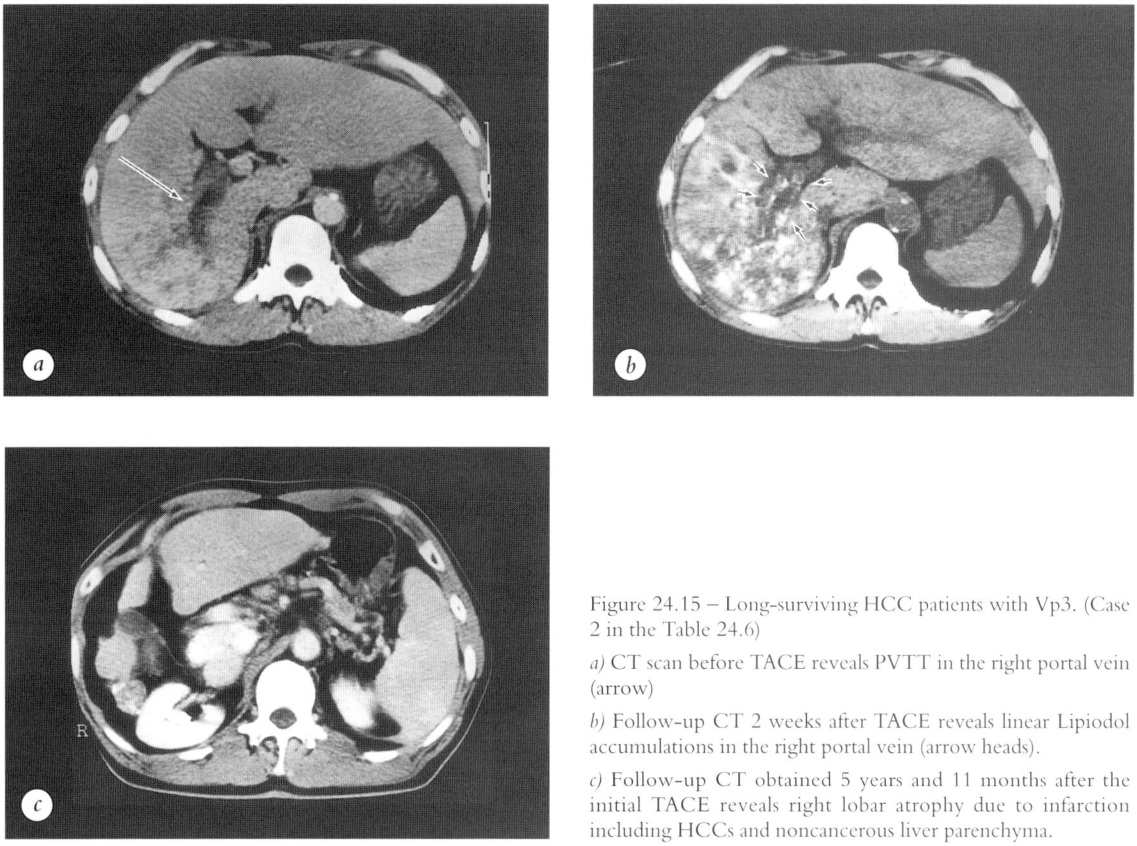

Figure 24.15 – Long-surviving HCC patients with Vp3. (Case 2 in the Table 24.6)

a) CT scan before TACE reveals PVTT in the right portal vein (arrow)

b) Follow-up CT 2 weeks after TACE reveals linear Lipiodol accumulations in the right portal vein (arrow heads).

c) Follow-up CT obtained 5 years and 11 months after the initial TACE reveals right lobar atrophy due to infarction including HCCs and noncancerous liver parenchyma.

Side-effects and major complications

Liver function tests in patients with PVTT after TACE demonstrate a marked elevation of liver enzymes, particularly serum GOT (glutamic oxaloacetic transaminase) and LDH (lactic dehydrogenase), which are mainly due to tumor necrosis after TACE.[36] This enzyme elevation can be as high as 20 to 30 times the preembolization level and lasts for 7 to 10 days in patients with PVTT. In some of our patients with PVTT, LDH increased to more than 10,000 units, but eventually returned to within normal limits. However, an increase in the total bilirubin level to above 3.0 mg/dl and GPT (glutamic pyruvic transaminase) dominant elevation (GPT » GOT) to as high as 30 or more times the preembolization level, along with a rapid decrease in serum albumin, are signs of hepatic failure induced by TACE.

REFERENCES

1. Ministry of Health and Welfare. *Annual report of demographic statistics in Japan*, 1989. Health and Welfare Statistics Association. Tokyo: 1990.
2. The Liver Cancer Study Group of Japan. Predictive factors for long term prognosis after partial hepatectomy for patients with hepatocellular carcinoma in Japan. *Cancer* 1994; **74**: 2772–80.
3. Takayama T, Makuuchi M, Hirohashi S, *et al* Malignant transformation of adenomatous hyperplasia to hepatocellular carcinoma. *Lancet* 1990; **336**:1150-3.
4. Nakashima T, Kojiro M. *Hepatocellular carcinoma. An atlas of its pathology*. Tokyo, Springer-Verlag, 1986; 117-32.
5. Sugihara S, Nakashima O, Kojiro M, *et al* The morphologic transition in hepatocellular carcinoma. A comparison of the individual histological features disclosed by ultrasound-guided fine-needle biopsy at autopsy. *Cancer* 1992; **70**: 1488-92.
6. Liver Cancer Study Group of Japan. Survey and follow-up study of primary liver cancer in Japan. Report 11. *Acta Hepatologica Japonica* 1995; **36**: 208-18 (in Japanese).
7. Kato T, Nemoto R, Mori H, *et al* Arterial chemoembolization with microencapsulated anticancer drug. An approach to selective cancer chemotherapy with sustained effects. *JAMA* 1981; **245**: 1123–7.

8. Breedis C, Young G. The blood supply of neoplasms in the liver. *Am J Pathol* 1954; **30**: 969–85.

9. Yamada R, Sato M, Kawabata M, *et al* Hepatic artery embolization in 120 patients with unresectable hepatoma. *Radiology* 1983; **148**: 397-401.

10. Okazaki M, Yamasaki S, Ono H, *et al* Chemoembolotherapy for recurrent hepatocellular carcinoma in the residual liver after hepatectomy. *Hepato-Gastroenterol* 1993; **40**: 320–3.

11. Sakurai M, Okamura J, Kuroda C. Transcatheter chemoembolization effective for treating hepatocellular carcinoma. A histopathologic study. *Cancer* 1984; **54**: 387-92.

12. Koganemaru F, Okazaki M, Higashihara H, *et al* Therapeutic effect of transcatheter hepatic arterial oily chemoembolization therapy for hepatocellular carcinoma: Analysis of 67 resected main tumor. *Intervent Radiol* 1994; **9**: 61-8 (in Japanese).

13. Kuroda C, Sakurai M, Monden M, *et al* Limitation of transcatheter arterial chemoembolization using iodized oil for small hepatocellular carcinoma: a study in resected cases. *Cancer* 1991; **67**: 81-6.

14. Uchida H, Ohishi H, Matsuo N, *et al* Transcatheter hepatic segmental arterial embolization using iodized oil mixed with an anticancer drug and gelfoam particles for hepatocellular carcinoma. *Cardiovasc Intervent Radiol* 1990; **13**: 140-5.

15. Higashihara H, Okazaki M, Koganemaru F, *et al* The devised transcatheter hepatic arterial chemoembolization for obtaining medical subsegmentectomy. *Cardiovasc Intervent Radiol* 1994; **17**: 21.

16. Rousselot LM, Grossi CE, Slattery J, *et al* Hepatic outflow occlusion during hepatic artery infusion with chemotherapeutic agents. *Cancer* 1964; **17**: 1979-85.

17. Okazaki M, Higashihara H, Koganemaru F, *et al* Intraperitoneal hemorrhage from hepatocellular carcinoma. Emergency chemoembolization or embolization. *Radiology* 1991; **180**: 647–51.

18. Okazaki M, Higashihara H, Koganemaru F *et al* A coaxial catheter and steerable guidewire used to embolize branches of the splanchnic arteries. *AJR* 1990; **155**: 405–6.

19. Nakamura H, Hashimoto T, Oi H, *et al* Iodized oil in the portal vein after arterial embolization. *Radiology* 1988; **167**: 415-7.

20. Ong GB, Chu EPH, Yu FYK, *et al* Spontaneous rupture of hepatocellular carcinoma. *Br J Surg* 1965; **52**: 123-9.

21. Nouchi T, Nishimura M, Maeda M, *et al* Transcatheter arterial embolization of ruptured hepatocellular carcinoma associated with liver cirrhosis. *Dig Dis Sci* 1984; **29**: 1137-41.

22. Hirai K, Kawazoe Y, Yamashita K, *et al* Transcatheter arterial embolization for spontaneous rupture of hepatocellular carcinoma. *Am J Gastroenterol* 1986; **81**: 275-9.

23. Kanai T, Hirohashi S, Upton MP, *et al* Pathology of small hepatocellular carcinoma: a proposal for a new gross classification. *Cancer* 1987; **60**: 810-9.

24. Chung JW, Park JH, Im JG, *et al* Pulmonary oil embolism after transcatheter oily chemoembolization of hepatocellular carcinoma. *Radiology* 1993; **187**: 689-93.

25. Matsui O, Kadoya M, Yoshikawa J, *et al* Small hepatocellular carcinoma: Treatment with subsegmental transcatheter arterial embolization. *Radiology* 1993; **188**: 79-83.

26. Park JH, Han JK, Chung JW, *et al* Superselective transcatheter arterial embolization with ethanol and iodized oil for hepatocellular carcinoma. *J Vasc Interv Radiol* 1993; **4**: 333–9.

27. Matsuo N, Uchida H, Nishimine K, *et al* Segmental transcatheter hepatic artery chemoembolization with iodized oil for hepatocellular carcinoma: Antitumor effect and influence on normal tissue. *J Vasc Interv Radiol* 1993; **4**: 543-9.

28. Kanazawa S, Wright KC, Kasi LP, *et al* Preliminary experimental evaluation of temporary segmental hepatic venous occlusion. Angiographic, pathologic, and scintigraphic findings. *J Vasc Interv Radiol* 1993; **4**: 759-66.

29. Choi BI, Kim HC, Han JK, *et al* Therapeutic effect of transcatheter oily chemoembolization therapy for encapsulated nodular hepatocellular carcinoma: CT and pathologic findings. *Radiology* 1992; **182**: 709-13.

30. Okazaki M, Moriyama N, Yamada T. Clinical evaluation of angiographic portal vein findings and operability in hepatocellular carcinoma. *Jpn J Gastroenterol* 1980; **77**: 758–67 (in Japanese).

31. Chuang VP, Wallace S. Hepatic artery embolization in the treatment of hepatic neoplasms. *Radiology* 1981; **140**: 51-8.

32. Okazaki M, Higashihara H, Koganemaru F *et al* Transcatheter arterial embolization for inoperable hepatocellular carcinoma. *Jpn J Clin Radiol* 1991; **36**:529–34 (in Japanese).

33. Kawasaki S, Makuuchi M, Kosuge T *et al* Systematic subsegmentectomy for hepatocellular carcinoma. In: Tobe T, Kameda H, Okudaira M *et al*, eds. *Primary liver cancer in Japan*. Tokyo: Springer–Verlag, 1992: 235–42.

34. Fujimitsu R, Okazaki M, Koganemaru F *et al* A long surviving hepatocellular carcinoma case (5 years 3 months) with tumor thrombus in the portal trunk treated by embolization. *Acta Hepatologica Japonica* 1990; **31**:93–8.

35. Okuda K, Mucha H, Yoshida T *et al* Demonstration of growing casts of hepatocellular carcinoma in the portal vein by celiac angiography. The thread and streaks sign. *Radiology* 1975; 117:303-9.

36. Shijo H, Okazaki M. Prediction of portal vein invasion by hepatocellular carcinoma. A correlations between portal vein tumor thrombus and biochemical tests. *Jpn J Clin Oncol* 1991; **21**:94–9.

25

Percutaneous ethanol injection

T Livraghi, S Lazzaroni, F Meloni, G Torzilli and C Vettori

The toxic effects of ethanol have been studied in animals[1-3] and confirmed in specimens resected from humans. Alcohol acts by diffusing within the neoplastic cells, which causes immediate dehydration of the cytoplasm, with consequent coagulation necrosis followed by fibrous reaction, and by entering the circulation, which induces necrosis of the endothelial cells and platelet aggregation with consequent thrombosis of the small vessels followed by neoplastic tissue ischemia.

Two features of HCC favor the toxic action of ethanol: hypervascularization and the difference in consistency between neoplastic and cirrhotic tissue. Since HCC neoplastic tissue is softer than the surrounding cirrhotic tissue, ethanol diffuses within it easily and selectively and, at the same time, hypervascularization ensures its uniform distribution within the rich network of neoplastic sinusoids.

Percutaneous ethanol injection (PEI) therapy in the treatment of liver tumors was devised independently at Chiba University in Japan and at Vimercate Hospital (Milan), in Italy. The first report in an international journal appeared in 1986.[4]

At our center, the grounds for introducing PEI were: 1) the good results of previous studies on percutaneous ethanol injection for the treatment of secondary hyperparathyroidism, by Solbiati *et al*,[5] and on percutaneous interstitial chemotherapy for the treatment of hepatic tumors, by the authors; [6] 2) US screening of a cirrhotic population which led to the detection of an increasing number of small HCC; 3) the lack of therapeutic options for these asymptomatic patients, because the resectability rate was low.

Today, 10 years after its introduction, PEI is one of the treatments most frequently offered to patients recruited at US screening.

PROCEDURE

Equipment

PEI is usually performed under US guidance, because this real-time control allows faster execution, precise centering of the needle on the target, continuous monitoring of ethanol distribution, and determination of the appropriate amount to inject each time.

Some authors prefer to use CT guidance.[7-8] In their experience, the advantage of CT is greatest in treating large tumors, where multiple needle placements may be necessary to ablate the lesion completely; in these cases, CT enables direct visualization of the area of tumor necrosis and identification of potentially untreated areas within the tumor. However, a major drawback of CT guidance remains the impossibility of checking in real-time the extent of ethanol diffusion.

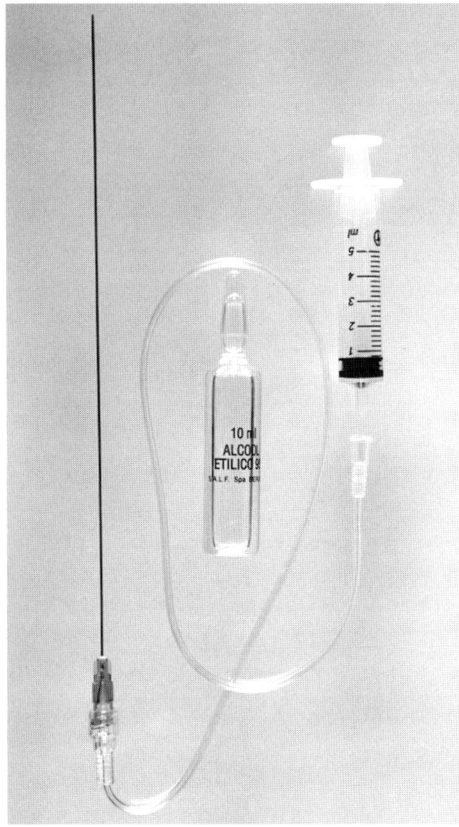

Figure 25.1 – Equipment for PEI

We use 3.5-MHz probes with a lateral guide attachment or with an incorporated guide that permits a perpendicular approach (see Figs. 19.1 and 19.2). We use sterile 95% ethanol and two types of needle: a 17.7 cm long, 22-gauge spinal needle (Becton-Dickinson, Rutherford, NJ, USA) or, more frequently, a 20 cm long, 21-gauge needle with a closed conical tip and three terminal side holes (PEIT needle, Hakko, Tokyo, Japan) (Fig. 25.1). Although this needle is more expensive, it has some important advantages: a) only one operator is required; b) a larger volume of

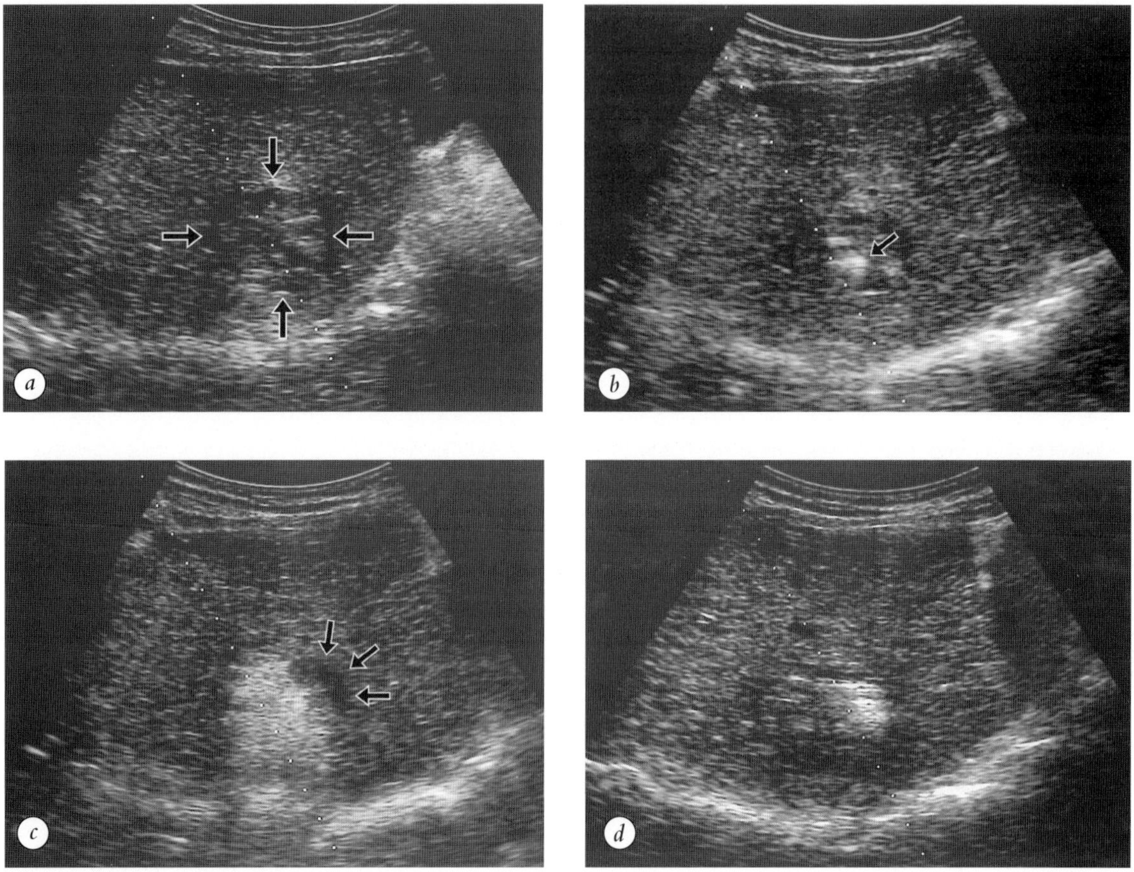

Figure 25.2 – Intercostal sonogram, with patient on the left side.

a) Before insertion of the needle, the lesion (arrows) was centered by the electronic guide system.

b) After insertion, needle tip was well detectable at the center of the lesion (arrow).

c) The area perfused was clearly seen as a patch of hyperechogenicity, with ethanol spreading within a radius of 3 cm around the tip; a semilunar peripheral area remained unperfused (arrows).

d) After some minutes a second injection was performed, centering the untreated tissue; being the first session, the rich neoplastic vascularization washed out the alcohol previously injected.

tissue can be treated in one session and so fewer injections are needed; c) there is less reflux of ethanol into the peritoneal cavity, which can cause pain, and so the procedure is more acceptable; d) the inconvenience of bending is minimized and so even small and deep-seated targets can easily be reached.

Technique

PEI is usually performed in several sessions in an outpatient department or, when HCC is more advanced, in a single session under general anesthesia.[9] We use the former for single HCC less than 4-5 cm in size or multiple HCC with 2-3 nodules less than 3 cm. We use it also for hyperplastic adenomatous nodules, usually small, considered precursors of HCC, the rationale being that resection of a lesion with no evidence of malignancy would not be acceptable either to surgeon or to patient.[10,11] We use the latter in other presentations provided that HCC, single or multiple, does not exceed 30-35% of liver volume, and when there is no neoplastic thrombosis in the main portal branches or in the hepatic veins. Either procedure can be repeated in the event of local recurrence or new lesions.

Multisession treatment

Patients should fast overnight, as a few develop nausea, through this is rare. Treatment is usually given without sedation and without local anesthesia. Some authors administer standard premedications for analgesia and sedation, and local anesthesia.

After local skin preparation with iodized alcohol, which also is used as contact medium, the optimal approach is chosen. Any lesion detected by US can be treated by PEI; however some locations are simpler to reach than others. For lesions in the right lobe, an intercostal approach with the patient on the left side is often preferred. During the insertion and withdrawal of the needle, the patient is asked to hold his breath; during the injection shallow breathing is required.

Alcohol 1 to 8 ml is injected per session, with one or more injections (in different areas) in the same session depending on ethanol distribution, patient compliance, lesion size, degree of vascularization, type of tumor, presence of septa and type of needle. When more than one injection is administered in one session, some minutes are allowed to elapse before the next to avoid a possible reflux of ethanol through the previous needle tract which is still open. The perfused area is clearly seen as a patch of hyperechogenicity (Fig. 25.2a-d). Ethanol is injected slowly and its diffusion checked in real-time on the monitor. Ethanol usually spreads within a radius of 2 to 3 cm around the tip of the needle to the periphery of the tumor except in the case of the sclerosing form in which the diffusion is not homogeneous. Injection is stopped when significant leakage outside the lesion is detected or when diffusion is not clearly visible and then resumed when conditions are right. Leakage is unusual, however, because the surrounding cirrhotic tissue is harder and ethanol tends to remain within the tumor. In the first sessions, when all tissue is viable, ethanol is easily washed out by the rich neoplastic blood supply; as long as ethanol is seen to disappear rapidly, injection is continued intermittently with small boluses until the ethanol pools in the lesion. As alcohol reflux may cause pain, the needle is left inside for 10 to 30 seconds after the injection, especially in superficial lesions, and then withdrawn slowly. If alcohol reflux is appreciated as a rapidly moving hyperechoic line along the needle path, withdrawal is stopped and resumed a few seconds later (Fig. 25.3).

The injection site is chosen before each session to ensure perfusion of areas considered not to have been treated previously. To facilitate this decision, we record every session on personal videotape and in a simple diagram. In all, each treatment generally takes approximately 10-20 minutes, and the patient rests in the waiting room for 1-2 hours. Treatment is usually given twice a week.

Treatment ends when the perfusion of the tumor is considered total. As a rule, using the multiholed needle, we treat lesions smaller than 2 cm in three to four sessions, lesions of 2 to 3.5 cm in four to eight sessions, and lesions of 3.5 to 5 cm in six to twelve sessions. The number of sessions is approximately twice the lesion diameter in centimeters. The total volume is not absolute and should be tailored to the patient. The duration of treatment may depend also on the goal, that is, whether to aim at a complete response or to be content with palliation. A complete, that is radical, response is sought when the HCC is single, free from intrahepatic metastases or portal infiltration, or when it is multinodular but apparently only midly aggressive. In such cases, if on checking for efficacy, neoplastic tissue is found to be still present, further sessions will follow until necrosis is complete. On the other hand, if the HCC presentation precludes radicality, the goal may be partial necrosis, that is, substantial enough to halt further growth for a time, and this sometimes lasts longer than expected. Another guideline for the total volume to inject is calculated according to the following equation, proposed by

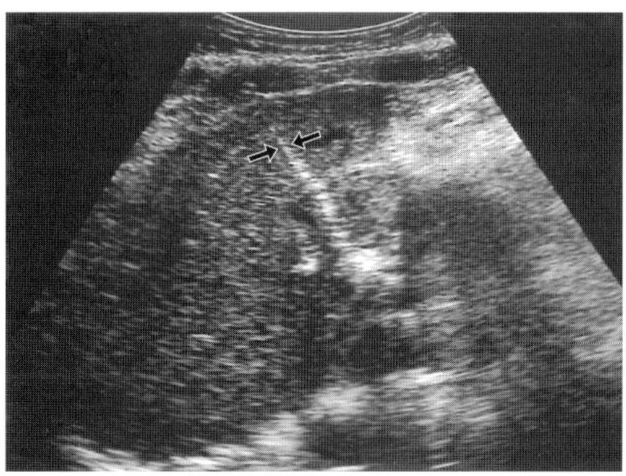

Figure 25.3 – A reflux of ethanol is seen as a hyperechogenic line along the needle path; in this case, withdrawal was stopped (arrows show the needle tip) and resumed a few seconds later, reducing possible pain.

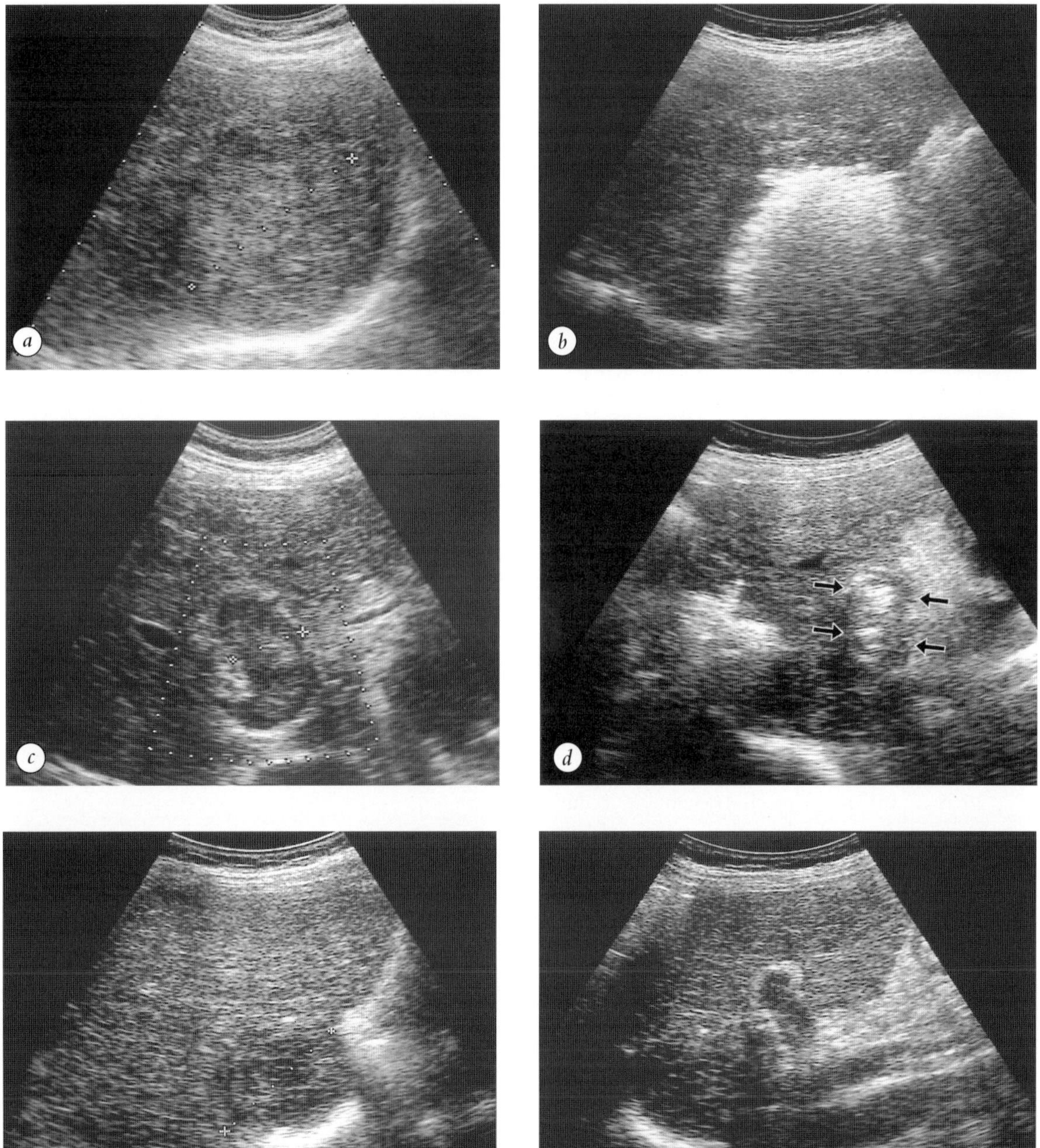

Figure 25.4 –

a) Subcostal sonogram showing a lesion, 6.7 cm in size, located in segment VIII, before "single session" PEI.

b) At the end of the treament (75 ml by 14 injections) the lesion appeared entirely hyperechogic and no significant leakage of ethanol was apparent outside the tumor. Although the perfusion of the tumor was considered total, the volume of ethanol injected was smaller than that of lesion.

c) In the same patient a neoplastic portal lobar thrombosis was present (markers).

d) During the "single session" procedure the thrombus also was treated with alcohol (arrows).

e,f) Clearly, in this case, the goal of PEI was only palliative. However, after one year, lesion *(e)* reduced in size (cm 5.3) and thrombus shrank *(f)*. The level of AFP decreased from 1380 to 6 ng/ml.

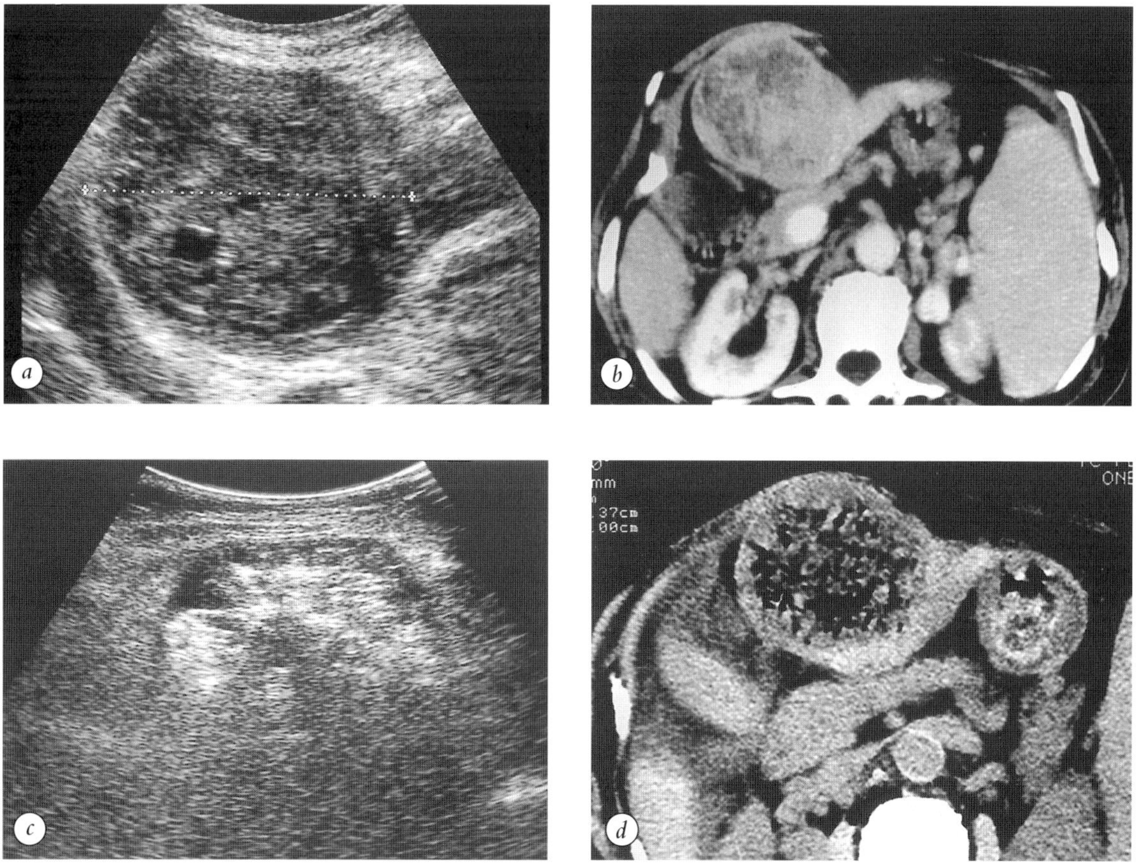

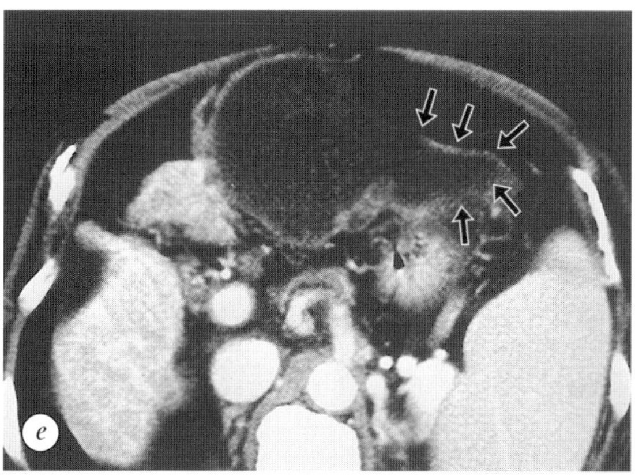

Figure 25.5 –

a,b) Transverse sonogram *a)* and CT *b)* showing lesion, 8.2 cm in size, superficially located at left lobe, before "single session" PEI.

c,d) Two days after treatment, a large amount of gas, recognizable on sonogram as hyperechogenic spots *c),* and on CT as high hypodense areas *d),* was present inside the lesion. Gas formation is due to necrotic changes and causes hyperpirexia.

e) One month after treatment, lesion appeared completely hypodense and devoid of enhancement, because of vascular occlusion. On imaging, a complete response was achievied. In this case also necrosis of the remnant non neoplastic tissue of the same segment occurred (arrows), causing epigastric pain lasting for one week.

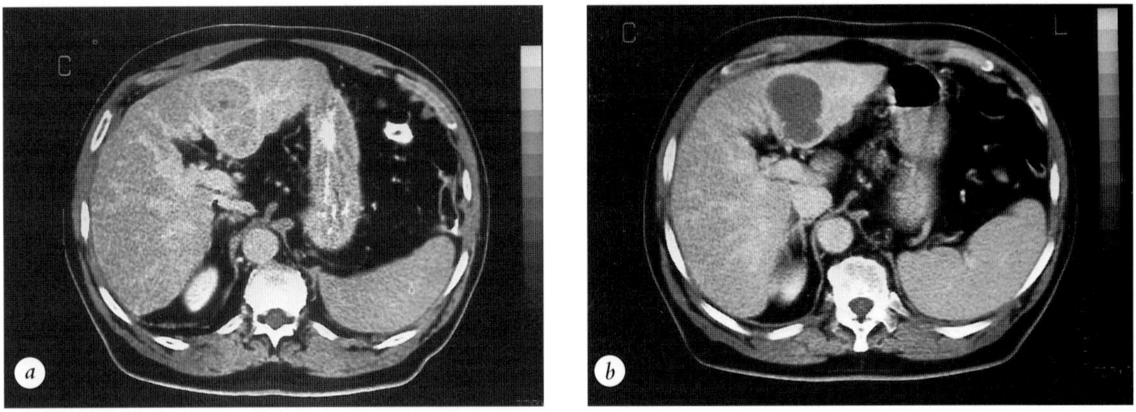

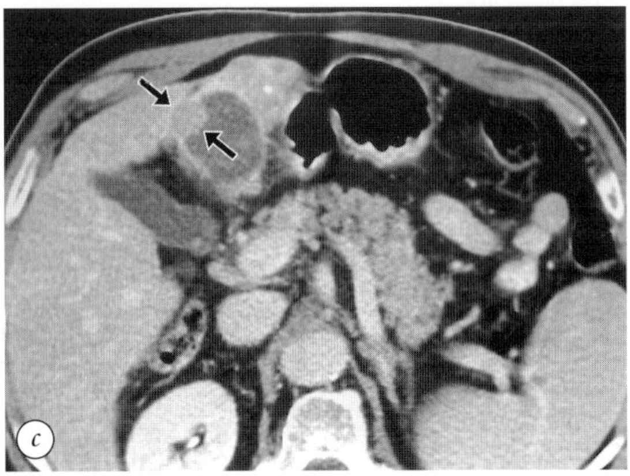

Figure 25.6 –

a) Lesion, 5.5 cm in size, located in left lobe, before "single session" PEI.

b) After six months no areas of enhancement were detectable inside the lesion, so the response was considered apparently complete.

c) After one year a small enhanced area due to local recurrence appeared at the periphery of the lesion (arrows).

Shiina *et al*: $V=4/3\pi(r+0.5)^3$ where V is the total volume of injected alcohol in milliliters and r is the radius of the tumors in centimeters.[12] The addition of 0.5 is intended to provide a safety margin, as it is assumed that some tissue surrounding the lesion should be destroyed to complete tumor necrosis. However, in our experience after "single session" PEI, a complete response was always obtained with a volume of ethanol smaller than that of the lesion, probably because the damage due to vessel thrombosis is greater than that obtained by intracellular diffusion, and the former needs less ethanol.

Because one of the shortcomings of multisession PEI, particularly in larger lesions in which the ethanol may be distributed unevenly, is that many sessions are necessary to complete the treatment, some modifications of the traditional technique have been introduced recently in order to shorten the treatment period or to extend the indications to more numerous and larger lesions. To ensure more homogeneous distribution of ethanol in the same session, Shiina *et al* inserted two or three needles at different sites before injection.[13] Using CT guidance, Redvanly *et al* increased the injected volume up to 40 ml per session for lesions larger than 3 cm in diameter.[14]

"Single session" treatment

"Single session" treatment is given under general anesthesia, endotracheal intubation and mechanical ventilation, since no limit is set on the volume of ethanol to be administered.[9] This technique suits operative requirement, i.e. it is possible to allow a period of controlled apnea or respiratory standstill with partial pulmonary inflation, if necessary. During the procedure patients receive fructose 1.6 diphosphate 1500 mg and gluthation 1200 mg by IV drip with the aim of reducing the systemic effects of alcohol by quickening its metabolism.

Care is taken to inject first the deepest portion of the lesion, then the central and lastly the superficial portions, the aim being to prevent any initial superficial spillage of ethanol from spoiling the view for subsequent injections. Care is also taken to avoid direct injection of ethanol into the hepatic veins, because too high and too sudden a concentration of ethanol in the blood could lead to prolonged hypoxemia with cardiopulmonary collapse.

Treatment ends when the tumor appears entirely hyperechogenic on the monitor (Fig. 25.4a,b,e). The time needed for the PEI procedure ranges from 20 to 50 minutes, depending on the number and size of the lesions. Up to now, the largest total quantity of ethanol injected has been 190 ml with 21 injections in a single tumor 14 cm in diameter. Gas is usually present in the lesion on the days immediately after PEI, particularly when a large amount of ethanol has been injected (Fig. 25.5a,d). As some complications do occur, caution is needed in patients with preexisting risk conditions.

Treatment of portal thrombosis

Treatment of neoplastic portal thrombosis is also possible even if only with palliative purpose[15] (Fig. 25.4c,d,f). Ethanol injection is generally performed when the thrombus is located segmentally or subsegmentally, with the aim of stopping its progression along the vessel to the main branches. A one-holed needle is precisely positioned in the thrombus and the alcohol usually diffuses selectively along it. Alcohol 1 to 2 ml is injected per session. In one patient who later received OLT, the segmental thrombus was completely necrotized. On the microscopic sections the neoplastic tissue and the layer of endothelial cells of the wall presented coagulative necrosis, whereas the muscular tunics were intact.

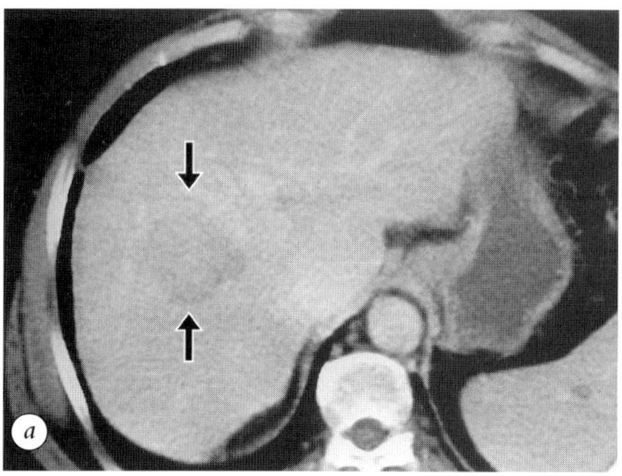

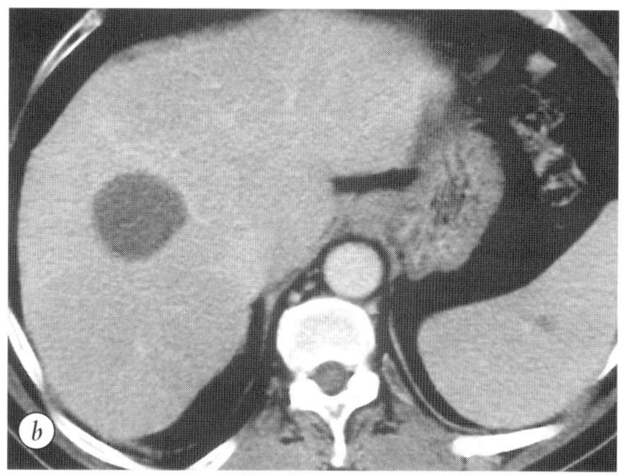

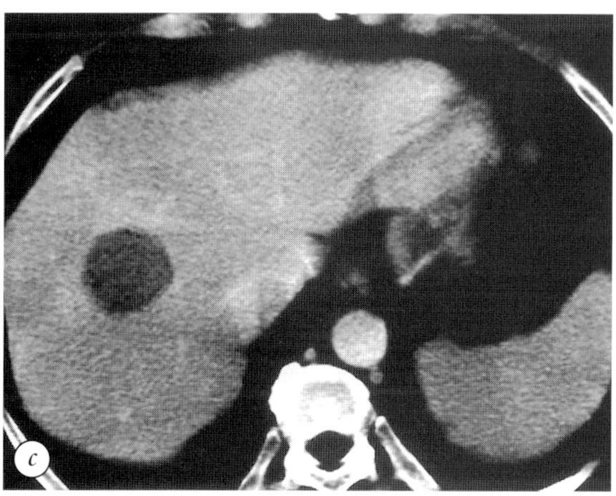

Figure 25.7 –

a) Lesion 4.4 cm in size located at the center of right lobe (arrows) before multi-session conventional PEI (8 sessions).

b) After one month, lesion appeared totally devoid of vascular supply because no areas of enhancement was recognizable and the response was considered apparently complete.

c) After 3 years, the complete response was confirmed.

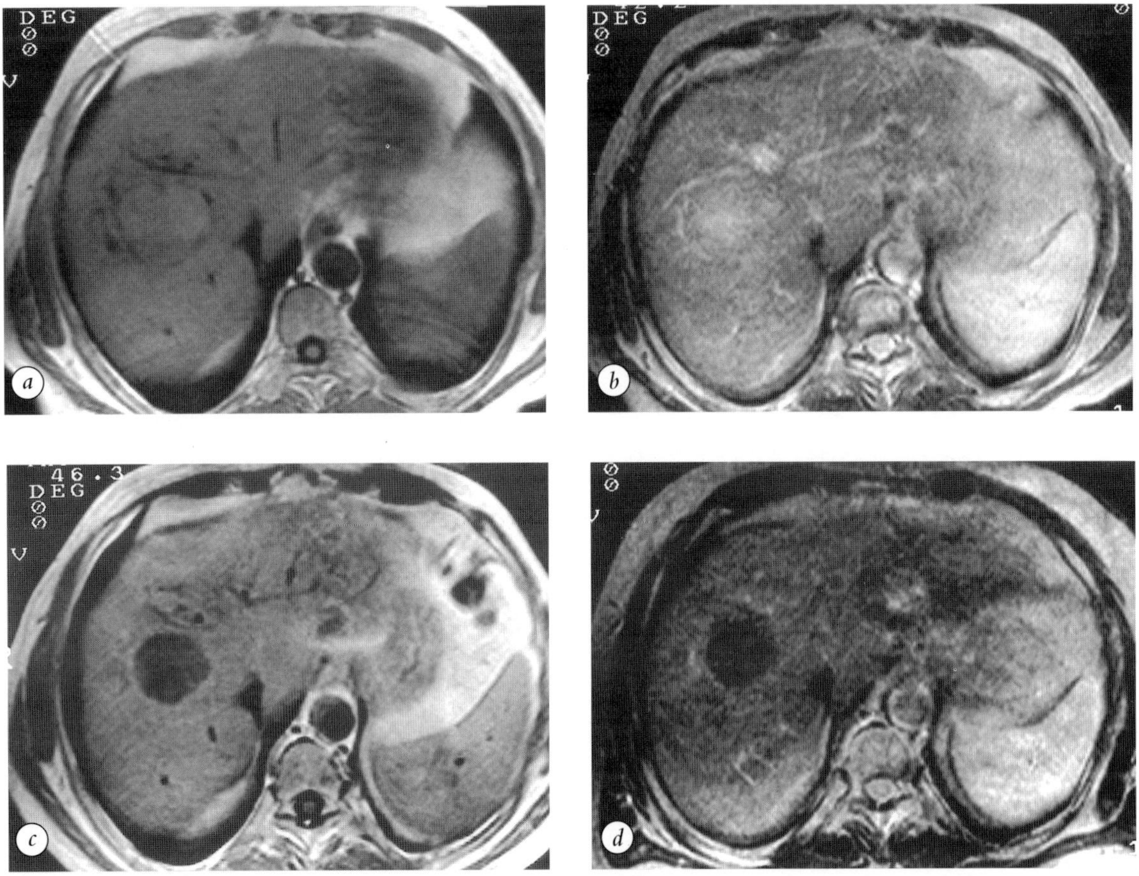

Figure 25.8 – Same case showed in Fig. 25.7, studied by MR.

a) Before PEI, lesion resulted isointense in T1-weighted scan, surrounded by a thin hyperintense halo.

b) In contrast enhanced T2 scan, lesion appeared lightly hyperintense .

c,d) After PEI, lesion became completely hypointense because it was devoid of vascular supply, confirming the CT pattern.

EVALUATION OF THERAPEUTIC EFFICACY

Short-term efficacy of PEI may be checked by percutaneous needle biopsy, imaging modalities and dosage of serum tumor markers.

Biopsy

Biopsy is performed with 21-22 gauge cutting needles, usually with two or three passes, care being taken to sample especially the peripheral areas. In our series it was always done at the beginning of PEI to study tissue and imaging changes in unresected lesions. Now we use needle biopsy only when imaging techniques are not sufficiently exhaustive, although false negatives are possible.

Imaging modalities

A combination of imaging techniques is used to evaluate the therapeutic response, i.e. to determine whether the tumor is completely necrotic or whether any neoplastic tissue persists (Figs. 25.4-10). These examinations are the same as those used for the initial workup and during the follow-up. They may include US, CT, MR and angiography. Patients are evaluated 1 month after PEI and then every 4-6 months. Because the examinations are many and some of them comparable, we do not do them all preferring to use routinely US and CT, and resort to the others or to biopsy only in case of doubt between complete and partial response. If, as is to be expected, the viable areas are very small and beyond present powers of resolution, they do not appear on imaging at the end

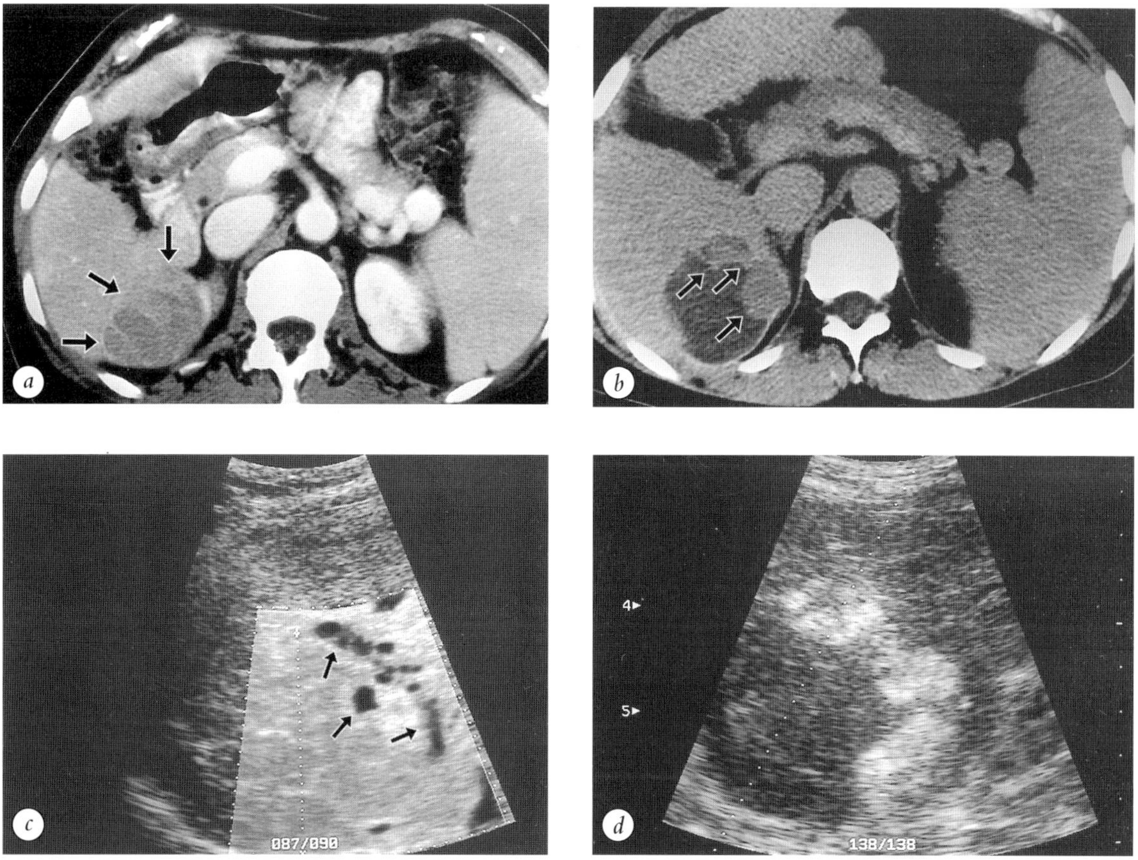

Figure 25.9 –

a) Lesion 6.7 cm in size located in right lobe (arrows), before "single session" PEI.

b) After one month persistence of enhanced areas was present at the periphery of the lesion (arrows).

c) Gray-power-Doppler scan (Idea, Esaote Biomedical, Italy) easily showed a rich vascularization (in black, arrows) inside the neoplastic areas.

d) Some sessions of conventional PEI were subsequently performed, using gray-power-Doppler for centering the target not easily recognizable by plain ultrasound. Ethanol spreaded selectively following the hypervascularized tissue.

of treatment, but become easily detectable on subsequent examinations because of the volume increase and/or the appearance of CT-enhanced areas.

We rate the imaging response complete when the CT scans show total disappearance of areas of enhancement within the lesion, when this finding is confirmed in the follow-up scans, and when the CT and US scans show no increase in tumor size. No enhancement means absence of a blood supply due to necrotic and fibrotic changes. The density after contrast medium of these changes generally ranges from 15 to 45 HU. Because these changes take up room, even when the response is complete, the lesions show only a small decrease in size. CT is performed with dynamic technique: 60 ml bolus (4 ml/s) followed by a rapid infusion (0.7 ml/s) of 80-130 ml depending on body weight. Two scans are done: the first begins 1 minute after the start of contrast administration and the second 15 minutes later. 1-cm thick sections are imaged and additional 5-mm sections when more precise details are needed. On US scans, all lesions show changes in their pattern, usually from hypoechogenicity to iso- or hyperechogenicity, and from iso- or hyperechogenicity to a marbled appearance; however US is not sufficiently reliable for recognizing areas that have remained viable.

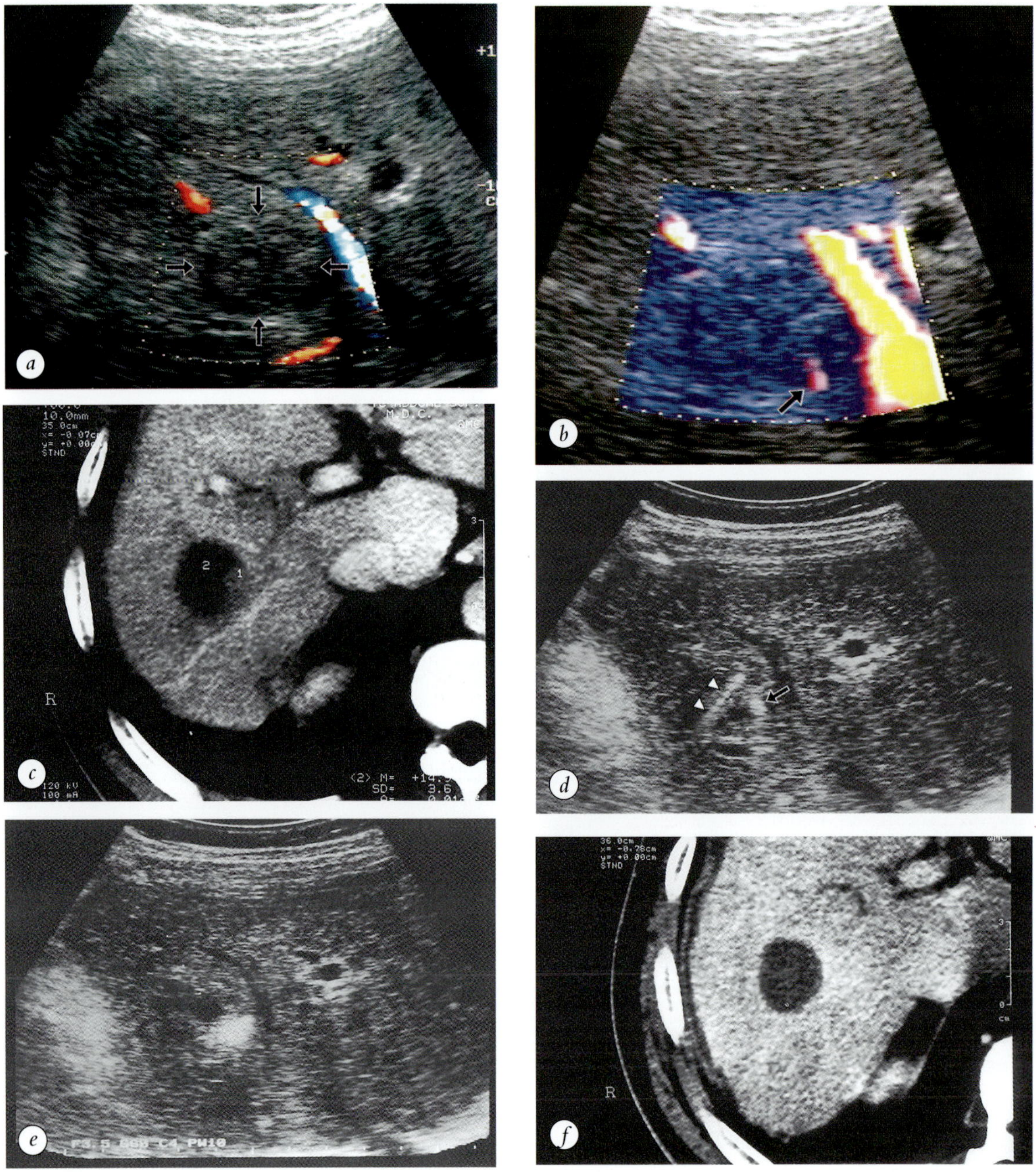

Figure 25.10 –

a) Single lesion 4.4 cm in size in right lobe (arrows) studied by color-Doppler after 7 sessions of PEI. No signals of vascularization (present at the baseline) were recognizable inside.

b) Power-Doppler was able to detect a small signal of vascularization at the periphery of the lesion (arrow).

c) In the same site CT confirmed a small area of enhanced viable tissue (mark 1). Density of this area was 54HU, while density of remnant necrotic area (mark 2) was 14 HU; on plain CT, density of all the lesion ranged from 12 to 19HU.

d) Following the indication supplied by power-Doppler, an additional treatment of PEI was performed, positioning the needle into the vascularized area (arrow). Arrow heads show needle artifact.

e) Immediately after the injection, the target was selectivley perfused by alcohol.

f) After 1-year, CT examination showed the complete disappearance of the enhanced viable tissue.

Color Doppler US is useful in the assessment of therapeutic efficacy, demonstrating residual arterial flow within the tumor.[16] Portions of the tumor in which Doppler signals are detected after PEI correspond to the enhancing areas seen on CT or MR scans. However, color Doppler should not be used as the final diagnostic test for establishing the outcome of PEI, because it does not detect the vascularization of small tumoral areas and because bolus-CT is more sensitive. Color Doppler is good enough for monitoring the response during the course of PEI treatment, because as long as the signals are still recognizable within the tumor further treatments should be administered, since the presence of residual tumor can be confidently assumed. But when no color Doppler signals are found after PEI, further evaluation with CT (or MR) imaging is still necessary to rule out false-negative diagnosis. Power Doppler is anyway more sensitive than color Doppler and color Doppler with echo-enchancers is more sensitive than power Doppler.

Both procedures are used during the follow-up for detecting the appearance of new lesions or local recurrences; US is better for the former and CT for the latter; however, more recently, spiral CT has increased the detection rate of conventional CT.

On MR imaging, HCC is usually isointense in T1- and hyperintense in T2-weighted scans; necrotic tissue shows low signal intensity on T2-images, whereas viable tissue remains hyperintense.[17] Contrast-enhanced T1-images are more accurate than unenhanced images.[18,19]

Angiography is not widely recommended because it is invasive and therefore not often repeatable; however, angiography is reliable for evaluating the efficacy of PEI, because the tumor stain disappears.

Tumor markers

Assay for tumor markers is done before, 1 month after PEI and every 4 months thereafter. AFP is the marker most commonly used, but this assay is useful only if AFP is initially elevated (>200 mg/ml) and normalizes after PEI. In reality, particularly when HCC is small (<5 cm), AFP is not elevated in 60-70% of cases.[20,21] When the imaging modalities show a complete response not followed by a large decrease in AFP levels, some undetected or not yet detectable neoplastic tissue is growing elsewhere. Moreover, an increase in AFP levels during the follow-up suggests a recurrent disease or new lesions.

Relatively new tumor markers are DCP and alpha-L-fucosidase. According to some studies assays for DCP and AFP combined are more sensitive than AFP alone both to HCC detection[22] and to tumor recurrence after surgery.[23] DCP may therefore be useful in the evaluation of the therapeutic efficacy of PEI. Alpha-L-fucosidase seems less closely correlated with tumor size than AFP.[24] We recently decided to determine the baseline values of all three markers, using only the elevated ones.

SIDE EFFECTS AND COMPLICATIONS

Multisession treatment

Most patients complain of mild pain during or immediately after the injection, but as a rule tolerate it and carry on their normal life. In our series no patients discontinued the treatment. Usually pain is confined to the injection site, but sometimes it is felt in the right shoulder or at the epigastric level. In our department, patients experiencing severe pain after the first session receive analgesics before subsequent sessions; about 1 patient in 20 needs analgesic drugs. Some authors prefer to inject a few milliliters of xylocaine before withdrawing the needle. Some cases of mild alcohol intoxication occurred in Asian patients. After the first sessions, when the necrosis of neoplastic tissue is greatest, patients may complain of fever, which lasts several days. Serum transaminases show no alteration or a mild and transient rise, sometimes accompanied by ascites. In a few patients, a limited chemical thrombosis in the tributary portal branch develops secondary to the ethanol injury, spontaneously disappearing within 1-2 months. None of these side effects requires treatment.

Among 1,623 patients collected by various authors, none died.[13,14,25-41] There has been an anedoctal report of one death due to a massive area of hepatic necrosis distant from the injection site and to myocardial infarction; however, no direct relation between PEI and myocardial infarction was demonstrated in this case.[42]

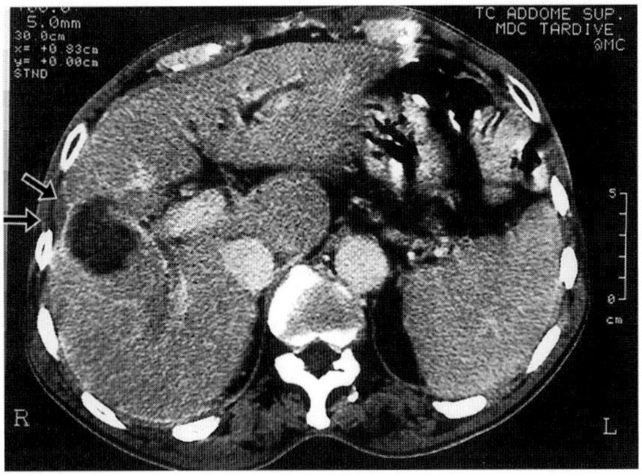

Figure 25.11 – Mild atrophy, manifested as concavity of the liver surface (arrows), was recognizable during follow-up.

Major complications are rare, ranging from 1.3 to 2.4%, and usually are treated conservatively. Complications that have been reported, in the above mentioned series or in case reports, include intraperitoneal hemorrhage, right pleural effusion, cholangitis or jaundice secondary to injury of bile ducts, liver abscess, hepatic infarction probably related to reflux of ethanol into portal vein branches, hemobilia, arterioportal shunt, shock.[43-45] With regard to neoplastic seeding along the needle track, only a few cases are reported, probably because the reflux of alcohol prevents this from happening.[46-51] Mild atrophy, manifested as concavity of the liver surface, or even segmental atrophy, can be detected with CT, particularly using arterial portography technique (Fig. 25.11), or MR. This change is due to a decreased portal blood flow, caused by organized thrombi, in the noncancerous liver parenchyma that surrounds the tumor being treated.[38,41]

"Single session" treatment

With larger volumes of ethanol per treatment session the complication rate increases. Some cases of alcohol intoxication are observed, but do not require treatment. The highest blood alcohol levels found immediately after treatment were 230 mg/100 ml, returning to normal within 24 hours. Abdominal pain is usually observed, lasting for 2-3 days. Hyperpyrexia always develops in patients who receive more than 50 ml of alcohol. Some transient and variable changes in transaminase, bilirubin, D-dimer, blood cells, platelets, hemoglobin, fibrinogen and haptoglobin are observed. These changes are due to hepatic necrosis, hemolysis and localized thrombosis. In our series of 111 treatments, one Child's C class patient died of hemorrhage from esophageal varices. Major complications included one hemorrhage requiring transfusion in a large superficially located tumor, one important liver decompensation in a Child's B class patient, one transient renal failure requiring some hemodialytic treatments and two chemical infarctions of a segment adjacent to the tumor, accompained by pain lasting for some days; minor complications included some modest hemorrhages and some transient liver decompensations.

The mortality was thus 0.9% and the major complications rate 4.5%.

CONTRAINDICATIONS

Contraindications related to general conditions are advanced cirrhosis or proneness to severe bleeding. We do not perform PEI when prothrombin time is less than 40% and platelets less than 40.000/mm.[3] Ascites is not a contraindication.

Contraindications depending on neoplastic presentation are: extrahepatic diffusion, presence of thrombosis in the main portal branches, large infiltrative (more than 30-35% by hepatic volume) or diffuse HCC. Shiina *et al* treated safely lesions protruding from the surface of the liver or near large vessels, and our experience bears out his claim (Fig. 25.5).[52]

In the presence of some risks such as marked portal and/or pulmonary hypertension, esophageal varices at risk of bleeding, enhanced fibrinolysis, cardiac ischemia and severe disorders of the electric conduction of the myocardium, large and superficial lesions associated with severe coagulation disorders, chronic renal failure, "single session" technique is contraindicated.

SURVIVAL RATES

Some PEI series include patients with 5-year survival rates.

The Chiba University group treated 112 patients, 93 of them with one, 16 with two and 3 with three lesions, all ≤3 cm in size. The 1,3,5-year survival rates were 96, 72, 51% for 60 Child's A patients, 90, 72,

48% for 33 Child's B patients, and 94, 25, 0% for 19 Child's C patients.[27]

Shiina treated 50 patients, with single or multiple lesions, ranging from 1.2 to 6.0 cm. The 1,3,5-year survival rates were 87, 62, 43%. Comparison of Child's A vs. Child's C ($p<0.0001$), size ≤3 cm vs. ≥4 cm ($p<0.0002$) and number ≤3 vs. ≥4 ($p<0.02$) yielded a significant difference.[53]

Tanikawa treated 217 patients, with lesions ≤3cm. The 1,3,5-year survival rates were 95, 73, 48%. In this series, the 5-year survival for Child's A patients only was 85%.[26]

We collected data for 746 patients treated by various Italian centers.[39] In patients with Child's A (n=293), B (n=149), or C (n=20) cirrhosis and single HCC 5 cm or smaller, the 1,3,5-year survival rates were 98, 79, 47%, 93, 63, 29%, and 64, 12, 0%, respectively. In patients with Child's A cirrhosis, the rates were 94, 68, 36% for multiple HCC (n=121), 85, 53, 30% for single HCC larger than 5 cm (n=28), and 90, 16, 0% for advanced HCC (n=16) (Fig. 25.12).

In our study, the high survival rate in patients with HCC > 5 cm should be accepted with caution both because of the small number of cases studied and because of a possible selection bias due to stricter enrolment but it is also conceivable that an HCC of this diameter, remaining single, has a less aggressive course. Therefore, it is too early to evaluate the survival of patients treated by the "single-session" treatment. In any case, most encapsulated lesions presented complete necrosis (up to 8.2 cm) or 80-90% necrosis, and infiltrating lesions 60-80% necrosis.

Advanced HCC, as expected, presented by far the worst prognosis; interestingly, the 16% 3-year survival rate is identical to that in the "mass reduction group" of Shiina *et al.*[13] The amount of necrosis obtained and the frequent lowering or even normalization of the baseline AFP point to an improvement in the prognosis (Fig. 25.4).

The main cause of death among Child's A patients was progression of HCC due to the appearance of new lesions, whereas among Child's C patients it was hepatic failure.

The 5-year new lesions rate reported by the Chiba group was 87%, by Shiina *et al* 64%, and by Tanikawa *et al.* nearly 100%. In our study it was 83%, 74% in patients with single HCC and 98% in patients with multiple HCC.

Local recurrence, i.e. increase in size or onset of enhanced areas inside the lesion treated by PEI, was 4% in Ebara *et al.*'s (in lesions <3 cm),[54] 7% in Shiina *et al.*'s (in lesions <4-5 cm) and 17% in our series (in lesions <5 cm). Many recurrences were treated again with PEI.

CONCLUSION

The rationale for using PEI includes the following:

1) Expanding form of HCC initially shows a regional growth, so a local therapy such as PEI may be applied.

2) US screening of cirrhotic populations allows detection of HCC at its initial stage, when the tumor size is small. In a study by Oka *et al*, 82% of the patients had HCC of less than 5 cm when the tumor was detected by US screening.[55]

3) Ethanol shows selective diffusion in HCC, because of its softer consistency and hypervascularity.

4) PEI carries no risk of loss or of important damage to the remaining parenchyma. In the days following treatment there may be a transient rise in transaminase levels but histologic examination has not shown important damage to healthy tissue at a distance from the treated lesion.[56] Whether the loss of healthy tissue due to multisegmental resection or the damage to the parenchyma involved in conventional TACE leads to a deterioration of liver function and a hastening of terminal failure is not established but is probable.[57,58]

5) PEI is safe. In the series published to date comprising 1,623 patients there was one fatality (0.06%) and the highest complication rate was 2.4%, most of the complications being treated conservatively. Near zero mortality for conventional PEI is in sharp contrast to the mortality for surgery which, although much lower than it used to be, is nonetheless a factor to be reckoned with, especially in centers with little experience. The most authoritative reports put mortality at 1.4% to 11% and the complication rate at up to 58%.[59-70] In this context it should be remembered that patients selected by US screening are symptom-free and even if not treated can expect to live for over a year.[71,72]

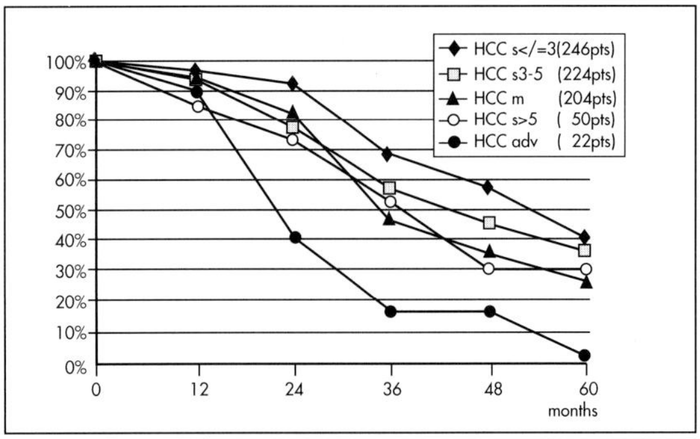

Months	0		12		24		36		48		60	
Stage HCC	% Cum. Survival	Pts	% Cum. Survival	Pts	%Cum. Survival	Pts	% Cum. Survival	Pts	% Cum. Survival	Pts	% Cum. Survival	Pts
s</=3	100	246	97	222	92	154	68	56	57	32	40	13
s3-5	100	224	94	197	77	126	57	57	45	30	37	12
m	100	204	94	170	82	117	47	40	36	17	26	9
s>5	100	50	85	38	73	26	53	11	30	3	30	3
adv	100	22	90	18	40	5	16	2	16	1	0	0

a

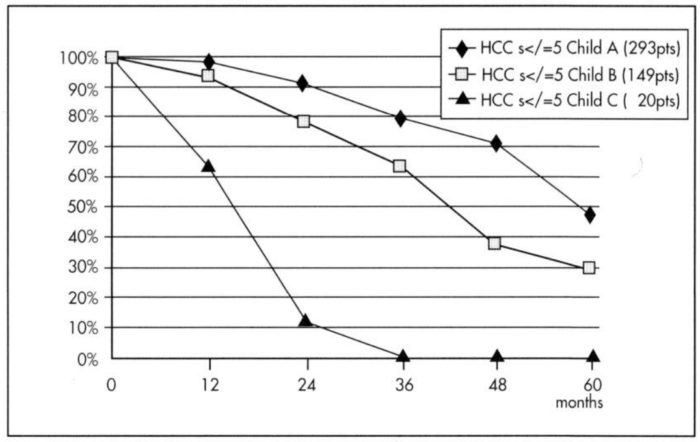

Months	0		12		24		36		48		60	
Stage HCC -Child	% Cum. Survival	Pts	% Cum. Survival	Pts	%Cum. Survival	Pts	% Cum. Survival	Pts	% Cum. Survival	Pts	% Cum. Survival	Pts
s</=5- Child A	100	293	98	260	91	179	79	117	70	77	47	20
s</=5- Child B	100	149	93	125	78	75	63	40	37	12	29	5
s</=5- Child B	100	20	64	12	12	1	0	0	0	0	0	0

b

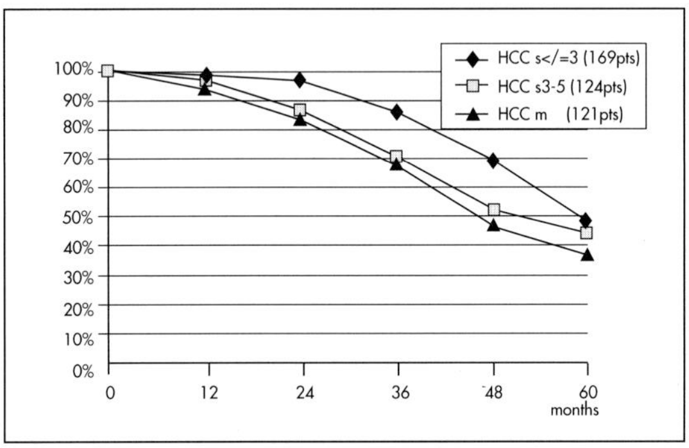

Months	0		12		24		36		48		60	
Stage HCC -Child	% Cum. Survival	Pts	% Cum. Survival	Pts	%Cum. Survival	Pts	% Cum. Survival	Pts	% Cum. Survival	Pts	% Cum. Survival	Pts
s</=3 - Child A	100	169	99	151	96	104	86	69	69	29	48	11
s 3-5 - Child B	100	124	97	109	86	75	70	50	51	20	44	9
m - Child B	100	121	94	101	83	67	68	41	46	16	360	9

c

Figure 25.12 –

a) Five-year cumulative survival curves stratified to HCC stage.

b) Five-year cumulative survival curves for patients with single HCC ≤5 cm in diameter stratified according to Child class.

c) Five-year cumulative survival curves for patients with Child A cirrhosis with single HCC <3 cm, single HCC 3-5 cm and multiple (up to 3 lesions) HCC.

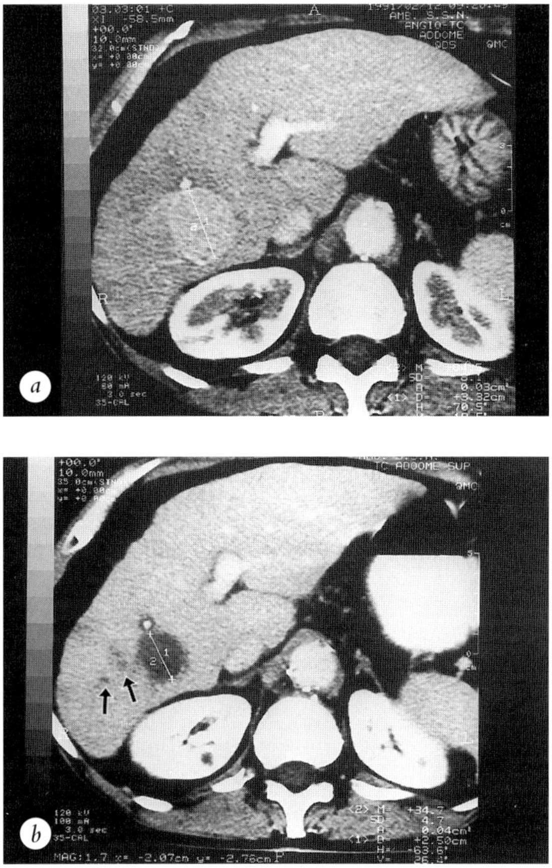

Figure 25.13 –

a) Lesion 3.3 cm in size before conventional PEI (6 sessions).

b) Six months after treatment, lesion reduced in size (2.5 cm) and was devoid of enhancement. However, small satellite lesions (arrows) appeared around the main lesion, probably present before treatment but not detectable.

6) PEI can easily be repeated when new lesions appear, as they do in the majority of patients followed for 5 years. The new lesion rate in the surgical series ranges from 67 to 100%,[50-70,73] in the PEI series from 64% to 100%. This fact, which has to be borne in mind in any evaluation of treatment, arises from the multifocal nature of HCC in cirrhotics.[73-76] It means that the first lesion to show up on the US scan usually is only the prelude to others and that surgery, even if it acts radically on the resected lesion, is usually only palliative not affecting the natural course of the disease. At Chiba University, the new lesion rate of two comparable groups of patients treated by surgery and PEI was the same.[27] As this reflects the natural history of the disease, the patient must be watched closely so that new lesions may be treated as and when they occur and are still small. With regard to this an advantage of PEI is that the patient is attended by the same operator both for diagnosis and treatment. Moreover, it is now possible to curb the course of the disease by "single-session" PEI even in some patients who could no longer be followed by conventional PEI.

7) PEI is a reproducible procedure, as shown by the results of different series, which were equivalent in terms of safety and survival.

8) The low cost, the accessibility of the necessary materials and the easy technique render PEI applicable everywhere, hence many, even outlying, hospitals can offer PEI without need for referral. Patients are treated in the outpatient clinic and many of them can carry on their normal life. An ordinary US scanner is sufficient. The material (needle, syringe, alcohol) costs little and is readily available. In Italy the cost is approximately $1,000 compared with $125,000 for OLT and $30,000 for liver resection.[39] In Japan, Kotoh reported an average cost of $759 for PEI (in out-patient department) and $27,105 for resection.[28] Since the number of patients per year contracting this disease in Japan is about 20,000[77] and in Italy 12,000,[78] cost can hardly be a secondary consideration.

9) Local therapeutic efficacy of PEI is high. Histopathologic examinations after surgical resection were specially carried out during the early stages of PEI development. Of the 37 lesions reported by different authors, ranging in size from 1.0 to 4.5 cm, 73% showed complete necrosis and the remainder showed more than 90% necrosis.[39] In our experience, six out of eight lesions (75%) presented a complete necrosis and the remainder approximately 90% necrosis. In a study designed to evaluate this, Shiina *et al*. demonstrated complete necrosis in 16 of 23 lesions (69.5%), 90% necrosis in six lesions and 70% necrosis in the remaining lesion.[56] Their histopathologic examination showed that the capsule and some of the surrounding tissue as well as the tumor itself had degenerated. Seeding of the cancer cells along the needle tracks was not encountered. In cases of incomplete necrosis, viable tissue remained in small nodules around the main lesion, along the edge of the lesion or in portions isolated by septa (Fig. 25.13).

10) Long-term results for PEI are fairly high. The overall 5-year survival rate in 628 patients with lesions ≤5 cm and compensated cirrhosis was 48%.[39]

There are no controlled studies of PEI *vs* no treatment but the same goes for surgery too. Nonetheless, as it has been clear from the start that PEI is effective and safe, a no-treatment arm has been considered unethical. Thus comparisons with no treatment are based on historical data. Of the two studies of untreated patients with comparable disease one presented a 5-year survival rate of 0% in 27 cases and the other 11% in 73 patients. [71,72]

In conclusion, the large number of patients enrolled in US screening programs has created a large demand for effective, safe, repeatable, low-cost treatment that can be offered at many centers. PEI substantially meets all these requirements. In the absence of randomized studies, on the strength of the results reported to date, PEI is indicated as treatment of choice for the majority of patients recruited by US screening, excluding candidates for OLT and for surgical resection. Regarding indications for surgery, recently the Liver Cancer Study Group of Japan has established predictive factors for prognosis.[79] By multivariate analysis the most predictive variables were in descending order: AFP levels, tumor size, number of tumors, age, stage of cirrhosis, surgical curability and portal involvement and, by univariate analysis, capsular infiltration , anatomical extent of the tumor and Edmondson-Steiner's classification. These values are of predictive significance for PEI too as has been demonstrated in the large studies.[13,26,39,40,54] But while surgery carries some peroperative mortality and morbility, which means that selection has to be tight in order to eliminate all factors that may adversely affect the prognosis, PEI is rarely accompanied by complications and so selection can be less rigid.

In practice, most patients should be managed as follows: early detection of HCC by US screening, treatment by PEI, follow-up by imaging and tumor markers, treatment by PEI of any new lesions.

REFERENCES

1. Burgener FA, Steinmetz SD. Treatment of experimental adenocarcinomas by percutaneous intratumoral injection of absolute ethanol. *Invest Radiol* 1986; **22**: 472-478
2. Kawano M. An experimental study of percutaneous absolute ethanol injection therapy for small hepatocellular carcinoma: effects of absolute ethanol on the healthy canine liver. *Gastroenterol Jpn* 1989; **24**: 663-669
3. Festi D, Monti F, Casanova S, *et al*. Morphological and biochemical effects of intrahepatic alcohol injection in the rabbit. *J Gastroenterol Hepatol* 1990; **5**: 402-406
4. Livraghi T, Festi D, Monti F, Salmi A, Vettori C. US-guided percutaneous alcohol injection of small hepatic and abdominal tumors. *Radiology* 1986; **161**:309-312
5. Solbiati L, Giangrande A, De Pra L, Bellotti E, Cantù P, Ravetto C. Percutaneous ethanol injection of parathyroid tumors under US guidance: treatment for secondary hyperparathyroidism. *Radiology* 1985; **155**: 607-610
6. Livraghi T, Baietta E, Matricardi L, Villa E, Lovati R, Vettori C. Fine needle percutaneous intratumoral chemotherapy under US guidance. *Tumori* 1986; **72**: 81-87
7. Redvanly RD, Chezmar JL. Percutaneous ethanol ablation therapy of malignant hepatic tumors using CT guidance. *Sem Interv Radiol* 1993; **10**:82-87
8. Lee MJ, Mueller PR, Dawson SL, *et al*. Percutaneous ethanol injection for the treatment of hepatic tumors: indications, mechanism of action, technique, and efficacy. *AJR* 1995; **164**: 215-220
9. Livraghi T,Vettori C, Torzilli G, Lazzaroni S, Pellicanò S, Ravasi S. Percutaneous ethanol injection of hepatic tumors: single-session therapy under general anesthesia. *AJR* 1993; **160**:1065-1069
10. Livraghi T, Sangalli G, Vettori C. Adenomatous hyperplastic nodules in the cirrhotic liver: a therapeutic approach. *Radiology* 1989; **170**:155-157
11. Livraghi T, Lazzaroni S, Meloni F, Torzilli G, Vettori C. Intralesional ethanol in the treatment of unresectable liver cancer. *World J Surg* 1995; **19**: 801-806
12. Shiina S, Tagawa K, Unuma T *et al*. Percutaneous ethanol injection therapy of hepatocellular carcinoma: analysis of 77 patients. *AJR* 1990; **155**:1221-1226
13. Shiina S, Niwa Y. Percutaneous ethanol injection therapy in the treatment of liver neoplasms. In: Howard E,ed. *Current techniques in interventional radiology*. Philadelphia: Cope C. 1994: 3.1-3.14
14. Redvanly RD, Chezmar JL, Strauss RM, Galloway JR, Boyer TD, Bernardino ME. Malignant hepatic tumors: safety of high-dose percutaneous ethanol ablation therapy. *Radiology* 1993; **188**:283-285
15. Livraghi T, Grigioni W, Mazziotti A, Sangalli G, Vettori C. Percutaneous ethanol injection of portal thrombosis in hepatocellular carcinoma: a new possible treatment. *Tumori* 1990; **76**:394-397
16. Lencioni R, Caramella D, Bartolozzi C. Hepatocellular carcinoma: use of color-Doppler US to evaluate response to treatment with percutaneous ethanol injection. *Radiology* 1995; **194:**113-118
17. Sironi S, Livraghi T, Del Maschio A. Small hepatocellular carcinoma treated with percutaneous ethanol injection: MR imaging findings. *Radiology* 1991; **180**:336-336
18. Bartolozzi C, Lencioni R, Caramella D, Mazzeo S, Ciancia EM Treatment of hepatocellular carcinoma with percutaneous ethanol injection: evaluation with contrast-enhanced MR imaging. *AJR* 1994; **162**: 827-832

19. Sironi S, De Cobelli F, Livraghi T *et al*. Small hepatocellular carcinoma with percutaneous ethanol injection: unenhanced and gadolinium-enhanced MR imaging follow-up. *Radiology* 1994; **192**: 407-412

20. Chen DS, Sung JL, Sheu JC *et al*. Serum α-fetoprotein in the early stage of human hepatocellular carcinoma. *Gastroenterology* 1984; **86**:1404-1409

21. Livraghi T, Sangalli G, Giordano F *et al*. 240 hepatocellular carcinomas: ultrasound features, tumor size, cytologic and histologic patterns, serum alpha-fetoprotein and HBsAg. *Tumori* 1987; **73**:507-512

22. Brunello F, Marcarino C, Pasquero P. The des-g-carboxyprothrombin for the diagnosis of hepatocellular carcinoma. *Ital J Gastroenterol* 1993; **25**: 9-12

23. Weitz IC, Liebman HA. Des-g-carboxy (abnormal) prothrombin and hepatocellular carcinoma: a critical review. *Hepatology* 1993; **18**: 990-997

24. Takahashi H, Saibara T, Iwamura S, *et al*. Serum alpha-L-fucosidase activity and tumor size in hepatocellular carcinoma. *Hepatology* 1194; **19**: 1414-1417

25. Sheu JC, Sung JL, Huang GT *et al*. Intratumor injection of absolute ethanol under ultrasound guidance for the treatment of small hepatocellular carcinoma. *Hepat-Gastroenterol* 1987; **34**:255-261

26. Tanikawa K. Multidisciplinary treatment of hepatocellular carcinoma. In: Tobe T, Kameda H, eds. *Primary liver cancer in Japan*. Tokyo: Springer-Verlag, 1992;327-334

27. Okuda K. Intratumor ethanol injection. *J Surg Oncol* 1993;**3** (suppl):97-99

28. Kotoh K, Sakai H, Sakamoto S *et al*. The effect of percutaneous ethanol injection therapy on small solitary hepatocellular carcinoma is comparable to that of hepatectomy. *Am J Gastroenterol* 1994; **89**:194-198

29. Seki T, Nonaka T, Kubota Y, Mizuno T, Sameshima Y. Ultrasonical guided percutaneous ethanol injection therapy for hepatocellular carcinoma. *Am J Gastroenterol* 1989; **84**:1400-1407

30. Borghetti M, Benelli G, Bonardi R. Trattamento mediante alcolizzazione percutanea ecoguidata di piccoli epatocarcinomi. *Radiol Med* 1991; **81**:502-509

31. Imari Y, Sakamoto S, Shiomichi S, *et al*. Hepatocellular carcinoma not detected with plain US: treatment with percutaneous ethanol injection under guidance with enhanced US. *Radiology* 1992; **185**:497-500

32. Kumada T, Nakano S, Takeda I *et al*. Treatment of small hepatocellular carcinoma. *Cancer Chem Pharmacol* 1992; **31** (suppl):25-29

33. Vilana R, Bruix J, Bru C, Ayuso C, Solé M, Rodés J. Tumor size determines the efficacy of percutaneous ethanol injection for the treatment of small hepatocellular carcinoma. *Hepatology* 1992; **16**:353-357

34. Hisa N, Ohkuma K, Fujikura Y *et al*. Percutaneous ethanol injection therapy for hepatic tumors. Results and technical considerations. *Sem Interv Radiol* 1993; **10**:27-34

35. Solmi L, Muratori R, Bertoni F, Gandolfi L. Echo-guided percutaneous ethanol injection in small hepatocellular carcinoma: personal experience. *Hepato-Gastroenterol* 1993; **40**:505-508

36. Onodera H, Ukai K, Nakano N *et al*. Outcomes of 116 patients with hepatocellular carcinoma. *Cancer Chemother Pharmacol* 1994; **33**:(suppl) 103-108

37. Horiguchi Y, Sekoguchi B, Imai H, *et al*. Treatment of choice for unresectable small liver cancer: percutaneous ethanol injection therapy or transarterial chemoembolization therapy. *Cancer Chemother Pharmacol* 1994; **33**: 111-114

38. Ito K, Honjo K, Fujita T, Awaya H, Matsumoto T, Matsunaga N. Enhanced MR imaging of the liver after ethanol treatment of hepatocellular carcinoma: evaluation of areas of hyperperfusion adjacent to the tumor. *AJR* 1995; **164**: 1413-1417

39. Livraghi T, Giorgio A, Marin G *et al*. Hepatocellular carcinoma and cirrhosis in 746 patients: long-term results of percutaneous ethanol injection. *Radiology* 1995; **197**:101-108

40. Lencioni R, Bartolozzi C, Caramella D *et al*. Treatment of small hepatocellular carcinoma with percutaneous ethanol injection. *Cancer* 1995; **76**: 1737-1746

41. Yoshikawa J, Matsui O, Kadoya M. Hepatocellular carcinoma: CT appearance of parenchymal changes after percutaneous ethanol injection therapy. *Radiology* 1995; **194**: 107-111

42. Taavitsainen M, Vehmas T, Kauppila R. Fatal liver necrosis following percutaneous ethanol injection for hepatocellular carcinoma. *Abdom Imag* 1993; **18**:357-359

43. De Sio I, Castellano L, Calandra M. Hemobilia following percutaneous ethanol injection for hepatocellular carcinoma in a cirrhotic patient. *J Clin Ultrasound* 1992; **20**:621-623

44. Koda M, Okamoto K, Miyoshi Y, Kawasaki H. Hepatic vascular and bile duct injury after ethanol injection therapy for hepatocellular carcinoma. *Gastrointest Radiol* 1992; **17**:167-169

45. Solinas A, Erbella GS, Distrutti E *et al*. Abscess formation in hepatocellular carcinoma: complications of percutaneous ultrasound-guided ethanol injection. *J Clin Ultrasound* 1993; **21**:531-533

46. Cedrone A, Rapaccini GL, Pompili M. Neoplastic seeding complicating percutaneous ethanol injection for treatment of hepatocellular carcinoma. *Radiology* 1992; **183**:787-788

47. Goletti O, De Negri F, Pucciarelli M *et al*. Subcutaneous seeding after percutaneous ethanol injection of liver metastasis. *Radiology* 1992; **183**:785-786

48. Zerbey AL, Mueller PR, Dawson SL, Hoover Jr HC. Pleural seeding from hepatocellular carcinoma: a complication of percutaneous alcohol ablation. *Radiology* 1994; **193**:81-82

49. Boland GW, Lee MJ, Dawson SL, Mueller PR. Percutaneous injection of ethanol in a patient with a solitary hepatocellular carcinoma. *AJR* 1993; **161**: 1071-1077

50. Cardinale L, Castiglione V. Disseminazione neoplastica sottocutanea lungo il tragitto dell'ago. *Radiol Med* 1995; **89**: 557-559

51. Shimada M, Maeda T, Saitoh A, Morotomi I, Kano T. Needle track seeding after percutaneous ethanol injection therapy for small hepatocellular carcinoma. *J Surg Oncol* 1995; **58**: 278-281

52. Shiina S, Tagawa K, Unuma T *et al*. Percutaneous ethanol injection therapy for neoplasm located on the surface of the liver. *AJR* 1990; **155**:507-509

53. Shiina S, Tagawa K, Niwa Y *et al*. Percutaneous ethanol injection therapy for hepatocellular carcinoma: results in 146 patients. *AJR* 1993; **160**:1023-1028

54. Ebara M, Kita K, Sugiura N. Therapeutic effect of percutaneous ethanol injection on small hepatocellular carcinoma: evaluation with CT. *Radiology* 1995; **195**: 371-377

55. Oka H, Kurioka N, Kim K *et al*. Prospective study of early

detection of hepatocellular carcinoma in patients with cirrhosis. *Hepatology* 1990; **12**:680-687

56. Shiina S, Tagawa K, Unuma T *et al*. Percutaneous ethanol injection therapy for hepatocellular carcinoma: a histopathologic study. *Cancer* 1991; **68**:1524-1530
57. Okuda K, Ohtsuki T, Obata H *et al*. Natural history of hepatocellular carcinoma and prognosis in relation to treatment. *Cancer* 1985; **56**:918-928
58. Groupe d'etude et de traitement du carcinome hèpatocellulaire. A comparison of lipiodol chemoembolization and conservative treatment for unresectable hepatocellular carcinoma. *N Engl J Med* 1995; **332**:1256-1261
59. Wu MC, Zhang XH, Chen H. Hepatic resection for primary liver cancer. *Chin Med J* 1986; **99**:175-180
60. Kawano N, Ohmori Y, Inoue O. Long-term prognosis of surgical patients with hepatocellular carcinoma. *Cancer Chem Pharmacol* 1989; **23**(suppl) :129-132.
61. Tang ZY, Yu YQ, Zhou XA. Surgery of small hepatocellular carcinoma. *Cancer* 1989; **64**:536-541
62. Yamanaka N, Okamoto E, Toyosaka. Prognostic factors after hepatectomy for hepatocellular carcinomas. *Cancer* 1990; **65**:1104-1110
63. Lai ECS, Ng IOL, You KT. Hepatic resection for small hepatocellular carcinoma: The Queen Mary Hospital experience. *World J Surg* 1991; **15**:654-659
64. Kanematsu T, Matsumata T, Shirabe K *et al*. A comparative study of hepatic resection and transcatheter arterial embolization for the treatment of primary hepatocellular carcinoma. *Cancer* 1993; **71**:2181-2186
65. Makuuchi M, Kosuge T, Takayama T *et al*. Surgery for small liver cancers. *Sem Surg Oncol* 1993; **9**:298-30
66. Sugioka A, Tsuzuki T, Kanai T. Postresection prognosis of patients with hepatocellular carcinoma. *Surgery* 1993;**113**:612-618
67. Takayasu T, Ino K, Yamaoka Y. Single nodular hepatocellular carcinoma: a clinicopathological study of 80 hepatectomized patients. *J Jpn Soc Cancer Ther* 1993; **28**:976-987
68. Izumi R, Shimizu K, Tohru II *et al*. Prognostic factors of hepatocellular carcinoma in patients undergoing hepatic resection. *Gastroenterology* 1994; **106**:720-727
69. Kawarada Y, Ito F, Sakurai H *et al*. Surgical treatment of hepatocellular carcinoma. *Cancer Chemother Pharmacol* 1994; **33**(suppl) :12-17
70. Kim ST, Kim KP. Hepatic resections for primary liver cancer. *Cancer Chemother Pharmacol* 1994;**33** (suppl) : 18-23
71. Ebara M, Ohto M, Sugiura N, Okuda K, Kondo F, Kondo K. Percutaneous ethanol injection for the treatment of small hepatocellular carcinoma: study of 95 patients. *J Gastroenterol Hepatol* 1990; **5**:616-626
72. Livraghi T, Bolondi L, Cottone M *et al*. No treatment, resection and ethanol injection in hepatocellular carcinoma: a retrospective analysis of survival in 391 cirrhotic patients. *J Hepatol* 1995; **22**:522-526
73. Adachi E, Maeda T, Matsumata T, Shirabe K, Kinukawa N, Sugimachi K, Tsuneyoshi M. Risk factors for intrahepatic recurrence in human small carcinoma. *Gastroenterology* 1995; **108**: 768-775
74. Cameron RG, Greig PD, Farber E *et al*. Small encapsulated hepatocellular carcinoma of the liver. *Cancer* 1993; **72**:2550-2559
75. Sheu JC, Huang GT, Chou HC *et al*. Multiple hepatocellular carcinomas at the early stage have different clonality. *Gastroenterology* 1993; **105**:1471-1476
76. Takenaka K, Adachi E, Nishizaki T *et al*. Possible multicentric occurrence of hepatocellular carcinoma: a clinicopathological study. *Hepatology* 1994; **19**:889-894
77. Okuda K. Epidemiology of primary liver cancer, in Tobe T, Kameda H, eds. *Primary Liver Cancer in Japan*. Tokyo: Springer, 1992;3-15
78. Bellentani S, Tiribelli C, Saccoccio G *et al*. Prevalence of chronic disease in the general population of northern Italy: the Dionysos study. *Hepatology* 1994; **20**: 1442-1449
79. The Liver Cancer Study Group of Japan. Predictive factors for long term prognosis after partial hepatectomy for patients with hepatocellular carcinoma. *Cancer* 1994; **74**: 2772-2780

26

Percutaneous radiofrequency ablation and related techniques

L Buscarini, S Rossi, E Buscarini and M Di Stasi

Many efforts have been made to improve the results obtained by PEI in HCC percutaneous ablation. Their aims in particular were:

a) to achieve a more reliable necrosis
b) to obtain complete tumor destruction in fewer sessions
c) to avoid complications related to alcohol

For these purposes, other chemical substances such as acetic acid [1], and hot saline [2] were employed. The procedure was the same as for PEI.

Percutaneous acetic acid injection

50% acetic acid solution was used; 1-2 ml for HCCs 1-2 cm in diameter and 2-3 ml for HCCs 2-3 cm in diameter were injected. One injection was performed in each session. The treatment was given twice a week and repeated two or three times for tumors less than 2 cm and three or four times for tumors 2-3 cm in diameter. 23 patients with single HCC in cirrhosis smaller than 2.6 cm in diameter were treated in this way. There was no evidence of viable HCC at post-treatment biopsies and CT scan; two nodules examined at surgical resection showed complete necrosis. No complications occurred.[1]

Percutaneous hot saline injection

20 cirrhotic patients with 23 HCC smaller than 2.8 cm were treated with injections of hot saline at a dose of 8-30 ml per session. The treatment was completed in 2-3 sessions, performed once a week. Post treatment examinations (CT, angiography) showed complete necrosis of the treated tumors. No complications occurred but in many instances after injection of 10 ml the patients complained of a burning pain, and the procedure had to be stopped. In follow up, ranging from 2 to 36 months, no recurrences were observed. [2]

No conclusions could be reached concerning these procedures due to the small number of patients; moreover experience remains limited to only a few centers.

Another kind of ablation has been attempted by using either low or high temperatures. Low temperature application (cryotherapy) however has been used only during surgery, as an intraoperative application described in chapter 27.

In constrast, a promising attempt in the treatment of HCC is represented by the use of percutaneous ablation by employing interstitial hyperthermia obtained either by radiofrequency energy or by laser. Finally a complex method is represented by focused ultrasound.

INTERSTITIAL HYPERTHERMIA

The interstitial hyperthermia can be obtained by laser or radiofrequency (RF) energy from a laser fiber, radiofrequency or microwave needle electrodes placed into a tissue.

These methods are based on electromagnetic radiation whose spectrum is divided into bands as follows: RF, infrared, visible light, ultraviolet light, x-rays and gamma rays.

Radiofrequency

RF waves are a band of electromagnetic radiation subdivided according to frequency into low frequency energy (to 300 KHz), intermediate (to 3 MHz), high frequency (to 300 MHz) and microwaves with a wavelength up to 1 mm and a frequency up to 2500 MHz.

The basic RF circuit is created when terminal outputs of the RF generator are connected to electrodes placed on the body, which becomes an element of the electric circuit. The active electrode is represented by a small area where the heat lesion is made; the dispersive electrode is a large area which does not produce heat (monopolar system).

The RF probe is not an electrocautery in which the probe is heated by passing current to its tip and heat flows from the tip to the tissue. With the RF technique an alternating current flows from the uninsulated tract of the active electrode to the tissue.

Ionic agitation is produced in the tissue around the electrode, as the ions attempt to follow the changes in direction of the alternating current. This ionic movement results in frictional heating, so that the tissue surrounding the electrode rather than the electrode itself is the primary source of heat. The difference between the heat generated by the RF current in the tissue surrounding the electrode tip and the heat lost through the vessels in the region is the real heat responsible for thermal lesion generation. The dimensions of the thermal lesion depend on the temperature around the needle tip (which in turn is bound to the radiofrequency output), from the dimension of the active electrode tip and on the exposure time. In the monopolar method the current flows symmetrically from the electrode, causing an ellipsoidal shaped lesion. If the current is too high the heating around the tip may be so intense to induce solidification and char formation which will quickly limit further current flow and heating. Moreover if the temperature exceeds 100°C there are scattered areas of explosive water vaporization, with an irregular shaped lesion larger than the desired volume.

Radiofrequency bipolar system

RF energy can be delivered between two electrode needles. A bipolar arrangement limits the current flow to a volume defined by the two electrodes, generating a bridging area of necrosis. The lesion produced by the bipolar method is greater than twice the size of the lesions produced by a single electrode; a critical factor in determining volume of necrosis is represented by the interelectrode distance. [3]

Microwave

When the wavelength is small relative to human body size the tissue behaves mainly as a dielectric material. The electric field will generate local currents with corresponding energy loss, both resistive and dielectric, that will show up as heat. Because dielectric is not uniform the field distribution inside the tissue is not predictable and therefore the heating of the tissue is not as predictable as with conduction heating. Tissue surrounding the electrode is coagulated in a spindle shape, starting from the base of the electrode.

Laser

The word is the acronym of Light Amplification of Stimulated Emission of Radiation. Laser is a source of energy in the form of light that possesses collimation, coherence and monochromaticity. These features enable transmission of very high energies through narrow quartz fibers in a predictable amount. Infrared radiation and visible light interact similarly to that described for RF energy with body tissue and since their wavelengths are so short, most of the energy is deposited in a small volume close to the source and converted to heat close to the fiber's distal end. The effect is that of a hot knife where tissue is burned at the point of contact. Secondary heating of the surrounding tissue occurs through heat conduction, amplifying the tissue destroying effects. Finally scattered light will spread in all directions and eventually it will be converted into heat by a large volume of tissue.

Radiofrequency interstitial thermal ablation

An Italian group was the first to propose the possibility of employing interstitial hyperthermia to percutaneous ablation of liver tumors.[4] In an experimental work performed on guinea pigs and pigs, liver thermal lesions were induced by using RF needle electrodes. The study showed that the volume of necrosis is related to the temperature, to the exposure time and to the needle caliber and the length of the exposed tract of the needle. The temperature was monitored by a thermistor located at the needle tip and was always maintained under 95 °C, in order to avoid boiling and the creation of irregular and possibly dangerous lesions. In the same work it was shown that the necrosis volume increased at a prefixed temperature with increases of exposure time up to 120 seconds. The thermal lesions appeared well demarcated with a thin reactive regenerative band with vascular neogenesis. The lesion appeared in an advanced fibrotic state on the 30th day. As the possibility of US monitoring of the needle electrode was shown in the same work, the authors' conclusion was: "...destruction of tumoral lesions inside the liver appears to be possible by applying an electrode needle...under US guidance".

The same results were communicated independently by a second group using an experimental model *in vitro*; the authors observed that US could monitor the thermal lesion as an hyperechoic zone, attributing the hyperechogenicity to the presence of microbubbles as the temperature was more then 100 °C.[5] However that this modification appeared even in cases treated by temperatures of about 90 °C is probably due to protein denaturation, and acute edema.

In successive *in vivo* experiments, a laser fiber introduced into pig liver under US guidance induced a hyperechoic cylindrical zone corresponding to the shape of the laser fiber tip, with an inconsistent thin hypoechoic rim, probably representing a mild cellular swelling. After 7-11 days the lesion appeared as a target lesion with a central hypoechoic cavity, due to vaporization. After 24-50 days the thermal lesion was represented by a small echogenic area with or without central cavity.[6] These results were confirmed by Bosman *et al*, who pointed out the good correlation between the dimension of the hyperechoic spot and the lesion observed histopathologically.[7]

Percutaneous radiofrequency interstitial thermal ablation (RITA) of HCC

Equipment and procedure

The RF delivery system used in published papers,[8-10] for the monopolar method was a RF-current generator (model RFG S Generator system, Radionics, Burlington, Massachusetts; ZoMed RF generator made by ZoMed International, Mountain View, California) with an active electrode and a discersive electrode; that for the bipolar method was the same ZoMed RF generator with two active electrode needles.[11] The generators have 480 KHz frequency with a maximum power of 26 RF-watt and are a source of RF-voltage through their output terminals which are connected to electrodes. The active electrodes have an insulated (by 0.1 mm thick plastic) stainless steel shaft 24-30 cm long and an exposed tip of prefixed length in Radionics models and of variable length (by moving the plastic covering) in ZoMed models. The tips contain one (Radionics) or two thermistors (ZoMed) that allow temperature monitoring in the tissue around the needle tip; the calibration is accurate to 0 ± 4°C at temperatures in the region of 90°C. The temperature appears on a display on the generator. Needle electrodes with an external diameter of 1.2, 1.3, 1.6 mm and exposed tips of 1 or 1.5 cm long have been used for the monopolar method; needle electrodes with an external diameter of 1.3 mm and exposed tips of 2 cm for bipolar.

The insertion of the electrode needles in the tumor is performed under US guidance, using a 3.5 MHz probe with a lateral biopsy apparatus for the monopolar method or with a multihole guide mounted on the transducer for the bipolar method. Needle access can be intercostal or subcostal.

The monopolar procedure is carried out by connecting the patient to the RF generator via a dispersive electrode; local anesthesia is performed from the insertion point at the skin to the peritoneum along the puncture line. Then after pricking the skin with a small lancet, the active electrode needle tip is introduced into the chosen area of the tumor, under US guidance. The power necessary to keep the temperature at the needle tip at 90°C for 120 seconds is delivered.

With a bipolar procedure local anesthesia along the two prefixed puncture lines is done as previously described. Two active needle electrodes directly connected to the RF generator are inserted into the tumor in parallel 2.0 cm apart, via the multihole lateral guide apparatus, under US guidance. A temperature of 90°C around the needle tips is maintained for 20 minutes.

The monopolar procedure described above makes a single thermal lesion with a volume that ranges from 1.0 to 1.8 cm^3;[4] the bipolar technique, a thermal lesion of about 8.0 cm^3.[11]

At each insertion, the tip of the needle is placed in the deepest part of the tumor. Multiple thermal lesions are created along the needle electrode's major axis by simply withdrawing the needle from the preceding thermal lesion, and reactivating the RF generator. When necessary, due to tumor size, multiple insertions of the needle electrodes are performed in all strategic points of the tumor.

In the above cited studies for tumors smaller than 3 cm in diameter a necrosis volume about twice the tumor volume was devised.[8-11]

Therapeutic efficacy assessment

The therapeutic efficacy of RITA[8-11] has been documented by dosage of serum AFP (when starting values were increased), by using either multiple US guided fine needle biopsies and imaging techniques such as dynamic CT and selective angiography.

Dynamic CT was considered negative if a completely unenhanced area was shown at the site of the treated tumor. Selective hepatic angiography was considered negative if signs of neoplastic vascularization (e.g. neovascularization; tumor stain) completely disappeared. If one post treatment investigation revealed residual tumor, additional treatment was undertaken.

In the patients with HCC follow-up included US every 2 months for 1 year, every 3 months in the second year, every 4 months thereafter; and AFP dosage and liver function tests every 4 months. Dynamic CT was performed after 1 year and then in cases of recurrence.

The patients treated by RITA had generally a solitary HCC in cirrhosis less than 3 cm of diameter. The treatment has been performed only in patients with high surgical risk or those refusing surgery or presenting recurrent tumors after surgery. From January 1989 to July 1995 the authors have treated 39 patients selected according to the following criteria: single HCC nodules not more than 3 cm in diameter; absence of portal vein thrombosis and or extrahepatic spread; blood clotting tests not severely impaired. 17 HCC nodules ranged from 1.0 to 2.0 cm in the greatest diameter and 24 from 2.1 to 3.0 cm. Moreover two patients with two HCC nodules who met all the other criteria were included. Tumors were located either in the anterior or posterior segments of the liver; 10 nodules were subcapsular.

As experimentally shown, an increasing homogeneous hyperechoic area, often with posterior acoustic shadow, appeared around the needle tip when the temperature reached 90°C. This US structural change, visible at every thermal lesion, diminished as soon as RF power was switched off; however, some enhancement in the treated zone persisted as long as 12 hours.

At the end of the treatment the US patterns of HCC were modified: usually the hypoechoic HCCs became isoechoic or hyperechoic areas; the iso-hyperechoic with hypoechoic rim became iso-hyperechoic, iso-hypoechoic, hypo-hyperechoic areas. (Fig. 26.1a–c).

Tumoral destruction was achieved in all cases, with normalization of AFP levels in cases where it was initially increased. Three patients who died from causes other than HCC underwent autopsy: five HCC treated nodules were analyzed and only one presented a minimum focus of viable cancer cells. The mean number of RITA sessions needed to obtain tumor destruction was 3.3 (1-8) but in the second part of the same study it decreased to 2.3 (1-5).

During follow-up the treated HCCs slowly diminished in size, becoming undetectable by US or appearing only as small hyperechoic areas or isoechoic areas with an hyperechoic rim or simply as non-homogeneous areas.

In a mean follow-up of 23 months (3-66) 16/39 (41%) patients had recurrences (local recurrences in 5% and new lesions in 36%). Most patients with recurrent tumors underwent new courses of effective RF treatment. In total 54 HCC nodules in 39 patients were treated during the study. No complications related to the treatment occurred, apart from the infrequent experience of transitory mild pain during performance of RITA, which disappeared soon thereafter. After the treatment, no patients had fever or pain; no increase in serum aminotransferases or decrease in hemoglobin level was observed.

During follow-up 11/39 (29.2%) patients died: five from hepatic failure due to advanced cancer; six from unrelated cancer causes. Three patients underwent autopsy. Five treated HCCs were analyzed; only one nodule 2 cm in diameter treated 13 months previously showed a 3 mm focus of viable cancer, the other nodules being undetectable (2) or completely necrotic (2).

Median survival time was 44 months.

Percutaneous microwave coagulation therapy (PMCT) of HCC

This technique is similar to that described for RITA but the needle electrode is inserted through a 14 gauge guiding needle. PMCT was employed in 18 patients with HCC not more than 2 cm in diameter (17 were not surgical candidates; one was operated on after PMCT).[12] The treatment was considered to be effective on the basis of US change confirmed by disappearance of contrast enhancement with CT and/or decreased intensity of the tumor with MRI. In all the patients, a mean number of 2.8 treatment sessions were carried out. In one case complete necrosis was confirmed during surgery. During follow-up ranging between 11 to 33 months recurrences occurred in 3 patients who were retreated with PMCT.

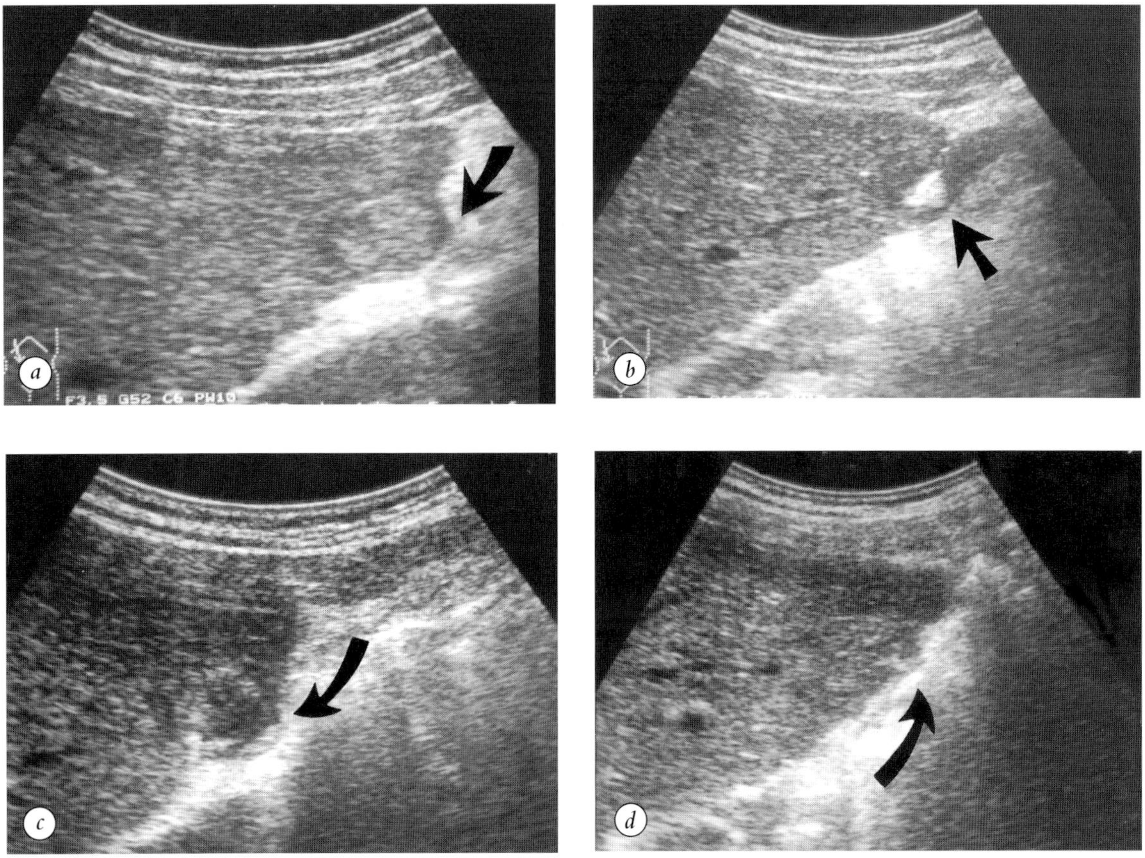

Figure 26.1

a) Sonography shows an iso-hypoechoic HCC nodule 2 cm in diameter located in the sixth liver segment. The tumor bulges into the liver margin (arrow).

b) Sonography shows a hyperechoic spot around the needle tip corresponding to a thermal lesion (arrow).

c) At the end of the RITA treatment sonography shows a hypoechoic with hyperechoic rim area in the sixth liver segment, smaller than the treated HCC (arrow).

d) One year after the end of the RITA course the treated HCC appears as a small liver margin deformity (arrow).

Another study involved 9 patients with HCC measuring 35-67 mm in diameter, in whom previously performed TAE had failed to induce a complete necrosis.[13] Multiple punctures and multiple microwave emissions were performed in various parts of the tumor by 2 sessions per week of PMCT. The treatment achieved complete tumor necrosis evaluated on the basis of dynamic CT in all patients, but in a mean follow-up of 6 months radiologic evidence of complete necrosis persisted only in five lesions.

The US modifications during PMCT are the same as described above for RITA. No complications are cited in either paper.

An isolated but interesting application of microwave therapy is represented by case of HCC proliferating in the bile duct. The microwave electrode was placed with a guide wire under fluoroscopic guidance. The treatment achieved a complete destruction of the intraductal mass and the patient was followed for 12 months without any recurrence.[14]

Interstitial laser photocoagulation (ILP)

The use of hyperthermia obtained by laser has been mostly applied to the treatment of liver metastases, with the possibility of complete tumoral destruction in several sessions.[15,16]

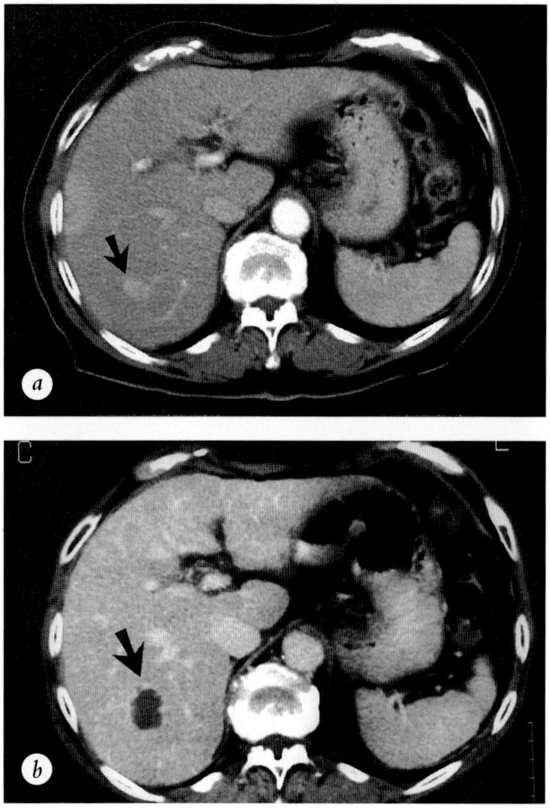

Figure 26.2

a) Dynamic CT shows a hyperdense area in the seventh segment (arrow) of the liver, due to HCC nodule.

b) After RITA dynamic CT shows a hypodense area in the site of the treated nodule (arrow), due to necrosis.

The method described by the authors can obviously be applied to HCC ablation, however only a few cases of HCC have been reported. The introduction of the laser fiber was performed under US guidance (as in the series of liver metastases). The US picture observed during the treatment is the same as that described in experiments and in clinical application for metastases. The occurrence of microbubbles is usual, as the temperature is more than 100 °C. However 5 patients with small HCC (not more than 4.2 cm in diameter) were treated with low-power laserthermia; that is, the power applied was low, achieving a temperature not higher than 80°C. Four patients had good results with complete necrosis of the tumor; 1 died 2 months after the treatment but the treated HCC was not described.[17] Only 1 case of HCC was treated by conventional laser showing a complete but transitory response, with local recurrence and new lesions in a short time.[18] No complications were observed in either experience.[17,18]

Focused ultrasound

High intensity focused ultrasound, when absorbed by the tumor, is partially transformed into heat, inducing rapidly and for a short time a tissue temperature of about 80°C, without heat diffusion. A second important effect is a mechanical one, represented by cavitation. The negative part of the US wave induces a depression within the biologic medium and intracellular water may enter in gaseous phase with microbubble formation. A sudden compression wave may provoke of the microbubbles with production of shock waves of high pressure with consequent damage of contiguous cells. The technique has been demonstrated in animal models.[19]

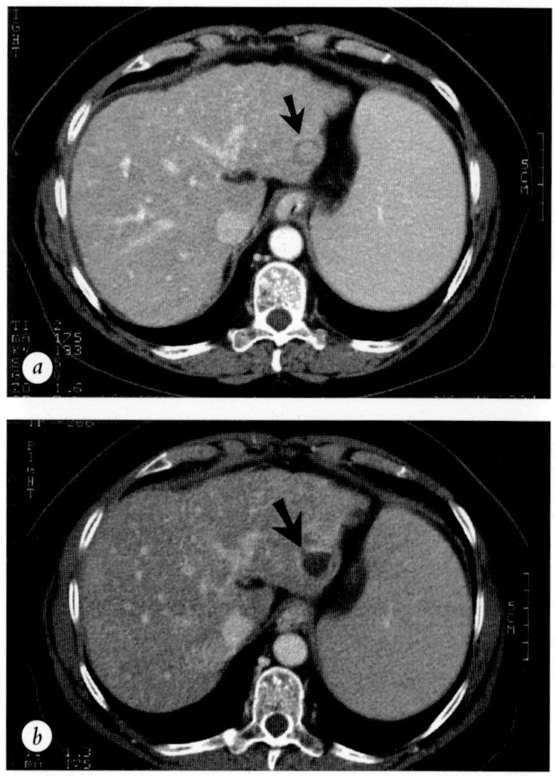

Figure 26.3

a) Basal dynamic CT shows a iso-hyperdense area in the second segment of the liver (arrow) due to HCC nodule.

b) After RITA in the site of the treated tumor appears a hypodense area due to induced necrosis (arrow).

CONCLUSION

Interstitial hyperthermia is a technique that can destroy liver tumors as demonstrated by US, US guided FNB, dynamic CT and selective angiography.

US is a good technique to guide the RF needle electrodes and to monitor the extent of necrosis but is not adequate to judge correctly the final result due to the impossibility of identifying persistent minimal tumor.

Even multiple FNBs can miss residual tumoral foci, because the information pertains to a very limited volume of liver; moreover the sampling of minute areas can be difficult. Therefore the role of dynamic CT in evaluating the response to treatment is very relevant (Figs. 26.2,a,b, 26.3a,b). In fact post-treatment nonenhancing CT images reflect tumor necrosis as shown by pathologic studies of resected tumors after TAE,[20] or PMCT.[12]

The effectiveness of RITA has been confirmed by pathologic study performed on surgical samples or on necropsy.

The presence in very few cases of tumor after the conclusion of the predetermined RF thermal ablation course can be related to the difficulty of placing the needles in all strategic points of the tumor. The same order of problems has been experienced with ILP of liver metastases.[15]

Follow-up of treated HCCs showed in some cases the appearance of multiple tumors some months after the conclusion of treatment due to underestimation of the disease extent at the time of staging. In fact, angiography and dynamic CT can miss about 20% of HCC less than 2 cm in diameter due to histologic-vascular features, as confirmed by the frequent presence of undetected tumor foci in cirrhotic explanted livers. In most of the treated HCCs recurrences are observed. Early recurrence (within 1 or 2 years of treatment) is mainly local, that is recurrence of the treated lesion; late recurrent tumors are new lesions which can arise in every segment of the liver. Local recurrence is the result of a lack of aggressiveness or thoroughness with the technique whereas new lesions are a part of the natural history of HCC in cirrhosis.

The total recurrence rate of HCC is similar after surgery, PEI or RF thermal ablation.

It is important to note that in the majority of HCCs with both local recurrence and new lesions, a new course of RITA or MPCT has been performed with good results.

The survival rate of HCCs treated with RITA is similar to that found in surgical series and in patients with small HCC treated with PEI. The satisfactory survival rate is, in part, related to strict follow-up, designed to detect and treat recurrences early.

RITA is a flexible technique: under laparoscopic guidance small liver tumors superficially located can be ablated.[21]

RITA and MPCT are safe and are unlikely to provoke venous thrombosis at the border of thermal lesions as experimentally shown, because the vessels eventually present induce a dispersion of heat. In contrast with some observations during treatment with RITA, no tissue microbubbles were observed because the temperature was maintained under 100°C. During some ILP exposures gas was identified in hepatic veins and in the heart with a risk for paradoxical air embolism in patients with interatrial defects.[22] The danger of bleeding with thermal ablation is reduced by the coagulative power of interstitial hyperthermia. In one case of subcapsular liver adenoma treated by RITA under laparoscopic control, no signs of bleeding were observed.

No tumor seeding along the needle track was seen either with RITA and MPCT in spite of the high number of punctures.

A percutaneous ablative therapy has to be effective and has to obtain a complete necrosis in a short time. The duration of therapy is a crucial point both for patient compliance and for economic reasons. For this purpose, the application of the bipolar technique,[11] and the study of new kinds of needles able to induce a larger volume of necrosis are very important and promising. The goal is to achieve destruction of a tumor of 3-4 cm in diameter in only one session and this is a realistic one.

REFERENCES

1. Hohnishi K, Ohyama N, Ito S, Fujiwara K. Small hepatocellular carcinoma: treatment with US-guided intratumoral injection of acetic acid. *Radiology* 1994; **193**: 747-752

2. Honda N, Guo Q, Uchida H, Ohishi H, Hiasa Y. Percutaneous hot saline injection therapy for hepatic tumors: an alternative to percutaneous ethanol injection therapy. *Radiology* 1994; **190**: 53-57

3. Chang RJ, Stevenson WG, Saxon LA Parker J. Increasing catheter ablation size by simultaneous application of radiofrequency current to two adjacent sites. *Am Heart J* 1993; **125**: 1276-1284

4. Rossi S, Fornari F, Paties C, Buscarini L. Thermal lesions induced by 480 KHz localized current field in guinea pig and pig liver. *Tumori* 1990; **76**: 54-57

5. McGahan JP, Browning PD, Brock JM, Tesluk H. Hepatic ablation using radiofrequency electrocautery. *Invest Radiol* 1990; **25**: 267-270

6. Dachman AH, Mc Gehee JA, Beam TE, Burris JA, Powell DA. US-guided percutaneous laser ablation of liver tissue in a chronic pig model. *Radiology* 1990; **176**: 129-133

7. Bosman S, Phoa SSK, Bosma A, Van Gemert MJC. Effect of percutaneous interstitial thermal laser on normal liver of pigs: sonographic and histopathological correlations. *Br J Surg* 1991; **78**: 572-575

8. Buscarini L, Fornari F, Rossi S. Interstitial radiofrequency hyperthermia in the treatment of small hepatocellular carcinoma: percutaneous guidance of electrode needle. In: Anderegg A, Despland PA, Henner H, Otto R, eds. *Ultraschall Diagnostik 91*. Heidelberg: Springer-Verlag, 1992: p 218-222

9. Rossi S, Fornari F, Buscarini L. Percutaneous ultrasound guided radiofrequency electrocautery for the treatment of small hepatocellular carcinoma. *J Intervent Radiol* 1993; **8**: 97-103

10. Rossi S, Di Stasi M, Buscarini E, Cavanna L, Quaretti P, Squassante L, Garbagnati F, Buscarini L. Percutaneous radiofrequency interstitial thermal ablation in the treatment of small hepatocellular carcinoma. *Cancer J Sci Am* 1995; **1**: 73-81

11. Rossi S, Di Stasi M, Buscarini E, Quaretti P, Garbagnati F, Squassante L, Paties CT, Silverman DE, Buscarini L. Percutaneous radiofrequency interstitial thermal ablation in the treatment of liver cancer. *AJR* 1996; **167**:759-768

12. Seki T, Wakabayashi M, Nakagawa T *et al*. Ultrasonically guided percutaneous microwave coagulation therapy for small hepatocellular carcinoma. *Cancer* 1994; **74**: 817-825

13. Murakami R, Yoshimatsu S, Yamashita Y, Matsukawa T, Takahashi M, Sagara K. Treatment of hepatocellular carcinoma: value of percutaneous microwave coagulation. *AJR* 1995; **164**: 1159-1164

14. Seki T, Kubota Y, Wakaba M *et al*. Percutaneous microwave coagulation therapy for hepatocellular carcinoma proliferating in the bile duct. *Dig Dis Sci* 1994; **39**: 663-666.

15. Amin Z, Donald JJ, Masters A *et al*. Hepatic metastases: interstitial laser photocoagulation with real-time US monitoring and dynamic CT evaluation of treatment. *Radiology* 1993; **187**: 339-347

16. Nolsoe C, Torp-Pedersen S, Burchart F *et al*. Interstitial hyperthermia of colorectal liver metastases with a US-guided Nd-YAG laser with a diffuser tip: a pilot clinical study. *Radiology* 1993; **187**: 333-337

17. Huang GT, Wang TH, Sheu JC *et al*. Low-power laserthermia for the treatment of small hepatocellkular carcinoma. *Eur J Cancer* 1991; **27**: 1622-1627

18. Dowlatshahi K, Bhattacharya AK, Silver B, Matalon T, Williams JW. Percutaneous interstitial laser therapy of a patient with recurrent hepatoma in a transplanted liver. *Surgery* 1992; **112**: 603-606

19. Prat F, Chapelon JY, El Fadil FA *et al*. Focused liver ablation by cavitation in the rabbit: a potential new method of extracorporeal treatment. *Gut* 1994; **35**: 395-400

21. Takayasu K, Moriyama N, Muramatsu Y *et al*. Hepatic arterial embolization for hepatocellular carcinoma: comparison of CT scan and resected specimens. *Radiology* 1984; **150**: 661-665

22. Buscarini L, Rossi S, Fornari F, Di Stasi M, Buscarini E. Laparoscopic ablation of liver adenoma by radiofrequency electrocautery. *Gastrointest Endoscopy* 1995; **41**: 68-70

23. Malone DE, Lesiuk L, Brady A, Wyman DR, Wilson BC. Hepatic interstitial laser photocoagulation: demonstration and possible clinical importance of intravascular gas. *Radiology* 1994;**193**: 233-237

27

Cryosurgery

X-D Zhou and Z-Y Tang

Cryosurgery is defined as the *in situ* destruction of abnormal tissue using subzero temperatures. The freezing of tissue was first used as early as 2500 BC as an anesthetic.

However, the first use of freezing techniques to destroy cancer was described in the middle part of the 1850s by James Arnott when he used iced saline solution to treat advanced carcinomas of the uterus, cervix and breast.[1] However, it was not until 1961 when Irving Cooper described a cryoprobe that circulated liquid nitrogen through an insulated metal sheath that modern cryosurgery became a reality. He also suggested that cryosurgery might be used to treat primary and metastatic hepatic cancer in the future. Currently, cryosurgery has achieved substantial stature in dermatology, proctology, gynecology, urology, and veterinary medicine, especially for diseases in easily accessible tissue.[1] Recently, encouraging trials using cryotherapy in the treatment of hepatic metastases have been published.[2-5] We have performed cryosurgery for 23 years and have previously demonstrated the pilot results of cryosurgery as a regional treatment for HCC in experimental systems and in humans.[6-15] In this chapter we review our cryosurgical experience and report the preliminary results of the potential efficacy of cryohepatectomy, cryosurgery followed by the resection of the frozen tumor, in reducing the recurrence and prolonging survival.

CRYOSURGERY

The optimal treatment of HCC is complete surgical excision of the tumors. At present, however, the resectability is low because of multiple tumor nodules involving both hepatic lobes, coexisting advanced liver disease, or the anatomical location of the tumor close to major vessels. Conservative treatments for HCC appear to be of limited efficacy. Therefore, we applied cryosurgery for treating unresectable HCC from June 1973.

Experimental cryosurgery[6,7]

Animal and tumor models

Group I consisted of rabbits, dogs and young cattle used in studies of cryosurgery of normal liver in order to observe the pathologic changes, safety, and physical condition during the operation. Group II was composed of hepatoma-22 solid tumors (in Kunming mice bearing human HCC) and S180 (pleomorphic cell) sarcomas; they were used to study the immunologic effects of cryosurgery.

Experimental methods

Animals in Group I were anesthetized and the liver was exposed through an upper midline incision. Cryosurgery of liver was applied in three ways: direct contact freezing using a plate-like probe 3-5 cm in diameter; penetration freezing via a trocar probe 0.3-0.4 cm in diameter; and spraying liquid nitrogen directly on the surface of liver. The duration of freezing was from 5-40 min. Needle thermocouples were placed onto the liver surface and inserted 1 cm deep near the center of the area of the liver to be frozen; temperature records were traced on a recorder. Probe temperature was maintained at a constant -180°C.

The probe was applied to the same site twice. After each freezing, thawing was allowed to proceed spontaneously, and then the abdominal incision was closed. In Group II animals, a 1 cm diameter probe was in contact with the tumor for 1-2 min so that the temperature of the tumor base could be cooled to -20°C. The tumor volume was measured periodically before and after cryosurgery; at the end, the growth rate of another implanted tumor was recorded.

Safety of hepatic cryosurgery

Two rabbits died of hypothermia during cryosurgery. Alanine aminotransferase rose to varying levels in the surviving animals immediately following cryosurgery and then returned to normal within 2 weeks. There were no significant changes in serum bilirubin after cryosurgery. During the operation, a crack in the hepatic capsule was occasionally observed with liquid nitrogen sprayed directly onto the surface of the liver or following insertion of the trocar probe into the liver parenchyma so that hemostasis was required. There was no evidence of rupture, delayed bleeding, or bile leakage after cryosurgery in any of the long-term survivors that were killed. The optimum effect was obtained after 12-14 min of freezing; only minor changes in temperature as well as in the frozen area were observed with prolongation of freezing. Tissue temperature at a 1 cm depth fell to -120°C, and the surface temperature to -155°C, during the 15-min period. The necrotic area was generally similar to the frozen area.

Pathologic changes

Necrosis of cellular structures was significant 6 h after cryosurgery, and infiltration by polymorphonuclear leukocytes, lymphocytes, and plasmacytes was seen at the border of the frozen area and normal tissue. One day after cryosurgery the hepatocellular structure was broken down in the frozen area, and capillaries, small bile ducts, and fibroblasts appeared around the margin of the frozen area; 3 days after cryosurgery a distinct, sharply circumscribed area of coagulative necrosis appeared in the frozen area, and 7 days after cryosurgery fibrous tissue developed gradually in the previously frozen area. Thirty days after cryosurgery the area of coagulative necrosis was found to have contracted, and 45 days after cryosurgery there was only thin white, scar tissue left in the previously frozen area, with normal surrounding liver.

Immunologic findings

After we froze hepatoma-22 solid tumors, the growth of the original tumors, as well as that of reimplanted tumors, was inhibited as compared with a control group (all $p<0.01$); this was considered to be a result of tumor-specific transplantation immunity induced by cryosurgery. Immunity was more significant 10 days after cryosurgery. The more completely the tumor was frozen, the stronger was the inhibition. There was no cross-immunity between hepatoma-22 solid tumors and S180 sarcomas.

Factors influencing freezing effects

DURATION OF FREEZING

According to our data, there is a balance between drop in temperature and extension of frozen area when the duration of freezing is 12-14 min. It was reported that a cryoprobe at a given temperature (-80 to -180°C) would produce 80%-90% of its maximum freezing effect within 15 min; however, the maximum effect would require approximately 2 h of freezing. Therefore, it is our opinion that for practical purposes 15 min is sufficient for each freezing.

REPETITIVE FREEZE-THAW CYCLES

It was demonstrated that the difference in the freezing rate between one and three cycles was highly significant ($p<0.01$). Repetitive freeze-thaw not only increases the volume of frozen tissue but also profoundly reduces the rate of thawing. Our experiments with hepatoma-22 after cryosurgery showed that the rate of tumor cure was enhanced (with one and two cycles it was 35% and 48% respectively).

BLOOD SUPPLY OF TISSUE

The experiments showed that the effects of one probe application with inflow occlusion approximated those of two to three freezes cycles without ischemia, and that the mean thawing time was increased by about 60% in the ischemic group.

Long-term results of clinical application[14,15]

We treated 145 patients with primary liver cancer (PLC) (HCC 142, cholangiocarcinoma 1, and mixed type 2). There were 41 cases (28.3%) with small tumors (up to 5 cm). Liver cirrhosis was present in 86.9% (126/145).

Indication

Cryosurgery for primary liver cancer was mainly indicated for patients with:

1) severe liver cirrhosis in whom liver resection, even limited resection, would be contraindicated;
2) residual tumor at the cut surface or in the rest of the liver after resection of the main tumor;
3) unresectable recurrent PLC after major hepatic resection.

Survival

The 1, 3, and 5-year survival rates were 69.2%, 49.2% and 34.8% respectively for the whole series, 91%, 76.5% and 64.2% respectively for the 41 patients with tumors up to 5 cm, and 59.9%, 35.7% and 17.3% respectively for the 104 patients with tumors over 5 cm.

Conclusion

Cryosurgery is a treatment in which tumors are frozen and then left *in situ* to be reabsorbed. Cryosurgery has certain merits in the treatment of HCC: it is a focal treatment, sparing more normal liver tissue than resection, thus allowing multiple lesions affecting both lobes of the liver to be treated. By piercing the liver with a trocar probe under intraoperative ultrasound guidance, even tumors deep within the hepatic parenchyma can be destroyed. In addition, there is some evidence that cryosurgery of a tumor has an added immunologic benefit by possibly sensitizing the patient to tumor antigen. Some reports have suggested that the distant metastases from cancer of the prostate might shrink in size in some individuals following cryosurgery. Regression of metastatic disease in the contralateral location has also been noted in some patients with lung cancer treated by cryosurgery.

Our results demonstrated that long-term control of HCC is achievable by cryosurgery, the 5-year survival rate being 34.8% for the whole series (n=145). This rate was much higher than that for other conservative treatments including radiotherapy, chemotherapy and/or Chinese herbs (1, 2, and 3 year survival rates were 6.6%, 1.1%, and 0%, respectively; n=117, 1976-1984), and much higher than those for non-treatment (1 year survival rate was 0%, n=29, 1976-1984).[16]

CRYOHEPATECTOMY

Recent advances in hepatic imaging and the monitoring of AFP in patients with cirrhosis have made it possible to detect HCC at an early stage. The number of hepatic resections, especially for small HCC, has increased greatly.[17-20] Moreover, improvements in surgical technique and perioperative care have resulted in lower operative morbidity and mortality rates in the most experienced centers.[21-23] However, long-term results after resection of HCC are still poor. The main reason for the poor prognosis is the high recurrence rate even after radical resection of small HCC.[24,25] Therefore, further improvement in long-term survival may depend on preventing the recurrence. Here we report the preliminary results of cryosurgery for HCC in reducing the recurrence rate and prolonging survival after the resection of HCC.

Patients

For entry into the current study, patients had to have a histologically verified HCC, a surgically verified resectable tumor, a tumor less than 8 cm in maximum diameter, and were undergoing cryosurgery followed by resection of the frozen tumor.

A total of 35 patients met all the above-mentioned criteria at the Liver Cancer Institute of Shanghai Medical University. The median age of the entire series was 47 years (range, 30-63 years), and the male-to-female ratio was 7.8:1.

Liver cirrhosis was present in 91.4% (32/35): macronodular cirrhosis (cirrhotic nodule ≥ 0.3 cm) accounting for 78.1% (25/32), and micronodular cirrhosis (cirrhotic nodule <0.3cm) 21.9% (7/32). Serum hepatitis B surface antigen (HBsAg) by reverse passive hemagglutination was observed in 77.1% (27/35). The size of the tumor ranged from 2 x 2 x 2 cm to 8 x 6 x 5.5 cm. Of the patients, 60.0% (21/35) had small tumors (≤5cm). The tumor was in the left lobe of the liver in 3 cases (8.6%), in the right lobe of the liver in 28 cases (80.0%), and bilateral in four cases (11.4%).

All 35 patients underwent local resection (any sublobar, however large) except 1 case with left lateral segmentectomy, all being radical resection, with cholecystectomy in 5 cases. In this series, radical resection meant complete removal of the tumor, with no grossly identifiable tumor emboli in the portal vein and no tumor residue in the remaining liver tissue or cut surface.

Pertinent abnormal findings were: AFP (>20ng/ml, radioimmunoassay) 74.3% (26/35); and gamma glutamyltranspeptidase (γ-GTP >10U, Orlowski method) 34.3% (12/35).

Technique

A right subcostal incision was used, either with an extension cranial to the xiphoid process or with a left subcostal extension for the resection of a left lobe tumor. The incision should be wide enough to permit the placement of an overshoulder retractor so that the right arch of the ribs can be retracted toward the ceiling.

The liver was examined by bimanual palpation and, recently, by intraoperative ultrasound. Cryoprobes of various sizes and shapes were used depending on the size and location of the tumor. Plate-like probes 3.5 cm in diameter were used for surface lesions. A trocar probe 6 mm in width and 7 cm in length was used for

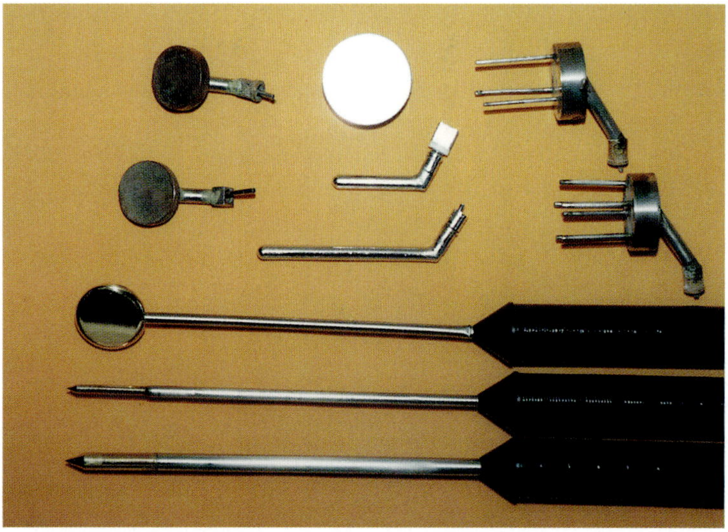

Figure 27.1 – Various cryoprobes

deeper lesions. Multiple penetrations (3 to 6 needles, each needle being 2.5 mm wide, 5 cm long) with a single cryoprobe (4 cm in diameter) were sometimes used for deeper lesions (Fig. 27.1). The probe and its handle were connected with a particular angle connector for treating tumors located in the right upper lobe of the liver. The probe was driven by a cryosurgical system (LD-2, Shanghai Institute of Technical Physics of the Academic Sinica) that circulated liquid nitrogen at -196°C through an insulated metal sheath. A probe temperature of -180°C was achieved by this system. Freezing was accomplished by placing the plate probe on the tumor surface with minimal pressure, or by placing the trocar probe into the tumor under ultrasound guidance with continuous monitoring of the freeze–thaw process by ultrasound. If a plate probe was used, care had to be taken to ensure good contact between the probe and the tissue to facilitate exchange of heat.

Recently, a new freezing system has been used (Cryogenic Technology Ltd. Ripley, UK) with 3 probes; a 5 mm and 10 mm diameter shaft, and a 3.5 cm diameter flat probe (Fig. 27.l). Two probes could be used simultaneouly. A few millimeters of the normal liver around the tumor was also frozen to ensure the completeness of cryofreezing. The time for each freezing was 15-20 min. Lesions that were too large to be frozen in a single application of the cryoprobe were treated by application of the probe to multiple sites, or by the simultaneous use of two freezing units. After cryosurgery, the frozen tumor was resected immediately by conventional technique. For control of bleeding during transection of the hepatic parenchyma, temporary occlusion of the portal pedicle was frequently used in our series.[22]

Routine perioperative medication was given. Liver function, serum AFP levels and US examination and/or CT scan were monitored preoperatively and postoperatively.

Survival and recurrence rates were calculated by the life-table method.

Physical conditions

The cryosurgical techniques provided a controllable and predictable area of necrosis. During the process of freezing, the white frosted appearance of the tissue gradually extended away from the side of the probe. The largest surface diameter of the frozen area was 7 cm when a 3.5 cm diameter plate-like probe was used. Freezing with the plate-like probe produced a roughly hemispherical lesion. The freezing depth relative to the surface diameter was approximately 1:2. The largest ice ball generated using the 6 mm trocar probe was 5-6 cm in diameter.

It is generally accepted that all of the cells in a frozen area, including the marginal zone, can be destroyed. Our previous data demonstrated that the frozen area is identical to the necrotic area.[6-7] Therefore, the gross frozen area might represent the necrotic area.

Safety

The postoperative course of cryohepatectomy in all of the 35 patients was uneventful, there being no operative mortality or severe complications. AFP decreased to normal (≤20 ng/ml) in 92.3% of the patients (24/26) with AFP-positive HCC. The animal studies showed that even the large blood vessels were frozen, and that rupture of the devitalized vessel wall did not occur. However, the common bile duct did not fare as well. Initially, edema of the wall caused partial luminal occlusion, and several days later stenosis developed. Among 13 dogs, one died of bile peritonitis following the development of a perforation in the duct wall. Therefore, great care should be exercized in treating HCC located near the hepatic hilum.[2]

Survival and recurrence rates

The 1, 3, and 5 year survival rates after cryohepatectomy were 100%, 83.3%, and 83.3%, repectively. These survival rates were better than those after conventional resection of small HCC (≤5 cm), the 1, 3, 5 year survival rates being 89.2%, 75.4%, and 63.8%, respectively.[17] The 1, 3, and 5 year recurrence rates after cryohepatectomy were 3.7%, 42.2%, and 42.2%, respectively. These recurrence rates seem better than those after conventional resection, the 1, 3, and 5 year recurrence rates being 15.0%, 45.4%, and 55.3%, respectively.[24]

Case reports

Case 1 — A 48-year-old man was picked up by AFP mass screening (>400 ng/ml). Hepatic angiography showed a 3 cm tumor in the middle hepatic lobe. He underwent surgery on June 15, 1979 and a small tumor 3.2 x 3 x 3 cm was found in the left middle hepatic lobe and without liver cirrhosis. Cryosurgery was carried out with a 3.5 cm probe which was in direct contact with the tumor for 20 min. The frozen area involved all the tumor and some surrounding normal liver tissue. The frozen tumor was resected with cholecystectomy. Pathologic examination revealed HCC. AFP returned to normal 1 month after resection and has remained negative. The patient is still alive and has been well for 16 years and 7 months.

Case 2 — A 54-year-old man was discovered by follow-up AFP for chronic hepatitis. He suffered from chronic liver disease for 16 years and his AFP had recently increased up to 280 ng/ml. Hepatic angiography showed a 3 cm tumor in the right lower portion of the liver. He underwent operation on August 6 1982 and a small tumor 3.5 x 3.5 x 4cm was found in the right lower lobe of the liver. Cryosurgery was performed with a 3.5 cm cryoprobe in direct contact with the tumor for 15 min, with two freeze-thaw cycles. The frozen area involved all the tumor and some surrounding normal liver tissue, and the frozen tumor was resected. HCC was confirmed by pathologic study. AFP declined to normal 1 month after resection and has remained negative. The patient has been in good health for 14 years and 4 months.

Electronmicroscopic findings

The frozen area appeared dark red immediately after thawing. Electronmicroscopic examination of the target area after cryosurgery showed cell necrosis and cell shrinkage in the center of the frozen area. In the necrotic cells, nuclear chromatin was seriously coagulated, but the nuclear membranes remained intact. Different sized vesicles and single or double membrane enclosed structures in which electron dense materials existed were the major contents in the cytoplasm, and were denatured endoplasmic reticulum and mitochondria. Plasma membranes in these cells had ruptured, so cell organelle outflow usually could be found in the sections (Fig. 27.2a).

In the area of the frozen tumor edge, the nuclei of hepatocytes were irregular in shape and contained pale chromatin. In their cytoplasm, obviously swollen mitochondria, some developing into large vesicles, were seen as well as an electron dense precipitation in other mitochonrial matrices. Rough endoplasmic reticulum was distributed around the mitochondria. Many small vesicles were swollen with smooth endoplasmic reticulum. The intact plasma membranes in adjacent hepatocytes were parallel to each other, and

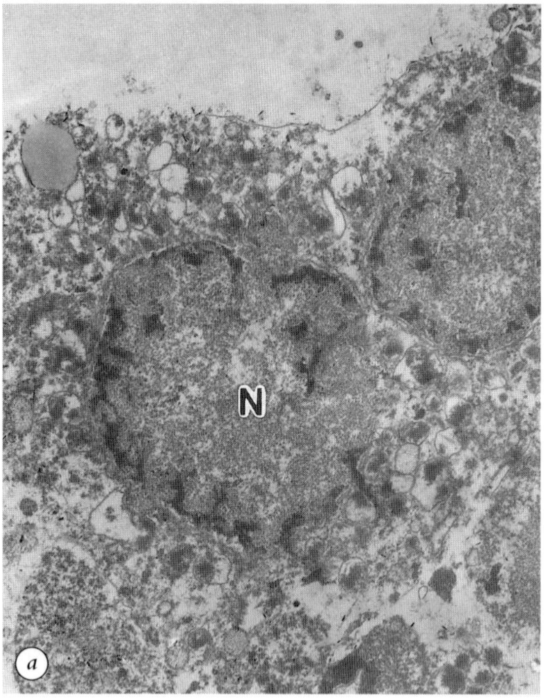

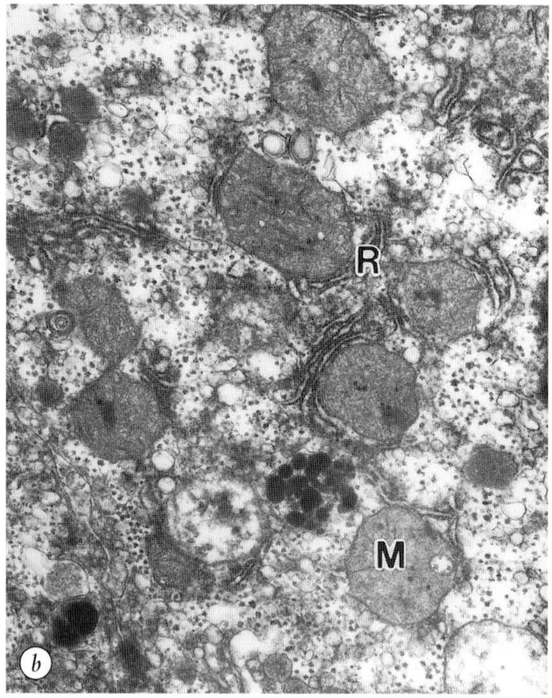

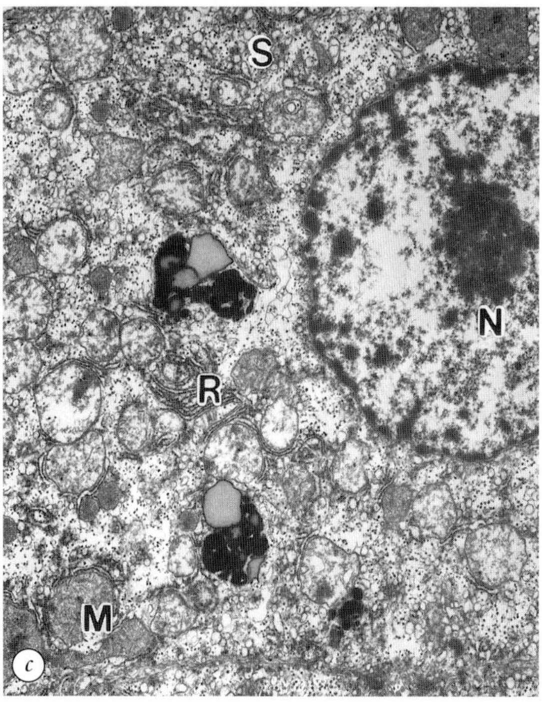

Figure 27.2 – Electronmicroscopic findings after cyrosurgery.

a) Frozen center of hepatocytes.

b) Frozen edge of hepatocytes.

c) Hepatocytes of 2mm from frozen edge.

N = Nucleus, M = Mitochondria, R = Rough endoplasmic reticulum, S = Smooth endoplasmic rediculum.

cell junctional structures such as demosomes were seen; in some places the small bile ducts were clearly observed (Fig. 27.2b).

In the area 2 mm from the frozen edge, the ultrastructural changes in hepatocyte were alleviated compared with the frozen edge itself, but mitochondrial swelling still appeared in the cytoplasm of hepatocytes (Fig. 27.2c).

Conclusion

Improvement in probe design and imaging technology now mean that superficial and deeply seated lesions within the liver can be treated with real time intraoperative ultrasound monitoring.[2-5] There is good correlation between the extent of the frozen area and the extent of the necrotic zone produced. The evolving and final area of frozen tissue can be seen sonographically in real time as an iceball generated around the cryoprobe.

In carcinoma of the breast, cryosurgery has been combined with surgical excision in a manner that may reduce the chance of spread of neoplastic cells during excision. When comparing cryosurgery with surgical excision with en bloc excision alone, a substantial protection against local recurrence of carcinoma of the mammary gland of the mouse was afforded.[26] Limited resection for HCC has been performed widely because most HCC is associated with severe cirrhosis. Cryohepatectomy for early HCC is potentially beneficial in causing selective necrosis of the cancer prior to excision and, therefore, may reduce the risk of iatrogenic cancerous diffusion and the recurrence of the cancer. Dead cancerous cells do not metastasize. Our preliminary results also demonstrated that the recurrence rates after cryohepatectomy seem better than those after conventional resection, the 5 year recurrence rate being 42.2% vs 55.3%.[24]

However, in our series most cryohepatectomy for HCC was done during the last 2 years. More time is needed to determine whether this procedure ultimately prevents recurrence of HCC.

ACKNOWLEDGEMENT

The authors thank Prof. Yi-Ping Ling, Department of Biophysics, Shanghai Medical University, for electronmicroscopic observation, and Dr. Bo-Heng Zhang, Dr. Yao Yu, Dr. Shu-Qun Cheng and Dr. Hul-Chuan Sun, Liver Cancer Institute for invaluable assistance in preparing the manuscript.

REFERENCES

1. Gage AA. Cryosurgery in the treatment of cancer. *Surg Gynecol Obstet* 1992; **174**:73-92
2. Onik GM, Atkinson D, Zemel R, Weaver ML. Cryosurgery of liver cancer. *Semin Surg Oncol* 1993; **9**:309-317
3. Ravikumar TS, Buenaventura S, Salem RR *et al.* Intraoperative ultrasonography of liver: Detection of occult liver tumors and treatment by cryosurgery. *Cancer Detect Prev* 1994; **18**: 131-136
4. Charnley RM, Doran J, Morris DL. Cryosurgery for liver metatases: a new approach. *Br J Surg* 1989; **76**:1040-1041
5. Kuramoto S, Kamegai T. Cryosurgery for the liver tumor (Abstr). *Cryobiology* 1978; **15**:710
6. Zhou XD, Tang ZY, Yu YQ *et al.* Cryosurgery for liver cancer: Experimental and clinical study. *Chin J Surg* 1979; **17**: 480-483
7. Zhou XD, Tang ZY, Yu YQ. Cryosurgery for hepatocellular carcinoma. In: Tang ZY, ed. *Subclinical Hepatocellular Carcinoma*. Beijing: China Academic Publishers & Berlin: Spring-Verlag, 1985; 107-119
8. Zhou XD, Tang ZY, Yu YQ, Ma ZC. Clinical evaluation of cryosurgery in the treatment of primary liver cancer. Report of 60 cases. *Cancer* 1988; **61**: 1889-1892
9. Zhou XD, Tang ZY, Yu YQ *et al.* Cryosurgery for primary liver cancer: A 15 year experience. *Cryo Supercondu* 1988; **16**:1-4
10. Zhou XD, Tang ZY, Yu YQ *et al.* A seventeen-year experience of cryosurgery for primary liver cancer. In: Stolar E, Turansky E, eds. *Cryomedicine*. Argentina: Montserrat SSC 1992; 79-85
11. Zhou XD, Yu YQ, Tang ZY *et al.* Cryosurgery for primary hepatic cancer of 87 patients. *Chin J Surg* 1992; **30**:335-337
12. Zhou XD, Yu YQ, Tang ZY, Weng JM, Ma ZC, Xu DB. An 18-year study of cryosurgery in the treatment of primary liver cancer. *Asian J Surg* 1992; **15**:43-47
13. Zhou XD, Tang ZY, Yu YQ *et al.* The role of cryosurgery in the treatment of hepatic cancer: a report of 113 cases.*Cancer Res Clin Oncol* 1993; **120**: 100-102
14. Zhou XD, Tang ZY, Yu YQ *et al.* Cryotherapy with liquid nitrogen for liver tumor. *J Practical Oncol* 1995; **10**:140-142
15. Zhou XD, Tang ZY, Yu YQ *et al.* Cryosurgery for liver tumor. In: Kawasaki S, Makuuchi M, eds. *Novel Regional Therapies for Liver Tumors.* Austin: RG Landes Company, Biomedical Publishers 1995; 187-196
16. Tang ZY, Yu YQ, Zhou XD. The changing role of surgery in the treatment of primary liver cancer. *Semin Surg Oncol* 1986; **2**:103-112
17. Zhou XD, Tang ZY, Yu YQ *et al.* Long-term results of surgery for small primary liver cancer in 514 adults. *J Cancer Res Clin Oncol* 1996; **122**: 59-62

18. Zhou XD. Advances in primary liver cancer research (Editorial comments). *Chin J Cancer Res* 1994; **6**: 1-2

19. Tang ZY. Results of treatment of primary liver cancer in China. *Reg Cancer Treat* 1992; **3-4**: 136-139

20. Makuuchi M, Kosuge T, Takayama T *et al.* Surgery for small liver cancer. *Semin Surg Oncol* 1993; **9**: 298-304

21. Zhou XD, Tang ZY, Yu YQ. Current management of hepatocellular carcinoma. *Hepato-Gastroenterol* 1991; **38** (suppl 1): 46-55

22. Zhou XD, Yu YQ, Tang ZY, Ma ZC. Results of liver resection for primary liver cancer. *J Hep Bil Pancr Surg* 1994; **2**: 118-122

23. Zhou XD, Yu YQ, Tang ZY. Advances in surgery for hepatocellular carcinoma. *Asian J Surg* 1994; **17**: 34-39

24. Zhou XD, Tang ZY, Yu YQ *et al.* Surgical treatment of recurrent hepatocellular carcinoma. *Hepato-Gastroenterol* 1993; **40**: 33,3-336

25. Zhou XD, Tang ZY, Yu YQ *et al.* Recurrence after resection of alphafetoprotein-positive hepatocellular carcinoma. *J Cancer Res Clin Oncol* 1994; **120**: 369-373

26. Rand RW, Rand RP, Eggerding F, DenBesten L, King W. Cryolumpectomy for carcinoma of the breast. *Surg Gynecol Obstet* 1987; **165**:392-396

BI Carr

28

Chemotherapy

BI Carr

You need not finish the task, nor are you free to desist from trying.

R. Tarfon. Avot B16

BIOLOGICAL CONSIDERATIONS

The hepatic artery

The portal vein supplies approximately 80% of oxygenated blood to the normal liver. By contrast, hepatocellular carcinomas (HCC) receive a similar percentage of their oxygenated blood from the hepatic artery and its branches. This functional difference in the blood supply, particularly to well vascularized tumors (those with a neovasculature), has led numerous investigators to deliver chemotherapy to the hepatic artery as a means of selectively delivering drugs to the tumors that are supplied by it. Although this method of drug delivery has been sanctioned by both instinct and usage, it also depends upon an enhanced relative hepatic uptake by the liver of the drug that is delivered by this route, and particularly by the assumption that the tumor will take up relatively more of the drug than the surrounding liver. Table 28.1 shows that the hepatic uptake of various drugs is critically dependent upon the blood flow rate. In addition, various drugs are taken up to a greater or lesser extent by the liver when they are delivered via a regional route and some drugs are taken up more efficiently than others (Table 28.1). On this basis, FUDR (5-fluorodeoxyuridine) would be the drug of choice for regional drug delivery. Unfortunately, there is little evidence that it has any useful activity against HCC. Interestingly, the same drugs mentioned in Table 28.1, which have a relative advantage for hepatic uptake are quite dependent upon a reduction in the hepatic arterial blood flow. Table 28.1 clearly shows great differences in the relative regional drug delivery advantage (RD) for five drugs when given at two different blood flow rates. This consideration is clearly important and as a consequence of which many investigators have tried to combine regional drug delivery with a slowing of the hepatic arterial blood flow by various hepatic artery occlusive agents (Table 28.8). In addition to a relative advantage in hepatic uptake, it is just as important for there to be a relatively greater uptake by the tumor than the liver. This is the idea behind delivery of chemotherapy into the hepatic artery. Unfortunately, as post chemotherapy monitoring of liver function tests shows, it is impossible to get a complete separation of chemotherapy delivered to the tumor from chemotherapy that is also delivered to the underlying liver. This is relatively unimportant for the treatment of metastatic tumors which metastasize and grow in an essentially normal liver. However, the liver that bears HCC is usually abnormal and therefore at a greater risk to damage. The normal liver is the organ par excellence for adapting to and detoxifying xenobiotic agents such as cancer chemotherapeutic drugs, which are usually cytotoxic agents. By contrast, the cirrhotic liver or the liver that has been damaged by chronic hepatitis has a greatly decreased ability to deal with such toxins.

Table 28.1– Regional drug delivery advantage (RD) for selected anticancer drugs at various regional blood flow rates (Q)

Drug	Q = 10 ml/min RD	Q = 1,000 ml/min RD
FUDR	2,501	26
5-Fluorouracil	401	5
BCNU	101	2
Doxorubicin	91	1.9
Cisplatin	41	1.4

Spread of HCC

There is a characteristic propensity for HCC to spread within the liver. This may occur across tissue planes as in the diffuse type of HCC, or via infiltration of the portal vein. Approximately 90% of HCCs greater than 5 cm diameter have microscopic invasion of the portal vasculature and almost 20% of HCCs less than 1 cm also have microscopic evidence of invasion of the portal vein, leading directly to spread within the liver.[1] In addition to this spread, the whole cirrhotic liver may be regarded as a pre-neoplastic organ, given the propensity of cirrhotic nodules to develop into HCC with time.[2] As a consequence, the whole liver of a patient with HCC may be regarded as being at risk from spread of tumor or for the development of additional primary foci of HCC.

Radiology

The evaluation of the patient with HCC needs to take into account the known tendency of HCC to spread within the liver. For this purpose, advances in radiologic techniques have shown that a number of procedures add to the information provided by the last generation of CT scanners.[3] Firstly, the new generation of helical (spiral) fast CT scanners when used in association with a fast bolus of dye, gives greater clarity and delineation of small tumors than the old type of CT scan. In addition, CT portography (or CT arteriography for the cirrhotic liver or the liver with portal hypertension) is capable of identifying more tumors and smaller tumors than conventional CT scanning alone (See Chapter 23). Clearly, if chemotherapy is to be directed into the relevant feeding hepatic artery that supplies a known tumor, it is important to know whether there are satellite lesions or contralateral lesions in the other lobe of the liver that might have been missed by conventional CT scanning techniques.

The patient with HCC usually has two diseases

Approximately 80% of HCCs arise on the basis of chronic hepatitis and/or cirrhosis. The cirrhosis may be caused by viral or non-viral aetiologies. This has significance for the radiologic evaluation of patients with HCC, since some of the smaller tumors with a poorly developed neovasculature may be difficult to distinguish from hyperplastic or cirrhotic nodules, and also because the underlying liver is diseased and this has quite specific consequences for the chemotherapist (see below).

Table 28.2 – International UICC (TNM) staging system for HCC

Stage	Group	Description
I	T1	Solitary HCC <2.0 cm, no vascular invasion
II	T2	Solitary HCC of any size without vascular invasion or multiple unilobar HCCs <2.0 cm without vascular invasion, or, solitary HCC <2.0 cm with vascular invasion.
III	T3	Single HCC >2 cm or multiple unilobar HCCs with vascular invasion
IV	T4	Bilobar HCCs, or major hepatic or portal vein invasion by tumor

SPECIAL PROBLEMS OF CHEMOTHERAPY FOR HCC

The chemotherapy of HCC is dominated by two factors: the need to deliver adequate doses of a suitable drug to the tumor on the one hand, and on the other, the sensitivity of the liver that has been damaged by cirrhosis to further damage inflicted by cytotoxic chemotherapeutic agents. The latter is the special province of the chemotherapist in dealing with HCC. It makes the management of HCC quite different from the management of metastatic tumors that have spread to (an otherwise normal) liver from extra-hepatic primary sites. The patient with HCC and cirrhosis presents problems to the oncologist that are peculiar to this disease type.

Hepatocellular damage from cirrhosis

1. Because the underlying liver that bears the HCC is damaged before the delivery of any chemotherapy, certain practical problems arise. Firstly, the hepatocellular damage of the underlying liver results in a decreased ability of the liver to metabolize xenobiotics and cancer chemotherapeutic agents. This leads to an increased half life of the chemotherapeutic agents in the blood stream, since the liver is unable to metabolize and excrete them with the same efficiency as the normal liver. Consequently, if cytotoxic drugs that have hepatic metabolism are given at the same doses as for a patient without cirrhosis, toxic side effects may be increased, particularly on the granulocyte and platelet precursors, resulting in bone marrow suppression.

2. Secondly, the chemotherapy has a direct effect on the underlying liver, since there is no means of separating the effects of the chemotherapy on the tumor from the effects of the chemotherapy that is delivered by the same vasculature to the surrounding liver. Basically, the normal liver that is involved with metastatic cancer can sustain similar doses of chemotherapy delivered into the hepatic artery as given intravenously. This is not true of diseased hepatocytes, which are more sensitive to damage by the same agents when given through the hepatic artery, since higher concentrations are delivered into the liver by this means. The diseased liver is thus at greater risk of further damage from regional

chemotherapy (and indeed also by systemic chemotherapy). Typically, we find that most patients with a bilirubin greater than 2.5 mg/ml cannot tolerate standard doses of chemotherapy when given into the hepatic artery. Indeed, the necessity for reducing the doses of chemotherapy in this circumstance is such that often only sub-therapeutic doses of chemotherapy can be given, with poor tumor responses as a result. As a consequence, such patients often die as much from their underlying liver disease as from their tumor. A failure to discriminate between these two causes of death has led to much confusion in the HCC literature, since reported overall survivals often do not discriminate between death from end-stage liver disease and death from tumor growth. This may have contributed considerably to the pessimism of physicians faced with a patient with HCC, in large part due to failure to carefully select those patients who can potentially benefit from chemotherapy, and whose livers are able to tolerate it.

Portal hypertension

1. Amongst the many results of portal hypertension, those that are of most concern to the chemotherapist include: hepato-fugal blood flow in the liver; esophageal and gastric varices; and the consequences of splenomegaly, namely granulocytopenia and thrombocytopenia. The existence of hepato-fugal flow in the liver of patients with cirrhosis means that some patients with HCC have a distorted arterial-vascular supply, so that chemotherapy delivered into the hepatic artery may be diverted into the portal system and away from the tumor. This is best observed at the time of tumor evaluation or at the time of first chemotherapy by hepatic angiography, when shunting of dye away from the tumor can clearly be seen. The delivery of regional chemotherapy into the hepatic artery under these circumstances is unlikely to be beneficial. In addition, for unknown reasons some HCCs do not have a tumor vasculature, and these tumors do not seem to respond to chemotherapy, as has been commented upon by many authors.

2. The increased back pressure that accompanies portal hypertension causes varices throughout the gastrointestinal system. Such patients can therefore have gastrointestinal bleeds, particularly from esophageal and gastric varices, even before they have any chemotherapy. Although there has been no published benefit of pro-active sclerosing or banding of esophageal varices prior to a bleed, it is our practice to sclerose or band varices of greater than 2+ size when observed during pre-chemotherapy endoscopic evaluation. Patients also have follow-up endoscopies at approximately 3-monthly intervals, to try to limit the complexity of dealing with these patients and their toxicities.

Gastric varices are extremely difficult to manage. They are not usually amenable to injection therapy, and shunting is not normally an option in the complex setting of advanced tumor. Although there is increasing experience with the TIPS procedure, we have experience with only two TIPS procedures in the presence of HCC, and both patients had dramatic increase in tumor growth in the 4 months that followed. In our experience therefore, the presence of bleeding gastric varices is a contraindication to chemotherapy.

3. Typically, patients with non-hepatic primary tumors who have a total white blood cell count of less than $3,000/cm^3$ or platelet count of less than $100,000/cm^3$ of blood have a relative contraindication to chemotherapy, and their low blood counts can be attributable to bone marrow involvement by tumor or prior chemotherapy or radiotherapy. By contrast, the patient with portal hypertension from cirrhosis commonly has a splenomegaly-associated WBC of less than $75,000/cm^3$, as a consequence of sequestration within the spleen. In this situation, the bone marrow is relatively normal. In our practice, we tend to ignore these low counts, in contrast to our practice with non-HCC patients who have other malignancies. The recent advent into routine clinical practice of granulocyte colony stimulating factor and granulocyte-macrophage colony stimulating factor means that we can, at will, increase the total white blood count to greater than $5,000/cm^3$ prior to chemotherapy and usually at any stage after chemotherapy. This has dramatically transformed the safety of giving chemotherapy in the setting of HCC and splenomegaly. Thrombocytopenia is also the frequent concomitant of portal hypertension with or without HCC. Clinical studies are already underway as a result of the cloning of thrombopoietin by several drug companies, which should have a major impact

in the future on the safety of managing patients with HCC by chemotherapy. At the moment, it is only available in the setting of clinical trials, but it is anticipated that it will soon be released for general use. In the interim, patients with HCC who have a platelet count above 50,000 cm^3 can usually be treated with cisplatin with or without embolization. However, it is much more difficult to use doxorubicin in this setting, since both granulocytopenia and thrombocytopenia are dose-limiting factors in the management of HCC patients with cirrhosis who might be treated with doxorubicin. For this reason, cisplatin with its limited mylo-suppressive activity compared to many other chemotherapeutic agents, as well as its activity againt HCC (below), is a particularly attractive drug for use in HCC patients.

Drug resistance

The idea that tumors can develop resistance to the cytocidal actions of many cancer chemotherapeutic drugs arose first from the studies of experimental leukemias in rodents, but was subsequently readily observed in human tumors such as breast cancer. In this situation, oncologists could often obtain a partial tumor response (shrinkage) with a first line of chemotherapy, but then the tumor often grew again. When they switched to different drugs, it was often quite difficult to obtain a subsequent response. This was thought to be due to the fact that tumor cells adapt to the environment of cytotoxic drugs by developing enhanced levels of various detoxification enzymes or enhanced levels of enzymes that are responsible for increasing efflux of drugs out of the cell, such as p-glycoprotein (products of multiple drug resistance genes 1 and 2, mdr1, mdr2). The biology of experimental chemical hepatocarcinogenesis, however, provides quite different evidence, namely that of primary drug resistance. It has been known for over 50 years, from the experiments of MacNider,[4a-c] that rodent livers exposed to a single dose of a hepatotoxin, and then subsequentally challenged with a second or third dose, experience much less hepatotoxicity than after the first dose. Some adaptive mechanism was clearly shown to occur. Further experiments showed that when rodents are treated with chronic hepatocarcinogens, the contained hepatocytes become quite resistant to the toxicity of a variety of hepatotoxins,[5] including many cancer chemotherapeutic agents.[6] This led to the idea that drug resistance may be an inherent characteristic of HCC, possibly as an adaptation to the chronic toxicity of chemical carcinogens (or possibly chronic viral carcinogenic damage also, although there are no experiments on this issue), and is not an adaptive process to the effects of cancer chemotherapy as seen in other tumors. The mechanistic basis of this has been studied for some time. Genes and/or enzymes that are involved in detoxification and are known to be increased in experimental chemical hepatocarcinogenesis and which therefore may be involved in the resistance of human HCC to cancer chemotherapy include:

1. gamma glutamyl transpeptidase
2. glutathione-S-transferase pi
3. epoxide hydrase
4. metaleothionein
5. heat shock cognate genes
6. cytochrome p450 genes
7. quinone reductase
8. multiple drug resistance gene family

Other factors are also important in the relative resistance of HCC to the cytocidal effects of cancer chemotherapy. These include the relative hypoxia at the center of large tumors, since the pecularities of the vasculature often impact on the ability of several chemotherapeutic drugs to access the center of a tumor. Also, hypoxia may interfere with the ability of a drug to act, particularly those drugs involved with redox cycling such as the quinone containing anthracyclene drugs such as doxorubicin (Adriamycin). The cell cycle is also very important in this regard. Many cancer chemotherapeutic agents only work on cells that are actively participating in the cell cycle, particularly in the sensitive DNA S phase of the cell cycle that typically lasts only a few hours. This has a practical consequence for the chemotherapist, since on any one day of the delivery of chemotherapy only a small percentage of the cells of a solid tumor will be in the S phase of the cell cycle during which many of the drugs work. This is one of the most important arguments against single shot chemotherapy for HCC, since very few solid tumors of any type respond dramatically to a single shot of any chemotherapy. It is particularly the case for HCC, where only recurrent administration of chemotherapy produces tumor shrinkage in most instances. The vagaries of the

Table 28. 3 – Staging of HCC patients.[10a-c]

Tumor size		Ascites		Albumin		Bilirubin	
>50%	<50%	(+)	(-)	<3 g/dl	>3 g/dl	>3 mg/dl	<3 mg/dl
of liver volume							
(+)	(-)			(+)	(-)	(+)	(-)

Stage I, all - ve; stage II, 1 or 2 +ve; stage III, 3 or 4 +ve

tumor vasculature may also be an important factor in the variability of results of cancer chemotherapy for HCC. Several factors need consideration here. Firstly, some large tumors may be fed by more than one hepatic arterial branch, and this may require administration of chemotherapy into either the proper hepatic artery or more than one major branch. In addition, the rims of large HCCs may have more than hepatic arterial blood supply, and portal vessels may feed these growing rims. Other arteries, including branches of the diaphragmatic artery, may feed some tumors, particularly those in which the hepatic artery has been damaged by repeated chemotherapy. Also the rims of large growing tumors may have an additional blood supply from the portal vein.

EVALUATION OF HEPATIC TOLERANCE TO CHEMOTHERAPEUTIC DRUGS

There are no standard criteria for identifying patients with poor liver function who are at risk of hepatic decompensation as a result of chemotherapy. We have assessed the use of MEGX and of ICG clearance for this purpose, but have not found any clear predictive value.[7] However, a greater than 30% change in the ICG 15 retention time after one or two chemotherapy treatments serves as a strong warning for us. In general, the baseline bilirubin level is as good a guide as any more sophisticated test. It is rare for a patient with a baseline bilirubin of greater than 3.0 mg/ml to be able to tolerate the full doses of chemotherapy that are normally necessary to achieve a tumor shrinkage. An important factor in minimizing hepatic decompensation has been the use of dose escalation (see below). In treating almost 300 patients with HCC by chemotherapy, I have found this to be the single most useful method for avoiding irreversible hepatocellular failure with chemotherapy.

In view of the importance of the two diseases in patients with HCC, namely the tumor and the cirrhosis, and the strong effect on survival of the underlying non-tumor hepatocellular damage, several groups have attempted a tumor classification system that takes account of the hepatic damage. Probably the two most useful are those of the Liver Cancer Study Group of Japan[8] (or the Child's[9] criteria for hepatic functional reserve) which take into account the level of serum bilirubin, albumin, the presence of ascites, and prothrombin time, and the system developed by Okuda *et al*,[10a-c] (Table 28.3) which includes the same criteria but in addition contains an assessment of the percentage of the liver occupied by tumor (greater than or less than 50%). Survival with more advanced stages of either of these classifications is greatly impaired, simply as a result of the severity of the underlying liver disease. These are important considerations when analyzing the results of any modality of treatment for HCC, since unlike other tumors, the underlying organ dysfunction profoundly affects overall survival. Since neither system takes into account unilober versus bilobar disease, nor presence, or absence of vascular invasion, I prefer the Child's classification for liver damage coupled with the international TNM staging system.

EVALUATION OF TUMOR RESPONSE

Criteria that have been used for tumor size and response to treatment in the past have included the size by CT scan, evaluation of the tumor extent by hepatic angiogram, and blood levels of alpha-fetoprotein or des gamma carboxy prothrombin (DCP or PIVKA2). The most useful and standard criteria are those that have been applied to almost all other solid tumors, namely the partial or complete response as evaluated by CT scan. By definition, a complete response is the disappearance of all evaluable disease by CT scan. A partial response (PR) is a 50% decrease in the product of two perpendicular diameters of tumor, usually as assessed by CT scan measurements. A decrease in a blood marker such as alpha-fetoprotein is not normally considered sufficient evidence of tumor response, since the markers may decrease before or independently of any change in tumor size, for reasons that are not entirely clear. In addition, we have found that the two blood markers, alpha-fetoprotein and PIVKA 2, may respond to chemotherapy independently of each other. A likely explanation is that the markers may be produced by different clones of tumor cells, reflecting the heterogeneity of solid human tumors. However, it is also our experience that some tumors appear to have little change in their size by CT scanning (stable disease) and yet the tumor markers can decrease to normal in association with the chemotherapy. Stablility can last for prolonged periods of time. The significance of this is not clear. We have recently biopsied the tumor of four such patients and have found only necrotic tissue from those same areas which were previously biopsy-positive for HCC. Whether this truly represents the conversion of HCC cells to only necrotic material as a result of the chemotherapy, or is a sampling artifact in which the needle on the second occasion only picked up non-viable cells, cannot be clarified with confidence at present. Following oncologic convention, such patients need to be regarded as 'stable disease', and should probably not be regarded as chemotherapy responders at present.

Some patients have diffuse tumors without well-defined boundaries, and their assessment is particularly difficult. Some of these tumors can be measured by nuclear magnetic resonance imaging (MRI), and some by a disappearance of the tumor vasculature, but these are very difficult tumors to objectively assess. Although the oily agent Lipiodol (ethiodol) has been used in many centers both for diagnosis and for the regional delivery of cancer chemotherapy agents, a change in the Lipiodol deposits by itself is often a difficult guide to tumor response, since the tumors are often heterogeneous with respect to Lipiodol uptake and there is also a tendency for the Lipiodol to disappear with time. In addition, many tumors are much more difficult to assess by CT scan when they contain Lipiodol. As a consequence, we do not use Lipiodol routinely. Typically, when we obtain a tumor shrinkage by chemotherapy, we see initially a decrease in the tumor blood markers, and then a decrease in the tumor neovasculature, followed by a decrease as evaluated by CT scan often by 2-3 months. However, once the tumor shrinkage is obtained, it can often last for several months, even in the absence of further chemotherapy.

Most objective responses of HCC to chemotherapy are only partial responses. The reason for this is unclear. If more than half of the tumor cells are killed and then reabsorbed by the scavenger system of the liver as a consequence of the chemotherapy, why not the rest of the cells in the tumor nodule? In several clinical trials, we have seen an average of about 50% of patients obtaining an objective partial response to the intra-hepatic arterial chemotherapy. However only 5 to 10% of patients obtained a complete response. Whether this is due to an inability of the tumor vasculature to provide access of the drug to all the tumor cells; to a heterogeneity in the vascular supply to tumors, particularly large ones; or to a heterogeneity of tumor cells with respect to drug resistance, is not clear at the moment, but worthy of investigation. We also have the impression that it is more difficult to obtain a partial response with a large as opposed to a small tumor nodule (greater than 10 cm maximum diameter versus less than 5 cm maximum diameter). Whether this also represents difficulties of getting chemotherapy drug into the center of the tumor or is because of differential supply of different parts of the tumor by different blood vessels is not yet determined. However, even a partial response is worth having. We now have many patients who have had a year of chemotherapy and a stable objective partial response and then have had their chemotherapy stopped. Many of these patients continue with stable disease for a year or more subsequent to cessation of their chemotherapy.

PORTAL VEIN THROMBOSIS

The characteristic tendency of HCC to invade the portal vein as assessed by histological means in the majority of HCCs[1, 11] has been to referred to above. This tendency is seen histologically on sections of pathological material in which HCC cells can be observed within the portal vasculature, and also macroscopically as portal vein thrombus on CT scan or by ultrasound. This is a major adverse prognostic sign both for long-term survival after resection and in particular after liver transplantation.

The idea behind delivery of chemotherapy through the hepatic artery is based both on the ability to apparently deliver higher hepatic doses of chemotherapy, as well as to deliver chemotherapy more selectively to the tumor than to the normal liver, since the underlying liver, fed mainly via the portal vein, is thought not to be so significantly impacted by hepatic arterial delivery of chemotherapeutic drugs. However, this assumption does not hold true in the presence of portal venous thrombosis. In the presence of portal venous thrombosis, chemotherapy, particularly chemotherapy with embolization into the hepatic artery, renders the relevant lobes of the liver susceptible to complete hepatic necrosis due to deprivation of both major feeding blood vessels - portal vein by thrombosis and hepatic artery by chemoembolization. As a consequence, the presence of portal venous thrombosis has been a traditional contraindication to the use of hepatic artery chemoembolization. However, it is not a contraindication to the delivery of chemotherapy without embolization to the hepatic artery. In addition, we have recently used biodegradable starch microspheres (Spherex) for vascular occlusion, and found no cases of hepatic decompensation as a result of the Spherex. Also, we have found several instances of reversal of portal venous thrombosis with restoration of blood flow in the portal vein in patients who had major tumor responses to the chemotherapy. Thus, portal vein thrombosis due to tumor growth is a potentially reversible process. Portal vein thrombosis does not seem to be an additional hazard to the delivery of chemotherapy either alone, or with Lipiodol (ethiodol) or Spherex. Quite possibly, it may not be a contraindication to the use of gelfoam embolization, if this can be delivered through a suitably-selective vascular approach.

Patients who are being considered for liver transplant have routine ultrasound-guided biopsies of portal vein thrombus, to determine if there are malignant cells in the thrombus. This is done because of the overridingly important adverse prognostic significance of this finding for HCC recurrence in patients for liver transplantation. The finding of portal vein thrombus due to malignant cell infiltration is thus a current exclusion criterion for treatment of HCC by liver transplantation.

ASSESSMENT OF THE HCC PATIENT FOR CHEMOTHERAPY

Biopsy

It is essential that all patients with a presumptive diagnosis of HCC who are being considered for chemotherapy have biopsy proof of HCC. Without proof of the diagnosis of tumor and the nature of the type of tumor, the choice of drugs becomes random and the analysis of any subsequent data becomes impossible. A core biopsy is always obtained at our institution from any hepatic mass, since fine needle aspiration biopsy sometimes produces insufficient tissue for tumor architecture. In addition, core biopsies provide additional tissue for special stains in case of doubt, or for detailed studies of molecular hepatology and drug resistance genes.

Sometimes a negative biopsy is obtained. In these cases, we perform a hepatic arteriogram and inject Lipiodol. One week later, after clearance of non-specifically retained Lipiodol, a subsequent post-Lipiodol CT scan is obtained. Lipiodol-containing nodules are then biopsied. The finding of Lipiodol on subsequent histologic staining for fat, using dyes such as Sudan red, is used as proof that the needle was actually in the biopsy nodule. A positive biopsy is therefore always of significance. However, a negative biopsy can indicate either that there was no tumor, or that the needle tip simply missed the tumor cells. The use of Lipiodol provides an adjunctive tool for decreasing this uncertainty.

Evaluation of tumor size

We always perform CT scan using fast bolus dye injection using helical (spiral) CT scanning, to obtain two dimensional measurements which can be used to formally assess partial responses. This is done with and without contrast, since some tumors are better seen on the non-contrast scans. The portal and the arterial phases of the CT scan are also assessed separately. In the small proportion of patients whose tumors are not assessable by CT scanning, ultrasound or MRI are done in addition. At the time of the first chemotherapy, a celiac angiogram and hepatic arteriogram are performed to assess the hepatic vasculature and the vessels feeding the tumor. In addition, evidence is sought for centrifugal blood flow and arterial-venous shunting. It should be noted that the hepatic arterial branch artery which feeds the tumor cannot always be assumed to be from the same side as the tumor on CT scanning. Sometimes a tumor on one side of the liver is fed predominantly by an artery from the contralateral hepatic arterial branch. A CT scan of the chest is performed to rule out lung metastases and a bone scan is routinely done to exclude bony involvement. Any bone scan lesion is subsequently evaluated by CT scan, or in the case of the spinal vertebrae, by MRI.

Evaluation of the underlying liver is performed by routine hematology, including complete blood count, differential white count and platelets, prothrombin time and PTT. Routine liver function tests are performed and an ICG clearance is done.

SAFETY TESTS FOR SPECIFIC CHEMOTHERAPY AGENTS

Patients who are scheduled to receive cisplatinum have a baseline creatinine clearance as well as blood electrolytes, calcium, and magnesium values; they all have a baseline audiogram for comparative follow-up audiology studies, since this is one of the most sensitive tests for neurological damage. Patients who are scheduled to have doxorubicin (Adriamycin) have a baseline EKG and MUGA heart scan. Normally, we use a 55% ventricular ejection fraction as a cut-off for doxorubicin administration. Patients with a prior history of angina or coronary artery disease are excluded from doxorubicin treatment. Patients with an elevated creatinine greater than 2.0 mg/ml, baseline hearing loss or neuropathy are normally given another drug such as carboplatinum instead of cisplatinum. Patients are rarely excluded from cisplatinum therapy based upon blood counts alone, unless the baseline platelet count is less than 30,000/cm^3. However, doxorubicin can cause such a profound myelosuppresson that we do not give it to patients with a baseline platelet count of less than 75,000/cm^3 or total white count of less than 3.5/cm^3.

CHEMOTHERAPY FOR HCC

The origin of cancer chemotherapy lay in the use of mustard gas by the armies of the first World War. This was secret military work until it was declassified in the early 1950s with the development of numerous nitrogen mustard analogs and the observation that animals treated with these drugs had diminished lymphoid systems. This realization led rapidly to the use in experimental and subsequently in clinical lymphoma and leukemia. After this, a whole generation of alkylating agents, that irreversibly caused a chemical cross-linking to the strands of DNA, were synthesized and tested. Examples of this type of agent include mechlorethamine (nitrogen mustard), cyclophosphamide, melphalan, and chlorambucil; the nitrosoureas BCNU, CCNU and methal CCNU; as well as dacarbazine and thiotepa. Subsequently, whole new classes of cytotoxic anti-cancer agents were developed including the antimetabolites, such as methotrexate, 5-fluorouracil, 6-thioguanine, mercaptopurine, cytosine arabinoside, and 5-azacydine; the antibiotics, such as actinomycin D, doxorubicin,daunorubicin, mitomycin C, mithramycin and bleomycins; the plant alkaloids such as vincristine and vinblastine; the podophyllotoxins such as VP 16 and VM 26; and miscellaneous drugs such as cisplatinum (cisplatin), carboplatinum, and the taxols (taxol and taxototere). Many of these agents are active only at specific parts of the cell cycle, particularly the antimetabolites. By contrast, the alkylating agents are largely cell-cycle non-specific. In addition to the chemotherapeutic cytotoxic drugs listed above, a variety of hormones have been employed in cancer therapy which do not appear to work in quite the same way as conventional chemotherapy and appear to be largely free of the cytotoxic side effects of the cancer chemotherapeutic drugs. These include the estrogens, the androgens, estrogen and androgen antagonists, prednisone and its derivatives, and the newer hormone receptor antagonists, including the androgen and estrogen receptor inhibitors. These have been used particularly for those tumors that are thought to be hormone sensitive or derived from hormone sensitive organs, such as the breast, prostate, pituitary, thyroid, and possibly the liver.

Route of chemotherapy drug administration

A large number of studies have shown essentially no reproducible objective tumor response rates for many of the common cancer chemotherapeutic agents when given by the intravenous route as single drugs

Table 28.4 – Intravenous chemotherapy for HCC: Single drugs minimal responses

Drug	References
5-FU	12, 14
Doxorubicin	15-18, 31
Mitoxantrone	19, 20
4-Epidoxorubicin	21, 22, 32
Idarubicin	23
VP 16 (etoposide)	24, 27, 31
Dichloromethotrexate	25, 26
Cisplatinum	20, 28, 29
Mitomycin C	30
Neocarzinostatin	32
M-AMSA (amsacrine)	33, 34
Acivicin	21
Ifosfamide	35
Alkylating agents (cylcophosphamide, mustards)	36,37

(Table 28.4). The low response rates are not reported in this table because of the high variability of reported results and confusion in the literature. However, there seems to be a general consensus that none of them has a more than 25% objective response rate in multiple studies, suggesting that they are of low value in the management of HCC. It is therefore of no surprise that combinations of these same ineffective drugs (Table 28.5) also have little activity when used together, since one of the principles of combining drugs is that they should have independent activity when used alone. The objective response rates for the

Table 28.5 – Intravenous chemotherapy for HCC: drug combinations minimal responses

Drugs	References
5-FU + Cytosine arabinoside	41
5-FU + Streptozotocin	39, 42
5-FU + Methyl CCNU	39, 42
5-FU + Mitomycin C	40
5-FU + Multiple drugs	38, 39, 48, 42
Doxorubicin +5-FU	48
Doxorubicin + Bleomycin	47
Doxorubicin + 5-Azacytidine	15
Doxorubicin + Mitomycin C	50
Doxorubicin + Multiple drugs	38, 42, 49
Doxorubicin + Interferon	45
Doxorubicin + Tamoxifen	44
Mitoxantrone + Interferon	46

Table 28.6 – Intra-hepatic arterial chemotherapy for HCC: Commonly used single agents: Responses below 30%.

Drug	References
Cisplatin	51- 53
Doxorubicin	12, 15, 54, 57
4-Epirubicin	58, 59, 68
Mitomycin C	61
FUDR (5-fluoro-deoxyuridine)	12, 56, 60
5-FU	54, 55, 123

drugs in Tables 28.4 and 28.5 are therefore generally low and are not considered to be useful when given intravenously for the management of patients with HCC. There is an enormous literature on this ineffective form of chemotherapy which has been well reviewed by Nerenstone *et al.*[13] The reader is referred to this excellent summary for details of individual studies on systemic chemotherapy. By contrast, several of the agents that appear to be quite ineffective when given by the intravenous route seem to have activity when given via the hepatic artery, particularly for the hypervascular tumors. The most commonly used drugs (Table 28.6) include doxorubicin, cisplatinum, mitomycin C, and to a lesser extent FUDR and possibly neocarzinostatin. Response rates are not in the table but references to the studies are given. This is because there are few studies with single agent chemotherapy given intra-hepatic arterially without some form of additional agents such as Lipiodol (ethiodol) or gelfoam. As a consequence, it is difficult to know what really are the response rates to these drugs. In addition, because much of this work has been done in countries where there is a lot of cirrhosis and chronic hepatitis in addition to HCC, the drugs have commonly been given at doses which would be considered sub-optimal for systemic use. Thus when low response rates have been found, it is difficult to know whether these are due to an inherent lack of sensitivity of the tumor to the action of the drug, or simply due to inadequate dosing. Some recent dose escalation studies have been undertaken in order to attempt to address this uncertainty. Although there have been many studies of intra-hepatic arterial therapy for metastatic tumor in an essentially normal liver, there is almost no literature on the tolerance of the cirrhotic liver to the commonly used cancer chemotherapeutic drugs.

Dosing and frequency of chemotherapy

The ideal dosing for any of the commonly used cancer chemotherapeutic agents has not been established. This is because there is a paucity[90, 53] of dose escalation studies of single agents when used without additional embolization material. However, commonly used doses for the most frequently employed drugs are: cisplatin 60 to 125 mg/m^2; doxorubicin 30-60 mg/m^2; mitomycin C 6-15 mg/m^2; and FUDR (5-fluoro-2-deoxy-beta-uridine, Floxidine) 0.2-0.3 mg/kg/day or approximately 100mg/m^2/day for 5 days. All drug treatments are repeated every 4-6 weeks, depending on the liver functions and the blood counts. All patients are required to have weekly liver function tests, electrolytes and complete blood count to determine the safety, frequency, and the amount of the next dose. Most patients have a decrease in the white count and platelets from 10 to 14 days after the chemotherapy, which returns to normal within 3-5 weeks after the previous dose of chemotherapy. Given the difficulty in judging a safe hepatic dose of any of the chemotherapeutic drugs when given to patients with Child's A and particularly with Child's Class B cirrhosis, we have adopted a simple empirical strategy that seems to be safe for most patients. The first dose of chemotherapy is given at approximately 50% of the calculated target dose. If there is no increase in the bilirubin beyond 1.5 x the baseline value and particularly no significant increase in the prothrombin time, then the dose is escalated on the second cycle to 75% of the target value. Third and subsequent doses are then given at 100% of the target value or more, depending upon the liver functions, but more importantly on the degree of myelosuppression. A total white count of 1.0/cm^3 or less and a nadir platelet count of 25,000/cm^3 or less would justify no further escalation of the dose of chemotherapy. For such nadir counts, we would typically decrease the doses of drugs by at least 25% on a subsequent cycle of chemotherapy. For the first 3 or 4 cycles of chemotherapy at least, the drug administration is repeated every 4-6 weeks, blood counts permitting. An ICG clearance is typically repeated after every third cycle, as are MUGA heart scans for patients being treated with doxorubicin, and creatinine clearance and audiograms for patients being treated with cisplatin. Once an objective partial response is obtained, we typically lengthen the period between cycles of chemotherapy to between once every 2 months and once every 3 months. After several months of stable disease, many patients can have their chemotherapy discontinued and maintain stable disease for several months thereafter. However, we usually obtain repeat CT scans every two to three months in such patients. Published doubling times of human HCC, which vary from 30 to 300 days, suggest that repeated dosing is necessary in order to ensure that most of the cells are eventually 'hit' at some point in the DNA synthesis phase of the cell cycle. Almost all other types of human cancer require multiple repeated treatments to effect partial responses, and human HCC is no different in this regard. Typically, we have found that patients require a minimum of four cycles of treatment before objective evidence of tumor shrinkage is obtained.

Combinations of intra-arterial chemotherapeutic drugs

Very few studies have been reported of combinations of cancer chemotherapeutic agents given alone without additional embolizing agents (Table 28.7). These include doxorubicin plus cisplatin, 5-FU plus mitomycin C; or FUDR, doxorubicin, cisplatin and leucovorin. Reported response rates have generally been higher than with single agents and appear to exceed 40% of the patients treated. Since the reported studies have often used the individual drugs at below the maximum tolerable dose that they might be used at if they had been given as single agents, it is difficult to know whether these combinations truly represent the maximum achievable response rates that might

Table 28.7 – Intra-hepatic arterial chemotherapy for HCC: Combination therapy

Regimen	Response	Reference
5-FU + Mitomycin C	50%	63
FUDR, Leucovorin, Doxorubicin + Cisplatin	41%	62
FUDR, Doxorubicin + Streptozotocin	10%	66
Doxorubicin + Cisplatin	52%	65
FUDR, Leucovorin, doxorubicin, cisplatin	61%	64

have been obtained with fewer agents used at maximum dosing. Some attempts have been made to reduce systemic toxicity after higher dose intra-hepatic arterial drug administration by use of blood chemo-filtration.[128,129] However, hepatotoxicity will limit this approach in the presence of cirrhosis.

Chemotherapy and hepatic arterial occlusion

A large number of studies have been performed with single or multiple cancer chemotherapeutic agents administered together with some form of hepatic arterial occluding agent. The agents most commonly employed with hepatic arterial occlusion (Table 28.8) include: the oily contrast medium Lipiodol (ethiodol), gelatin sponge particles (Gelfoam), and to a lesser extent, degradable starch microspheres (Spherex), which were developed because they are rapidly degraded by plasma amylases and therefore may be safer than Gelfoam; and the irreversible agent polyvinyl alcohol foam (Ivalon). The difficulty with using Ivalon is that since it is irreversible, it is likely to be dangerous in the presence of any form of portal venous thrombosis and because of the irreversible nature of the obstruction, multiple dosing of chemotherapy cannot easily be given. Several recent papers have suggested a rather clever use of autologous tissues, especially the patient's own clotted blood for embolization, but this has not yet come into general usage. Another recently introduced approach for the reversible inhibition of hepatic artery blood flow is that of degradable starch microspheres (Spherex), which are broken down by serum amylases with a half life of approximately 20 minutes. The idea is to introduce a safer form of hepatic artery occlusion than Gelfoam, and recent indications are that it can be safely used even in the presence of portal vein occlusion without causing hepatic decompensation. Recently, other procedures have been devised for the selective hepatic uptake and retention of delivered chemotherapy including microcapsulation of drugs such as mitomycin C; and the use of liposomes, which have so far only been used with doxorubicin and daunorubicin and have been given intravenously.

Table 28.8 – Agents used for hepatic arterial occlusion in HCC

1, Lipiodol (Ethiodol) contrast medium
2. Gelatin sponge particles (Gelfoam[R])
3. Polyvinyl alcohol foam (Ivalon[R])
4. Degradable starch microspheres (Spherex[R])
5. Microcapsules of anticancer drugs
6. Autologus tissue
(e.g. blood clot, muscle, fat, fascia lata)
7. Miscellaneous:
Collagen (Angiostat)
Detachable balloons
Steel coils
Isobutyl-2-cyanoacrylate

Probably the most widely used agent for vascular occlusion has been Lipiodol (ethiodol). This is retained within the hepatic artery for variable periods of time, from hours to weeks. Since it is an oily substance, it needs to be mixed with chemotherapeutic agents together with an emulsifying agent such as lecithin, since otherwise the chemotherapy and Lipiodol separate and the benefits of Lipiodol addition disappear. The actual mechanism of its supposed benefits are unclear, but probably its most useful effect is to retain part of the chemotherapy at the site of the tumor vascular bed, rather than all being washed through and into the general circulation. We have never seen any hepatic decompensation as a result of its use. It seems to be a safer, but less effective means of reducing hepatic arterial blood flow than Gelfoam. Many protocols combine the two agents. Since these comprise the majority of the literature on chemoembolization, the effects of multiple drugs alone without the Lipiodol and Gelfoam cannot be assessed. The precise function of any of the embolizing procedures and how they might add to the effects of the chemotherapy is unclear at the present time. Possible mechanisms include a slowing of the blood flow, resulting in increased uptake of regionally delivered drug; the opening of previously closed vascular channels to the tumor, allowing more chemotherapy to directly access the tumor; effects on the permeability of the neovasculature, again permitting increased delivery of drug to the tumor site; and increased retention of drugs at the tumor site by mixing the drug with a locally retained agent. Several studies have addressed the issue of the effect of embolization alone on the tumor, without addition of chemotherapy (Table 28.9a). These have been done as part of randomization studies, or by studying the effect of surgically induced de-arterialization or surgically induced arterial ligation. Gelfoam alone appears to induce necrosis and some responses, as does surgical de-arterialization, which presumably acts by the same mechanisms of simple physical obstruction of the hepatic arterial flow to the tumor. These procedures are dangerous in the presence of more than mild degrees of hepatocellular dysfunction, such as Child's B or C cirrhosis, and in the presence of portal vein thrombus. They are therefore not suitable for the majority of non-resectable patients. However, some authors have claimed that the chemotherapy together with the embolization does not add to what can be achieved by embolization alone. The problem with these claims is that the chemotherapy has normally been given at low or possibly sub-therapeutic doses, so that its effects cannot be assessed. Also, many patients, as stated above, cannot be given embolization anyway because of their poor liver function. A clear clinical trial, comparing maximally-tolerated chemotherapy given intra-hepatic arterially, versus Gelfoam alone, versus Gelfoam plus the same dose of chemotherapy has never been done, so that this issue has yet to be resolved.

There is an extensive literature on single or multiple agent chemotherapy together with Lipiodol. Many of the papers do not give objective response rates, therefore unfortunately cannot be assessed. Table 28.9b gives a selection of those papers where response rates or survival have been given. There is a wide range from 20 to 50% response rate. Most series do not report more than 30% 2-year survival, and in almost all of them there is no distinction made between death from tumor or death from progressive liver disease. Thus, it is difficult to discern whether treatment failures are due to failure of the chemotherapy on the cancer, or failure of the underlying organ from progressive end-stage liver disease. It may be, therefore, no matter how successful the chemotherapy ultimately proves to be, there may be no escaping the need for liver transplantation once organs become more freely available.

A large number of studies have been reported in which patients have been treated with single or combinations of drugs together with Gelfoam embolization with or without additional Lipiodol (Table 28.9). Overall, doxorubicin (Adriamycin) and derivatives do not appear to give particularly impressive response rates either with Lipiodol or Gelfoam. It is anyway a particularly difficult drug to give in the presence of portal hypertension and splenomegaly, since the low baseline blood counts are further depressed by doxorubicin, making it extremely difficult if not impossible to give satisfactory doses of chemotherapy. Several studies report on the effects of cisplatin with response rates ranging from 16% for a fixed dose of drug to 65% for higher doses of drug (Table 28.9). Cisplatin is particularly attractive for the management of HCC patients because of its reduced myelo-toxicity, although after more than a dozen treatments, many patients get high tone hearing deficits and paraesthesiae. Although it has the potential for nephrotoxicity, aggressive hydration and disresis normally prevent this, particularly when given with the addition of intravenous thiosulfate. In the first decades after its introduction, cisplatin was associated with profound nausea and emesis. However, multiple recent studies with combination high doses of antiemetics, particularly the combination of dexamethasone, metoclopramide and ondansetrone (5-HT3 receptor antagonists) have revolutionized the control of nausea. As a consequence, most of our patients have two or less emetic episodes in the 24 hours after cisplatin therapy. The old fears associated with patient rejection of their chemotherapy because of profound or prolonged nausea have thus essentially disappeared from the oncologic scene. While several studies have employed mitomycin C, it is a difficult drug to use because it is often associated with prolonged and profound thrombocytopenia

Other embolizing agents that have been used include microcapsulation of drug, Spherex, microfibrillar (Angiostat) collagen and autologous tissues such as blood clot. Only small numbers of reports are currently available on any of these modalities, so that their contribution is not clear. Some reports include occlusion of both the hepatic artery as well as the portal vein.[133] In addition, several groups have assessed ethanol injection plus chemoembolization, with results similar to each clone.[134-136]

Experience of intra-hepatic arterial chemotherapy for unresectable HCC at the University of Pittsburgh

The majority of our patients are unresectable, as is the general experience. The mean age was 56 years with

Table 28.9– Intra-hepatic arterial chemotherapy and blood flow obstruction for HCC*

Regimen	Partial Responses	Survival		References
a) Embolization alone				
Lipiodol alone	6%	n/a		67
Gelfoam alone	67%, 62%	39% 2 yr; 33% 3 yr		80, 89, 127
Surgical de-arterialization	n/a	10-15% 1 yr		68
Gelfoam + Steel coils	81%	38% 2 yr		
b) Lipiodol + Chemotherapy				
Doxorubicin	15% necrosis			67
Epirubicin vs	42%	35%	2 yr	74
Epirubicin alone	12%	0%	yr	
Doxorubicin**	48%, 0%	29%	2 yr	68
Epirubicin	n/a	Median	48 days	69
Doxorubicin, Epirubicin, or cisplatin	n/a	38%	2 yr	70
SMANCS (Neocarzinostatin, styrene)	46%	47%	2 yr	71
FUDR or Doxorubicin	66%; 27%	46%, 28%	1 yr	72
Epirubicin	14% (estimate)	Mean	6 months	73
Cisplatin + Doxorubicin	61%			65
Cisplatin	38%, 47%			74,75
c) Gelfoam (+/- Lipiodol) + Chemotherapy				
Doxorubicin, Mitomycin C, 5-FU	67%	Median	14 months resp 6 months non-resp.	78
Doxorubicin, Mitomycin C, Cisplatin	24%	Median	7 months	82
5-FU	14%	20%	2 yr	89
Cisplatin	68%; 22%	26%; n/a	2 yr	80,90
Cisplatin or Doxorubicin	38% or 11%	45%, 35%	2 yr	99
Cisplatin	65%	Median	8 months	88
Doxorubicin	n/a; 43%	30%	2 yr	81,125
Doxorubicin vs 0	33%	24%, 31%	1 yr	83
Doxorubicin vs Epirubicin	15%, 18%	44%	2 yr	86
Cisplatin	16%	38%	2 yr	77
Doxorubicin + Mitomycin C	n/a	53%, 13% Uni, Bilobar	3 yr	76
d) Other embolising agents				
Mitomycin C Microcapsules vs	28%	19%	1 yr	84
Mitomycin C + gelfoam	59%	52%	1 yr	
Mitomycin C + blood clot	n/a	100%	2 yr	85
Cisplatin + aclarubicin microspheres	50%	64%	2 yr	87
Cisplatin + Spherex	62%	Median	11 months	131,132
Mitomycin C, Dox, FUDR + Ivalon	54%	Median	6 months	78
vs same drugs, without Ivalon	78%	Median	6 months	

*Selected studies; ** Dependent on lipiodol uptake; n/a, not available the majority being Caucasian (Table 28.10). Approximately one third of our patients each had an underlying chronic HBV or chronic HCV, 8% had both HBV and HCV, 12% had alcoholic liver disease, and 28% of patients had no hepatitis. 71% of our patients had an associated cirrhosis and 53% had more than three separate tumor nodules identifiable by CT scan. Importantly, almost 60% also had CT scan evidence of portal venous invasion. Many of these also had biopsy-proof of the invasion via the percutaneous needle technique of portal vein biopsy (see above), and the majority also had bilobar tumors.

In addition to the 320 patients treated with chemotherapy in the years 1990 to 1995, an additional 39 patients were untreated by any modality because they refused or because of a bilirubin greater than 3.0 mg/dl. Their median survival was 4.5 months. Of the 320 patients who embarked upon regional chemotherapy, 54 patients or 17% refused or could not tolerate three cycles of chemotherapy for various reasons (excluding those who received liver transplants during their planned chemotherapy treatments). Their median survival was 7.0 months. 266 patients were evaluable for tumor response by virtue of receiving three or more chemotherapy cycles of treatment. They were treated on three chemotherapy trials (Table 28.11). These included doxorubicin plus cisplatin versus doxorubicin plus cisplatin plus Lipiodol; doxorubicin plus cisplatin plus Spherex (degradable starch microspheres), a phase I/phase II trial; and a cisplatin dose escalation study. In addition, a variety of patients were ineligible for any of these studies and were treated with cisplatin and doxorubicin 'off study'. Overall, 64% had objective partial responses or better. The survival of these 266 patients is also shown in Table 28.11C. There is a major difference in survival between responders and non-responders. However, even responders had a frustrating 24% 2-year survival. Approximately 40% of these responders died of progressive hepatic decompensation from their cirrhosis and not because of tumor progression. This indicates that control of the tumor alone is insufficient for increasing patient survival in this large category of HCC patients. Possibly the most important impact of liver transplantation in the future will be on those patients whose tumors respond to chemotherapy, since the liver transplantation can then take care of the underlying disease. A randomized study of liver transplantation plus or minus chemotherapy for advanced stages TNM 3 and 4 HCC is thus badly needed.

Table 28.10 – 320 unresectable HCC patients personally treated with 1/hepatic artery chemotherapy 1990-1995. University of Pittsburgh.

Mean Age (SD)	56± 13 years
Sex:	
M:F	1.5:1
Race:	
Caucasian	72%
Middle Eastern	10%
Oriental	13%
Negro	5%
Concomitant hepatitis:	
B	30%
C	27%
B&C	8%
Negative, no known cirrhosis	28%
Alcoholism	12%
Unknown	5%
Concomitant cirrhosis:	
Yes	71%
No	27%
Unknown	2%
Number of tumors:	
1	26%
2	21%
>3	53%
Portal venous invasion	59%
Lobar involvement:	
Unilobar	24%
Bilobar	76%

FIBROLAMELLAR HCC

Several short reports have appeared in the literature on the chemotherapy of fibrolamellar HCC. There is no convincing evidence that objective tumor response rates can be achieved with any of the drugs that have been tried for adult type HCC when given systemically. There is hardly any literature on intra-hepatic arterial chemotherapy with sizable numbers of patients. We have treated 18 patients over the last 6 years with either intra-venous 5-FU and folinic acid, or intra-hepatic arterial doxorubicin plus cisplatin. Only three minor responses were seen. There is thus a need for new drugs in the management of this relatively slowly growing tumor of young people.

METASTATIC HCC

No single or combination chemotherapy regimen has been shown to give reproducible response rates in excess of 20% of the patients when given intravenously for HCC confined to the liver. It is thus no surprise that no currently available chemotherapy protocol is thought to be useful for metastatic HCC. Patients with extra-hepatic HCC should therefore be treated with new agents in the setting of experimental clinical protocols.

NON-CHEMOTHERAPY DRUGS AND NOVEL APPROACHES

Hepatocyte growth control

The essence of cytotoxic chemotherapy, which has dominated the management of non-resectable tumors of all types since its introduction in the early 1950s, has been that of cell killing. The ideal has been the selective poisoning of tumor cells with the relative sparing of the normal cells. However, to the extent that the metabolism of normal and tumor cells has been found in the main to be frustratingly similar, few drugs have been developed that have been able to exploit biochemical or pharmacological differences between normal and tumor cells. The main difference has depended upon growth rate, since tumor cells have tended to grow faster than normal cells, or to have a slower death rate (apoptotic). The delivery of nonspecific cytotoxins into the blood stream has resulted in death of tumor cells and damage to many normal cell types. The assumption has been made that because of the enhanced growth rate of the tumors, they would be more sensitive to cell poisoning and would recover less quickly than normal cells. To a large extent, this expectation has been realized and cytotoxic chemotherapy has become part of the standard armamentarium of practising clinical oncologists. However, the cancers for which chemotherapy has unambiguously contributed to an extension of life span have been limited to relatively rare ones and include Burkitt's lymphoma, choriocarcinoma, acute lymphocytic leukemia of childhood, Hodgkin's disease, testicular teratocarcinoma, Wilm's tumor, Ewing's sarcoma, Rhabdomysarcoma, and retino-blastoma. Cancers in which chemotherapy has produced objective response rates in a high proportion of patients have included small cell carcinoma of the lung, breast cancer, anal cancer, and ovarian cancer. Even in those cases where greater than 50% of the patients experience objective partial responses, such as in metastatic breast cancer, the contribution of chemotherapy to survival is still controversial. The disappointing contribution of increasingly aggressive doses of combinations of chemotherapy to the enhancement of response rates has led to a re-evaluation of the limitations of chemotherapy and the search for alternative approaches. The latter have always included a biologically based approach to the problem of growth control and its loss during the carcinogenic process.

A great deal of work has been done on experimental chemical hepato-carcinogenesis and on the genes, growth factors and hormones that interplay to control normal hepatocyte growth and the changes in those controls during the carcinogenic process. Several growth factors have been implicated in normal hepatocyte growth and include transforming growth factor alpha, epidermal growth factor, hepatocyte growth factor, insulin, IGF-II (insulin-like growth factor), heparin binding growth factor (basic FGF), angiotensin, neurotensin, endothelian, vasoactive intestinal polypeptide, HSS (hepatocyte stimulatory substance), and ALR (augment of liver regeneration), as well as the cells of the immune system, particularly natural killer (NK) cells. It is also increasingly clear that specific interactions between hepatocytes and their matrix are important in regulating the hepatocyte response to growth factors. Indeed the matrix may even control the availability and release of some growth factors. Some of the matrix components that have been best studied include the collagens, fibronectin, and the laminins. There is already evidence for an increased expression of TGF alpha and IGF-II in experimental and clinical HCC. In addition, it is clear that hepatocyte growth factors are also balanced by the effect of hepatocyte growth inhibitors in maintaining quiescence and in regulating growth. Amongst the best studied inhibitors are transforming growth factor beta (TGF beta), the activins, the vitamin Ks and probably prothrombin. Additional factors that may be important in the control of hepatocyte growth include the interleukins, the interferons, and the products of various genes such as the tumor suppressor gene p53 and the Rb (retinoblastoma) gene. The relatively high male to female gender ratio of human HCC in cirrhosis

Table 28.11 – 320 patients with unresectable HCC: 1990-1995
Chemotherapy data: University of Pittsburgh

a)	Untreated patients (refused or bilirubin >3.0 mg/dl) (Additional to 320 patients)	39 patients
	Untreated patients survival (median)	4.5 months
b)	Patients tolerating <3 chemotherapy cycles	54/320 (17%)
	Survival of patients not tolerating chemotherapy (median)	7.0 months
c)	266 Evaluable patients:	
	Objective (CT) responses (PR & CR)	64%

Evaluable patient survival	**Years**		
	1	**2**	**3**
Responders	68%	24%	15%
Non-Responders	17%	0%	0%

d)	Chemotherapy regimens	1) Doxorubicin & Cisplatin ± Lipiodol
		2) Doxorubicin & Cisplatin + Spherex (DSM)
		3) Cisplatin dose escalation

PR = partial response; CR = complete response

(only) has led to the idea that the sex steroids may also play a role in the control of growth. As a consequence, both androgenic and estrogenic hormones have been studied for their effects on growth control in cells, in animals and in humans. Recently, the observation that one of the most useful blood markers for HCC is the immature prothrombin, des gamma carboxy prothrombin (DCP) or PIVKA-II (protein-induced by vitamin K absence) has led to direct experimental evidence that compounds of the vitamin K family may have growth regulatory and hepatoma inhibitory actions, since the DCP or PIVKA-II is produced because of a defect in the metabolism of vitamin K in HCC. Clinical trials are currently ongoing to assess the usefulness of vitamin K in the management of experimental and clinical HCC. More importantly, novel vitamin Ks with up to 200 fold greater growth inhibitory potency than naturally-occurring K1 are currently at the stage of experimental testing. The era of gene therapy has resulted from the ability to identify and clone various genes that are thought to be important in the regulation of growth control. The plausibility of this type of therapy has arisen with the ability to incorporate these genes into vectors that can then be administered into patients by direct injection into the tumor or through the blood supply with homing into the liver. An example of this is the experimental use of wild type p53, given the large spectrum of p53 mutations in human HCC. The next few years will almost certainly see an increase in the studies of novel growth factors or growth factor inhibitors, or growth factor receptor modifying drugs, as new knowledge concerning hepatic growth control becomes translated into experimental clinical drug designs.

Two hormones in particular have been the subject of clinical trials in HCC. These are tamoxifen, an estrogen antagonist, and the androgen antagonists luprolide and flutamide. Tamoxifin has been in clinical use for many years as an essentially non-toxic modifier of breast cancer, particularly in post-menopausal women. Its advantage is that it is easy to give (by tablets), relatively cheap and safe. However, as so often, an initial encouraging report of its activity in HCC has been followed up by conflicting reports of its effectiveness. Indeed, even the initial report did not actually show tumor responses, but only suggested enhanced patient survival, which is normally a consequence of tumor responses. The emerging consensus is that even though it is easy to give, it probably does not contribute to responses in HCC. If it affects survival, possibly it does so by actions on the cirrhosis. The pronounced gender bias of HCC in favor of males in cirrhosis has led to the idea that an inhibition of the male hormone pathway should impact HCC growth, at least in males. However, a large randomized study from a European collaborative group (EORTC) has unfortunately not provided support for the activity of at least two drugs in this category (Table 28.12).

The idea that the immune system has an important role in controlling the growth of cancer cells or at least in interfering with the development of cancers (immune surveillance) has led to a long history of attempts to boost the immune system in patients who have a variety of cancers. The only cancers for which there is encouraging evidence for this have been melanoma and renal cancer. However, several studies have focused on using the interferons (alpha or beta) in human HCC. Only one study has given encouraging evidence for this, but at extremely high doses that would not be tolerated by most Western patients. A variety of studies have begun to appear in the use of the interleukins, particularly IL-2 and IL2 with or without lymphocyte activated killer (LAK) cells (Table 28.12). So far the results using immunotherapy have not been encouraging, but with refinements in technique and potency of immune modulation, further trials will undoubtedly appear.

In addition to the use of gene therapy to replace the activity of suppressed genes that are thought to be important in growth control, or to induce the activity of genes that are thought to be important in suppressing growth control (above), two other approaches are worthy of mention. These are the drugs that are thought to be involved in the modification of drug resistance, and the idea of neovascular endothelium as a target for chemotherapy. Several genes are thought to be important in the phenotype of drug resistance, particularly the multiple drug resistance gene (p-glycoprotein). Various experimental strategies have already started to appear in an attempt to suppress the proteins of this gene family. In addition, several agents such as quinidine, verapmil and the phenothiazines, that are known to modify the membrane activities associated with drug transport, have also been involved in clinical trials. The immune suppressive drugs cyclosporin A and

Table 28.12 – Non-cytotoxic therapies

	References
Hormones, nutrients, gene therapy	
Tamoxifen	91-94, 124
LH-RH analog+ Tamoxifen (anti-estrogen)	95
LH-RH analog+ Flutamide (anti-androgen)	
Nilutamide (anti-androgen)+1- LH-RH analog	96
Cyproterone acetate (anti-androgen)	97
Vitamins K	115, 116, 119
Gene therapy: Wild type p53, Rb	117, 118, 120, 126
Immune modulation	
Interferons	45, 99, 101, 102
Interferon as chemopreventive	100
Interferons + chemotherapy	103, 104
IL-2+ melatonin	105
IL-6	106
LAK cells +1- IL-2	121, 122
Radiation	
Conformal external beam radiation	107
^{131}1- Anti-ferritin antibody	108, 109
^{131}I- Lipiodol	110, 111
^{90}Yttrium microspheres	112, 114

FK506 are also known to modify experimental drug resistance and have been the subject of clinical trials in several tumor types. Finally, many tumor types have been documented to induce a neovasculature which is thought to be important in the enhanced oxygen and metabolite requirements that accompany the enhanced tumor growth. This is particularly well-studied at a clinical level in the case of HCC, for which a neovascularization is characteristic and is associated with the majority of (but not all) HCCs. If the continued HCC growth is dependent upon the growth of the neovasculature, then the neovasculature itself is a legitimate and rational target for controlling the HCC growth, which is dependent upon it. Recently, the normal and carcinogen-altered endothelial cells of many tumor types have been the subject of cell biological and molecular studies, particularly with a view to understanding their growth characteristics and their responses to known growth factors and hormones such as basic FGF (fibroblast growth factor) and VEGF (vascular endothelial growth factor), TGF beta, and alpha-V, beta-3 integrin. Compounds of the heparin family are already known to have endothelial growth inhibitory actions, and recently reports have appeared on heparin analogs that retained their endothelial growth inhibitory effects without having the associated anti-coagulant activities. If they also work *in vivo* on human HCC, they may prove to be an important and exciting addition to the chemotherapeutic options.

LIVER TRANSPLANTATION AND HCC: WE STILL NEED IT

One of the major problems of the management of HCC patients is that many of their tumors arise on the basis of an already dysfunctional liver. Even with the best chemotherapeutic regimens, a good proportion of patients, particularly those with a bilirubin greater than 3.0mg/ml cannot tolerate any form of chemotherapy. There is thus an important need for non-cytotoxic chemotherapeutic agents, as listed in the previous section. However, even in the circumstance in which major tumor responses can be induced by chemotherapy, patient survival is still limited by the progressive liver disease of the underlying cirrhosis, which is the presumptive causal factor in the generation of the HCC. Up to now, liver transplantation has had its greatest impact on the management of small HCCs, particularly on those of less than 5 cm without vascular invasion accompanied by cirrhosis, which could not easily be resected because of the underlying cirrhosis. As aggressive chemotherapy for HCC becomes more successful, the problem of dealing with the underlying cirrhosis will remain. Once more donor livers become available, then it will be important to transplant HCC patients whose tumors have had a major response to chemotherapy. Increased organ availability will likely occur either through advances in xeno-transplantation or in the ability to split donor livers into several liver fragments that could be transplanted into several recipients. It is predicted that those patients with advanced-stage non-metastatic HCC who have had an objective partial tumor response to chemotherapy should be the next category of patients whose survival will be enhanced by liver transplantation. To this author's mind, the most rational next step is to determine if a chemotherapy-induced major tumor response coupled to a subsequent liver transplantation might not enhance the survival of these patients, most of whom do not survive beyond 2 years at present. On account of the underlying cirrhosis, we still have to consider liver transplantation in the management of advanced stage HCC, and as with so many other tumors before it, the best management of HCC will probably be multimodality therapy, with either resection plus chemotherapy or liver transplantation plus chemotherapy for those patients whose tumors arise on the basis of cirrhosis – the majority.

CONCLUSION

Most patients with HCC in countries in which there is no surveillance program, usually present in an advanced and unresectable stage. The main treatment is therefore likely to be some form of medical management. For tumors greater than 3 cm or multifocal tumors, this is still likely to be chemotherapy or some form of hormonal therapy in the future. Most surgery for non-minimal disease as well as all chemotherapy is constrained by the presence of two diseases, namely the HCC and the cirrhosis. It is the cirrhosis that usually limits both modalities of treatment. The majority of patients with HCC do not die of their HCC *per se*, but of the underlying cirrhosis and end-stage liver disease, although this can be exacerbated by growth of diffuse type HCC. Future results of clinical trials need to clearly indicate whether survival is diminished by hepatocellular failure due to the underlying chronic liver disease or from tumor growth.

Although a great many studies of the effects of chemotherapy on HCC have been performed, no clear survival advantage has so far been claimed for the effects of chemotherapy. In part this may be due to patient selection, since so many patients die of underlying liver disease, which is usually not specified in overall survival results. Also, most studies of intra-hepatic arterial chemotherapy have tended to use lower doses of chemotherapy than would have been used for systemic use. The probability is that most patients in these clinical studies received suboptimal dosing of drug. As a result, many drugs that are thought to have been minimally effective may only be so described based upon suboptimal dosing. For several of our most commonly used drugs, the optimal dose in non-cirrhosis and in Child's A or B stage cirrhosis has not really been defined. It is thus no surprise that when mixtures of drugs are put together at suboptimal doses, they show no advantage over single drugs. Thus, there is an important need to define the optimal (maximum tolerated) dose of each of the commonly used drugs, in normal liver and in Child's A and B stage cirrhosis, as a preliminary to putting combinations of drugs together. Since the tolerance to chemotherapy and the survival of the patient is clearly related to the stage of cirrhosis, it is important in future cancer chemotherapy clinical trials to separate the responses to chemotherapy and particularly of survival stratified by Child's or other staging system of chronic liver damage, otherwise non-comparable patients are lumped together. Given that more aggressive intrahepatic arterial chemotherapy with or without embolization seems to be resulting in consistent response rates of greater than 40% in series from several institutions in the last few years, it might be expected that this would have a positive impact on survival. In order to show this, it will probably be best to concentrate on those patients with the least advanced underlying liver disease, such as non-cirrhotics and patients with Child's A cirrhosis. With the large number of prognostic variables and the huge differences in reported response rates to various drugs and drug combinations, probably for the reasons given above, patients should probably only be treated within the confines of a clinical trial. This is particularly true of metastatic disease for which nothing at present seems to work.

Several studies have suggested that embolization does not add to chemotherapy and that chemotherapy does not add to embolization. These two modalities probably work through different mechanisms and in theory should be additive if not synergistic. Several possible explanations could be given for the failure thus far to show additive advantages of the combination, including the use of sub-therapeutic doses of chemotherapy and the achievement of maximum responses with either modality alone. Although it is assumed from the higher reported response rates, that intra-hepatic arterial chemotherapy is superior to intravenous chemotherapy, there has not been a randomized trial to actually prove the point, and this is needed. Also, there needs to be a randomized trial of intra-hepatic arterial chemotherapy, given at optimal doses compared to embolization alone, compared to embolization plus the same doses of chemotherapy, in patients with excellent liver function. Only then can we answer some of the important questions which can and should be answered with the modalities currently available. As with so many other tumors, optimal results will probably result from multi-modality therapy with some form of neoadjuvant or adjuvant chemotherapy coupled with surgery, in the form of resection or transplantation. The latter has the great advantage of having the potential for curing the underlying liver disease.

REFERENCES

1. Ohto M, Kondo F, Ebara M. Pathology diagnosis and treatment for small liver cancer. In: Tobe T *et al.* (eds) *Primary Liver Cancer in Japan* 1992; Springer-Verlag, Tokyo and New York pp:
2. Shiratori Y, Shiina S, Imamura M, *et al.* Characteristic difference of hepatocellular carcinoma between hepatitis B and C viral infection in Japan. *Hepatology* 1995; **22**:1027-1033.

3a. Matsui O, Takashima T, Kadoya M, *et al.* Dynamic computed tomography during arterial portography: the most sensitive examination for small hepatocarcinomas. *J Comput Assisted Tomagr* 1985; **9**:19-24.

3b. Baron RL. Understanding and optimizing use of contrast material for CT of the liver. *Am J Radiol* 1994; **163**: 323-331.

4a. MacNider, WdB. A study of the acquired resistance of fixed tissue cells morphologically altered through processes of repair. III. The resistance to chloroform of a naturally-acquired atypical type of liver epithelium occurring in senile animals. *J Pharm Exp Ther* 1936; **56**: 383-387.

4b. MacNider WdB. A study of the acquired resistance of fixed tissue cells morphologically altered through processes of repair. IV. Observations on the resistance to the toxic action of chloroform. *J Pharm Exp Ther* 1937; **59**: 393-398.

4c. Haddow A. Cellular inhibition and the origin of cancer. *Acta Union Inter Contra Cancer* 1938; **3**: 342-352.

5a. Farber Parker S, Gruenstein M. The resistance of putitive premalignant liver cell populations, hyperplastic nodules to the acute cytotoxic effects of some hepatocarcinogens. *Cancer Res* 1976; **35**: 3279-3287.

5b. Judah DL, Legg RF, Neal GE. Development of resistance to cytotoxicity during aflatoxin carcinogenesis. *Nature* 1977; **265**: 343-345.

6. Carr BI, Laishes BA. Carcinogen-induced drug resistance in rat hepatocytes. *Cancer Res* 1981; **41**: 1715-1719.

7. Cattano CG, Carr BI. Is ICG clearance predictive of acute hepatic intolerance to intra-arterial cancer chemotherapy? *Hepatology* 1991; **14**: 890.

8. Liver Cancer Study Group of Japan. The general rules for clinical and pathological study of primary liver cancer. *Jpn J Surg* 1989; **19**: 98-129.

9. Child CG,Turcotte J. In: Child CA (ed) *The Liver and Portal Hypertension*. Philadelphia. WB Saunders, Co. 1965, p602.

10a. Okuda K, Ohnishi K. Prognosis of hepatocellular carcinoma. In: Okuda K, Ishak KG (eds) *Neoplasms of the Liver.* Springer-Verlag, Tokyo and New York 1987, pp: 407-415.

10b. Okuda K, Ohtsuki T, Obata, *et al.* Natural history of hepatocellular carcinoma and prognosis in relation to treatment: study of 850 patients. *Cancer* 1985; **56**: 918-928.

10c. Okuda K, Obata H, Nakajima Y *et al.* Prognosis of primary hepatocellular carcinoma. *Hepatology* 1984; **4**: 3S-6S.

11. Dodd GD, Carr BI. Percutaneous biopsy of portal vein thrombus: a new staging technique for hepatocellular carcinoma. *Am J Radiol* 1993; **161**: 229-223.

12. Al-Sarraf M, Go T, Kithier K *et al.* Primary liver cancer: a review of the clinical features, blood group, serum enzyme, therapy and survival of 65 cases. *Cancer* 1974; **33**: 574-582.

13. Nerenstone SR, Ihde DC, Friedman MA. Clinical trials in primary hepatocellular carcinoma: current status and future directions. *Cancer Treat Rev* 1988; **15**: 1-31.

14. Luporini G, Labianca R, Pancera G. Medical treatment of hepatocellular carcinoma. [Review] *J Surg Oncol* 1993; (Suppl) **3**:115-118.

15. Olweny CL, Katonge-Mbidde E, Bakendeka S *et al.* Further experience in treating patients with hepatocellular cancer in Uganda. *Cancer* 1985; **46**: 2717-2722.

16. Sciarrino E, Simonetti R, LeMoli S *et al.* Adriamycin treatment for hepatocellular carcinoma: Experience with 109 patients. *Cancer* 1985; **56**: 2751-2754.

17. Chlebowski RT, Brzechwa-Adjukiewica A, Cowden A *et al.* Doxorubicin (75 mg/m^2) for hepatocellular carcinoma: Clinical and pharmacokinetic results. *Cancer Treat Rep* 1984; **68**: 487-491.

18. Ihde DC, Kane RC, Cohen MH *et al.* Adriamycin therapy in American patients with hepatocellular carcinoma. *Cancer Treat Rep* 1977; **61**: 1385-1387.

19. Colleoni M, Buzzoni R, Bajetta E, Bochicchio AM, Bartoli C, Audisio R, Bonfanti G,Nole F. A phase II study of mitoxantrone combined with beta-interferon in unresectable hepatocellular carcinoma. *Cancer.* 1993. **72(11)**: 3196-201.

20. Falkson G, Ryan LM, Johnson LA,*et al.* A randomized phase II study of mitoxantrone and cisplatin in patients with hepatocellular carcinoma: An ECOG study. *Cancer* 1987; **60**:2141-2145.

21. Falkson G, Lipsitz S, Borden E, Simson I, Haller D. Hepatocellular carcinoma. An ECOG randomized phase II study of beta-interferon and menogaril. *Am J Clin Oncol* 1995; **18(4)**:287-92.

22. Hochster H, Green M, Spyer J *et al.* 4-Epidoxorubicin (epirubicin); activity in hepatocellular carcinoma. *J Clin Oncol* 1985; **11**:1535-1540.

23. Cheng E, Chun H, Schiff C *et al.* Phase II trial of 4-demethoxydaunoribicin (DMDR) in patients with primary liver carcinoma. *Proc Am Clin Oncol* 1985; **4**:88-

24. Yoshino T, Okazaki N, Yoshino M *et al.* Phase II trial of etoposide in patients with hepatocellular carcinoma by the Tokyo Liver Cancer Study. *Jpn J Clin Oncol* 1989;**19**:120-

25. Tester W, Donhower R, Eddy J *et al.* Evaluation of weekly escalating doses of dichloromethotexet in patients with hepatocellular carcinoma and other solid tumors. *Cancer Chemother Pharmacol* 1982;**8**:305-310.

26. Vogel C, Adamson R, DeVita V *et al.* Preliminary clinical trials of diachlorametatrexate (NSC-29630) in hepatocellular carcinoma. *Cancer Chemother Rep* 1972;**56**:249-258.

27. Melia WM, Wilkinson M, Portmarin BC, *et al.* Hepatocellular carcinoma in the non-cirrhotic liver: a comparison with that complicating cirrhosis. *Q J Med* 1984;**211**:391.

27. Cavalli F, Rozencweig M, Goldhirsch A, Hansen HH. Phase II study of oral VP-16-213 in hepatocellular carcinoma. *Eur J Cancer Clin Oncol* 1981;**17**:1079-1082

30. Cheirspula A, Leelasthekaul S, Auethaveekiat V *et al.* High dose mitomycin C: activity in hepatocellular carcinoma. *Cancer Chemother Pharmacol* 1989;**24**:50-

31. Melia WM, Johnson PG, Williams R. Induction of remission in hepatocellular carcinoma. *Cancer* 1983;**51**:206-210.

32. Falkson G, Von Hoff D, Klaasen D *et al.* A Phase II study of neocarzinostatin (NSC-157365) in malignant hepatoma. ECOG group pilot study. *Cancer Chemother Pharmacol* 1980;**4**: 33-36.

33. Falkson G, Koetzer B, Klaasen D. Phase II study of m-AMSA in patients with primary liver cancer. *Cancer Chemother Pharmacol* 1981;**6**:127-129.

34. Bukowski R, Legha S, Saiki J *et al.* Phase II trial of m-AMSA in hepatocellular carcinoma; a Southwest oncology group study. *Cancer Treat Rep* 1982;**66**:1651-1652.

35. Thongprasert S, Klunkin K, Phornphuthul K *et al.* Phase II study of ifosfamide in hepatoma. *Eur J Clin Oncol* 1988;**24**: 1795-

36. South African Primary Liver Cancer Research Group malignant hepatoma-controlled therapeutic trials. *S African Med J* 1967; **41**:309-314.

37. Plengvanit U, Viranuvanuvatti V. Treatment of primary carcinoma of the liver with nitrogen mustard and prednisolone. *Am J Gastroenterol* 1964;**42**:521-528.

38. Bezwoda WR, Weaving A, Kew M *et al.* Combination chemotherapy of heaptocellular cancer: comparison of adriamycin + VM26 + 5-fluorouracil with mAMSA + VM26 + 5-fluorouracil. *Oncology* 1987; **44**: 207.

39. Falkson G, Moertel CG, Lavin P *et al.* Chemotherapy studies

in primary liver cancer. *Cancer* 1978;**42**:2149-2156.

40. Umsawasdi T, Chainuvati T, and Viranuvatti V. Combination chemotherapy of hepatocellular carcinoma with 5-fluorouracil and mitomycin-C. *Proc Am Assoc Cancer Res* 1978;**19**:193-

41. Gailani S, Jolland J, Falkson G *et al*. Comparison of treatment of metastatic gastrointestinal cancer with 5-fluorouracil to a combination of 5-FU with cytosine arabinoside. *Cancer* 1972; **29**: 1308-1313.

42. Falkson G, MacIntyre JM, Moertel CG *et al*. Primary liver cancer: An Eastern cooperative oncology group trial. *Cancer* 1984; **54**: 970-977.

43. Choi TK, Lee NW, Wong J. Chemotherapy for advanced hepatocellular carcinoma. *Cancer* 1984; **53**: 401-405.

44. Melia WM, Johnson PJ, Williams R. Controlled clinical trial of doxorubicin and tamoxifen versus doxorubicin alone in hepatocellular carcioma. *Cancer Treat Rep* 1987; **71**: 1213.

45. Colleoni M, Nole F, Di Bartolomeo M, de Braud F, and Bajetta E. Mitoxantrone in patients affected by hepatocellular carcinoma with unfavorable prognostic factors. *Oncology* 1992; **49(2)**:139-142.

45. Feun LG, Savaraj N, Hung S *et al*. A phase II trial of recombinant leukocyte interferon plus doxorubicin in patients with hepatocellular carcinoma. *Am J Clin Oncol* 1994;**17(5)**:393-345.

47. Ravry MR, Omura GA, Bartolucci AA. Phase II evaluation of doxorubicin plus bleomycin in hepatocellular carcinoma. *Eur J Cancer Clin Oncol* 1981;**7**:275-280.

48. Baker L, Kaiki J, Jones S *et al*. Adrimycin and 5-fluorouracil in the treatment of advanced hepatoma; a Southwest Oncology Group Study. *Cancer Treat Rep* 1977;**61**:1595-1597.

49. Oon C, Hepatoma and Liver Study Research Group. Clinical studies in Asian patients with unresectable primary hepatocellular carcinoma treated by adriamycin and prednisoline alone or in combination with 5-fluorouracil, vincristine and prednisone. *Singapore Med J* 1978;**19**:192-204.

50. Al-Idrissi H, Ibrahim E, Satir A *et al*. Primary hepatocellular carcinoma in the Eastern province of Saudia Arabia; treatment with combination chemotherapy using 5-fluorouracil, adriamycin and mitomycin C. *Hepatogastroenterology* 1982;**32**:8-10.

51. Kajanti M, Rissanen P, Virkkunen P *et al*. Regional intra-arterial infusion of cisplatin in primary hepatocellular carcinoma. *Cancer* 1986;**58**:2386-2388.

52. Onohara S, Kobayashi J, Itoh Y *et al*. Intra-arterial cisplatinum infusion with sodium thiosulfate protection and angiotensin 2 induced hypertension for treatment of hepatocellular carcinoma. *Acta Radiologica* 1988;**29**:197-202.

53. Carr BI. Escalating cisplatin doses by hepatic artery infusion for advanced stage hepatocellular carcinoma. *Proc Am Soc Clin Oncol* 1996;**15**:432-

54. Doci R, Bignami P, Bozzetti F *et al*. Intra-hepatic chemotherapy for unresectable hepatocellular carcinoma. *Cancer* 1988; **61**:1983-1987.

55. Ramming K, Sparks F, Eilber F *et al*. Hepatic artery ligation and 5-fluorouracil infusion for metastatic colon carcinoma and primary hepatoma. *Am J Surg* 1976;**132**:236-240.

56. Wellwood J, Kady B, and Oberfield R. Treatment of primary liver cancer; response to regional chemotherapy. *Clin Oncol* 1979;**5**:25-31.

56. Ando K, Hirai K, KuboY. Intra-arterial administration of epirubicin in the treatment of non-resectable hepatocellular carcinoma. *Cancer Chemother Pharmacol* 1987;**19**:183-189.

57. Urist M, Balch C. Intra-arterial chemotherapy for hepatoma using adriamycin administered via an implantable infusion pump. *Proc Am Soc Clin Oncol* 1984;**3**:148.

59. Epirubicin study group for HCC. Intra-arterial administration of epirubicin in the treatment of nonresectable hepatocellular carcinoma. *Cancer Chemother Pharmacol* 1987; 19: 183-189.

60. Reed M, Vitkevicius V, Al-Sarraf M *et al*. The practicality of chronic hepatic artery infusion therapy of primary and metastatic hepatic malignancies. *Cancer* 1981;**47**:402-409.

61. Kinami Y and Miyazaki I. The super selective and the selective one shot methods for treating inoperable cancer of the liver. *Cancer* 1978;**41**:1720-1727.

62. Patt YZ, Charnsangavej C, Lawrence D*et al*.. Hepatic arterial infusion of FUDR, leucovorin, adriamycin and platinol (FLAP): effective palliation for non-resectable hepatocellular cancer. *Proc Am Soc Clin Oncol* 1992;**11**:474-

63. Miura T. Treatment of hepatic cancer by hepatic artery infusion chemotherapy. *Cancer Chemother Pharmacol* 1989;**23**: S1212-S122.

65. Carr BI, Iwatsuki S, Baron R *et al*. Prospective randomized study of intra-hepatic artery for chemotherapy with cisplatin and doxorubicin with or without lipiodol for advanced stage hepatocellular carcinoma. *Proc Am Soc Clin Oncol* 1993;**12**: 668-

66. Shildt R, Baker L, Stuckey W. Hepatic artery infusion with 5-FUDR adriamycin and streptozotocin in unresectable hepatoma. *Proc Am Soc Clin Oncol* 1984;**3**:150-

67. Takayasu K, Shima Y, Muramatsu Y *et al*. Hepatocellular carcinoma: treatment with intra-arterial iodized oil with and without chemotherapeutic agents. *Radiology* 1987;**162**:345-351.

68. Kanematsu T, Furuta T, Takenaka K *et al*. A 5-year experience of lipiodolization: Selective regional chemotherapy for 200 patients with hepatocellular carcinoma. *Hepatology* 1989; **10**:89-102.

69. Madden MV, Krige JE, Bailey S, *et al*. Randomised trial of targeted chemotherapy with lipiodol and 5-epidoxorubicin compared with symptomatic treatment for hepatoma. *Gut* 1993; **34(11)**:1598-600.

70. Bronowicki JP, Vetter D, Dumas F *et al*. Transcatheter oily chemoembolization for hepatocellular carcinoma. A 4-year study of 127 French patients. *Cancer* 1994;**74**:16-24.

71. Konno T. Targeting chemotherapy for hepatoma: arterial administration of anticancer drugs dissolved in Lipiodol. *Eur J Cancer* 1992;**28**:403-409.

72. Yamashita Y, Takahashi M, Shinzato J, Bussaka H, Bab Y, and Oguni T. Evaluation of oil-soluble FUDR ester for transcatheter arterial treatment of hepatomas. *Ann Oncol* 1992;**3**:367-370.

73. Higashi S, Shimizu M, Nakashima T *et al*. Arterial-injection chemotherapy for hepatocellular carcinoma using monodispersed poppy-seed oil microdroplets containing fine aqueous vesicles of epirubicin. *Cancer* 1995;**75**:1245-1254.

74. Yoshikawa M, Saisho H, Ebara M *et al*. A randomized trial of intrahepatic arterial infusion of 4'-epidoxorubicin with Lipiodol versus 4'-epidoxorubicin alone in the treatment of hepatocellular carcinoma. *Cancer Chemother Pharmacol* 1994; **33**: S149-52.

75. Shibata J, Fujiyama S, Sata T *et al*. Hepatic arterial injection chemotherapy with cisplatin suspended in an oily lymphographic agent for hepatocellular carcinoma. *Cancer* 1989; **10**:89-102.

76. Taniguchi K, Nakata K, Kato Y *et al*. Treatment of hepatocellular carcinoma with transcatheter arterial emoblization. *Cancer* 1994;**73**:1341-1345.

77. Tinchet J-C*et al*.. A comparison of lipiodol chemoembolization and conservative treatment for unresectable hepatocellular carcinoma. *N Engl J Med* 1995; **332(19)**:1256-61 and Editorial pp:1294-1296.

78. Patt YZ, Charansangave C, Boddie A *et al*. Treatment of hepatocellular carcinoma with hepatic arterial fluoxuridine, doxorubicin, and mitomycin C with or without hepatic artery embolization. *Reg Cancer Treat* 1989;**2**:98-104.

79. Bruix J, Castells A, Montanya X *et al*. Phase II study of transarterial emoblization in European patients with hepatocellular carcinoma: a need for controlled trials. *Hepatology* 1994;**20**: 643-650.

80. Chang JM, Tzeng WS, Pan HB, Yang CF, Lai KH. Transcatheter arterial emoblization with or without cisplatin treatment of hepatocellular carcinoma. A randomized controlled study. *Cancer* 1994;**74**:2449-2453.

81. Vetter D, Wenger J-J, Bergier J-M *et al*. Transcatheter oily chemoembolization in the management of advanced hepatocellular carcinoma in cirrhosis: results of a western comparative study in 60 patients. *Hepatology* 1991;**13**:427-433.

82. Venook AP, Stagg RJ, Lewis BJ *et al*. Chemoembolization for hepatocellular carcinoma. *J Clin Oncol* 1990;**8**:1108-1114.

83. Pelletier G, Roche A, Ink O *et al*. A randomized trial of hepatic artery chemo-embolization in patients with unresectable hepatocellular carcinoma. *J. Hepatol*. 1990;**11**:181-184.

84. Ohnishi K, Tsuchiya S, Nakayama T *et al*. Arterial chemoembolization of hepatocellular carcinoma with mitomycin C microcapsules. *Radiology* 1984;**152**:51-55.

85. Gunji T, Kawauchi N, Ohnishi S *et al*. Treatment of hepatocellular carcinoma associated with advanced cirrhosis by transcatheter arterial chemoembolization using autologous blood clot. *Hepatology* 1992;**15**:252-257.

86. Watanabe S, Nishioka M, Ohta Y *et al*. Prospective and randomized controlled study of chemoembolization therapy in patients with advanced hepatocellular carcinoma. *Cancer Chemother Pharmacol* 1994;**33**:S93-S96.

87. Beppu T, Ohara C, Yamaguchi Y *et al*. A new approach to chemoembolization for unresectable hepatocellular carcinoma using aclarubicin microspheres in combination with cisplatin suspended in iodized oil. *Cancer* 1991;**12**:2555-2560.

88. Sasaki Y, Imaoka S, Kasugai H *et al*. A new approach to chemoembolization therapy for hepatoma using ehtiodized oil, cisplatin, gelatin sponge. *Cancer* 1987;**60**:1194-1203.

89. Lin D, Liaw Y, Lee T *et al*. Hepatic arterial embolization in patients with unresectable hepatocellular carcinoma: A randomized controlled trial. *Gastroenterology* 1988;**94**:453-456.

90. Feun LG, Reddy KR, Yrizarry JM *et al*. A Phase I study of chemoembolization with cisplatin and lipiodol for primary and metastatic liver cancer. *Am J Clin Oncol* 1994;**17**: 405-410.

92. Farinati F, Salvagnin M, Mariana N *et al*. Unresectable hepatocellular carcinoma: a prospective controlled trial with tamoxifen. *J Hepatol* 1990;**11**:297-301.

92. Manesis EK, Giannoulis G, Zoumboulis P *et al*. Treatment of hepatocellular carcinoma with combined suppression and inhibition of sex hormones: a randomized controlled trial. *Hepatology* 1995;**21**:1535-1542.

93. Friedman MA, Demanes DJ and Hoffman PG. Hepatomas: Hormone receptors and therapy. *Am J Med* 1982;**73**:362-365.

94. Engstrom PF, Levin B, Moertel CG, Schutte A. A Phase II trial of tamoxifen in hepatocellular carcinoma. *Cancer* 1990;**65**: 2641-2643.

95. Castell SA, Bruix J, Bru C *et al*. Treatment of hepatocellular carcinoma with tamoxifen: A double blind placebo-controlled trial in 120 patients. *Gastroenterology* 1995;**109**:917-922.

96. Bleiberg H, Grimaldi C, Gay F *et al*. Double blind clinical trial of anti-androgen therapy vs placebo in unresectable hepatocellular carcinoma. *Proc Am Soc Clin Oncol* 1993;**12**:193-

97. Forbes A, Wilkinson ML, Igbal MJ *et al*. Response to cyproterone acetate treatment in primary hepatocellular carcinoma is related to four in three 5a-dihydrotestorone. *Eur J Cancer Clin Oncol* 1987;**23**:1659-1664.

98. Lai CI, Lau JY, Wu PC, Ngan H *et al*. Recombinant interferon-alpha in inoperable hepatocellular carcinoma: a randomized controlled trial. *Hepatology* 1993;**17**:389-394.

99. Kasugai H, Kojima J, Tatsuta M *et al*. Treatment of hepatocellular carcinoma by transcatheter arterial emoblization combined with intraarterial infusion of a mixture of cisplatin and ethiodized oil. *Gastroenterology* 1989;**97**:965-1971.

100. Nishiguchi S, Kuroki T, Nakatani S *et al*. Randomized trial of effects of interferon alpha on incidence of hepatocellular carcinoma in chronic active hepatitis C with cirrhosis. *Lancet* 1995; **346**:1051-1055.

101. Gastrointestinal Tumor Study Group: A prospective trial of recombinant human interferon alpha 2 in previously untreated patients with hepatocellular carcinoma. *Cancer* 1990;**66**:135-139.

102. Sachs E, Di Bisceglie AM, Duscheiko GM *et al*. Treatment of hepatocellular carcinoma with recombinant leuocyte interferon: a pilot study. *Br J Cancer* 1985;**52**:105-110.

103. Lotz JP, Grange JD, Hannoun L *et al*. Treatment of unresectable hepatocellular carcinoma with a combination of human recombinant alpha-2b interferon and doxorubicin: results of a pilot study. *Eur J Cancer* 1994; **30A**: 1319-25.

104. Kardinal CG, Moertel CG, Wie HS *et al*. Combined doxorubicin and alpha-interferon therapy of advanced hepatocellular carcinoma. *Cancer* 1993;**71(7)**:2187-90.

105. Aldeghi R, Lissoni P, Barni S *et al*. Low-dose interleukin-2 subcutaneous immunotherapy in association with the pineal hormone melatonin as a first-line therapy in locally advanced ormetastatic hepatocellular carcinoma. *Eur J Cancer* 1994;**30A(2)**:167-170.

106. Matsuda Y, Kawata S, Nagase T *et al*. Interleukin-6 in transcatheter arterial embolization for patients with hepatocellular carcinoma. *Cancer* 1994;**73**:53-57.

107. Robertson JM, Lawrence TS, Dworzanin LM *et al*. Treatment of primary hepatobiliary cancers with conformal radiaiton therapy and regional chemotherapy. *J Clin Oncol* 1993;**11**: 1286-1293.

108. Order SE, Stillwagon SB, Klein JL *et al*. Iodine 131 antiferritin, a new treatment modality in hepatoma: a radiation therapy oncology group study. *J Clin Oncol* 1985;**3**:1573-1582.

109. Order S, Pajak T, Leibel S *et al.* A randomized prospective trial comparing full dose chemotherapy to I antiferritin: an RTOG study. *Int J Radiat Oncol Biol Phys* 1991;**20**:953-

110. Bretagne J-F, Raoul J-L, Bourguet P *et al.* Hepatic artery injection of I-131-labeled lipiodol. *Radiology* 1988;**168**:547-550.

111. Yoo HS, Park CH, Suh JH *et al.* Radioiodinated fatty acid esters in the management of hepatocellular carcinoma: preliminary findings. *Cancer Chemother Pharmacol* 1989;**23**:S54-S58.

112. Lau W-Y, Leung W-T, Ho S *et al.* Treatment of inoperable hepatocellular carcinoma with intra-hepatic arterial yttrium-90 microspheres: a Phase I and II study. *Brit J Cancer* 1994;**70**: 994-999.

113. Houle S, Yip T-C K, Shepherd FA *et al.* Hepatocellular carcinoma: pilot trial of treatment of Y-90 micropsheres. *Radiology* 1989;**172**:857-860.

114. Andrews JC, Walker SZ, Ackermann RJ *et al.* Hepatic radioembolization with yttrium-90 containing glass micropsheres: preliminary results and clinical follow-up. *J Nuclear Med* 1994;**35**:1637-1644.

115. Wang Z, Wang M, Finn F, and Carr BI. Growth inhibitory effects of vitamins K and their actions on gene expression. *Hepatology* 1995;**22**:876-882.

116. Nishikawa Y, Carr BI, Wang M *et al.* Growth inhibition of hepatoma cells induced by vitamin K and its analogs. *J Biolog Chem* 1995; **270**: 28,304-28,310.

117. Nigro JM, Baker SJ, Preisinger AC *et al.* Mutations in the p53 gene occur in diverse tumor types. *Nature* 1989; **324**: 705-708.

118. Liu T-J, El-naggar AK, McDonnell TJ. Apoptosis induction mediated by wild-type p53 adenoviral gene transfer in squamos cell carcinoma of the head and neck. *Cancer Res* 1995; **55**:3117-3122.

119. Carr BI, Wang Z, Virji MA, and Piper M. Vitamin K inhibits hepatoma cell growth in vitro and in patients. *Proc Am Assoc Cancer Res* 1996;**37**:1485.

120. Ferry N, Duplessis O, Houssin D *et al.* Retroviral-mediated gene transfer into hepatocytes in vivo. *Proc Natl Acad Sci USA* 1991;**88**:8377-

121. Komatsu T, Yamauchi K, Furukawa To, Obata H. Transcatherer arterial injection of autologous lymphokine-activated killer (LAK) cells into patients with liver cancers. *J Clin Immunol* 1990;**10**:167-

122. Onishi S, Saibara T, Fujikawa M *et al.* Adoptive immunotherapy with lymphokine-activated killer cells plus recombinant interleukin 2 in patients with unresectable hepatocellular carcinoma. *Hepatology* 1989;**10**:349-353.

123. Toyoda H, Nakano S, Kumada T *et al.* The efficacy of continuous local arterial influsion of 5-fleurouricill through and inplanted reservoir for a severe advanced hepatocellular carcinoma. *Oncol* 1995;**52**:295-299.

124. Martinez Cerezo FJ, Donoso TA, Donoso L *et al.* Controlled trial of tomoxifen in patients with advanced hepatocellular carcinoma. *J Hepatol* 1994;**20**:702-706.

125. Stuart K, Stokes K, Jenkins *et al.* Treatment of hepatocellular carcinoma using doxorubicin/ethoidized oil/gelatin powder chemoembolization. *Cancer* 1993;**72**:125:33202-3209.

126. Huber BE, Richards CA, and Krenitsky TA. Retroviral-mediated gene therapy for the treatment of hepatocellular carcinoma: an innovative approach for cancer therapy. *Proc Nat Acad Sci USA* 1991;**88**:8039-8043.

127. Kawai S, OkamuraJ, Ogawa M *et al.* Prospective and randomized clinical trial for the treatment of hepatocellular carcinoma—a comparison of lipiodol transcatheter arterial embolization with and without adriamycin. *Cancer Chemother Pharmacol* 1992; Suppl. 1: S1.

128. Curley SA, Newman M, Dougherty TB *et al.* Complete hepatic and venous isolation and extracorporeal chemofiltration as a treatment for human hepatocellular carcinoma: A Phase I study. *Ann Surg Oncol* 1994;**1**:389-399.

129. Poo W-J, Salem R, Pollak J *et al.* Hemodynamically-isolated hepatic perfusion of high dose doxorubicin in patients with advanced liver tumors; a Phase I/II study. *Proc Am Soc Clin Oncol* 1996;**15**:494-

130. Saltz L, Murphy B, Kemeny N *et al.* A Phase I trial of intrahepatic verapamil and doxorubicin. *Cancer* 1994;**74**:2757-2764.

131. Carr BI, Orons P, Zajko P *et al.* Spherex (degradable starch microspheres): a novel and safe embolizing agent in the management of hepatocellular carcinoma (HCC). *Proc Am Soc Clin Oncol* 1994;**13**:605-

132. Taguchi T, Ogawa N, Bunker B *et al.* The use of degradable starch microspheres (Spherex) with intra-arterial chemotherapy for the treatment of primary and secondary liver tumors—results of a Phase III clinical trial. *Reg Cancer Treat* 1992;**4**:161-165.

133. Nakao N, Miura K, Takahashi H *et al.* Hepatocellular carcinoma: combined hepatic, arterial, and portal venous embolization. *Radiology* 1986;**161**:303-307.

134. Tateishi H, Kinuta M, Furukawa J *et al.* Follow-up study of combination treatment (TAE and PEIT) for unresectable hepatocellular carcinoma. *Cancer Chemother Pharmacol* 1994;**33**:S119-S123.

135. Kato T, Saito Y, Niwa M. Combination therapy of transcatheter chemoembolization and percutaneous ethanol injection therapy for unresectable hepatocellular carcinoma. *Cancer Chemother Pharmacol* 1994;**33**:S115-S118.

136. Tanaka K, Okazaki H, Nakamura S *et al.* Hepatocellular carcinoma: treatment with a combination therapy of transcatheter arterial emoblization and percutaneous ethanol injection. *Radiology* 1991;**179**:713-717.

29

Radiotherapy

M Ryu, A Yasuhisa, T Nagashima,
K Isono and T Ogino

Radiotherapy has been of limited value in treating HCC, mostly because of the tumor's radioresistance and radiation hepatitis.[1-5] At first, because radiotherapy was carried out for extreme advanced cancer only, HCC was regarded as a radioresistant tumor. With advances in image diagnostics, however, determination of the exact location of the cancer lesion and irradiation limited to a small field have become possible. Therefore, it would seem appropriate to re-evaluate the use of radiotherapy for HCC. The development of effective new therapy for HCC with portal vein embolus is necessary too. We have carried out radiotherapy for HCC as part of a multidisciplinary therapy.[6,7]

PROCEDURE

All patients were treated with external beam radiation by photon. The radiation field was established by means of US and CT, and confined to the necessary minimum the maximum was 7.5 cm x 14 cm. In other patients, the radiation fields were restricted to less than 8 cm x 8 cm. Radiotherapy was performed at a dose of 50 Gy (equivalent to a time dose fractionation factor (TDF) of 80). For the treatment of patients with HCC with portal vein embolus, TAE was carried out prior to radiotherapy.

US and CT were performed before and after radiotherapy and imaging findings were compared. The response for the main tumor was defined by the following criteria. A partial response (PR) was defined as an estimated decrease in tumor size of 50% or more. A minor response (MR) was defined as an estimated decrease in tumor size of 25% to 49%. A no change (NC) was defined as no significant change. A progressive disease (PD) was defined as an estimated increase of more than 25% in the extent of the lesion. The PR for portal vein embolus was defined a as decrease in the size of tumor embolus or amelioration of portal blood flow.

The radiation effect was evaluated histologically according to Ohoshi and Shimosato's grade:[8] Grade 0 was defined as no change in the irradiated cancer; Grade I as cancer cells remaining viable with minimal effect of radiation; Grade II as more than half of the cancer cells remaining viable; Grade III as more than half of the cancer cells showing degeneration and/or necrosis; Grade IV as no viable cancer cells remaining.

EXPERIENCE AT CHIBA UNIVERSITY

Patients

We treated 75 patients with HCC from 1983 to 1995. We carried out radiotherapy for the main tumor without portal vein embolus in 16 patients, portal vein embolus in 46 patients, hepatic vein embolus in 5 patients and bone metastasis in 8 patients.

Results

1. Imaging findings.
   i) Effect on the main tumor (Table 29.1).

      Out of 11 patients who could be evaluated, 6 patients (55%) showed PR, 3 patients (27%) showed MR and 2 patients showed NC. Fig. 29.1 shows that the tumor has become indistinct, the right lobe is atrophied and the left lobe shows compensatory hypertrophy.

   ii) Effect on portal vein embolus (Table 29.2).

      Out of 29 patients, 22 patients showed PR (76%), 5 patients showed NC, and 2 patients showed PD. Fig. 29.2 shows that tumor embolus in the main trunk of the portal vein subside after radiotherapy.

Table 29.1– The effect of radiotherapy on the main tumor as measured by imaging

Response	Number of patients (%)
PR	6 (55%)
MR	3 (27%)
NC	2 (18%)
Total	11 (100%)

PR= partial response; MR= minor response; NC= no change

Table 29.2– The effect of radiotherapy on portal vein embolus as measured by imaging

Response	Number of patients (%)
PR	22 (76%)
MR	5 (17%)
NC	2 (7%)
Total	26 (100%)

PR= partial response; MR= minor response; NC= no change

Table 29.3 – Effect of radiotherapy on the main tumor according to histologic finding

Ohoshi Shimosato's grade[8]	Number of patients (%)
Grade I	1 (12.5%)
Grade II	7 (87.5%)
Grade III	0
Grade IV	0
Total	8 (100%)

Table 29.4 – The effect of radiotherapy on the tumor embolus in portal vein according to histologic finding

Ohoshi Shimosato's grade[8]	Number of patients (%)
Grade I	1 (20%)
Grade II	2 (40%)
Grade III	1 (20%)
Grade IV	1 (20%)
Total	5 (100%)

Table 29.5 – Effect of radiation dose

Radiation dose	Number of patients	Grade			
		I	II	III	IV
TDF ≥80	9	0	7	1	1
TDF <79	4	2	2	0	0

Table 29.6 – Patient characteristics

	Irradiated group	Non-irradiated group	x2 test
Sex			
Male	24	20	NS
Female	2	2	
Age	57.96	56.34	NS
Tumor occupying extent <49%	10	6	NS
≥50%	16	17	
Liver function			
Child-Pugh A	8	6	
Child-Pugh B	12	11	NS
Child-Pugh C	6	6	

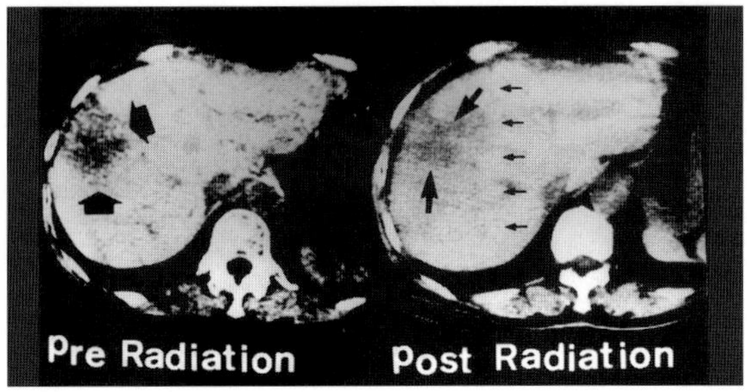

Figure 29.1 – Tumor has become indistinct, right lobe atrophied and left lobe shows compensatory hypertrophy.

2. Histologic findings.
   i) Effect on the main tumor (Table 29.3).

   Out of 8 patients, 7 patients (87.5%) showed Grade II. No patient showed complete necrosis and cancer cells remained viable. Fig. 29.3 shows marked degeneration and necrosis in more than half of the cancer cells but viable cells also remain.

   ii) Effect of radiotherapy on portal vein embolus (Table 29.4).

   Two patients showed Grade II, 1 patient showed Grade III and 1 patient showed Grade IV. In total 4 patients out of 5 showed good response including 2 patients with total necrosis of portal vein embolus. Another patient who was given irradiation less than TDF 70, showed Grade I. Fig. 29.4 shows complete necrosis of the irradiated tumor embolus.

   iii) The effect of radiotherapy on bone metastasis.

   Both patients showed good response for bone metastasis. 1 patient showed Grade IV.

   iv) Effect in radiation according to radiation dose (Table 29.5).

   Nine patients underwent radiotherapy with a radiation dose greater than TDF 80 and radiation effect was confirmed in all patients. Out of 4 patients who underwent radiotherapy with a radiation dose less than TDF 79, 2 patients showed Grade I.

3. Survival of patients with HCC with portal embolus.

   Out of comparable 48 patients with HCC with tumor embolus in the main portal vein,

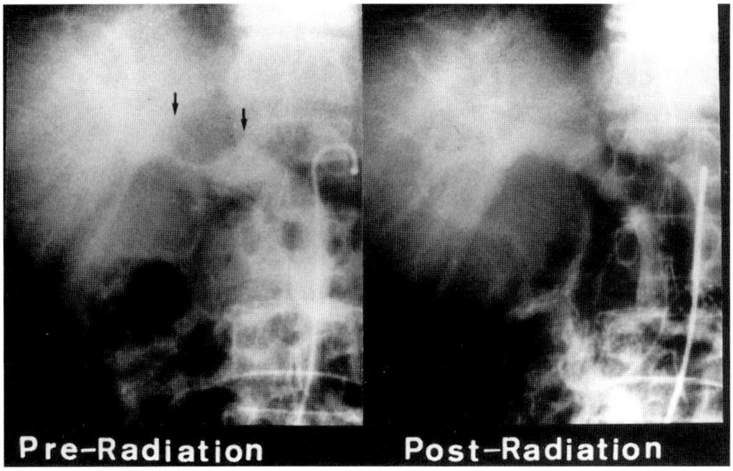

Figure 29.2 – Tumor embolus in main trunk of the portal vein subsided after radiotherapy.

26 patients underwent radiotherapy (irradiated group) and 22 patients underwent another therapy (non-irradiated group). A retrospective comparison study between both groups was performed. Both groups were similar with regard to sex, age, tumor extent, and liver function (Table 29.6).

The survival of the irradiated group was significantly better than that of the non-irradiated group; mean survival was 545 days and 106 days respectively. 2-year survival was 18% in the irradiated group but no patient in the non-irradiated group survived. (Fig. 29.5).

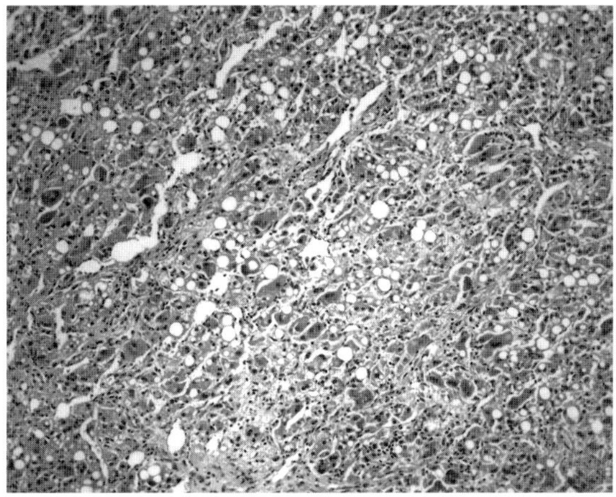

Figure 29.3 – Marked degeneration and necrosis in more than half of the cancer cells occured.

EXPERIENCE AT NATIONAL CANCER CENTER HOSPITAL EAST

Patients

We treated 25 patients until 1995. We carried out radiotherapy on the main tumor without portal vein embolus in 4 patients, portal vein tumor embolus in 15 patients, and bone metastasis in 6 patients. The patients who underwent radiotherapy to the main tumor had received several medical treatments previously and the radiotherapy was performed to treat recurrent lesions.

Results

All patients treated for the main tumor died within 1 year. The 2-year survival of 15 patients who underwent radiotherapy to portal vein tumor embolus was 19%. Patients with bone metastasis showed good response and relief of pain their 2-year survival was 66 %.(Fig. 29.6)

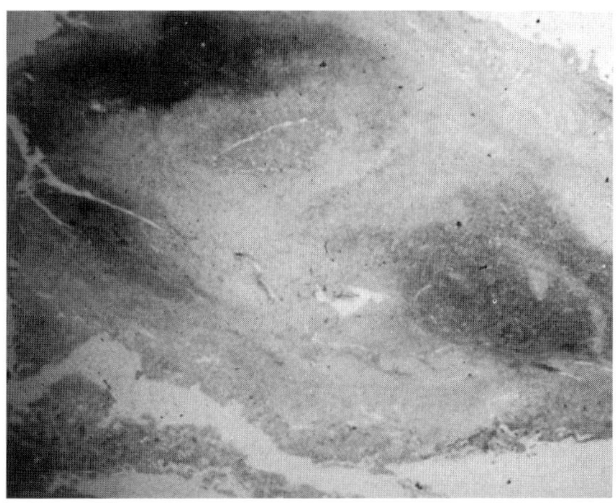

Figure 29.4 – Complete necrosis of the irradiated tumor embolus.

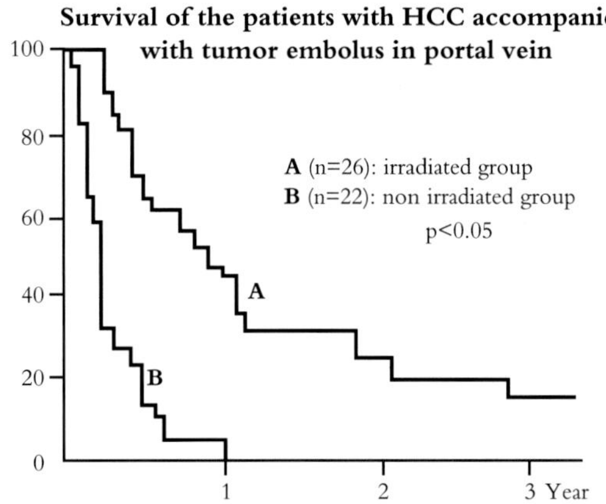

Figure 29.5 – Survival of the patients with HCC accompanied with portal embolus.

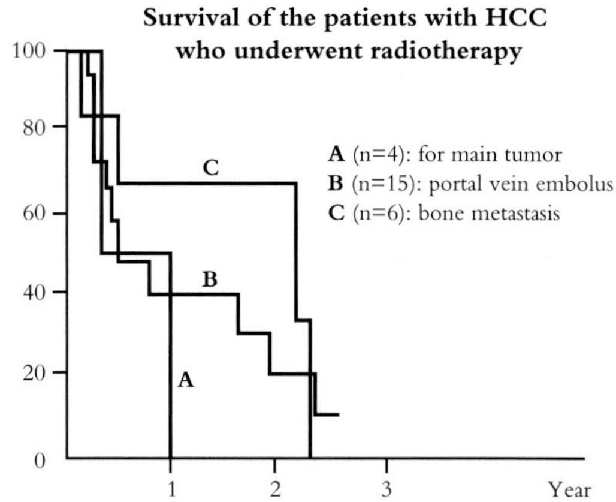

Figure 29.6 – Survival of the patients who underwent radiotherapy

CONCLUSION

Reports of radiation therapy for HCC are few. Phillips & Murakami[1] carried out radiotherapy for 32 patients with HCC in 1960. They reported that no anticancer effect was seen under 2000 rad, but some effect was found in more than half of the patients who received doses exceeding 2000 rad, however one patient died of radiation nephritis. El-Domeri *et al*[2] in 1971 carried out irradiation with 1200-3600 rad on 31 patients. All patients died within 6 months. There was no benefit compared with the non-treatment group and they concluded that radiotherapy for HCC was not effective. Cochrane *et al*[5] in 1977 also compared the anticancer effect of radiotherapy and chemotherapy for HCC and reported that radiotherapy was not effective. Niblett[9] in 1979 reported that radiotherapy for HCC alleviated symptoms but did not improve the survival rate. Ingold *et al*[3] reported that histologic changes in the liver after irradiation were bleeding and congestion in the sinusoid, degeneration and fat vacuoles in hepatocytes and later interstitial fibrosis. Lewin & Millis[4] reported that radiation hepatitis occurred by obstruction of the intrahepatic minor vascular system. It seemed that liver was a radiosensitive organ and up to the present radiotherapy has not been widely used in treating liver cancer.

However, in the past, radiotherapy was performed for far advanced HCC[9,10] and the irradiated field was very wide including whole liver irradiation. Because radiotherapy with wide irradiation field for far advanced liver cancer caused liver failure, radiotherapy for HCC was also invalidated.

Through development of image diagnostics and radiation exposure apparatus, radiotherapy has been performed safely and precisely. We reported the usefulness of radiotherapy for HCC in clinical practice in 1986.[6,7] Nagashima[11] reported that mouse hepatoma MH129-p disappeared after irradiation of 45 Gy and that radiation sensitivity for HCC was moderate experimentally.

Takara *et al*[12] reported in 1986 that tumor stain by angiography decreased after radiotherapy and atrophy of the irradiated liver occurred after radiation therapy. They concluded that patients with inoperable HCC smaller than 10 cm in size without liver cirrhosis are good candidates for radiotherapy.

We reported that a radiation dose of 50 Gy is necessary to treat HCC. Uno *et al*[13] reported that a total dose of 50 Gy seemed to be well tolerated by patients without liver cirrhosis and with liver cirrhosis of Child-Pugh A. Notsumata *et al*[14] performed radiotherapy over 50 Gy in patients with unresectable advanced HCC. They concluded that radiotherapy was useful to treat advanced HCC.

Radiation hepatitis can occur in the irradiated liver, so the radiation field should be minimized. To perform radiotherapy safely, it is necessary to evaluate liver function. Radiotherapy should be performed on selected patients according to their liver function.

Nagashima *et al*[6] reported that no severe change of liver function was seen in patients with HCC treated with a small irradiated field. They reported that only 1 patient who underwent radiotherapy with a field of 7.5 cm x 14 cm showed severe change of liver function and there was a marked increase from 10% to 36.6% in the value of indocianin green retention after 15 minutes. The patients with poor liver function such as liver cirrhosis or Child-Pugh C are not candidates for radiotherapy.

The anticancer effect of irradiated HCC occurs not only directly but also from fibrosis of irradiated circumferential liver and occlusion of the intrahepatic small vascular system due to radiation angitis. The candidate for radiotherapy for HCC is the patient with HCC that TAE and PEI cannot ameliorate. Repeated TAE sometimes obstructs the hepatic artery and additional TAE cannot be performed. The patient with hypovascular HCC larger than 3 cm is also a good candidate for radiotherapy.

It is debated whether radiotherapy for HCC improves survival. Uno *et al*[13] reported that median survival of 17 patients who underwent radiotherapy was 13.8 months, and 1-year and 3-year survival rates were 38.8% and 9.8%, respectively. Uno *et al*[13] concluded that pretreatment liver function affected the survival rate after radiation therapy. Nerenstone *et al*[15] reviewed the use of radiotherapy for HCC and they concluded that it did not improve the survival rate. Farmer *et al*[16] concluded that radiotherapy should be used as a palliative treatment only in carefully selected patients.

It is very difficult to treat the patient with HCC accompanied by tumor embolus in the main trunk of the portal vein. Because the feeding arteries of the tumor embolus are few, treatment is not completed by TAE. In 1987, Nagashima *et al*[6,7] reported that radiotherapy was valid for patients with HCC accompanied by tumor embolus. The effect of radiotherapy on tumor embolus was confirmed by imaging and pathologically in their studies. In our retrospective study, survival of patients with HCC who underwent radiotherapy was significantly better than that of patients who underwent another therapy. But because this study was not a prospective randomized study, we cannot prove whether radiotherapy contributes to survival improvement.

Radiotherapy for bone metastasis was also effective in our experience. Forbes *et al*[17] also reported that radiotherapy was helpful in the control of symptomatic bone metastasis. Pain related to bone metastasis disappeared after radiotherapy. If the main cancer of HCC could be treated sufficiently, radiotherapy for bone metastasis increases the probability of survival improvement too.

In conclusion, therapy for HCC is an effective and useful modality. The radiation dose necessary for treatment is 50 Gy. The radiation field range should be minimized to reduce irradiation of non-cancerous lesions of the liver. Radiotherapy is effective not only for the main tumor but also for tumor embolus and bone metastasis. Prospective randomized study is necessary to show whether radiotherapy increases survival of patients with HCC.

REFERENCES

1. Phillips R, Murakami K. Primary neoplasmas of liver. Results of radiation therapy. *Cancer* 1960; **13**: 714-720
2. El-Domeri AA, Huvos AG, Goldsmith HS, Foote FW. Primary malignant tumors of the liver. *Cancer* 1971; **27**:7-11
3. Ingold JA, Reed GB, Kaplan HS, *et al*. Radiation hepatitis. *Am J Roentgenol Radium Ther Nucl Med* 1965;**93**:200-208
4. Lewin K, Millis RR: Human radiation hepatitis. A morphologic study with emphasis on the late changes. *Arch Pathol* 1973; **96**:21-26
5. Cochrane AM, Murray-Lyon IM, Brinkley DM, Williams R: Quadruple chemotherapy versus radiotherapy in treatment of primary hepatocellular carcinoma. *Cancer* 1977; **40**:609-614
6. Nagashima T, Ryu M, Mukai M, Kikuchi T, Ariga T, Koh Z, Yamamoto Y, Odaka M, Satou H, Tsunemoto H, Utility of radiotherapy in primary liver cancer. *Southeast Asian J Surg* 1986; **9**:137-142
7. Nagashima T, Ryu M, Mukai M, Ariga T, Koh Z, Amano H, Furukawa T, Maruyama T, Yamamoto Y, Odaka M, Isono K, Arimizu N, Uematsu S, Ishikawa T. Therapy of hepatocellular carcinoma complicated with intravascular tumor emboli - Effectiveness of radiotherapy for tumor emboli (in Japanese with English abstract) *Kanzou* 1987; **28**:735-744
8. Shimosato Y, Ohoshi S, Baba K. Histopathological evaluation of radiotherapy and chemotherapy for carcinomas. *Jpn J Clin Oncol* 1971; **1**:19-35
9. Niblett JS. Radiation-treatment of hepatoma to Papua New Guinea. *Aust Radiol* 1979; **23**:242-247
10. Friedman MA, Volberding PA, Cassidy MJ, *et al*. Therapy of hepatocellular cancer with combined intrahepatic arterial chemotherapy and whole liver irradiation. *Ann Acad Med* 1980; **9**: 260-263
11. Nagashima T. The study on radiotherapy for hepatocellular carcinoma. (in Japanese with English abstract) *Nippon Act Radiol*. 1989; **49**:1141-1151

12. Takara K, Ohto M, Yoshikawa M, Ebara M, Okuda K, Itami J, Arimizu N. Clinical and pathological study of irradiation therapy in 24 patients with hepatocellular carcinoma (in Japanese with English abstract) *Jpn J Gastroenterol* 1986; **83**:1473-1482

13. Uno J, Itami J, Shiina T, Toita T, Serizawa S, Kato H, Hatano K, Arimizu N. Radiation therapy in patients with unresectable hepatocellular carcinoma. (in Japanese with English abstract) *J Jpn Soc Cancer Ther* 1992; **27**:1842-1847

14. Notsumata K, Okazaki A, Yokoyama T, Yamazaki T, Ito M, Sakurai Y, Takasu S, Abe T, Ikegami F, Yamaguchi K. Radiotherapy for advanced hepatocellular carcinoma. (in Japanese with English abstract) *Kanzou* 1992; **33**: 611-616

15. Nerenstone SR, Ihde DC, Friedman MA. Clinical trials in primary hepatocellular carcinoma: current status and future directions. *Cancer Treat Rev* 1988; **15**:1-31

16. Farmer DG, Rosove MH, Shaked A, Busuttil RW. Current treatment modalities for hepatocellular carcinoma. *Ann Surg* 1994; **219**:236-247

17. Forbes A, Williams R. Chemotherapy and radiotherapy of malignant hepatic tumors. *Bailliere's Clinical Gastroenterology* 1987; **1**:151-169

30

Multimodality treatments

S Lazzaroni and T Livraghi

Ultrasound screening, in use for some years now in many countries for monitoring patients at high risk of hepatocellular carcinoma (HCC), while not so far showing any proven gain in cost-benefit terms,[1] has led to the recruitment of growing numbers of candidates for curative treatment alternatives to surgery. Now that data are available on several modes of treatment, it is possible to say that:

1. In the case of HCC, unlike most other digestive tract cancers, early diagnosis is not synonymous with radical treatment. HCC may frustrate the radical purpose of surgical resection in two ways: by early vascular invasion, responsible for intrahepatic micrometastases, demonstrated by pathologic evidence but not detectable by any diagnostic investigation, and by its multifocal origin, inherent in the fact that HCC is a whole-organ disease.[2] Therefore no treatment, however extensive and aggressive, can ensure radicality except orthotopic liver transplantation (OLT), and this only if total hepatectomy precedes the extrahepatic migration of neoplastic cells or an associated treatment can sterilize metastatic microfoci already there. It is thus not surprising that even resection, certainly the most radical of the options on offer,[3-6] carries a high recurrence rate,[7-11] which rises as follow-up goes on. Nonetheless, surgery, if properly applied and expertly performed, is bound to remain the gold standard for locoregional treatments. In other words, no other locoregional therapy, present or future, can deliver a higher success rate, although it may equal this provided that it can ensure complete necrosis of the lesion. This is confirmed by the survival rates, practically equivalent to those of resection, as shown by the percutaneous ethanol injection (PEI) and segmental transarterial chemoembolization (segmental TACE) series.[12-18]

2. To date there are no sure parameters by which to predict the biologic behavior of an early small lesion through the wide spectrum of growth, invasion and multifocality of HCC. A search has been made for prognostic markers[8-11,19] but these are not always unequivocal across the various series and often they cannot be determined in a pretreatment work-up.

3. No treatment, excepting in some measure OLT, can ignore the constant association between HCC and chronic liver disease (in the main cirrhosis), which requires that the functional reserve be spared as far as possible, since the long term outcome of a treatment, which is anyway not permanently curative, is the result of a tightrope act between ability to treat the cancer and the cost, in terms of liver damage, to achieve it. Thus, in practice, cirrhosis and its severity are a constant prognostic indicator of any treatment.[3]

4. Chemotherapy has little effect on HCC, as is the case with other digestive tract cancers.[3,5,6] This "primary" resistance can be broken by means of special drug concentration strategies, like intra-arterial infusion, coupling with iodized oil, transient stoppage of the arterial flow with embolizing agents. As these methods are flow-dependent, their efficacy cannot be quantified beforehand, since it is correlated with two interconnected variables, namely: the volume of the tumor blood supply and, within the peculiar two-way hepatic flow system, the variable contribution of portal venous flow which, though usually minor for HCC, may be increased by various arterioportal communications to become actually predominant for early unencapsulated lesions and for capsular and extracapsular infiltrations.[20-25]

In the light of these considerations it is reasonable to say that, excluding OLT, which is hardly likely to make any substantially greater contribution to the treatment of HCC - due to the shortage of organs, its high social and organizational cost and often older patient age - it is an illusion to expect single treatments to deliver an improvement in success rates beyond what can be accomplished through refinements in procedures and more targeted patient selection. This "unsurmountable limit" to therapeutic efficacy has stimulated, alongside the search for new procedures, efforts to devise a philosophy of treatment whereby the benefits of individual therapies can be combined to produce better end-results.[3-26] Hence the emergence of a multimodal strategy with its four configurations:

a) *neoadjuvant therapy:* a "major" (surgical) treatment is backed up or consolidated by "minor" treatments (Table 30.1);

b) *combined therapy:* two equally effective therapies are combined to ensure synergy (Table 30.2);

c) *multistep therapy:* several treatments are given in succession in response to disease resumption and changes in presentation, progression of cirrhosis, advancing patient age, inefficacy of previous therapy or delay of surgery (Table 30.3);

d) *besides therapy:* treatments of scant, doubtful or unproven efficacy used in association with or in addition to proven therapies in the context of trials or in patients for whom no other treatment is possible or indicated (Table 30.4).

Any multimodal strategy must take into account the importance to survival of correcting risk factors for the cirrhotic patient, such as esophageal varices, and of promptly detecting and adequately treating the complications of cirrhosis.

NEOADJUVANT THERAPIES

In this sphere most progress has been made in presurgical chemoembolization on the basis of the following rational premises: a) seeding of neoplastic cells in the course of surgery must be limited in order to prevent intrahepatic recurrence and extrahepatic spread; b) any neoplastic microfoci already present but not removable surgically because they are not demonstrable must be sterilized; c) the tumor mass should be debulked to permit or facilitate resection.

The effects on survival and on tumor recurrence have not, however, lived up to expectations in initially resectable HCC. Indeed, the undoubted advantage of cytoreduction has been accompanied by an unexpected and paradoxical facilitation, instead of reduction, of neoplastic seeding secondary to surgical manipulation.[3,27,28] Pathologic reports on surgical specimens and on livers explanted in the course of OLT have shown that non segmental TACE, the only form indicated and practised at the presurgical stage, even when lesions are small, more often than not produces only partial necrosis;[13,20,21,29,30] this, whether spontaneous or induced, is thought to explain the higher incidence of intra- and extra-hepatic recurrences after resection, by diminishing cell cohesion.[27] Any sterilizing effect that TACE may exert on the final outcome was not foreseeable, since neoplastic foci are known to be portal flow-dependent.[22,25]

A different unforeseeable combination of such opposite effects, according to series, may account for the discordance among the data on the value of presurgical TACE, some retrospective studies on small lesions reporting a benefit[27,31,32] and others similar or lower disease-free survival rates in treated patients.[33-36] However, when stringent patient selection criteria were applied[27] or the study was randomized and prospective,[28] the data were concordant. So now it may be concluded that preoperative TACE must be avoided in initially resectable HCC because it not only fails to improve the survival rate or lower the recurrence rate but also complicates subsequent resection, at least in large HCC, making it

Table 30.1 – Neoadjuvant and adjuvant therapies

Preoperative TACE
Preoperative Cytoreduction
Pre- and Post-OLT Chemotherapy
Pre-OLT TACE

Table 30.2 – Combined therapies

TACE	+	PEI
PEI	+	TACE
TACE	+	TPEI

Table 30.3 – Multistep therapies

Resection	➡ Resection	➡ PEI	➡ TACE	➡ OLT
PEI	➡ PEI	➡ TACE	➡ OLT	
TACE	➡ TACE	➡ PEI	➡ OLT	
OLT	➡ TACE	➡ PEI		

Table 30.4 – Besides therapies

Tamoxifen
Interferon
LAK Cells
Interleukin-2
^{131}I polyclonal antiferritin antibodies
^{131}I Iodized Oil

longer and more laborious; this is due to the presence of tough adhesions between tumor and neighboring organs caused by the necrosis-induced inflammation, adhesions that may also facilitate tumor spread by contiguity.[28]

Since debulking, however effected, is advantageous *per se*, if it is sufficient to allow resection of initially unresectable HCC, it may extend the curative effects of surgery to otherwise inoperable patients, provided that the baseline hepatic functional reserve is sound and is not significantly worsened by the debulking, and that operative mortality is minimal and surgery curative. The need for several factors to converge in the patient is what limits this multimodal approach. Some surgeons[37,38] have nonetheless achieved high long term survival rates in patients who at first laparotomy were not rated candidates for resection due to the extent of the disease, when they were able - after intensive debulking combined with two or three modalities among ligation of the hepatic artery, intra-arterial and systemic chemotherapy, radiotherapy, radioimmunotherapy, immunotherapy, PEI, cryotherapy and laser therapy – to secure complete tumor removal. Since some of these patients were certainly not cirrhotic or at all events had a residual liver function that could withstand such a therapeutic assault, these results are not reproducible in a general population of cirrhotics. Absence of vascular invasion, a single neoplastic focus, presence of a capsule and location in the right lobe or close to the hilum proved to be favorable prognostic factors.[38]

On analyzing the survival rates after OLT for HCC, we find that they vary greatly according to tumor stage, even when the lymph nodes are intact and there is no extrahepatic spread. Lesion size and number, bilobar lesions and vascular invasion are also predictive of recurrence.[39-44] In other words, neoplastic cells migrate outside the liver early, depending on disease presentation, and, if they survive total hepatectomy, they reimplant on the liver graft or grow at other sites, helped by an impaired immunosurveillance.[45] Presumably it is not explantation of the liver that determines tumor spread so much as surgical resection, since the organ is removed en bloc, protected by exclusion of the drainage vessels. It is therefore reasonable to suppose that it is the early and repeated migration of cells beforehand, due to the peculiar portal vascular invasiveness of HCC, that is the primary event which later triggers recurrence when immunosuppressive therapy lessens the natural control of tumor cells. For the same reason, recurrence after OLT is early and speedy.[46] Since this undesirable effect is the inevitable price for combating graft rejection, the only possible way of preventing tumor recurrence is to sterilize the cells that have survived the hepatectomy and migrated. This form of chemotherapy, necessarily systemic rather than regional, is far from standardized in timing, drugs and dosage, but it seems to offer promising results on long term survival.[6,31,47-50] However, the benefit has to be confirmed in randomized prospective trials in order to avoid, as with preoperative TACE, giving useless or even harmful treatment for longer than necessary. And there are anyway other open questions.

First of all, we need to establish which patients are likely to benefit from this treatment rather than lay down a general indication. It is in fact possible that in initial HCC, that is in pTNM stages I and II, chemotherapy is of no value, because there is little or no risk of recurrence at these stages,[2,39,44,51] or that, since vascular invasion may be present even at stage II, chemotherapy might be started if the pathologic evidence is positive. The need to restrict the indication arises from the increased risk of toxicity in these patients both before OLT, because of reduced liver function secondary to cirrhosis and coexisting leukocyte and platelet deficiency from hypersplenism, and after OLT, when, despite normalization of liver function and of drug clearance, the associated immunosuppressive therapy and antibiotic prophylaxis enhance bone marrow toxicity.[50] Furthermore, as has happened with chemotherapy for other cancers, there is a high risk of reactivating hepatitis B in a severe form, given the state of immunosuppression,[50] a risk that could be obviated simply by excluding HBsAg subjects from this approach.

Another open question is the timing and duration of treatment. The schedules so far tried envisage preoperative and more often than not also postoperative chemotherapy for periods ranging from a few months to a year. The latter seems to be the more obvious option, for several reasons: firstly, the longer duration might offset the necessarily lower dose; secondly, it must be advantageous to reduce the systemic burden of tumor cells surviving hepatectomy to a minimum;

thirdly, even a minute quantity of tumor cells unscathed by the previous systemic treatment or migrating in the course of operation would stand a stronger chance of implanting and growing after OLT because of the immunosuppressive therapy.

As to the choice of chemotherapeutic agent, opinions differ because no one drug has emerged as provenly more effective on HCC. This tumor is known often to express the multidrug resistance gene product p-glycoprotein, which induces drug resistance by transporting it outside the cell.[45,50,52,53] Hence systemic chemotherapy has always yielded disappointing results. At all events it would seem to be more effective in association with OLT, both because microscopic neoplastic disease might be a better target than a macroscopic one[45] – especially after the growth acceleration induced by surgical debulking of the tumor and by immunosuppression[50] – and because cyclosporin, used to prevent rejection, might be capable of blocking the activity of the multidrug resistance gene.[45,50] Doxorubicin alone,[50] or in association with cisplatinum[48] has been used more often than mitoxantrone[49] or adriamycin-fluorouracil association.[31] Pre-OLT TACE alone[6] or with adjuvant chemotherapy[31] has also been tried, but its real impact on survival, over and above that due to the strict patient selection in these studies, has yet to be proved.[6]

COMBINED THERAPIES

Locoregional treatments other than surgical resection may fail to fulfil the ever desirable aim of complete necrosis of the treated lesions through insufficient distribution of the destructive agent. This failure has been demonstrated in the pathologic evidence from patients who later underwent resection or total hepatectomy. Total necrosis of a single lesion attacked by a single therapy was obtained in not more than 80% of cases either after PEI or after segmental TACE.[13,16,20,29] In line with this datum, treatment was followed by local recurrence in 20 to 40% of cases on average.[13,16,17,54] Pathologic studies further revealed that neoplastic disease is often understaged by imaging,[20,21,30] which anyway has to be done for the execution of PEI and segmental TACE, because of frequent early cell migration to the capsule, outside it and within small portal blood vessels, or because of latent multifocality. Hence the need to combine treatments in the attempt to remedy the weakness of each.

With this aim in mind attempts have been made to combine TACE and PEI.[29,55-57] Ethanol, though highly effective on HCC because of its intrinsic capacity to spread preferentially in the softer neoplastic tissue and to thrombose small vessels, may be prevented from diffusing by the presence of intracapsular septa, by an increased consistency of the tumor, and by the excessive volume to be perfused, with the result that it leaves cellular residues that form the core of subsequent recurrences. TACE, on the other hand, although regional in scope and therefore providing a larger distribution bed, has less local effect, and so its efficacy on a single lesion is unpredictable. And yet analysis of the results of the combination shows no advantage over PEI alone, at least when the lesions are few and small, since the total percentages of necrosis, recurrence rates and survival curves proved to be much the same.[29,55] On larger lesions, on the other hand, the success rate of the combination was higher than for TACE alone.[55,56] The reason for this is thought to be that pretreatment with TACE reduces tumor volume, thereby facilitating the subsequent diffusion of ethanol, even in large lesions. However, there has been no comparison with PEI alone, which might have yielded similar results, since a large number of lesions and large size, which used to be constraints on PEI because of the large quantities of ethanol to be injected and the unduly long course of treatment, can now be overcome with the one-shot technique. This is certainly more invasive and aggressive than multisession PEI, but it carries lower complication rates than TACE.[54,58] With regard to the possibility that chemoembolization may exert a favorable effect on any neoplastic microfoci or on capsular, extracapsular or vascular invasion by the tumor, it is thought to be unlikely because these lesions are portal flow-dependent and hence resistant to arterial treatment. A possible extension of the destructive effect might be obtained with high-dose iodized oil (more than 10 ml), enough to cause an overflow from the hepatic artery into the portal vein via arterioportal communications.[24] This approach has not been tried in association with PEI, partly because despite a presumed greater effectiveness there is the greater parenchymal toxicity, great enough to contraindicate lobar or regional administration, and partly because PEI alone has proved capable of destroying these neoplastic infiltrations, if located in the areas in which the injected ethanol has been distributed.[29] Lastly, it is hard to detect by ultrasonography imaging (US) and treat by PEI the areas left viable after TACE, because they present no US-imageable structural changes. This necessitates extensive treatment of the lesion with ethanol also. To overcome this difficulty, the reverse sequence has been tried, ie PEI followed by TACE, a course supported by the fact that pre-TACE angiography provides a means of testing the efficacy of PEI; furthermore, the chemoembolizing agent is likely to be more concentrated in a tumor mass reduced by PEI. There are, however, no known studies in this field, in particular none to find out whether this combination is superior to PEI alone.

There are better premisses for effectiveness in the combination of TACE with TPEI (transportal ethanol injection), because in a given area of the liver, segment or lobe, the arterial and portal flows are interrupted successively.[59] Furthermore, ethanol can exert a direct action on the lesions accessible by the portal route, which initially escape imaging. The TACE-TPEI combination produces what may be called a chemical segmentectomy, that is to say the tumor and any intrasegmental micrometastases are totally destroyed by parenchymal overnecrosis rather than by a targeted action on a segment or lobe. This is proved by the marked rise in the indices of cytolysis to the point of frank fulminating hepatitis with liver failure and death from right portal embolization. Since therapeutic effectiveness correlates closely with damage to liver function, it is essential to improve the cost-benefit ratio by identifying the correct timing of TPEI and TACE. The point is that the closer they are in time the greater the efficacy and the damage, whereas the longer portal embolization is delayed the greater the recovery of function, arterial occlusion being gradually reversible, but the greater the survival of neoplastic foci. The way out is to resort to successive TACE, which is potentiated by the permanent abolition of the portal flow. Actually, this combined approach can yield results similar to those of surgical segmentectomy but it has the same limitations and risks as well as benefits. Scrupulous patient selection is therefore mandatory, hingeing on the extent of the neoplastic disease and the functional reserve of the liver in order not to bring on liver failure. It has to be said that, although this procedure is less invasive than surgical resection, it is complex and not easily reproducible.

MULTISTEP THERAPIES

Even when a treatment is potentially curative, as with surgical resection, permanent cure is rarely, if ever, achieved. In other words, the tumor recurs, as is clear from all the case series, whether surgical, TACE or PEI, chiefly because HCC is a whole-organ disease, due to the precancerous state that is cirrhosis, still not correctible except by means of OLT, and secondarily because the marked tendency to early vascular invasion enables neoplastic microfoci to survive and develop even when total hepatectomy has removed the condition of precancerosis. Consequently retreatment is an obligate step in the history of this cancer, except in those cases that, being very early, can be permanently cured by OLT.

The pretreatment strategy must take into account the following points. First, recurrence signifies persistence of disease, however curative the previous treatment may have been in intention. It is therefore reasonable to opt for a less aggressive and less invasive therapy. Although a re-resection provenly affords better survival rates than no treatment,[60,61] there are today no grounds for resorting to it. Reoperation may fail due to extensive adhesions between organs and to the development of vessels secondary to the first operation and/or to portal hypertension.[62] In addition, it is not popular with patients, has a social and economic cost, carries a further risk and is likely to decrease the hepatic reserve. It has to be remembered that although the patient was previously eligible for surgery, the recurrence may occur several years later and the favorable conditions present earlier may no longer be so, given older age, onset of other diseases that carry a surgical risk and, most importantly, worsening cirrhosis. Since the pathogen, in most cases viral, persists, the functional reserve is bound to decrease gradually. The final argument against reoperation is the frequent finding that, although close follow-up of resected patients allows early diagnosis – especially if US, which is limited by the sequelae of earlier surgery, is backed by other imaging techniques – the disease often assumes a different presentation even when the original HCC was monofocal and well circumscribed. It has in fact been demonstrated that the most common pattern of recurrence in surgical series, certainly the best staged locoregional therapy, is multinodular and more often than not affects both lobes. Common too is portal vascular invasion and, especially in patients with these characteristics, the incidence of distant metastases – to lung, bone and adrenal glands – is fairly high. For these reasons recurrence later complicates a second resection.[63] This being so, surgery is gradually giving way to TACE and PEI even in a surgical environment. Chemoembolization was the first used extensively in postsurgical recurrences, demonstrably improving survival *vs* no treatment in retrospective series.[62] Since, as emphasized earlier, the disease is most often multifocal when it represents, this treatment option would seem to be rational. On the other hand, there is room for reservations considering that recent randomized studies have failed to show a benefit on survival, notwithstanding a positive trend, in patients who have had repeated TACE for inoperable HCC, due to a worsening of liver function that outweighs the advantage of tumor growth inhibition.[64] On the strength of this evidence it would seem legitimate to extend this reasoning to the recurrences after surgery, because liver function has already been reduced by the previous resection and the progression of cirrhosis. If this were true, it would lead to the conclusion that PEI, whether multisession or single-session, might be the treatment of choice for surgical recurrences, since it certainly, for the same degree of efficacy as TACE, is capable of preserving the functional reserve. A randomized study comparing PEI and TACE is nevertheless needed in support of this choice.

OLT might also have a curative role in recurrences after resection,[65] as after PEI and TACE too, as long as the prognostic factors – like small size, single focus, no vascular invasion, no lymph node or extrahepatic metastases – that have proved to have a favorable influence on survival are present. If this were confirmed on large numbers, beyond the few reports on perhaps only slow-growing HCC,[44] this multistep approach might shift the OLT option from the time of cancer diagnosis to the time of recurrence, at least in patients whose cirrhosis is not too severe for them to be eligible for transplantation. This approach would widen the indications of resection and other locoregional therapies like TACE and PEI, which would thus become the first choice even in candidates for transplantation. This postponement would have the undoubted advantage of deferring OLT, an event that is anyway fraught with uncertainty, risks and complications, and of sequels like immunosuppressive treatment. However, before approving this approach, though it is usually applied in practice due to the shortage of donors, we need to be able to show that postponement of OLT does not jeopardize its outcome by allowing the tumor to evolve to a more adverse presentation or stage. The search for and identification of negative prognostic markers might be of help here.

As the wait for OLT may be long in practice, pretreatment with TACE or PEI, although *per se* unnecessary and unavailing, may be a rational choice by halting or at least curbing tumor growth. It would, moreover, have a neoadjuvant function in that it would not only reduce tumor volume but also might prevent cell migration and vascular invasion. With its regional action, TACE would seem preferable to PEI in this indication, partly because it can be combined with angiography, a study essential to pre-OLT staging. However the pathologic evidence from explanted liver pretreated with TACE shows that this treatment is only partially effective, since it has no effect on small satellite nodules, depending as they do on portal flow, and since the complete objective response it low, under 40%, because the small neoplastic nodules, that characterize the stages of patients ideal for OLT, have little or no blood supply. Furthermore, as these patients are often candidates for OLT because of advanced cirrhosis, TACE may precipitate liver failure, making it necessary to put the patient on the emergency list for OLT. For these reasons, PEI might be a valid alternative at least for some patients, even though it perhaps carries the risk of seeding. In other cases TACE might be given first, followed by PEI, for visible lesions not impregnated with iodized oil.[30] In these pre-OLT indications there are nonetheless no studies showing the value of TACE or PEI or of their association.

A graft recurrence is most likely to arise when the tumor is at an advanced stage before hepatectomy. Although the current tendency to confine OLT to the lowest stages and the use of neoadjuvant therapy may help to limit the risk of recurrence, the risk is there for up to 2 years after hepatectomy. Unfortunately in these cases the treatment strategy is complicated by the tumultuous rate of neoplastic growth,[46] despite systemic chemotherapy, and by the frequent concomitance of metastases – especially to the lung – because of iatrogenic immunosuppression. If the disease is confined to the liver graft, TACE might offer some benefit because the restored liver function might enable the patient to tolerate the hepatic toxicity of chemoembolization. A second OLT in these patients does not seem justified on ethical grounds either, unless there has been a relapse of cirrhosis, later complicated by "*de novo*" tumor. In such an event the decision to reimplant is subject to quantification of the risk of a further recurrence of viral infection.

Recurrences arising after nonsurgical locoregional therapy include not only new lesions but also local recurrences, since radicality cannot be guaranteed. The next treatment, except in patients who might benefit from deferred OLT, is much the same as before. In effect, at least for PEI because it is easily repeated and well tolerated, patients receive what is really multistep treatment, which, by combining multisession and single-session treatments, continues in courses for some years in the attempt each time to induce a remission of the disease, as with chemotherapeutic treatment of hematological cancers. And, as with the latter, it is often not easy to identify the stage of the disease and hence the moment at which the treatment can no longer bring even minimal benefit. Whether this chronic treatment of HCC has any real impact on patient survival, in addition to its purely psychologic effect, is very hard to establish and probably in some cases it has none. However, rational or not, the therapist sometimes does not know how to stop when confronted by an informed patient determined to go on, given the simplicity and low cost of the treatment.

For TACE too treatment is usually given in sessions, though fewer because of the greater cumulative toxicity or because it is not feasible due to vascular damage. In such cases, if the disease is still limited, treatment switches to PEI. Otherwise, if the disease has become multifocal or diffuse, TACE may be given in place of PEI.

BESIDES THERAPIES

A systemic means of combating a cancer that eludes locoregional treatment is an attractive aim that has long been pursued. Given their different and additional effect, systemic substances are used in association with locoregional modes of treatment or even alone as palliatives, singly or combined, in patients for whom the former are considered inappropriate. These treatments are classified by mechanism of action as hormono- or immunotherapy.

Among hormonal substances tamoxifen, a nonsteroidal antiestrogen used in the treatment of breast cancer, has been tried in HCC with the aim of slowing growth, following the discovery of estrogen receptors in hepatocytes also.[66,67] After nonrandomized trials supplied contradictory results regarding the value of its use, alone or in combination with other hormones or chemotherapeutic drugs,[68-72] a recent double blind controlled trial *vs* placebo showed no benefit on survival or on quality of life or on growth and progression of the tumor in patients with advanced HCC. It is therefore concluded that tamoxifen has no place in the treatment of HCC patients.[73] Extrapolating the results of single-drug therapy, there is no longer any justification for its association with locoregional treatments.

Immunotherapy is supported by a stronger rationale than hormonal therapies in the treatment of HCC in cirrhotic patients, since interferon has already proved its worth in controlling the hepatitis viruses implicated in oncogenesis while interleukin-2 by the systemic route corrects the activity of Lymphokine Activated Kill (LAK) cells, which destroy neoplastic hepaticells *in vitro*, and which is often depressed in HCC patients.[5] Unfortunately these modes of treatment, alone or in association with chemotherapeutic drugs, have likewise failed to yield satisfactory results and their use is not justified outside the research setting on account of the complexity of the procedures and the high cost.[3,5,6] With regard to interferon, alpha or beta, no clinical efficacy has been proved in advanced HCC.[74,75]

^{131}I polyclonal antiferritin antibodies have been tried in association with chemo- and radiotherapy both in inoperable HCC[76,77] and as a neoadjuvant,[37,38] but here again, given the unimpressive results, the side effects and the complexity of the procedure, this therapy can have no place in the routine treatment of HCC.[3,6]

An internal radiation therapy can also be achieved coupling ^{131}I with iodized oil intra-arterially, when chemoembolization is contraindicated because of portal vein thrombosis or previous portacaval shunt. Preliminary results seem to be promising. In fact the ^{131}I -iodized oil is retained within the tumor thrombi being arterially vascularized and thus one might expect ^{131}I-iodized oil to act upon the thrombus itself. Survival rate was statistically higher after this therapy *versus* medical support in advanced HCC in a prospective randomized trial.[78] However the low numbers of patients studied and the advanced stage of disease could represent a bias. Therefore further studies are necessary to validate this therapeutic approach, although this technique is interesting because it can be used in association with other modalities in the treatment of HCC with portal vein thrombosis.

CONCLUSION

In sum, since single treatments for HCC, including the latest ones, are still unsatisfactory, notwithstanding early diagnosis by means of extensive screening of patients at risk, the attempt to step up the response to treatment through a multimodality strategy is both logical and necessary.

Several experimental and clinical trials have been conducted but, despite the favorable premises, not all have provided evidence of efficacy. Preoperative TACE, hormonal and immunologic therapies have failed in this objective and it looks as if the same applies to the combination of TACE with PEI.

The outlook is better for pre-OLT chemotherapy, for preoperative cytoreduction, for the combination of TACE with TPEI and for multistep PEI in recurrences. However, only future randomized prospective trials can supply the final word on the value of these combinations.

Despite the concentrated efforts of all kinds of therapists – surgeons, interventional radiologists, radiotherapists, gastroenterologists, oncologists and immunologists – the results obtained to date even with multimodality approaches, as for single therapies, have achieved only partial success against this cancer that looms over the cirrhotic patient.

REFERENCES

1. Colombo M, De Franchis R, Del Ninno E *et al.* Hepatocellular carcinoma in Italian patients with cirrhosis. *N Engl J Med* 1991; **325**:675-80
2. Selby R, Kadry Z, Carr B, Tzakis A, Madariaga J, Iwatsuki S. Liver transplantation for hepatocellular carcinoma. *World J Surg* 1995; **19**:53-58
3. Farmer DG, Rosove MH, Shaked A, Busuttil RW. Current treatment modalities for hepatocellular carcinoma. *Ann Surg* 1994; **219**:236-247
4. Colombo M. Hepatocellular carcinoma in cirrhotics. *Semin Liver Dis* 1993; **13**:374-383
5. Colleoni M, Gaion F, Liessi G, Mastropasqua G, Nelli P, Manente P. Medical treatment of hepatocellular carcinoma: any progress? *Tumori* 1994; **80**:315-326
6. Venook A. Treatment of hepatocellular carcinoma: too many options? *J Clin Oncol* 1994; **12**:1323-1334
7. Belghiti J, Panis Y, Farges O, Benhamou JP, Fekete F. Intrahepatic recurrence after resection of hepatocellular carcinoma complicating cirrhosis. *Ann Surg* 1991; **214**:114-117
8. Adachi E, Maeda T, Matsumata T *et al.* Risk factors for intrahepatic recurrence in human small hepatocellular carcinoma. *Gastroenterology* 1995; **108**:768-775
9. The Liver Cancer Study Group of Japan. Predictive factors for long term prognosis after partial hepatectomy for patients with hepatocellular carcinoma in Japan. *Cancer* 1994; **74**:2772-2780
10. Yamanaka N, Okamoto E, Toyosaka A *et al.* Prognostic factors after hepatectomy. *Cancer* 1990; **65**: 1104-1110
11. Jwo SC, Chiu JH, Chau GY, Loong CC, Lui WY. Risk factors linked to tumor recurrence of human hepatocellular carcinoma after hepatic resection. *Hepatology* 1992; **16**:1367-1371
12. Livraghi T, Bolondi L, Buscarini L *et al.* No treatment, resection and ethanol injection in hepatocellular carcinoma: a retrospective analysis of survival in 391 patients with cirrhosis. *J Hepatol* 1995; **22**:522-526
13. Livraghi T, Giorgio A, Marin G *et al.* Hepatocellular carcinoma and cirrhosis in 746 patients: long term results of percutaneous ethanol injection. *Radiology* 1995; **197**:101-108
14. Livraghi T, Bolondi L, Lazzaroni S *et al.* Percutaneous ethanol injection in the treatment of hepatocellular carcinoma. *Cancer* 1992; **69**:925-929
15. Kotoh K, Sakai H, Sakamoto S *et al.* The effect of percutaneous ethanol injection therapy on small solitary hepatocellular carcinoma is comparable to that of hepatectomy. *Am J Gastroenterol* 1994; **89**:194-198
16. Matsui O, Kadoya M, Yoshikawa J *et al.* Small hepatocellular carcinoma: treatment with subsegmental transcatheter arterial embolization. *Radiology* 1993; **188**:79-83
17. Nishimine K, Uchida H, Matsuo N *et al.* Segmental transarterial chemoembolization with Lipiodol mixed with anticancer drugs for nonresectable hepatocellular carcinoma: follow-up CT and therapeutic results. *Cancer Chemother Pharmacol* 1994; **33**(suppl): 60-68
18. Onodera H, Ukai K, Nakano N *et al.* Outcomes of 116 patients with hepatocellular carcinoma. *Cancer Chemother Pharmacol* 1994; **33**(suppl): 103-108
19. Lencioni R, Bartolozzi C, Caramella D *et al.* Treatment of

small hepatocellular carcinoma with percutaneous ethanol injection. *Cancer* 1995; **76**:1737-46

20. Higuchi T, Kikuchi M, Okazaki M. Hepatocellular carcinoma after transcatheter hepatic arterial embolization. *Cancer* 1994; **73**:2259-67
21. Choi BI, Kim HC, Han JK *et al*. Therapeutic effects of trans - catheter oily chemoembolization therapy for encapsulated nodular hepatocellular carcinoma: CT and pathologic findings. *Radiology* 1992; **182**:709-713
22. Kuroda C, Sakurai M, Monden M *et al*. Limitation of trans-catheter arterial chemoembolization using iodized oil for small hepatocellular carcinoma. A study in resected cases. *Cancer* 1991; **67**:81-86
23. Ackerman NB. Experimental studies on the circulatory dynamics of intrahepatic tumor blood supply. *Cancer* 1972; **29**:435-442
24. Oi H, Kim T, Kishimoto H, Matsushita M, Tateishi H, Okamura J. Effective cases of trancatheter arterioportal chemoembolization with high-dose iodized oil for hepatocellular carcinoma. *Cancer Chemother Pharmacol* 1994; **33**(suppl): 69-73
25. Wakasa K, Sakurai M, Kuroda C *et al*. Effect of transcatheter arterial embolization on the boundary architecture of hepatocellular carcinoma. *Cancer* 1990; **65**:913-919
26. Tanikawa K. Multidisciplinary treatment of hepatocellular carcinoma. In: Tobe T, Kameda H, eds. *Primary liver cancer in Japan*. Tokyo, Japan: Springer-Verlag, 1992; 327-334
27. Adachi E, Matsumata T, Nishizaki T, Hashimoto H, Tsuneyoshi M, Sugimachi K. Effects of preoperative trans-catheter hepatic arterial chemoembolization for hepatocellular carcinoma. The relationship between postoperative course and tumor necrosis. *Cancer* 1993; **72**:3593-8
28. Wu C-C, Ho Y-Z, Lin Ho W, Wu T-C, Liu T-J, P'eng F-K. Preoperative transcatheter chemoembolization for resectable large hepatocellular carcinoma: a reappraisal. *Br J Surg* 1995; **82**:122-26
29. Shiina S, Tagawa K, Niwa Y *et al*. Percutaneous ethanol injection therapy for hepatocellular carcinoma: results in 146 patients. *AJR* 1993; **160**:1023-1028
30. Spreafico C, Marchiano A, Regalia E *et al*. Chemoembolization of hepatocellular carcinoma in patients who undergo liver transplantation. *Radiology* 1994; **192**:687-690
31. Bismuth H, Morino M, Sherlock D *et al*. Primary treatment of hepatocellular carcinoma by arterial chemoembolization. *Am J Surg* 1992; **163**:387-394
32. Yu Y-Q, Xu D-B, Zhou X-D, Lu J-X, Tang Z-Y, Mack P. Experience with liver resection after hepatic arterial chemoembolization for hepatocellular carcinoma. *Cancer* 1993; **71**:62-65
33. Monden M, Okamura J, Sakon M *et al*. Significance of transcatheter chemoembolization combined with surgical resection for hepatocellular carcinomas. *Cancer Chemother Pharmacol* 1989; **23**(suppl): 90-95
34. Nagasue N, Galizia G, Kohno H *et al*. Adverse effects of preoperative hepatic artery chemoembolization for resectable hepatocellular carcinoma: a retrospective comparison of 138 liver resections. *Surgery* 1989; **106**:81-86
35. Nagasue N, Kohno H, Uchida M. Evaluation of preoperative transcatheter arterial embolization in the treatment of resectable primary liver cancer. *Semin Surg Oncol* 1993; **9**: 327-331
36. Hwang T-L, Chen M-F, Lee T-Y, Chen T-J, Lin D-Y, Liaw Y-F. Resection of hepatocellular carcinoma after transcatheter arterial embolization. Re-evaluation of the advantages and disadvantages of preoperative embolization. *Arch Surg* 1987; **122**:756-759
37. Sitzmann JV, Abrams R. Improved survival for hepatocellular carcinoma with combination surgery and multimodality treatment. *Ann Surg* 1993; **217**:149-154
38. Tang Z-Y, Yu Y-Q, Zhou X-D *et al*. Cytoreduction and sequential resection for surgically verified unresectable hepatocellular carcinoma: evaluation with analysis of 72 patients. *World J Surg* 1995; **19**:784-789
39. Yokoyama I, Todo S, Iwatsuki S, Starzl TE. Liver transplantation in the treatment of primary liver cancer. *Hepato-Gastroenterol* 1990; **37**:188-193
40. Iwatsuki S, Starzl TE, Sheahan DG *et al*. Hepatic resection versus transplantation for hepatocellular carcinoma. *Ann Surg* 1991; **214**:221-229
41. Bismuth H, Chiche L, Adam R, Castang D, Diamond T, Dennison A. Liver resection versus transplantation for hepatocellular carcinoma in cirrhotic patients. *Ann Surg* 1993; **218**:145-151
42. McPeake JR, O'Grady JG, Zaman S *et al*. Liver transplantation for primary hepatocellular carcinoma: tumor size and number determine outcome. *J Hepatol* 1993; **18**:226-234
43. McPeake J, Williams R. Liver transplantation for hepatocellular carcinoma. *Gut* 1995; **36**:644-646
44. Ringe B, Pichlmayr R, Wittekind C, Tusch G. Surgical treatment of hepatocellular carcinoma: experience with liver resection and transplantation in 198 patients. *World J Surg* 1991; **15**:270-285
45. Gores GJ, Steers JL. Progress in orthotopic transplantation for hepatocellular carcinoma. *Gastroenterology* 1993; **104**:317-320
46. Yokoyama I, Carr B, Saitsu H, Iwatsuki S, Starzl TE. Accelerated growth rates of recurrent hepatocellular carcinoma after liver transplantation. *Cancer* 1991; **68**:2095-2100
47. Pichlmayr R, Weimann A, Ringe B. Indicatons for liver transplantation in hepatobiliary malignancy. *Hepatology* 1994; **20**:33S-40S
48. Carr BI, Selby R, Madriaga J, Iwatsuki S, Starzl TE. Prolonged survival after liver transplantation and cancer chemotherapy for advanced-stage hepatocellular carcinoma. *Transpl Proc* 1993; **25**:1128-1129
49. Cherqui D, Piedbois P, Vavasseur D *et al*. Liver transplantation with combined adjuvant treatment in hepatocellular carcinoma (abstract). *HPB Surg* 1993; **6**: 121
50. Stone MJ, Klintmalm GBG, Polter D *et al*. Neoadjuvant chemotherapy and liver transplantation for hepatocellular carcinoma: a pilot study in 20 patients. *Gastroenterology* 1993; **104**:192-202
51. Cummings OW. Disease recurrence after orthotopic liver transplantation. *Semin Diagn Pathol* 1993; **10**:292-301
52. Arias IM, Multidrug resistance genes, p-glycoprotein, and the liver. *Hepatology* 1990; **12**:159-165
53. Huang C, Wu M, Xu G *et al*. Overexpression of the MDR1 gene and P-glycoprotein in human hepatocellular carcinoma.

J Natl Cancer Inst 1992; **84**:262-264

54. Livraghi T, Lazzaroni S, Meloni F *et al*. Intralesional ethanol in the treatment of unresectable liver cancer. *World J Surg* 1995; **19**:801-806
55. Tanaka K, Nakamura S, Numata K *et al*. Hepatocellular carcinoma: treatment with percutaneous ethanol injection and transcatheter arterial embolization. *Radiology* 1992; **185**:457-460
56. Tateishi H, Kinuta M, Furukawa J *et al*. Follow-up study of combination treatment (TAE and PEIT) for unresectable hepatocellular carcinoma. *Cancer Chemother Pharmacol* 1994; **33**(suppl): 119-123
57. Bartolozzi C, Lencioni R, Caramella D, Falaschi F, Cioni R, Di Coscio G. Hepatocellular carcinoma: CT and MR features after transcatheter arterial embolization and percutaneous ethanol injection. *Radiology* 1994; **191**:123-128
58. Livraghi T, Vettori C, Torzilli G, Lazzaroni S, Pellicano S, Ravasi S. Percutaneous ethanol injection of hepatic tumors: single-session therapy under general anesthesia. *AJR* 1993; **161**:1065-1069
59. Yamakado K, Hirano T, Kato N *et al*. Hepatocellular carcinoma: treatment with a combination of transcatheter arterial chemoembolization and transportal ethanol injection. *Radiology* 1994; **193**:75-80
60. Han C, Meng-Chao W. Reoperative primary liver cancer. *Chinese Med J* 1987; **100**:795
61. Lange IF, Leese T, Castaing D, Bismuth H. Repeat hepatectomy for recurrent malignant tumors of the liver. *Surg Gynecol Obstet* 1989; **169**:119
62. Takayasu K, Muramatsu Y, Moriyama N *et al*. Clinical and radiologic assessments of the results of hepatectomy for small hepatocellular carcinoma and therapeutic arterial embolization for postoperative recurrence. *Cancer* 1989; **64**:1848-1852
63. Takayasu K, Wakao F, Moriyama N *et al*. Postresection recurrence of hepatocellular carcinoma treated by arterial embolization: analysis of prognostic factors. *Hepatology* 1992; **16**:906-911
64. Groupe d'etude et de traitement du carcinome hepatocellulaire. A comparison of Lipiodol chemoembolization and conservative treatment for unresectable hepatocellular carcinoma. *N Engl J Med* 1995; **332**:1256-61
65. Koneru B, Cassavilla A, Bowman J, Iwatsuki S, Starzl TE. Liver transplantation for malignant tumors. *Gastroenterol Clin North Am* 1988; **17**:177
66. Friedman MA, Demanes DJ, Hoffmann PG. Hepatomas: hormone receptors and therapy. *Am J Med* 1982; **73**:362-365
67. Nagasue N, Ito A, Yukaya H, OgawaY. Estrogen receptors in hepatocellular carcinoma. *Cancer* 1986; **57**:87-91
68. Melia WM, Johnson PJ, Williams R. Controlled clinical trial of doxorubicin and tamoxifen versus doxorubicin alone in hepatocellular carcinoma. *Cancer Treat Rev* 1987; **71**:1213-1216
69. Engstrom PF, Levin B, Moertel CG, Schutt A. A phase II trial of tamoxifen in hepatocellular carcinoma. *Cancer* 1990; **65**:2641-1643
70. Farinati F. Salvagnini M, De Maria N *et al*. Unresectable hepatocellular carcinoma: a prospective controlled trial with tamoxifen. *J Hepatol* 1990; **11**:297-301
71. Martinez-Cerezo FG, Tomas A, Donoso L *et al*. Controlled trial of tamoxifen in patients with advanced hepatocellular carcinoma. *J Hepatol* 1994; **20**:702-706
72. Manesis EK, Giannoulis G, Zoumboulis P, Vafiadou I, Hadziyannis SJ. Treatment of hepatocellular carcinoma with combined suppression and inhibition of sex hormones: a randomized, controlled trial. *Hepatology* 1995; **21**:1535-1542
73. Castells A, Bruix J, Bru C *et al*. Treatment of hepatocellular carcinoma with tamoxifen: a double-blind placebo-controlled trial in 120 patients. *Gastroenterology* 1995; **109**:917-922
74. Kardinal CG, Moertel CG, Wieand HS *et al*. Combined doxorubicin and alpha-interferon therapy of advanced hepatocellular carcinoma. *Cancer* 1993; **71**:2187-2190
75. Colleoni M, Buzzoni R, Bajetta E *et al*. A phase II study of mitoxantrone combined with Beta-interferon in unresectable hepatocellular carcinoma. *Cancer* 1993; **72**:3196-3201
76. Order SE, Stillwagon GB, Klein JL *et al*. Iodine 131 antiferritin, a new treatment modality in hepatoma: a radiation therapy Oncology Group study. *J Clin Oncol* 1985; **3**: 1573-1582
77. Order SE, Pajak T, Leibel S *et al*. A randomized prospective trial comparing full dose chemotherapy to 131 I antiferritin: an RTOG study. *Int J Radiat Oncol Biol Phys* 1991; **20**:953-963
78. Raoul JL, Guyader D, Bretagne JF *et al*. Randomized controlled trial for hepatocellular carcinoma with portal vein thrombosis: intra-arterial Iodine-131-iodized oil versus medical support. *J Nucl Med* 1994; **35**:1782-1787

31

Therapeutic guidelines

T Livraghi, M Makuuchi and L Buscarini

In countries where US (and AFP) screening of the at risk population is practised, early diagnosis of HCC is possible while elsewhere, apart from the odd incidental finding, diagnosis is not made until the disease is already advanced. The time of diagnosis governs the type of treatment offered: possibly curative when diagnosis is early, palliative when diagnosis is late. The range of treatment options is fairly wide and the choice is not always easy, given the number of variables to be assessed. Economic resources and the expertise available at each center are other factors that may play a not inconsiderable part in the choice of treatment.

Before going into the various aspects of the different treatments, we need to state some fundamental premises for the evaluation and hence management of the patient. The first premise concerns the survival of the untreated patient, the second the multifocality of HCC and the third the factors affecting prognosis.

SURVIVAL OF THE UNTREATED PATIENT

The effectiveness of most interventions is assessed on inter-group comparisons or on histologic evidence whereas the impact on survival has not been demonstrated by randomized studies but was measured against historic data. Therefore selection bias cannot altogether be ruled out. The survival studies usually taken as points of reference fall into two groups: those relating to patients in whom the disease was not advanced, and therefore likely to be amenable to curative treatment, and those in whom the disease was advanced.

The first group includes the studies of Tang, Ebara and Livraghi.[1-3] Tang *et al*[1], whose work covered 12 patients rated comparable to patients treated surgically, with a single HCC ≤5 cm, reported 1, 2, 3 and 4 year survival rates of 66, 41, 10 and 0% respectively. The study of Ebara *et al*[2], relating to 22 patients with a single HCC ≤3 cm of every Child's class, yielded 1, 2 and 3 year survival rates of 90, 55 and 12% respectively; presumably the Child class A patients fared better than the group as a whole. The work of Livraghi *et al*[3] (including the series previously published by Barbara *et al* and Cottone *et al*)[4,5] comprised 116 patients with a single HCC ≤5 cm, 73 of Child class A and 43 of class B, with 1, 2, 3 and 5 year survival rates of 86, 51, 26 and 11% and 65, 22, 13 and 0% respectively; of the 73 Child class A patients 47 were deemed potentially operable and the survival rates in this group were 89, 51 and 30% at 1, 2 and 3 years respectively. The latter data, given the number of patients and their stratification, may be held the most reliable to date as the standard for comparison with the results of radical treatment.

The second group includes the studies of Okuda and Calvet.[6,7] Okuda *et al*[6] whose series of 229 patients comprised 33 stage I, 134 stage II and 62 stage III cases (see Chapter. 21), reported mean survival rates of 8.3, 2.0 and 0.7 months respectively. Calvet *et al*[7], studying 206 patients, reported a median survival of 10.9 months in the first group, 3.9 in the second and 1 month in the third. Interestingly, survival proved to be substantially equivalent in the two studies and so the rates can safely be taken as benchmarks for the results of treatment given to patients with advanced disease.

There are no studies on patients with "intermediate" HCC. One possible point of reference might be the study published by the Groupe d'Etude et de Traitement du Carcinome Hepatocellulaire[8] comparing an intra-arterial therapy against 49 controls, whose 1, 2 and 3 year survival rates were 43, 26 and 15% respectively.

MULTIFOCALITY

It is now known, though only confirmed a few years ago, that HCC should be considered an organ disease, since it is provenly multicentric in origin.[9-11] The implication of this fact, which must always be borne in mind in patient management, is that the only treatment likely to afford permanent cure is OLT.[12] A recent study by Adachi *et al* in which it was possible to select 102 patients who had undergone resection for a single HCC <3 cm without venous invasion and without intrahepatic metastases, thus excluding recurrences from the resected tumor, demonstrated new lesions in 67% of the cases at 5 year follow-up.[13] Higher percentages, up to 100%,[14] have emerged from numerous other surgical studies, which often included local recurrences. Interestingly, in the study of Adachi *et al*, the factors associated with the highest new recurrence rate stemmed from the underlying liver disease, that is, an active inflammation and a low albumin level, and not from the tumor *per se*.

Table 31.2 – Therapeutic Options

Surgical	Intra-arterial	Interstitial	Systemic	Radiant
Resection	TAE	PEI	Chemotherapy	External
OLT	CA	Radiofrequency	Hormone therapy	Internal
	TAE + CA	Hot saline	Immunotherapy	
	Lip + TAE + CA	Acetic acid		
	Lip + CA	Microwaves		
	seg - Lip + TAE + CA	Cryo		

CA= Chemotherapeutic Agents

PROGNOSTIC FACTORS

The search for predictive factors has led, through more far-reaching knowledge of the disease, to more appropriate patient management. Better assessment has made possible the accurate selection of patients, thereby safeguarding them from useless or even harmful interventions. For example, it is not only advances in surgical technique and in postoperative care but also the exclusion of patients with adverse predictive factors that have ensured great improvements in survival in surgical series over the years. It is understood that these factors may vary depending on the type of treatment. For example, while portal thrombosis is always deleterious whatever the treatment, replicating hepatitis B is an adverse factor more particularly for OLT. Clearly, there cannot always be rigid criteria for exclusion for a given treatment on the grounds of one or more adverse factors, if the patient stands to get some benefit from it. However, the greater the risk for the patient, the more careful selection must be, especially if alternative therapies carrying less risk and lower cost are available. The best known prognostic factors have nearly always been identified by means of multivariate analysis, even though the results are sometimes discordant. These factors, on which the various staging schemes are based (Chapter. 21), are listed in Table 31.1, classified according to whether they depend on the underlying liver disease or the tumor. Recent studies have identified some prognostic factors evaluated by optical microscopy, as Ag NOR, PCNA, Ki 67 and nucleo-cytoplasmic ratio (see addendum); however these studies need further confirmation.

Table 31.1 – Adverse Prognostic Factors

Liver Function	Tumor
Ascites	Vascular invasion
Bilirubin >1.8	Intrahepatic metastases
GOT >35	Extrahepatic metastases
Child's grade B and C	Lymphnodes involvement
Advanced age (>65)	Increasing size (>5)
Albumin <30	Increasing number (≥2)
Bromosulphalein >30	Toxic syndrome
Severe active hepatitis	Capsule infiltration
Blood urea nitrogen >20	Low differentiation
	Infiltrating type
	AFP >200
	DCP positivity

THERAPIES

The options open today are listed in Table 31.2 under the following headings: surgical, interstitial, intra-arterial, systemic and radiant. We now consider the indications, survival rates and complications of each.

Partial resection

The indications range from an ideal situation, that is, one in which the patient of <65 years is Child's A with a single HCC <3 cm, with capsule intact, at an easily accessible site to cases in which resection has to be very extensive because of an HCC at any stage of locoregional disease requiring vascular reconstruction due to portal and inferior vena cava tumor thrombi and resection of intrahepatic metastases in both lobes. Resection is feasible in both situations but both the operative risk and long term survival differ when major adverse prognostic factors are present. In one series of 225 patients encompassing both situations peroperative mortality was 2.4% in the better cases and 21% in the worse and the corresponding 3 year survival rates 100% and 35% respectively.[15]

In 1838 patients collected from 15 series with a single HCC ≤5 cm and well compensated cirrhosis the 5 year survival rates ranged from 33 to 64% with a mean of 51%, peroperative mortality from 1.4 to 11% with a mean of 7% and a complications rate of up to 58%.[16-30]

The Liver Cancer Study Group of Japan reported the factors affecting long term survival of 1167 patients submitted to partial hepatectomy.[31] In this study multivariate analysis indicated that significant prognostic indicators were AFP level, tumor size, number of tumors, accompanying cirrhosis, age, surgical curability and portal involvement; univariate analysis indicated HBsAg positivity, capsular infiltration, anatomic extent of the tumor, a 1 cm cancer-free margin, Edmondson classification and habitual alcohol intake.

OLT

The Paris Consensus Conference of 1994[32] produced the following conclusions: *"It is difficult to offer liver transplantation to all patients with primary malignant liver tumors, given the uncertain long term benefit in some cases. This is in particular the case with a patient with large malignant tumors or multinodular tumors. It is also difficult to determine which patients with smaller tumors are likely to benefit from transplantation: even though good results can be obtained, they must be compared with those of other methods such as excision, alcoholization and chemoembolization. In conclusion, liver transplantation in patients with primary liver cancer must be thoroughly evaluated by taking into account the likely midterm and long term benefits"*. The following guidelines were then proposed: any type of extrahepatic spread is a contraindication to OLT, an unresectable tumor at UICC stage II a *favorable* indication, and a UICC stage III or IV tumor a *borderline individual decision*.[33] However, the selection criteria at the leading centers were somewhat discordant. The Pittsburgh group, despite their significantly better survival rates for OLT at every tumor stage (in stage II 5 year survival 75% *vs* no year survival after resection), stated that: *"It is impractical and even fraudulent to recommend that all HCCs in the cirrhotic liver should be treated by liver transplantation. It is equally incorrect to exclude the patients with HCC from liver transplantation when the malignancy is confined to the liver. The treatment of choice for HCC confined to the liver is subtotal hepatic resection when it is anatomically and functionally feasible. Liver transplantation is the treatment of choice for HCC confined to the liver when the hepatic functions are poor and/or the HCC cannot be removed by subtotal hepatic resection"*.[34]

The King's College London team considers OLT to be the treatment of choice for Child's classes B and C with a single HCC <8 cm and, given the high incidence of satellite and multifocal lesions found in explanted liver but not diagnosed by imaging in the work-up for OLT, probably also for Child's class A with single HCC <8 cm.[35]

The group from Hôpital Paul Brousse Paris state that: *"OLT for HCC should be avoided for large (>3 cm) lesions with three or more nodules and should be restricted to small lesions (<3 cm) with one or two nodules, the group that until now was thought to be indicated for resection,"*[36] while the team from Hannover resorts to OLT only *"in the nonresectable situation, because of anatomical and functional restrictions"*.[37]

It is worth noting that despite the general consensus against OLT in advanced HCC because of the near certainty of recurrence, a few cases of this type with long disease-free survival were reported in some of the series.

In 66 patients collected from 4 series with HCC ≤5 cm and even advanced cirrhosis, 5 year survival ranged from 60 to 75% with a mean of 65%.[33-38] Peroperative mortality in 236 of the cases collected from 6 series ranged from 5 to 32% with a mean of 12%.[33-38]

Tumoral factors statistically significant as negatively influencing survival were bilobar involvement, the presence of vascular invasion, positive surgical margin, and the presence of lymph node metastases.[38]

The chief problem with OLT is the shortage of donors. In Italy alone the number of new cases of HCC is estimated at around 12,000 a year whereas in the whole of Europe the number of OLT performed in 1994 (from the European Liver Transplant Registry) for neoplastic disease in general was 196 with a tendency to decline in the past few years (from 213 in 1990). In Japan, where the number of new cases is around 20,000 a year, OLT is not performed.

PEI (and other interstitial treatments)

The range of indications for PEI is becoming wider than for surgery. Indeed, while for some years only patients with up to three small (<3 or <5 cm) lesions were treated, and this still applies at many centers, with the introduction of the "single session" procedure under general anaesthesia, or at any rate with the injection of larger quantities of ethanol, even patients with a greater number of lesions, including those of >10 cm, are now being treated. Clearly, the aim of treatment will be radical removal or palliation according to tumor stage.

In 737 patients with a single HCC <5 cm and moderate cirrhosis collected from 5 series, the 5 year survival rate ranged from 44 to 61% with a mean of 47%.[22,39-42] The mortality attributable to conventional PEI across the 1623 published cases was 0.06% and for single session PEI 0.8% while the corresponding major complications rates were up to 2.4 and 3.6% (see Chapter 25).

Other percutaneous interstitial therapies such as radiofrequency, acetic acid, hot saline and microwaves (see Chapter 26) have broadly the same indications as PEI, although, as they are more recent, further confirmation is needed. Cryotherapy is an interstitial therapy but it is given after laparotomy because of the large diameter of the probe, using IOUS for guidance. For this reason it is less widely performed than PEI, even though the indications are the same and the results comparable (see Chapter 27).

Intra-arterial therapies

Intra-arterial therapy has the widest range of indications and, since the principal one is a multifocal tumor, the commonest situation, it is also the one most often used. Over the years several variants of Yamada *et al*'s original procedure based on the administration of gelatin sponge particles (TAE)[43] have been proposed; the most widely used involves the injection in several sessions of a mixture of Lipiodol and chemotherapeutic agents, as a rule doxorubicin, and gelatin sponge particles. There is, however, some considerable uncertainty about which is really the best procedure. Recent reports are conflicting. While Nakamura *et al*[44] and Uchida *et al*[45] claim that the addition of Lipiodol contributes greatly to prolonging survival, a prospective trial of Hatanaka *et al*[46] showed equal survival in patients who did not receive Lipiodol; likewise a randomized study of Chang *et al*[47] showed that the addition of chemotherapeutic agent (cisplantin) did not enhance the therapeutic effect. The effectiveness of the treatment is proved by histologic studies,[48-51] and by survival studies comparing the results with historic data.[52-55]

Surprisingly, the only two randomized studies failed to show a statistically significant gain in the treated patients despite a proven reduction of tumor growth.[8,56] In the more recent study 1 and 2 year survival rates were 62 and 37% respectively in the treated group and 43 and 26% in the untreated, with a relative risk of death in the latter group of 1.3. The investigators reported that *"Lipiodol chemoembolization has numerous side effects, requires hospitalization and is expensive. Since it did not markedly improve survival, we do not believe its use can be recommended."* However, since *"tumor size decreased in more than half the patients who received TACE and increased in more than half the patients assigned to conservative management"*, they concluded that *"Lipiodol chemoembolization may be beneficial in a more select group of patients, but factors predictive of a response to this treatment, without the development of side effects, have yet to be determined"*. The fact that most of the patients enrolled in these two studies had alcoholic liver disease might account for the disappointing results but only supposing a better response to intra-arterial therapy of the HCC on posthepatitic liver disease, as occurs in the majority of Japanese patients. However, in a French nonrandomized comparative multicenter trial in which each treated patient was closely matched with an untreated patient, both with prevalent alcoholic liver disease, the 1, 2 and 3 year probabilities of survival were 64, 38 and 27% respectively in the former group and 18, 6 and 5% in the latter.[57] A more likely explanation of the disappointing results is the rather aggressive approach adopted, namely four sessions with an interval of 2 months, with consequent deterioration of liver function in some patients and earlier liver failure. This is a major side effect seen in earlier studies.[58-61]

Bruix *et al*[60] draw attention to another aspect of intra-arterial therapy, that is, since this is nearly always a palliative intervention, *"the reactivation of this disease may counteract the potential benefit of the initial response to treatment. In fact, the main difference in survival between the treated and the mathematical control group is observed after 6 and 12 months, indicating that successful TAE is able to diminish the first-year deaths but not act thereafter, when the tumor grows again"*; these investigators go on to conclude that *"although the patients are classified as being at an intermediate stage, some patients would probably really benefit from treatment and in others TAE would be useless or even deleterious. To unequivocally ascertain whether TAE is an effective treatment for HCC prospective placebo-controlled studies including a large number of patients carefully stratified according to the functional status of the liver and evolutionary stage of the neoplasm are mandatory. Our data provide the rationale and ethical basis for conducting and designing these trials, which, in addition to assessing the effects on survival, may also show that initial tumor necrosis induced by TAE may reduce the incidence or delay the onset of symptoms or life-threatening complications. If these secondary goals of treatment are demonstrated, despite the absence of a noteworthy effect on survival, TAE will still have a role as as a palliative treatment for HCC"*.

Studies designed to identify factors that might predict the success of treatment have recently been published.[46,57,61-63] The overall treatment mortality rate is around 2%.

Segmental TAE has broadly the same indications as segmental resection and PEI. As treatment has been confined to one segment and in some cases to one subsegmental area, this treatment presents no short term complications or the problems of long term liver function deterioration that mark conventional intra-arterial therapies.

The 5 year survival rate among 173 patients collected from two series of patients with HCC <5 cm whose cirrhosis was not advanced ranged from 33 to 53% with a mean of 44%.[64,65] In comparison, among 640 patients from 5 series with the same disease presentation treated with conventional TAE the 5 year survival rate ranged from 9 to 32% with a mean of 13%.[61,66-68] The reason for the large difference is that segmental TAE inflicts much greater damage on neoplastic tissue with a significantly lower rate of local recurrence.[69] Some technical improvements such as occlusion of the hepatic vein which drains the tumor-bearing segment have further enhanced therapeutic effectiveness.[70] (see Chapter 24)

A new arterial option that promises well involves the injection of OK 432 and fibrinogen.[71]

Systemic chemotherapy

To date systemic therapies have been used only in patients with advanced HCC. Regardless of regimen, that is, either single-drug or combination chemotherapy, response rates have not exceeded 30% and survival has not been affected. Furthermore, in one randomized study doxorubicin, considered one of the potentially most active drugs, not only failed to prolong survival but also caused fatal complications due to cardiotoxicity in 18% of the patients.[72] Possible explanations for the refractoriness of HCC to the cytotoxic drugs currently in use include the inducible overexpression of the multidrug-resistance gene product p-glycoprotein, which transports doxorubicin out of the cell conferring drug resistance,[73,74] or tumor heterogeneity.[75] On the other hand, some workers have observed that with a rather aggressive pre- and post-OLT approach the recurrence rate dropped;[76,77] the explanation could be that cyclosporin may block the activity of the multidrug-resistance gene, thereby enhancing the effectiveness of doxorubicin.[78]

The administration of immunotherapeutic drugs, with or without chemotherapeutic agents, has yielded similarly disappointing results.[79]

With regard to hormonal therapy, the promising results of one randomized study using tamoxifen have not been confirmed.[80] In fact, in a recent study by Castells *et al*[81], in which 120 patients were enrolled and carefully stratified, the 1 and 2 year survival rates were 51 and 27% respectively compared with 43 and 29% in the untreated group; furthermore, there were no differences in the probability of disease progression or baseline performance maintenance during follow-up.

Radiation treatment

Attempts with conventional radiation therapy have yielded disappointing results. Severe adverse effects on the liver and other organs have prevented irradiation of sufficient quantity and duration. More recently, the administration of 50 Gy to patients without severe cirrhosis has yielded an improvement in survival: the mean survival of the irradiated patients was 545 days vs 106 in the untreated group (see Chapter 29). In another study, using proton beams at doses of 50-87 Gy, there was a "main reduction" in 92% of the cases without major complications.[82] If these results were confirmed by other studies, new options would be open to patients excluded from conventional therapies.

To allow higher tumor doses and to limit undesiderable side effects a procedure for intra-arterial irradiation has been proposed. In a prospective study in which one group of patients with portal thrombosis treated with iodized oil injections was compared with controls receiving medical support, survival was significantly longer in the first group.[83]

CHOICE OF TREATMENT

HCC is a tumor of multifocal origin that grows on chronic liver disease. The liver disease, if aggressive, may kill before the tumor. This being so, it is clear that only OLT, if available, can offer permanent cure, and then only when the tumor is at an early stage. Unfortunately, since demand hugely exceeds supply, OLT is at present often not an option. No other treatment can do more than prolong survival as far as possible, and in variable measure.

The choice among available treatments ought to have been based on controlled trials of these one by one *versus* no treatment, after which, once a gain in survival was established, on trials comparing the various possibilities. Unfortunately yet again, the data on the survival of untreated patients with a "curable" HCC stem from a few uncontrolled studies. While on the one hand, according to strictly scientific criteria these data should not be taken as a standard, on the other, the setting up of a randomized trial of treated *vs* untreated patients would be ethically unacceptable. In fact, several surgical teams have reduced their peroperative mortality to under 3% and have learnt to select patients accurately according to the predictive factors. At the same time treatments such as PEI and segmental TAE have proved beyond doubt to be effective and almost risk-free. But studies comparing the various treatments, even when conducted at the same center, were not randomized.

In the three studies comparing OLT and partial resections OLT yielded distinctly better results: in two[34,35] 3 year survival was 56% *vs* 0% and 63% *vs* 33%; in the third it was 49% *vs* 52%, but with a significant difference in disease-free interval.[36]

Table 31.3 – Single HCC ≤5 cm: Results

Therapy	Number of patients	Survival(%) 3 years	Survival(%) 5 years	Peroperative Mortality(%)
OLT	66	72	65	12
Resection	1838	71	51	7
PEI	737	74	47	0
TAE-TACE	640	43	13	2
seg-TACE	155	72	44	0

Of the four studies comparing partial resection with intra-arterial therapies, all studies vitiated by selection bias penalizing the latter, three showed better results with resection[84-86], the 3 year survival rates being 64% *vs* 31%, 85% *vs* 38% and 74% *vs* 50%, and one with TAE with 64% *vs* 47%.[87]

In the four studies comparing resection with PEI the 3 year survival rates were broadly equivalent,[3,22,88,89] that is, 79% *vs* 80%, 78% *vs* 87%, 88% *vs* 78% and 44% *vs* 55%. In the second study[22], cited by the Reports on Projects of the Comprehensive Ten-year Strategy of Cancer Control sponsored by the Ministry of Health and Welfare of Japan, the 5 year survival rates favored resection, i.e. 58% *vs* 47%; in this study resection was also compared stage for stage with TAE, which presented 3 and 5 year survival rates of 42% and 13% respectively. In the fourth study[89] the cohort of patients who received PEI presented significantly poorer liver function.

For comparison, the mean (n1 x % + n 2 x % + n ^{x} x %/total number) of results for single HCC <5 cm together with the collective data presented in this chapter are given in Table 31.3.

These data call for detailed analysis. The small difference in 3 and 5 year survival after OLT reflects the fact that recurrences, whether neoplastic or viral, develop, when they do, within the first 3 years; once over this hurdle, most patients may be regarded as cured. Contrariwise, all patients who received another treatment can only present progression of the neoplastic disease with the onset of new lesions (and of local recurrences in the case of non surgical treatment) and, of course, also of the cirrhosis. It is rather puzzling that the results of resection should be so similar to those of PEI and of segmental TAE when it by definition ensures removal and PEI and TAE both do so in only about 70% of cases. In our view,

HCC STAGING CARD

Name .... Age 63 Sex [X] M [ ] F Date ....

Associated Diseases	//		
Previous Therapies of HCC	//		
Etiology	HBsAg+ (active / inactive / HDV)	**anti-HCV+**	other ( )
	1	2	3
ESOPHAGEAL VARICES	absent	**low risk**	high risk
CHILD'S CLASS	**A**	B	C
GRADING	**well differentiated**	moderately differentiated	poor differentiated
TYPE	**nodular**	infiltrating	diffuse
NUMBER	**1**	2-3	> 3 ( )
SIZE	< 2 cm	**2.1 - 5 cm**	> 5.1 ( )
LOCATION	1 segment (6)	> 1 segment ( )	bilobar ( )
TUMOR INVASIVENESS	**absent**	local	IM
VASCULAR INVASION (P.V.B)	**absent**	local	diffuse
NM	**0**	N+	M+
AFP	**< 20 ( )**	21-200 ( )	> 200 ( )

P = portal veins, V = hepatic veins, B = bile ducts, IM = intrahepatic metastases (satellites)

Note ....

Figure 31.1

HCC STAGING CARD

Name .... Age 66 Sex [ ] M [ ] F Date ....

Associated Diseases	//		
Previous Therapies of HCC	//		
Etiology	**HBsAg+** (**active** / inactive / HDV)	anti-HCV+	other ( )
	1	2	3
ESOPHAGEAL VARICES	absent	**low risk**	high risk
CHILD'S CLASS	A	**B**	C
GRADING	well differentiated	**moderately differentiated**	poor differentiated
TYPE	nodular	**infiltrating**	diffuse
NUMBER	1	2-3	**> 3 (5)**
SIZE	< 2 cm	**2.1 - 5 cm**	> 5.1 ( )
LOCATION	1 segment ( )	> 1 segment ( )	**bilobar** ( )
TUMOR INVASIVENESS	absent	**local**	IM
VASCULAR INVASION (P.V.B)	absent	**local**	diffuse
NM	**0**	N+	M+
AFP	< 20 ( )	21-200 ( )	**> 200 ( )**

P = portal veins, V = hepatic veins, B = bile ducts, IM = intrahepatic metastases (satellites)

Note ....

Figure 31.2

the small difference arose from insufficiently careful selection of patients for resection (underestimate of some adverse predictive factors; removal of too much non neoplastic tissue, which may have hastened liver failure; inaccurate staging; peroperative mortality not low enough in a few series), which affected the overall results. The excellent success rates in recent series made up of carefully selected patients bear out this interpretation.

By way of example, some case reports are reviewed in the light of the staging card presented in Chapter 21.

Figure 31.1 shows the common case of a patient diagnosed in the course of US screening, that is, one with an early HCC. Age, moderate cirrhosis, scant aggressiveness of the tumor and the segment affected all suggest resection as the treatment of choice. A change in any of these factors could lead to a different choice. If the patient were 10 years older, the increase in operative risk might contraindicate surgery in favor of PEI or segmental TAE. If the cirrhosis were class C, treatment of any kind might bring little benefit and might cause harm. If the tumor were in segment 8 and deepseated, resection would be indicated only at centers capable of ensuring low peroperative mortality (<3%) and morbidity. If the patient were 10 years younger, OLT, if available, might be the treatment most likely to afford long survival, and the only choice if the patient were Child's class C. If segmental portal thrombosis or intrahepatic metastases were present, any treatment could only halt the evolution of the neoplastic disease for a time; in this case resection affords better guarantee of local radicality in the face of an anyway short life expectancy and of some risk due to the mandatorily more extensive tissue removal. On the other hand, PEI, segmental TAE, intra-arterial injection of ^{131}iodine iodized oil and radiotherapy reduce the mass of the main lesion with some chance of retarding the growth of the thrombus but none has any certain significant impact on survival. If the patient had five lesions, conventional chemoembolization is the treatment most indicated, although single-session PEI may often yield good results. In the five-lesion situation there are anecdotal reports of long survival with OLT, even though success would not be expected. When called upon to take a decision regarding a patient who would otherwise die within a few years, this course has to be considered.

To sum up, the possible combinations are many and so it is not easy to lay down strict rules for the management of patients whose HCC is not advanced. This means that the most opportune treatment has to be decided in the light of each individual patient's characteristics, evaluating every variable, of the expertise available at each center and of the economic resources of the national health service.

Figure 31.2 gives the profile of a patient diagnosed as having an advanced HCC. Although no other therapies are available at the moment, systemic therapies are not a justifiable option except in clinical trials. Even so, it is not rare for there to be a tacit agreement between patient and doctor, when the patient insists on treatment and the doctor finds it easier to comply with his wishes.

REFERENCES

1. Tang ZY, Yu YQ, Zhou XD, *et al.* Surgery of small hepatocellular carcinoma. Analysis of 144 cases. *Cancer* 1989; **64**: 536-541
2. Ebara M, Ohto M, Shinagawa T, *et al.* Natural history of minute hepatoocellular carcinoma smaller than three centimeters complicating cirrhosis. A study in 22 patients. *Gastroenterology* 1986; **90**: 289-298
3. Livraghi T, Bolondi L, Buscarini L, *et al.* No treatment, resection and ethanol injection in hepatocellular carcinoma: a retrospective analysis of survival in 391 patients with cirrhosis. *J Hepatol* 1995; **22**: 522-526
4. Barbara L, Benzi G, Gaiani S, *et al.* Natural history of small untreated hepatocellular carcinoma in cirrhosis: a multivariate analysis of prognostic factors of tumor growth rate and patient survival. *Hepatology* 1992; **16**: 132-137
5. Cottone M, Virdone R, Fusco G, *et al.* Asymptomatic hepatocellular carcinoma in Child's A cirrhosis. A comparison of natural history and surgical treatment. *Gastroenterology* 1989; **96**: 1566-1571
6. Okuda K, Ohtsuki T, Obata H, *et al.* Natural history of hepatocellular carcinoma and prognosis in relation to treatment. Study of 850 patients. *Cancer* 1985; **56**: 918-928
7. Calvet X, Bruix J, Ginés P, Bru C, Solé M, Vilana R, Rodés J. Prognostic factors of hepatocellular carcinoma in the West: a multivariate analysis in 206 patients. *Hepatology* 1990; **12**: 753-760
8. Groupe d'Etude et de Traitement du Carcinome Hépatocellulaire. A comparison of Lipiodol chemoembolization and conservative treatment for unresectable hepatocellular carcinoma. *N Engl J Med* 1995; **332**: 1256-1261
9. Sheu JC, Huang GT, Chou Hc, *et al.* Multiple hepatocellular carcinomas at the early stage have different clonality. *Gastroenterology* 1993; **105**: 1471-1476
10. Takenaka K, Adachi E, Nishizaki T, *et al.* Possible multicentric occurence of hepatocellular carcinoma: a clinicopathological study. *Hepatology* 1994; **19**: 889-894
11. Oda T, Tsuda H, Scarpa A, Sakamoto M, Hirohashi S. Mutation pattern of the p53 gene as a diagnostic marker for multiple hepatocellular carcinoma. *Cancer Res* 1992; **52**: 3674-3678
12. McPeake J, Williams R. Liver transplantation for hepatocellular carcinoma. *Gut* 1995; **36**: 644-646
13. Adachi E, Maeda T, Matsumata T, Shirabe K, Kinukawa N, Sugimachi K, Tsuneyoshi M. Risk factors for intrahepatic recurrence in human small hepatocellular carcinoma. *Gastroenterology* 1995; **108**: 768-775
14. Belghiti J, Panis Y, Farges O, Benhamou JP, Fekete F. Intrahepatic recurrence after resection of hepatocellular carcinoma complicating cirrhosis. *Ann Surg* 1991; **214**: 114-117
15. Ozawa K, Takayasu T, Kumada K, *et al.* Experience with 225 hepatic resections for hepatocellular carcinoma over a 4-year period. *Am J Surg* 1991; **161**: 677-682
16. Wu MC, Zhang XH, Chen H. Hepatic resection for primary liver cancer. *Chin Med J* 1986; **99**: 175-180
17. Kawano N, Ohmori Y, Inoue O. Long-term prognosis of surgical patients with hepatocellular carcinoma. *Cancer Chemother Pharmacol* 1989; **23**(suppl): 129-132
18. Tang ZY, Yu YQ, Zhou XA. Surgery of small hepatocellular carcinoma. *Cancer* 1989; **64**: 536-541
19. Yamanaka N, Okamoto E, Toyosaka A, *et al.* Prognostic factors after hepatectomy for hepatocellular carcinomas. *Cancer* 1990; **65**: 1104-1110
20. Lai ECS, Ng IOL, You KT. Hepatic resection for small hepatocellular carcinoma: the Queen Mary Hospital experience. *World J Surg* 1991; **15**: 654-659
21. Kanematsu T, Matsumata T, Shirabe K, *et al.* A comparative study of hepatic resection and transcatheter arterial embolization for the treatment of primary hepatocellular carcinoma. *Cancer* 1993; **71**: 2181-2186
22. Makuuchi M, Kosuge T, Takayama T, *et al.* Surgery for small liver cancers. *Semin Surg Oncol* 1993; **9**: 298-304
23. Sugioka A, Tsuzuki T, Kanai T. Postresection prognosis of patients with hepatocellular carcinoma. *Surgery* 1993; **113**: 612-618
24. Takayasu T, Ino K, Yamaoka Y. Single nodular hepatocellular carcinoma: a clinicopathological study of 80 hepatectomized patients. *J Jpn Soc Cancer Ther* 1993; **28**: 976-987
25. Izumi R, Shimizu K, Tohru II, *et al.* Prognostic factors of hepatocellular carcinoma in patients undergoing hepatic resection. *Gastroenterology* 1994; **106**: 720-727
26. Kawarada Y, Ito F, Sakurai H, *et al.* Surgical treatment of hepatocellular carcinoma. *Cancer Chemother Pharmacol* 1994; **33**(suppl): 12-17
27. Kim ST, Kim KP. Hepatic resections for primary liver cancer. *Cancer Chemother Pharmacol* 1994; **33**(suppl): 18-23
28. Arii S, Tanaka J, Yamazoe Y, *et al.* Predictive factors for intrahepatic recurrence of hepatocellular carcinoma after partial hepatectomy. *Cancer* 1992; **69**: 913-919
29. Yoshimi F, Nagao T, Inowe S, *et al* Comparison of hepatecto-

my and transcatheter arterial chemoembolization for the treatment of hepatocellular carcinoma: necessity for prospective randomized trial. *Hepatology* 1992; **16**: 702-706

30. Sasaki Y, Imaoka S, Masutani S, *et al*. Influence of coexisting cirrhosis on long-term prognosis after surgery in patients with hepatocellular carcinoma. *Surgery* 1992; **112**: 515-521
31. The Liver Cancer Study Group of Japan. Predictive factors for long term prognosis after partial hepatectomy for patients with hepatocellular carcinoma in Japan. *Cancer* 1994; **74**: 2772-2780
32. Consensus statement on indications for liver transplantation: Paris, June 22-23, 1993. *Hepatology* 1994; **20**: 635-685
33. Pichlmayr R, Weimann A, Ringe B. Indications for liver transplantation in hepatobiliary malignancy. *Hepatology* 1994; **20**: 33S-40S
34. Iwatsuki S, Starzl T, Sheahan DG, *et al*. Hepatic resection versus transplantation for hepatocellular carcinoma. *Ann Surg* 1991; **214**: 221-229
35. Tan KC, Rela M, Ryder SD, *et al*. Experience of orthotopic liver transplantation and hepatic resection for hepatocellular carcinoma of less than 8 cm in patients with cirrhosis. *Br J Surg* 1995; **82**: 253-256
36. Bismuth H, Chiche L, *et al*. Liver resection versus transplantation for hepatocellular carcinoma in cirrhotic patients. *Ann Surg* 1993; **218**: 145-151
37. Romani F, Belli LS, Rondinara GF, *et al*. The role of transplantation in small hepatocellular carcinoma complicating cirrhosis of the liver. *J Am Coll Surg* 1994; **178**: 379-384
38. Selby R, Kadry Z, Carr B, Tzakis A, Madariaga JR, Iwatsuki S.Liver transplantation for hepatocellular carcinoma. *World J Surg* 1995; **19**: 53-58
39. Okuda K. Intratumor ethanol injection. *J Surg Oncol* 1993; **3**(suppl): 97-99
40. Shiina S, Tagawa K, Niwa Y, *et al*. Percutaneous ethanol injection therapy for hepatocellular carcinoma: results in 146 patients. *AJR* 1993; **160**:1023-1028
41. Tanikawa K. Multidisciplinary treatment of hepatocellular carcinoma. In: Tobe T, Kameda H, eds. *Primary liver cancer in Japan*. Tokyo, Japan: Springer-Verlag, 1992; 327-334
42. Livraghi T, Giorgio A, Marin G, *et al*. Hepatocellular carcinoma and cirrhosis in 746 patients: long-term results of percutaneous ethanol injection. *Radiology* 1995; **197**: 101-108
43. Yamada R, Nakatsuka H, Nakamura K, *et al*. Transcatheter arterial embolization therapy in 29 patients with various malignancies. *J Jpn Coll Angiol* 1978; **18**: 563-571
44. Nakamura H, Mitani T, Murakami T, *et al*. Five-year survival after transcatheter chemoembolization for hepatocellular carcinoma. *Cancer Chemother Pharmacol* 1994; **33**(suppl): 89-92
45. Uchida H, Matsuo N, Nishimine K, Nishimura Y, Sakaguchi H, Ohishi H. Transcatheter arterial embolization for hepatoma with lipiodol. Hepatic arterial and segmental use. *Sem Intervent Radiol* 1993; **10**: 19-26
46. Hatanaka Y, Yamashita Y, Takahashi M, *et al*. Unresectable hepatocellular carcinoma: analysis of prognostic factors in transcatheter management. *Radiology* 1995; **195**: 747-752
47. Chang JM, Tzeng WS, Pan HB, Yang CF, Lai KH. Transcatheter arterial embolization with or without cisplatin treatment of hepatocellular carcinoma. *Cancer* 1994; **74**: 2449-2453
48. Hsu HC, Wei TC, Tsang YM, Wu MZ, Lin YH, Chuang SM. Hostologic assessment of resected hepatocellular carcinoma after transcatheter hepatic arterial embolization. *Cancer* 1986; **57**: 1184-1191
49. Nakamura H, Tanaka T, Hori S, Yoshioka H, Kuroda C, Okamura J, Sakurai M. Transcatheter embolization of hepatocellular carcinoma: assessment of efficacy in cases of resection following embolization. *Radiology* 1983; **147**: 401-405
50. Choi BI, Kim HC, Han JK, *et al*. Therapeutic effect of transcatheter oily chemoembolization therapy for encapsulated nodular hepatocellular carcinoma: CT and pathologic findings. *Radiology* 1992; **182**: 709-713
51. Higuchi T, Kikuchi M, Okazaki M. Hepatocellular carcinoma after transcatheter hepatic arterial embolization. *Cancer* 1994; **73**: 2259-267
52. Okuda K, Ohtsuki T, Obata H, *et al*. Natural history of hepatocellular carcinoma and prognosis in relation to treatment: study of 850 patients. *Cancer* 1985; **56**: 918-928
53. Sato Y, Fujiwara K, Ogata I, *et al*. Transcatheter arterial embolization for hepatocellular carcinoma: benefits and limitations for unresectable cases with liver cirrhosis evaluated by comparison with other conservative treatments. *Cancer* 1985; **55**: 2822-2825
54. Vetter D, Wenger JJ, Bergier JM, Doffoel M, Bockel R. Transcatheter oily chemoembolization in the management of advanced hepatocellular carcinoma in cirrhosis: results of a Western comparative study in 60 patients. *Hepatology* 1991; **13**: 427-433
55. Chang JM, Tzeng WS, Pan HB, Yang CF, Lai KH. Transcatheter arterial embolization with or without cisplatin treatment of hepatocellular carcinoma. *Cancer* 1994; **74**: 2449-2453
56. Pelletier G, Roche A, Ink O, *et al*. A randomized trial of hepatic arterial chemoembolization in patients with unresectable hepatocellular carcinoma. *J Hepatol* 1990; **11**: 181-184
57. Bronowicki JP, Vetter D, Dumas F, *et al*. Transcatheter oily chemoembolization for hepatocellular carcinoma. A 4-year study of 127 French patients. *Cancer* 1994; **74**: 16-24
58. Miyoshi S, Minami Y, Kawata S, *et al*. Changes in hepatic functional reserve after transcatheter embolization of hepatocellular carcinoma: assessment by maximal removal rate of indocyanine green. *J Hepatol* 1986; **6**: 332-336
59. Khan KN, Nakata K, Kusumoto Y, *et al*. Evaluation of nontumorous tissue damage by transcatheter arterial embolization for hepatocellular carcinoma. *Cancer Res* 1991; **51**: 5667-5671
60. Bruix J, Castells A, Montanya X, *et al*. Phase II study of transarterial embolization in European patients with hepatocellular carcinoma: need for controlled trials. *Hepatology* 1994; **20**: 643-650
61. Taniguchi K, Nakata K, Kato Y, Sato Y, Hamasaki K, Tsuruta S, Nagataki S. Treatment of hepatocellular carcinoma with transcatheter arterial embolization. *Cancer* 1994; **73**: 1341-1345
62. Mondazzi L, Bottelli R, Brambilla G, *et al*. Transarterial oily chemoembolization for the treatment of hepatocellular carcinoma: a multivariate analysis of prognostic factors. *Hepatology* 1994; **19**: 1115-1123
63. Urata K, Matsumata T, Kamakura T, Hasuo K, Sugimachi K. Lipiodolization for unresectable hepatocellular carcinoma: an analysis of 205 patients using univariate and multivariate analysis. *J Surg Oncol* 1994; **56**: 54-58

64. Matsui O, Kadoya M, Yoshikawa J, *et al.* Small hepatocellular carcinoma: treatment with subsegmental transcatheter arterial embolization. *Radiology* 1993; **188**: 78-93

65. Nishimine K, Uchida H, Matsuo M, *et al.* Segmental transarterial chemembolization with lipiodol mixed with anticancer drugs for nonresectable hepatocellular carcinoma: follow-up CT and therapeutic results. *Cancer Chemother Pharmacol* 1994; **33**(suppl): 60-68

66. Nakao N, Kamino K, Miura K, Takayasu Y, Onnishi M, Miura T. Transcatheter arterial embolization in hepatocellular carcinoma: a long-term follow-up. *Radiat Med* 1992; **10**:13-18

67. Uchida H, Matsuo N, Nishimine K, Nishimura Y, Sakaguchi H, Ohishi H. Transcatheter arterial embolization for hepatoma with lipiodol. Hepatic arterial and segmental use. *Sem Intervent Radiol* 1993; **10**: 19-26

68. Kanematsu T, Matsumata T, Shirabe K, *et al.* A comparative study of hepatic resection and transcatheter arterial embolization for the treatment of primary hepatocellular carcinoma. *Cancer* 1993; **71**: 2181-2186

69. Murakami R, Yoshimatsu S, Yamashita Y, Sagara K, Arakawa A, Takahashi M. Transcatheter hepatic subsegmental arterial chemoembolization therapy using iodized oil for small hepatocellular carcinomas. Correlation between lipiodol accumulation and local recurrence. *Acta Radiologia* 194; **35**: 576-580

70. Higashihara H, Okazaki M, Koganemaru F, *et al.* The devised transcatheter hepatic arterial chemoembolization for obtaining medical subsegmentectomy. *Cardiovasc Intervent Radiol* 1994; **17**:21

71. Kanai T, Monden M, Sakon M, *et al.* New development of transarterial immunoembolization (TIE) for therapy of hepatocellular carcinoma with intrahepatic metastases. *Cancer Chemother Pharmacol* 1994; **33**(suppl): 48-54

72. Lai C, Wu P, Chang G, *et al.* Doxorubin versus no antitumor therapy in inoperable hepatocellular carcinoma. A prospective randomized trial. *Cancer* 1988; **62**: 479-483

73. Arias IM. Multidrug resistance genes, gamma-glycoprotein and the liver. *Hepatology* 1990; **12**: 159-165

74. Huang C, Wu M, Xu G, *et al.* Overexpression of the MDR1 gene and gamma-glycoprotein in human hepatocellular carcinoma. *J Natl Cancer Inst* 1992;**84**: 262-264

75. Dexter DL, Leith JT. Tumor heterogeneity and drug resistance. *J Clin Oncol* 1986;**4**: 244-257

76. Carr B, Starzl TE, Iwatsuki S, Van Thiel D. Aggressive treatment for advanced HCC: high response rates and prolonged survival. *Hepatology* 1991; **14**: 103A

77. Stone MJ, Klintmalm GBG, Polter D, *et al.* Neoadjuvant chemotherapy and liver transplantation for hepatocellular carcinoma: a pilot study in 20 patients. *Gastroenterology* 1993; **104**: 196-202

78. Sommeveld P, Mooter K. Reversal of drug-resistance by cyclosporin A in a patient with acute myelocytic leukemia. *Br J Haematol* 1990; **75**: 208-211

79. Colleoni M, Gaion F, Liessi G, Mastropasqua G, Nelli P, Manente P. Medical treatment of hepatocellular carcinoma: any progress? *Tumori* 1994; **80**: 315-326

80. Farinati F, Salvagnini M, de Maria N. Unresectable hepatocellular carcinoma: a prospective controlled trial with tamoxifen. *J Hepatol* 1990; **11**: 297-301

81. Castells A, Bruix J, Bru C, *et al.* Treatment of hepatocellular carcinoma with tamoxifen: a double-blind placebo-controlled trial in 120 patients. *Gastroenterology* 1995; **109**: 917-922

82. Matsuzaki Y, Osuga T, Saito Y, *et al.* A new effective, and safe therapeutic option using proton irradiation for hepatocellular carcinoma. *Gastroenterology* 1994; **106**: 1032-1041

83. Raoul JL, Guyader D, Bretagne JF, *et al.* Randomized controlled trial for hepatocellular carcinoma with portal vein thrombosis: intra-arterial iodine-131-iodized oil versus medical support. *J Nucl Med* 1994; **35**: 1782-1787

84. Ohnishi K, Tanabe Y, Ryu M, *et al.* Prognosis of hepatocellular carcinoma smaller than 5 cm in relation to treatment: study of 100 patients. *Hepatology* 1987; **7**: 1285-1290

85. Monden M, Sakon M, Gotoh M, *et al.* Selection of therapeutic modalities for hepatocellular carcinoma in patients with multiple hepatic lesions. *Cancer Chemother Pharmacol* 1992; **31**(suppl): 38-44

86. Kanematsu T, Matsumata T, Shirabe K, *et al.* A comparative study of hepatic resection and transcatheter arterial embolization for the treatment of primary hepatocellular carcinoma. *Cancer* 1993; **71**: 2181-2186

87. Yoshimi F, Nagao T, Inoue S, *et al.* Comparison of hepatectomy and transcatheter arterial chemoembolization for the treatment of hepatocellular carcinoma: necessity for prospective randomized trial. *Hepatology* 1992; **16**: 702-706

88. Kotoh K, Sakai H, Sakamoto S, Nakayama S, Satoh M, Morotomi I, Nawata H. The effect of percutaneous ethanol injection therapy on small solitary hepatocellular carcinoma is comparable to that of hepatectomy. *Am J Gastroenterol* 1994; **89**: 194-198

89. Castells A, Bruix J, Bru C, *et al.* Treatment of small hepatocellular carcinoma in cirrhotic patient: a cohort study comparing surgical resection and percutaneous ethanol injection. *Hepatology* 1993; **18**: 1121-1126

ADDENDUM

MICROSCOPIC PREDICTIVE FACTORS

Recent studies have identified some prognostic factors, evaluated by optical microscopy.

The prognostic significance of the number of argyrophilic nucleolar organizer regions (Ag NORs), which has been suggested to correlate with cellular activity and the aggressiveness of malignancy, was evaluated in 89 patients undergoing curative resection.[1] The silver-staining technique was applied to surgically resected specimens to indicate Ag NORs. The survival rate of the patients with a high number (>3.04) of Ag NORs was significantly worse than those with a low number (≤3.04) of Ag NORs when determined by univariate analysis. Moreover, after having divided the patients with and without portal vein invasion, the predictive value of the Ag NORs number was investigated and multivariate analysis showed that the number of Ag NORs was a significant prognostic indicator in patients without portal vein invasion.

Proliferating cell nuclear antigen (PCNA), a nuclear protein synthesized in the G1/S phase of the cell cycle and related to cell proliferative activity, was studied in a group of 72 patients having HCC surgically resected.[2] Tumor and non-tumor tissues were selected from each case and stained immunohistochemically with PCNA antibody. Tumor and non-tumor PCNA scores were assessed by counting the positive staining nuclei per 1000 cells. When the tumors were stratified into two group with a PCNA score ≤200 and a PCNA score >200, those patients with a PCNA score ≤200 had significantly longer disease-free survival and actual survival rates than those with a score >200. In another study[3] immunohistochemical staining of PCNA was examinated as a proliferative marker in 114 cases of HCC and the relationship between PCNA labeling index and the positivity of des-gamma carboxy prothrombin investigated. PCNA labeling index positively correlated with plasma des-gamma carboxy prothrombin levels; furthermore, patients des-gamma carboxy prothrombin positive with a high PCNA labeling index showed the highest incidence of tumor thrombus of the portal vein and intrahepatic metastasis and the lowest recurrence freedom rate.

Ki 67 antigen expression, one of the most widely studied proliferation associated markers, was examined using immunohistochemical staining with monoclonal antibody MIB 1 in a group of 72 patients having HCC surgically resected.[4] Tumor and non-tumor scores were assessed by counting the positive staining nuclei per 1000 cells. The tumor scores were found to be significantly higher in less differentiated tumors (Edmondson grade III-IV) than in well differentiated ones (Edmondson grade I-II). When the tumors were stratified in two groups with a score ≤20 and >20, those patients with a score ≤20 had significantly longer disease-free survival than patients with scores >20.

Finally, the relationship between the morphometric indices of atypism and the postoperative survival rate were evaluated in a group of 84 cases of HCC treated by hepatic resection.[5] The mean survival time was significantly longer for cases with a nucleocytoplasmic ratio of 0.28 or more, and was significantly longer for cases with a coefficent of variance of nuclear form factor of less than 5.5% than for cases with a coefficent of more than 5.5%. These trends were remarkable in the stage III cases and in the cases treated by relatively non-curative hepatic resection.

All the above mentioned indices seem to be potentially valuable prognostic factors in patients with HCC, however they need further confirmation

REFERENCES

1. Shimizu K, Izumi R, Ii T, *et al.* Prognostic significance of nucleolar organizer regions in hepatocellular carcinoma. *Hepatology* 1995; **21**: 393-397
2. Ng IO, Na J, Lai EC, *et al.* Prognostic significance of proliferating cell nuclear antigen expression in hepatocellualr carcinoma *Cancer* 1994;**73**:2268-2274
3. Suehiro T, Matsumata T, Itasaka H, Taketomi A, Yamamoto K, Sugimachi K. Des-gamma-carboxy prothrombin and proliferative activity of hepatocellular carcinoma. *Surgery* 1995; **117**: 682-691
4. Ng IO, Na J, Lai EC, Fan ST, Ng M. Ki-67 antigen expression in hepatocellular carcinoma using monoclonal antibody MIB1. A comparison with proliferating cell nuclear antigen. *Am J Clin Pathol* 1995; **104**: 313-318
5. Kawai Y, Takeshige K, Nunome M, *et al.* Prognosis after hepatic resection in patients with hepatocellular carcinoma, estimated on the basis of the morphometric indices. *Cancer Chemother Pharmacol* 1994; **33**(suppl): 24-28

PART V
FIBROLAMELLAR HCC

32

Fibrolamellar hepatocellular carcinoma: pathology, diagnosis and therapy

MD Simms, DH Stephens, JW Charboneau, DM Nagorney and KP Batts

In the late 1970s and early 1980s several reports appeared in the literature describing the unique pathologic and clinical characteristics of fibrolamellar hepatocellular carcinoma (FL-HCC).[1–3] FL-HCC represents an uncommon but distinct clinical and pathologic variant of the more frequent HCC, occurring in cirrhotic patients.[4] Affected patients tend to be adolescents or young adults, without underlying liver disease (hepatitis or cirrhosis), and with normal serum AFP levels. Unlike HCC, which is three to four times more prevalent in males than females by a factor of three to four, FL-HCC has no predilection for either sex.[2,3,5-10] In addition, FL-HCC is felt by most authors to be more amenable to surgical resection and carries with it a more favorable prognosis. The pathology, diagnosis, and therapy of FL-HCC are reviewed.

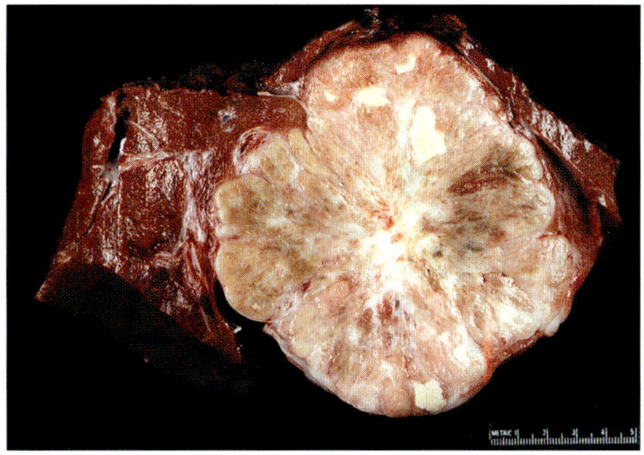

Figure 32.1 – Fibrolamellar carcinoma of liver – typical gross appearance. Tumors are typically single, large, circumscribed, and lobulated, and frequently demonstrate a central stellate scar. The background liver is normal, as usual.

PATHOLOGY

Gross

FL-HCC usually occurs as a single, firm, tan-white, well-circumscribed but unencapsulated, lobulated mass in a background of normal liver. Most tumors are large, with a range of 4 to 17 cm and weighing up to 3600 g.[11] While 55-65% of tumors are solitary,[2,5,6,9,21] multiple hepatic tumors, generally in the form of a dominant mass with small satellite lesions in the adjacent liver parenchyma, may also be seen. An isolated report of a multicystic FL-HCC exists.[12] Diffuse liver involvement has not been reported to our knowledge. Some authors have noted an unusually frequent involvement of the left hepatic lobe.[2]

An interesting feature of FL-HCC is the presence of a central, stellate scar reminiscent of that seen in focal nodular hyperplasia (FNH) (Fig. 32.1). The scars appear to be found in a minority of tumors but interestingly may be seen in metastically involved lymph nodes as well. While elements of FNH may occasionally be seen in the periphery of FL-HCC,[13] these may represent a secondary reaction to local perfusion abnormalities[14] rather than the benign precursor for FL-HCC as proposed by some.[15]

Microscopic

The two hallmark histologic features of FL-HCC are large polygonal neoplastic hepatocytes with abundant eosinophilic cytoplasm, and lamellar bands of dense connective tissue lying between nests and cords of the neoplastic hepatocytes (Fig. 32.2).[2] The abundant eosinophilic cytoplasm is due to numerous mitochondria. The collagenous lamellae consist of plate-like stacks of connective tissue of variable thickness. Collagens I, III, and V are the dominant forms and are most likely produced by stromal fibroblasts.[16] The lamellae are usually not seen uniformly throughout the entire tumor, but in most cases more than 50% of the tumor will show lamellar fibrosis. If lamellar fibrosis involves only a small portion of the tumor, the remaining clinical and pathologic features (see below) should be carefully evaluated to ensure one is dealing with a true FL-HCC rather than a mimicking HCC.

While distinguishing HCC from FL-HCC is usually straightforward using these two "major" criteria, ambiguous cases exist. In our experience, all FL-HCC cases will demonstrate obvious macronuclei such that we feel that their presence should be regarded as a third "major" criterion for diagnosis.[17]

In addition to prominent macronucleoli, nuclei typically demonstrate prominent intranuclear cytoplasmic invaginations and peripheralized chromatin. Mitotic activity is typically low (3 or less mitoses per 10 high power fields). In addition to abundant mitochondria, a number of other cytoplasmic features are seen. Pale bodies (Fig. 32.2b) are clear, round cytoplasmic structures, which appear to represent aberrant intracytoplasmic bile canaliculi lined by microvilli.[11] Dense bodies are darkly eosinophilic,

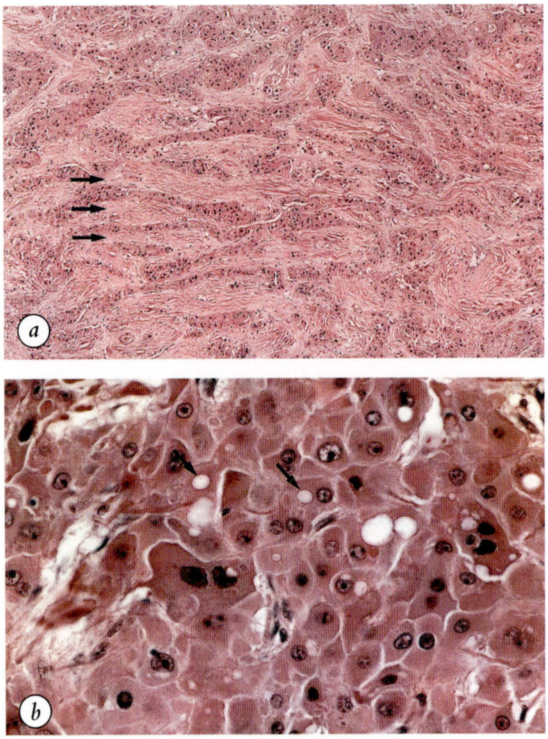

Figure 32.2 – FL-HCC, histopathology.

a) Bands of plate-like "lamellar" collagen can be seen (arrows) separating cords of neoplastic hepatocytes with abundant eosinophilic cytoplasm. (H&E, x40).

b) The neoplastic hepatocytes contain abundant eosinophilic cytoplasm, prominent macronucleoli, and pale bodies (arrows) which likely represent intracytoplasmic bile canaliculi. (H&E, x240)

PAS-positive structures which are AFP and alpha-1-anti-trypsin negative.[2] Bile plugs are common but fat is uncommon.

Histochemistry

The majority of FL-HCC will show stainable copper and copper-protein complexes, in contrast to HCC. Immunohistochemically, keratin profiles, and uniform alpha-1-antitrypsin positivity are similar to HCC. Polyclonal antisera to carcino embryonic antigen (CEA) will frequently reveal abnormally large, distorted bile canaliculi, some of which appear to be intracytoplasmic as noted above.[18] Like HCC, monoclonal antibodies against CEA will fail to show cytoplasmic positivity. AFP immunoreactivity is uniformly absent.

Ultrastructure: The major cytoplasmic feature of FL-HCC is the presence of abundant mitochondria (Fig. 32.3a). One may also see intracytoplasmic bile canaliculi (Fig. 32.3b).[18] There is general agreement that FL-HCC is of hepatocytic origin, although the presence of neurosecretory granule-like structures has been noted and has in the view of some suggested an element of neuroendocrine differentiation.[19]

DIAGNOSIS

Clinical presentation

Most patients afflicted with FL-HCC present with a palpable abdominal mass or abdominal pain, or weight loss and cachexia.[2,3,7,9] The duration of symptoms is quite variable, with a reported range of less than 1 month to 40 months.[2,9,23] Several large

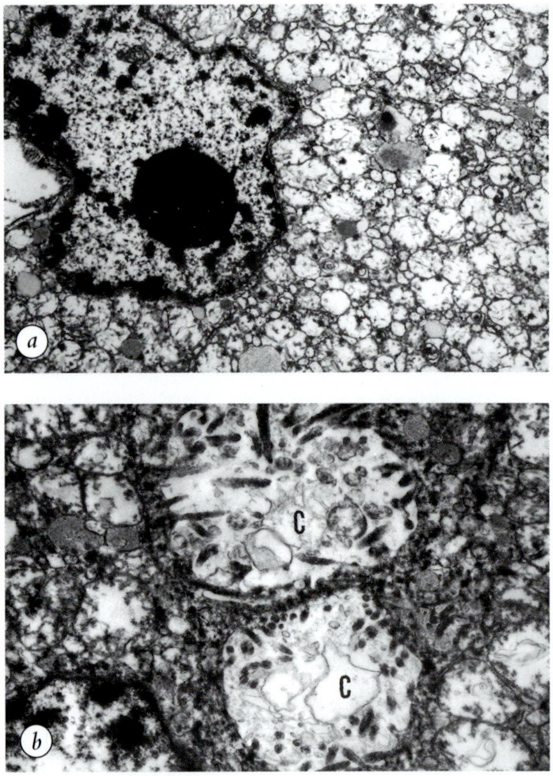

Figure 32.3 – FL-HCC, transmission electron microscopy.

a) The nucleus contains a single, macronucleolus and peripheralized chromatin and the cytoplasm contains abundant mitochondria. (x3000).

b) In this cell, two intracytoplasmic bile canaliculi, (C) lined by microvilli are present. (x10,000).

series report patient mean age at time of diagnosis between 20 and 26 years, with a range of 5 years to 75 years.[2,3,5-10] Unlike HCC, there is no association between liver cirrhosis and FL-HCC. Therefore, presentation with signs of acute liver decompensation such as bleeding varices or hepatic encephalopathy is distinctly uncommon. Rarely, presentation with gynecomastia secondary to increased aromatization of circulating androgens by the liver tumor has been reported.[24,25]

A significant distinction between FL-HCC and HCC with regard to laboratory tests is the serum AFP. While it is very common for serum AFP to be elevated in patients with HCC, and often this serves as a presumptive diagnosis of HCC (values >500 ng/ml), it is rare for this marker to be elevated in most patients with FL-HCC.[2,26,28-30] Exceptions to this rule, however, have been reported.[6,22] Mild to moderate elevation of serum transaminase and serum alkaline phosphatase is common. Serum neurotensin and vitamin B12 binding capacity have been shown to be elevated in patients with FL-HCC; however, these two assays have limited specificity in distinguishing between FL-HCC and HCC and the sensitivities of these measures are not determined.[31-33] There may be a role in following these values to assess response to therapy if initially elevated at the time of diagnosis.[34]

Diagnostic imaging

Diagnostic imaging plays an important role in the workup and differential diagnosis of any suspected hepatic mass. The imaging findings of FL-HCC often provide information strongly suggestive of the diagnosis. Definitive diagnosis usually requires histologic confirmation. Computed tomography (CT), ultrasonography (US), magnetic resonance imaging (MRI), and angiography have all been utilized in the imaging of FL-HCC.

Both unenhanced and intravenous (IV) contrast-enhanced CT images are valuable in the evaluation of a hepatic mass, particularly a vascular lesion such as FL-HCC. On unenhanced CT, FL-HCC appears as a large hypoattenuating mass lesion relative to surrounding hepatic parenchyma (Fig. 32.4). Most tumors are solitary but some have small satellite nodules[9,21]. A case of multi-focal FL-HCC has been reported.[35] Surface lobulation is common.[22] Fibrotic

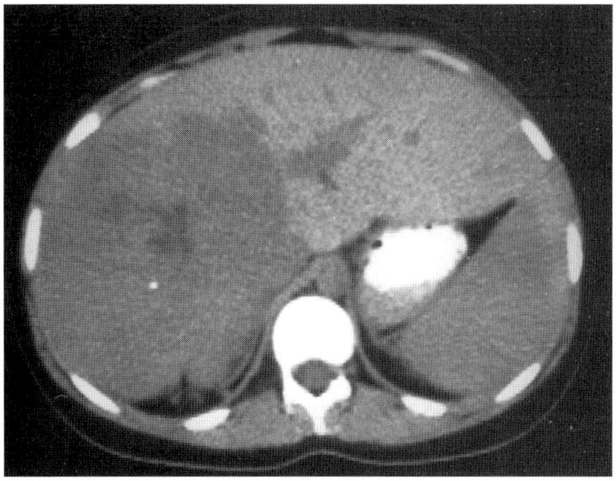

Figure 32.4 – FL-HCC — Unenhanced CT image showing a large solitary hypoattenuating lobulated mass occupying the right liver lobe. Note the central scar and central punctate calcification.

scar or central necrosis will demonstrate low attenuation relative to the remainder of the mass and has been reported in 20-50% of cases.[22,29] Unenhanced CT is helpful in displaying calcific foci within the tumor, which can occasionally be confused with vascular structures on contrast-enhanced images. Punctate calcification has been reported in 40-60% of cases of FL-HCC[22,36] and is less commonly seen in untreated HCC.[23,26,37] As previously noted, FL-HCC occurs in an otherwise normal liver, in contradistinction to HCC, which often arises in a cirrhotic liver. It is therefore useful to note overall appearance of the liver size and contour and to assess for evidence of portal venous hypertension. A cirrhotic liver will often show a nodular contour or discrepant hypertrophy of the caudate lobe and lateral segment of the left lobe.

Attention to delivery of IV contrast material is important for the evaluation of any focal liver mass lesion. Assuming helical or fast scanning is available, one can best appreciate the vascular nature of FL-HCC by obtaining dual phase (arterial and portal) contrast enhancement. While the majority of these tumors are large, one can optimally image the extent of the mass and possibly detect small satellite lesions during the vascular phases of IV bolus contrast material enhancement. The non-necrotic and non-fibrotic components of the tumor show contrast enhancement and typically undergo notable enhancement, often appearing hyperattenuating relative to

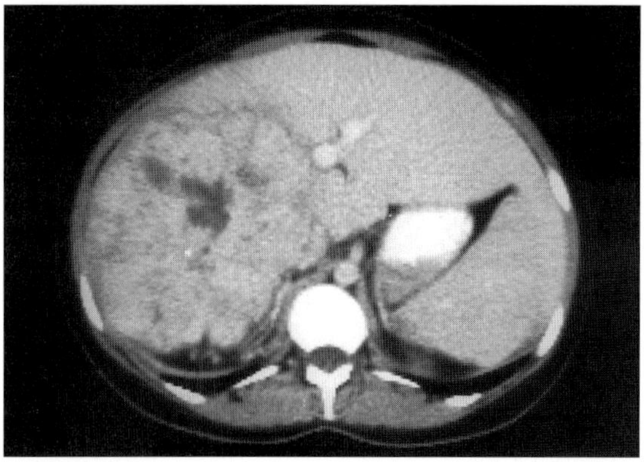

Figure 32.5 – FL-HCC – Contrast material enhanced CT image showing the central scar more clearly. Most of the tumor has become nearly isodense with the normal hepatic parenchyma.

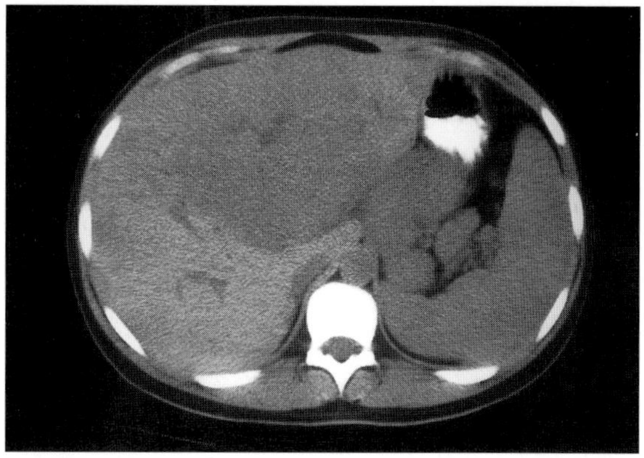

Figure 32.6 – FL-HCC – Unenhanced CT image showing a large tumor in the left liver with a large nodal mass in the gastrohepatic ligament and metastatic involvement of the left adrenal gland.

normal liver. After the peak vascularized enhancing phase, the vascular tumor may appear isoattenuating relative to normal liver parenchyma and will be visible only secondary to mass distortion and the presence of central scar, necrosis, or calcification (Fig. 32.5). Other secondary effects include intrahepatic biliary ductal dilatation and evidence of major venous obstruction or thrombosis. Regional lymphadenopathy and other evidence of metastatic disease in the upper abdomen can also be evaluated with CT (Fig. 32.6).

With regard to resectability, a tumor is considered resectable if it is technically possible to excise the entire mass, leaving tumor free margins and enough residual liver to support life. Tumors involving the main portal vein, proper hepatic artery, or central intrahepatic biliary tree are usually considered unresectable. In one study tumors were correctly staged as resectable or unresectable in 75% of cases using CT.[22]

The sonographic appearance of FL-HCC can be variable. US usually demonstrates a large solitary mass that may be isoechoic, hyperechoic, or of mixed echo texture relative to normal hepatic parenchyma. Sonography is often able to show the hyperechoic central scar (Fig. 32.7) and echogenic foci with distal acoustic shadowing representing punctate calcification. In one published series,[22] the central scar was identified in 3 (60%) of 5 cases of FL-HCC, with calcification demonstrated in 4 (80%) of five tumors. Another series,[36] reporting the imaging findings in 10 cases of FL-HCC, found that the central scar was identified sonographically in only 1 (33%) of 3 patients, whose tumors had a central scar identified on CT. In this same study, calcification was seen sonographically in only 1 (25%) of 4 patients. Dilatation of the biliary tree and major venous invasion or thrombosis can be demonstrated with US and color Doppler. To date, the color Doppler findings of FL-HCC have not been specifically reported. It is conceivable that color Doppler would show a vascular mass with avascular regions representing the central scar or necrotic tumor. While both CT and US are capable of detecting regional lymphadenopathy and distant metastatic disease, overall CT is the favored imaging modality.[22] US is very useful in those patients in whom the use of contrast material is contraindicated.

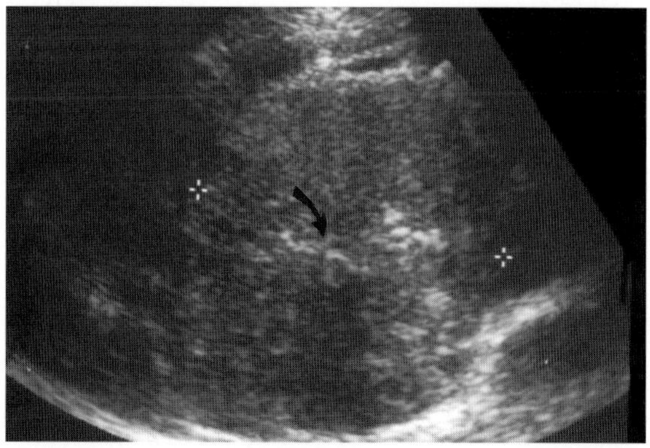

Figure 32.7 – FL-HCC – Ultrasound image showing mixed echogenicity mass containing a central echogenic scar (arrow).

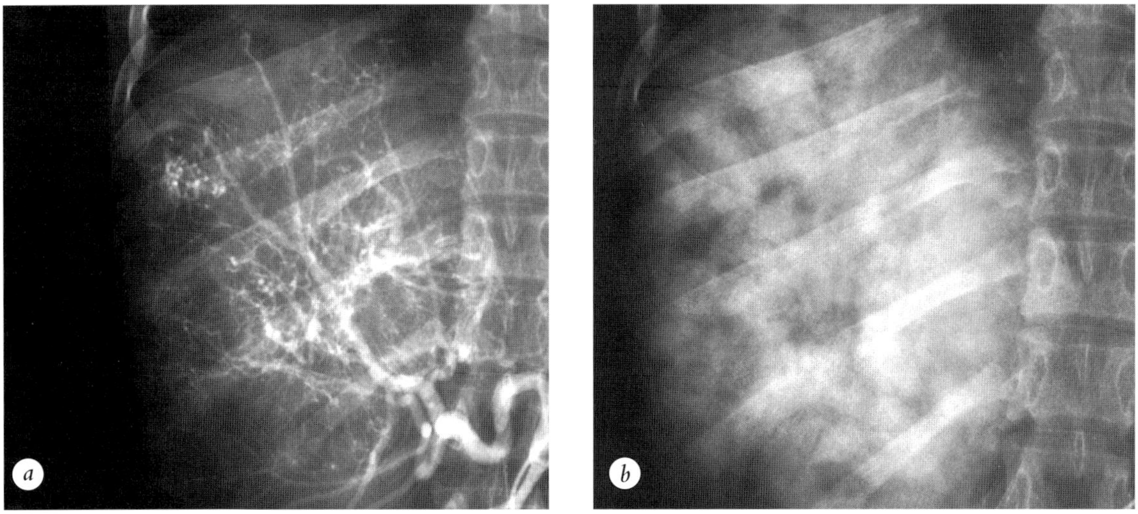

Figure 32.8 – FL-HCC — Angiography.

a) Arteriogram with celiac artery injection shows large hypervascular mass.

b) Late-phase arteriogram shows the central scar as a hypovascular region.

Angiography is an excellent tool for defining hepatic arterial and portal venous anatomy. FL-HCC is a hypervascular tumor with an intense parenchymal stain (Fig. 32.8a). The central scar appears as a hypovascular region (Fig. 32.8b). While enlarged feeding vessels are common, arterial-portal venous or arterial-hepatic venous shunting is notably absent, having been described in only one case.[38] Angiography can sometimes display intrahepatic tumor not seen on CT[22] and offers the surgeon preoperative evaluation of the hepatic vasculature.

Experience with the MRI appearances of FL-HCC has been relatively limited. Initial experience showed FL-HCC to be predominantly of low signal on T1-weighted spin echo (T1SE) images and of increased signal intensity on T2-weighted intensity spin echo (T2SE) images (Fig. 32.9). The central scar, if present, was shown to be of low signal intensity on both T1- and T2-weighted spin echo images. Following IV administration of gadolinium-DTPA (Gd-DTPA), the tumor shows diffuse heterogenous enhancement with no enhancement of the central scar.[24]

FNH shares several radiologic features with FL-HCC. Obviously differentiation between these two pathologies is of great clinical significance with FL-HCC resulting in aggressive surgical management and FNH benign neglect. Both FNH and FL-HCC are well-defined, well-vascularized tumors that often have a central scar. Initial reports with CT suggested distinguishing FNH based on vascular enhancement of the central scar favoring FNH.[39] This occurs in the early arterial vascular phase and is easily missed with conventional scanning. The non-fibrotic portion of FNH usually appears more homogenous than that of FL-HCC, and FNH tends to be a smaller tumor usually measuring less than 5 cm in diameter.[40] The scar or non-enhancing central portion of FL-HCC tends to be larger. With Technetium 99m sulfur colloid scintigraphy, FNH will usually show uptake equal to or greater than normal liver parenchyma due to the presence of Kupffer cells. FL-HCC does not take up this radiopharmaceutical. However, approximately 30-40 % of FNH show no uptake of Technetium 99m sulfur colloid.

With MRI, increased signal intensity on T2SE within the central scar was felt to be a reliable distinguishing feature of FNH.[41-44] However, a more recent report[45] describes a case of FL-HCC which displayed signal characteristics consistent with FNH.

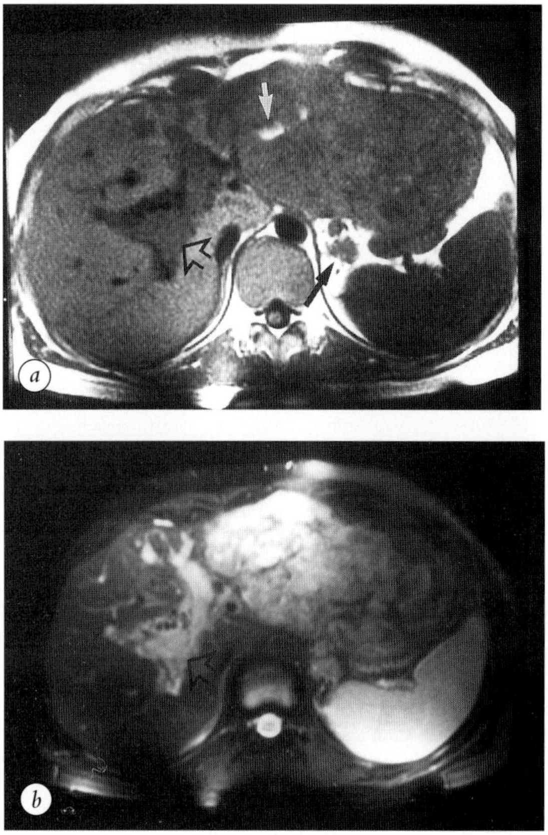

Figure 32.9 – FL-HCC, MRI.

a) T1-weighted

b) and T2-weighted

Spin echo images show large heterogeneous mass occupying the left liver lobe. Tumor is relatively isointense on T1-weighted image and hyperintense on T2-weighted image. Evidence of recent hemorrhage is seen on T1-weighted image (white arrow). Extensive tumor thrombus is present in portal veins (open arrows). adrenal mass is also identified (black arrow).

Specifically, the tumor was isointense with liver on T1SE and T2SE and the central scar was hyperintense on T2SE. In addition, the central scar showed enhancement on images obtained after IV administration of Gd-DTPA. The pathologic basis for scar hyperintensity on T2SE images and Gd-DTPA enhanced images was the demonstration of multiple vascular channels within the dense collagenous scar. It does appear, as with CT, that the enhancement pattern is more homogenous with FNH than FL-HCC. Whether this feature holds true for smaller FL-HCC tumors is unclear. Therefore, while certain MRI features may by highly suggestive of FNH as opposed to FL-HCC, they are not pathognomonic. Depending on clinical circumstances, serial imaging follow-up has been suggested.[24] In those cases that show no uptake on Technetium 99m sulfur colloid scintigraphy, caution must be exercized. Percutaneous or surgical biopsy is usually required for definitive diagnosis. As noted in the pathology section, elements of FNH may be found in the periphery of FL-HCC.[13] Inadequate tissue sampling may yield a diagnosis of FNH delaying the definitive diagnosis of FL-HCC and potentially eliminating an opportunity for a curative resection.

THERAPY

The mainstay of therapy for FL-HCC is surgical resection. Several studies have shown increased resection rates and improved 5-year survival statistics for patients with FL-HCC as compared with patients who have HCC,[6,9] although the natural history of FL-HCC is not known. Moreover, prolonged survival for patients with advanced tumor stage and metastatic disease is not rare.[34] These findings have supported the clinical impression that FL-HCC is a less aggressive malignancy with a more favorable prognosis if treated with potentially curative liver resection.

Published series have shown overall 5-year survival rates of between 25 and 63% for both resectable and unresectable tumors with median survival rates between 21 and 45 months.[3,6,8] Reported resection rates have ranged between 47 and 100%.[2,3,5,6,9,46] Five-year survival after resection has ranged between 40 and 65%, with median survival between 33 and 50 months.[2,3,5,6,8,46] In fact, long-term survival of 14 years with recurrent disease after initial resection has been reported.[3] In contrast, 5-year survival rates of 0 to 26% with median survival of 4 to 7 months are typically reported for HCC.[47] Some authors hypothesize that differences in resectability rates may account for the differences in survival rates between FL-HCC and HCC in non-cirrhotic patients.[6,8,9] Interestingly, expansile rather than infiltrating local growth characteristics of FL-HCC with infrequent vascular invasion or multicentricity may account for the increased resectability rate in many reports. However, a retrospective single institution comparison of resected FL-HCC versus HCC showed no difference in survival by disease stage, suggesting that reported "improved" survival for FL-HCC may result from resection of early stage lesions.[5] A recent report evaluating stage of disease at the time of presentation and results of aggressive surgical management[35] found 70% (7 of 10) of patients to have extrahepatic tumor at the time of diagnosis. Seventy percent of patients underwent curative resections including 4 with lymph node metastases. All patients who had resection with intent to cure experienced tumor recurrence. Other series report recurrence rates of 42 to 67%.[2,3,8] Recurrence was detected within 6 to 18 months in 6 of 7 patients and in 1 patient at 66 months postoperatively. This suggests that frequent follow-up imaging in these patients is warranted to detect early recurrence.

For patients with unresectable FL-HCC and no evidence of metastatic disease, orthotropic liver transplantation (OLT) is a therapeutic option. While results are inferior to those with standard surgical resection, OLT offers patients longer survival than without operative treatment. Median survival is reported in one study to be 8 months; and 3 years in another series with a 5-year survival rate of 37.5%.[9,46] Of note, 5-year survival is similar between patients with FL-HCC and HCC.[46]

Chemotherapy offers patients with unresectable FL-HCC improved survival compared to the poor prognosis of patients with non-resectable HCC. In one reported series, median survival for patients with FL-HCC treated with Adriamycin (doxorubicin) alone or doxorubicin and streptozocin was 24 months compared to 3 months for patients with HCC.[10] Another series showed median survival of 8 months with chemotherapy and 4 months without chemotherapy.[6] These results lend support to the notion that the prognosis for FL-HCC is better than for HCC, not only on the basis of resectability, but also due to the biologic behavior of the neoplasm and response to chemotherapy.

Additional non-surgical therapies for patients with unresectable FL-HCC include ethanol ablation, cryoablation, and transcatheter oily chemoembolization. Experience with these techniques is limited. In a recent report, 3 patients underwent seven courses of transcatheter oily chemoembolization. One patient experienced stabilization of tumor size and in 2 patients, there was a decrease in tumor size allowing for subsequent hepatic resection.[48]

REFERENCES

1. Peters RL. Pathology of hepatocellular carcinoma. In: Okuda K, Peters R, eds. *Hepatocellular Carcinoma* 1976; 107-168 John Wiley & Sons
2. Craig JR, Peters RL, Edmondson HD, Omata M. Fibrolamellar carcinoma of the liver: a tumor of adolescents and young adults with distinctive clinicopathologic features. *Cancer* 1980; **46**: 372-379
3. Berman MM, Libbey NP, Foster JH. Hepatocellular carcinoma: polygonal cell type with fibrous stroma - an atypical variant with a favorable prognosis. *Cancer* 1980; **46**: 1448-1455
4. Rolfes DB. Fibrolamellar carcinoma of the liver. In Okuda K, Ishak KG, eds. *Neoplasms of the liver.* New York 1987, Springer Verlag
5. Ringe B, Wittekind C, Weimann A, Tusch G, Pichlmayr R. Results of hepatic resection and transplantation for fibrolamellar carcinoma. *Surg Gynecol Obstet* 1992; **175**: 299-305
6. Wood WJ, Rawlings M, Evans H, Lim CNH. Hepatocellular carcinoma: importance of histologic classification as a prognostic factor. *Am J Surg* 1988; **155**: 663-666
7. Berman MA, Burnham JA, Sheahan DG. Fibrolamellar carcinoma of the liver: an immunohistochemical study of nineteen cases and a review of the literature. *Hum Pathol* 1988; **19**: 784-794
8. Soreide O, Czerniak A, Bradpiece H, Bloom S, Blumgart L. Characteristics of fibrolamellar hepatocellular carcinoma: a study of nine cases and a review of the literature. *Am J Surg* 1986; **151**: 518-523
9. Nagorney DM, Adson, MA, Weiland LH, Knight CD Jr, Smalley SR, Zinsmeister AR. Fibrolamellar hepatoma. *Am J Surg* 1985; **149**: 113-119
10. Ihde DC, Matthews MJ, Makuch RW, McIntire KR, Eddy JL, Seff LB. Prognostic factors in patients with hepatocellular carcinoma receiving systemic chemotherapy. *Am J Med* 1985; **78**: 399-406
11. Craig JR, Peters RL, Edmondson HA. Tumors of the liver and intrahepatic ducts. *AFIP Fascicle* 1989; **26**:171-179
12. Pombo F, Rodriguez E, Arnal-Monreal F. Multicystic fibrolamellar hepatocellular carcinoma – CT appearance. *Clin Imag* 1993; **17**: 67-69
13. Saul S, Titelbaum DS, Gansler TS, *et al.* The fibrolamellar variant of hepatocellular carcinoma. Its association with focal nodular hyperplasia. *Cancer* 1987; **60**: 3049-3055
14. Hodgson HJF. Fibrolamellar cancer of the liver.*Hepatology* 1987; **5**: 241-247
15. Vecchio FM, Fabiano A, Ghilandia G, Manna R, Massi G. Fibrolamellar carcinoma of the liver: the malignant counterpart of focal nodular hyperplasia with oncocytic change. *Am J Clin Path* 1984; **81**: 521-526
16. Nerlich AG, Majewski S, Hunzelmann N, *et al.* Excessive collagen formation in fibrolamellar carcinoma of the liver: a morphological and biochemical study. *Modern Pathol* 1992; **5**(5): 580-585

17. Burgart LJ, Martinez CJM, Batts KP. Fibrolamellar carcinoma - importance of using a strict definition. *Modern Pathol* 1994; **7**(1): 129A (abstract)

18. Snover DC. *Biopsy Diagnosis of Liver Disease*. Williams & Wilkins, Baltimore, 1992; pp.246-247

19. deDavila MTG, Gonzalez-Crussi F, Mangkornkanok M. Fibrolamellar carcinoma of the liver in a child: ultrastructural and immunohistochemical aspects. *Ped Pathol* 1987; **7**:319-331

20. Wanless IR, Mandsley C, Adams R. On the pathogenesis of focal nodular hyperplasia of the liver. *Hepatology* 1985; **5**:1194:1200

21. Titelbaum DS, Burke DR, Meranze SG, Saul SH. Fibrolamellar hepatocellular carcinoma: pitfalls in nonoperative diagnosis. *Radiology* 1988; **167**: 25-30

22. Brandt DJ, Johnson CD, Stephens DH, Weiland LH. Imaging of fibrolamellar hepatocellular carcinoma. *AJR* 1988; **151**: 295-299

23. Farhi DC, Shikes RH, Murari PF, Silverberg SG. Hepatocellular carcinoma in young people. *Cancer* 1983; **52**: 1516-1525

24. Corrigan K, Semelka RC. Dynamic contrast-enhanced MR imaging of fibrolamellar hepatocellular carcinoma. *Abdom Imag* 1995; **20**: 122-125

25. McColskey JJ, Germain-Lee El, Perman JA, Plotnick LP. Gynecomastia as a presenting sign of fibrolamellar carcinoma of the liver. *Pediatrics* 1988; **82**: 379-382

26. Lack EE, Neave C, Vawter G. Hepatocellular carcinoma: review of 32 cases in childhood adolescence. *Cancer* 1983; **52**: 1510-1515

27. Farhi DC, Shikes RH, Murari PJ, Silverberg SG. Hepatocellular carcinoma in young people. *Cancer* 1983; **52**: 1516-1525

28. Francis IR, Agha FP, Thompson NW, Keren DF. Fibrolamellar hepatocarcinoma: clinical, radiologic, and pathologic features. *Gastrointest Radiol* 1986; **11**: 67-72

29. Friedman AC, Lichtenstein JE, Goodman Z, Fishman EK, Siegelman SS, Dachman AH. Fibrolamellar hepatocellular carcinoma. *Radiology* 1985; **157**: 583-587

30. Adam A, Gibson N, Soreide O, Hemingway AP, Carr DH, Blumgart LH, Allison DJ. *Clin Radiol* 1986; **37**: 355-358

31. Collier NA, Weinbren K, Bloom SR, Lee YC, Hodgson HJ, Blumgart LH. Neurotensin secretion by fibrolamellar carcinoma of the liver. *Lancet* 1984; **1**: 538-540

32. Wood JR, Melia WM, Wood SM, *et al.* Neurotensin and hepatocellular carcinoma [letter]. *Lancet* 1984; **1**: 538-540

33. Paradinas FJ, Melia WM, Wilkinson ML, *et al.* High serum vitamin B12 binding capacity as a marker of the fibrolamellar variant of hepatocellular carcinoma. *Br Med J Clin Res* 1982; **285**: 840-842

34. Rosen CB, Nagorney DM. Fibrolamellar and less aggressive hepatocellular carcinomas. In: Terblanch J, ed *Hepatobiliary Malignancy*. Boston: Little Brown & Company, 1994:203-214.

35. Stevens WR, Johnson CD, Stephens DH, Nagorney DM. Fibrolamellar hepatocellular carcinoma: stage at presentation and results of aggressive surgical management. *AJR* 1995; **164**: 1153-1158

36. Soyer P, Roche A, Levesque M, Legmann P. CT of fibrolamellar hepatocellular carcinoma. *J Comput Assist Tomogr* 1991; **15**(4): 533-538

37. Darlack JJ, Moskowitz M, Kattan KR. Calcifications in the liver. *Radiol Clin North Am* 1980; **18**: 209-219

38. Wong LK, Link DP, Frey CF, Ruebner BH, Tesluk H, Pimstone NR. Fibrolamellar hepatocarcinoma: radiology, management, and pathology. *AJR* 1982; **139**: 172-175

39. Mathieu D, Bruneton JN, Drouillard J, Pointreau CC, Vasile N. Hepatic adenomas and focal nodular hyperplasia: dynamic CT study. *Radiology* 1986; **160**: 53-58

40. Powers C, Ros, PR, Stoupis C, Johnson WK, Segel KH. Primary liver neoplasms: MR imaging with pathologic correlation. *RadioGraphics* 1994; **14**: 459-482

41. Titelbaum DS, Hatabu H, Schiebler ML, Kressel HY, Burke DR, Saul SH. Fibrolamellar hepatocellular carcinoma: MR appearance. *J Comput Assist Tomogr* 1988; **12**: 588-591

42. Mattison GR, Glazer GM, Quint LE, Francis IR, Bree RL, Ensminger WD. MR imaging of hepatic focal nodular hyperplasia: characterization and distinction from primary malignant tumors. *AJR* 1987; **148**: 711-715

43. Lee MJ, Saini S, Hamm B, *et al.* Focal nodular hyperplasia of the liver: MR findings in 35 proved cases. *AJR* 1991; **145:** 317-320

44. Shamsi K, DeSchepper A, Degryse H, Deckers F. Focal nodular hyperplasia of the liver: radiologic findings. *Abdom Imag* 1993; **18**: 32-38

45. Hamrick-Turner JE, Shipkey FJ, Cranston PE. Fibrolamellar hepatocellular carcinoma: MR appearance mimicking focal nodular hyperplasia. *J Comput Assist Tomogr* 1994; **18**(2): 301-304

46. Iwatsuki S, Starzl TE, Sheahan DG, *et al.* Hepatic resection versus transplantation for hepatocellular carcinoma. *Ann Surg* 1991; **214**: 221-229

47. Que FG, Nagorney DM. Hepatocellular carcinoma: a western perspective. *Dig Surg* 1995; **12**: 45-52

48. Soyer P, Roche A, Rougier P, Levesque M. Nonresectable fibrolamellar hepatocellular carcinoma: outcome of 4 cases treated by intra-arterial chemotherapy. (French) *J Belge Radiol* 1992; **75**(6): 463-468

Index

A

D

E

H

I

N

O

P

Q

R

S

U

V

W

X

Y

Z